ISSN: 1360-8592   4 issues per year

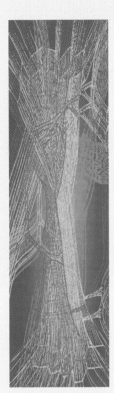

Journal of Bodywork and Movement Therapies

Practical issues in musculoskeletal function, treatment and rehabilitation

Editor: Leon Chaitow

- Renowned editorial team
- Includes peer-reviewed articles, editorials, summaries, review and technique papers
- Professional guidance for practitioners and teachers of physical therapy, osteopathy, chiropractic, massage, Rolfing, Feldenkrais, yoga, dance and others

Subscribe Online: www.elsevierhealth.com/journals/jbmt

Elsevier Science, 32 Jamestown Road, London NW1 7BY, UK
Tel: +44 (0)20 8308 5790   •   Fax: +44 (0)20 7424 4258
Email: journals@elsevierhealth.com   •   Call toll free in the US: 1-877-839-7126

ELSEVIER SCIENCE

Clinical Application of Neuromuscular Techniques

In loving dedication to Sasha and Kaila.

For Churchill Livingstone:

Editorial Director: Mary Law
Project Development Manager: Katrina Mather
Project Manager: Jane Shanks
Design Direction: George Ajayi

Clinical Application of Neuromuscular Techniques

Volume 1 – The Upper Body

Leon Chaitow ND DO
Senior Lecturer, University of Westminster, London, UK

Judith Walker DeLany LMT
Lecturer in Neuromuscular Therapy, Director of NMT Center,
St Petersburg, Florida, USA

Forewords by

John Lowe MA DC
Board Certified: American Academy of Pain Management; Director of Research,
Fibromalgia Research Foundation, Tulsa, Oklahoma, USA

Benny F Vaughn LMT ATC CSCS
Clinic Director and Senior Instructor, Sports Therapy and Performance Center,
Fort Worth, Texas, USA

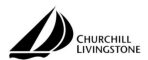
CHURCHILL
LIVINGSTONE

EDINBURGH LONDON NEW YORK OXFORD PHILADELPHIA ST LOUIS SYDNEY TORONTO 2000

CHURCHILL LIVINGSTONE
An imprint of Elsevier Limited

First published 2000
  Reprinted 2001, 2002, 2003 (twice), 2005, 2007

ISBN-13: 978-0-443-06270-4
ISBN-10: 0-443-06270-6

British Library Cataloguing in Publication Data
A catalogue record for this book is available from the British Library

Library of Congress Cataloging in Publication Data
A catalog record for this book is available from the Library of Congress

Note
Medical knowledge is constantly changing. As new information becomes available, changes in treatment, procedures, equipment and the use of drugs become necessary. The editors, contributor and the publishers have taken care to ensure that the information given in this text is accurate and up to date. However, readers are strongly advised to confirm that the information, especially with regard to drug usage, complies with the latest legislation and standards of practice.

ELSEVIER   your source for books, journals and multimedia in the health sciences

www.elsevierhealth.com

Working together to grow
libraries in developing countries

www.elsevier.com | www.bookaid.org | www.sabre.org

ELSEVIER   BOOK AID International   Sabre Foundation

Printed in China
C / 08

The publisher's policy is to use **paper manufactured from sustainable forests**

Contents

List of boxes

Forewords

The most common introductory sentence authors of book forewords use is: 'I am honored to write this Foreword.' At the risk of sounding trite, I must begin this Foreword in the same way. I do so, however, with slight displeasure. The displeasure does not arise from my using a threadbare expression. Instead, it arises from my failure to think of a sentence that conveys something more superlative than honor, something that expresses the unique honor of writing the Foreword to a book that is sorely needed by soft tissue practitioners of all disciplines and destined to become their preeminent resource. An appropriate superlative is especially needed in that the book is the pinnacle publication of Leon Chaitow, eminent and prolific author and soft tissue authority, and Judith DeLany, leading pioneer of neuromuscular therapy, and acclaimed author, lecturer, and educator. For lack of a fitting superlative, let me simply say that *Clinical Application of Neuromuscular Techniques, Vol.1* is a momentous work, almost more than one would expect even from authors of the stature of Chaitow and DeLany. I am privileged to have the opportunity to comment on some of the extraordinary merits of the book.

Both Chaitow and DeLany contributed to all parts of the book, but their relative contributions to different parts varied. Yet the book, through and through, is a collaboration in which the authors richly integrate European neuromuscular technique with American neuromuscular therapy. In so doing, they provide a detailed and comprehensive description of this clinical approach to soft tissue pain and dysfunction, designated 'NMT'.

The first 10 chapters cover the scientific and academic background of NMT, its history, and its clinical principles. Many clinicians have less interest in such subjects than they do instructions on assessment and treatment techniques. However, the valuable material in these chapters will hold the attention of even the most practical-minded clinician. Consider for a moment the basic science material the authors present. They frequently weave clinically relevant insights through the text. When they present information on an anatomical structure, for example, the reader whose main interests are clinical will quickly see the information's practical pertinence. The reader will do so because the authors, at short intervals, thread in attention-holding descriptions of how stresses may alter the anatomical structure, impairing its ability to serve its normal function. And often, they entwine through the text clinical methods useful in restoring anatomical integrity and normal function. Then, deftly, they return to the anatomy, carrying the reader's attention with them. Hence, the reader sees a tapestry formed of interwoven basic science and clinical threads, crafted to provide a scientifically based understanding of material that has the utmost practical relevance.

The reader's understanding of the information is made even easier by the authors' use of comprehension aids. They have included an abundance of photographs, drawings and diagrams that clarify subjects they cover in the text. In addition, with tables and bulleted statements, they have distilled the key points of the text so that they are perfectly clear. These aids will be especially useful for students in grasping the essentials of NMT, and for busy practitioners who need quick reminders.

The scope of the material in these first 10 chapters is as remarkable as the authors' presentation of it. To my knowledge, journal publications on soft tissue treatment span back at least two hundred years. In the past twenty years, however, the number of publications has increased precipitously. Many of these newer publications are reports of research findings that expand our understanding of the nature and dynamics of the soft tissues, disorders they are heir to, and treatments that can correct the disorders. A vast body of published literature now exists. I personally know how tough it is to read enough of the new publications to keep abreast of the expanding understanding of the soft tissues. In view of this difficulty, Chaitow's and DeLany's wide coverage of these subjects seems all the more impressive. I know of no other book that so comprehensively and intelligibly summarizes this literature as does *Clinical Application of Neuromuscular Techniques, Vol. 1.*

Chaitow and DeLany devote the last four chapters of the book to specific clinical applications of NMT. In these chapters, they describe the treatment methods they have found most useful in their clinical experiences. The authors show fair-minded courtesy toward advocates of techniques they do not describe; they qualify that practitioners may also find these other techniques useful. The value of the book is heightened by their limiting descriptions of clinical applications to techniques they have personally found useful. This means that the techniques they describe are not those they intellectually *hope* practitioners will find of value; they are ones the authors *know* are of practical value, having found them to be so in their own clinical practices. However, by saying that the authors limit their descriptions of techniques, I do not mean to imply that the book contains a paucity of information on techniques. On the contrary, the authors describe a vast array of treatment techniques. These include variations on muscle energy technique, positional release technique, myofascial release technique, hydrotherapy, acupressure, lymphatic drainage, mobilization, stretching, and more. In fact, I have never before seen a book that contains precise and detailed descriptions of such a wide diversity of soft tissue techniques.

In the chapters on clinical applications, the authors cover many disorders involving pain and dysfunction of the cervical spine, cranium, shoulder, arm, hand, and thorax. But they cover far more than soft tissue assessment and treatment technique. For example, they describe spinal joint dysfunction, how to evaluate it, and its relation to the soft tissues. They also describe a host of orthopedic, neurological, and articular tests. These tests are not new to traditionally trained chiropractors, physiatrists, and physical therapists. But what will be novel for many such practitioners is the authors' approach to the tests from a soft tissue perspective. This will prove a refreshing shift in perception for many traditionally trained practitioners.

For the disorders included in these chapters, the authors provide a wide range of treatment options. Among these are rehabilitation methods. They also describe proper precautions and make suggestions for avoiding or overcoming obstacles to patients' improvement or recovery.

To me, something that has limited the clinical success of many soft tissue practitioners is their failure to address biochemical, and to a lesser extent, psychosocial factors that affect (directly or indirectly) the soft tissues of their patients. Thus, some soft tissue practitioners see their professional domain as limited to manual examination and direct manual treatment of the soft tissues. When considering what may be contributing to a patient's soft tissue pain and dysfunction, these practitioners address only biomechanical factors, such as faulty posture, excessive repetitive motion, or deconditioning of muscles and connective tissues.

This compartmentalized-type practice is the opposite from a holistic, integrative practice – one that embraces safe and effective treatments, no matter what methods they involve or who provides them. Chaitow and DeLany herald this approach, explaining that soft tissue practitioners can achieve the best clinical results with most patients by addressing all classes of factors that may be adversely affecting a patient's soft tissues. They insightfully note, '. . . there is a constant merging and mixing of fundamental influences on health and ill health', and they explain the value of 'clustering etiological factors' when trying to make sense of a patient's clinical problems. They describe adverse interactive effects of biomechanical factors (such as overuse and trauma), biochemical factors (such as toxicity, nutritional deficiencies, and endocrine imbalances), and psychosocial factors (such as anxiety and depression). The advantage of this interactive approach, they write, is that it helps focus the practitioner's attention on factors that are amenable to change, thus enabling a more satisfactory therapeutic outcome. The book is a superb example of holistic, integrative philosophy in health care.

Through the years that I have taught soft tissue diagnosis and treatment, I have often wished for the ideal book to recommend – one that satisfies both academic interests and, at the same time, within a holistic conceptual framework, provides guidance in comprehensive assessment and the application of a wide range of soft tissue techniques. That book, *Clinical Application of Neuromuscular Techniques, Vol. 1,* now exists, and I strongly recommend it. I have no doubt that soon it (and its forthcoming companion, Vol. 2) will be the standard informational resource of students, teachers, and practitioners whose main clinical concern is the health of their patients' soft tissues.

Oklahoma 2000   Dr John C Lowe

Finally, a textbook that truly integrates science and the artful skill of 'hands on' therapy! Leon Chaitow and Judith DeLany have organized a wonderfully comprehensive view of the effective clinical applications of neuromuscular techniques.

These two authors, both of whom are practising clinicians, share their decades of patient care experience along with detailed scientific evidence and explanation of pain and soft tissue dysfunction. They include many practical examples of therapeutic intervention for conditions frequently encountered by the practitioner. For the practitioner who wishes to have a comprehensive model of care to address soft tissue challenges, this textbook goes above and beyond. The views, experience, and research of Chaitow and DeLany offer an understandable model that scientists and practitioners alike will find stimulating and encouraging.

I have been a clinical practitioner since 1975, specializing in the prevention, treatment, and care of athletic and occupational soft-tissue maladies. This is the first textbook that has pulled it all together in an intelligible and compelling format. From Chaitow's description of the fascial system and the causes of pain to DeLany's description of the precise neuromuscular techniques for specific regions of patient complaints, the mystery of neuromuscular phenomena is made clear. By following the model outlined by the authors, results with even the most stubborn soft tissue pain are attainable by the skilled practitioner.

This textbook has taken special emphasis to utilize techniques of expression that help the reader to understand biomechanical principles of the body's complexities and their relationship to the biochemical factors that contribute to pain and dysfunction. Notwithstanding the psychosocial implications that can challenge the practitioner, this textbook delivers superb guidelines and instruction with supported scientific basis.

The authors utilize fundamental science to create fundamental knowledge to build a better understanding of pain and dysfunction. This evidence supports the tremendous benefit that patients can gain from sound clinical application of neuromuscular techniques and therapy.

I am impressed by the authors' efforts to integrate science with the art of health care. This is especially critical for patients suffering from chronic pain due to common conditions that have not responded to many conventional standards of care. This textbook has been long overdue, not because this information did not exist before, but because it did not exist in one book in a comprehensive and understandable format.

Any practitioner who is interested in providing patient care that can make a difference would be wise to invest their study time in this text. It will help you to make sense out of a higher standard for patient care and getting results and resolution for many of the common challenges we all face daily in our practices. Congratulations Leon Chaitow and Judith DeLany on a job well done and well needed. Thank you.

Texas 2000   Benny F Vaughn

Preface

The clinical utilization of soft tissue manipulation has increased dramatically in recent years in all areas of manual health-care provision. The authors believe that a text which integrates the safe and proficient application of some of the most effective soft tissue techniques is both timely and necessary. The decision to write this book was therefore based on a growing awareness of the need for a text which describes, in some detail, the clinical applications of neuromuscular techniques in particular, and soft tissue manipulation in general, on each and every area of the musculoskeletal system.

There are numerous texts communicating the features of different manual therapy systems (osteopathy, chiropractic, physical therapy, manual medicine, massage therapy, etc.) and of modalities employed within these health-care delivery systems (high-velocity thrust techniques, muscle energy techniques, myofascial release and many, many more). There are also excellent texts which describe regional problems, say of the pelvic region, temporomandibular joint or the spine, with protocols for assessment and treatment, often described from a particular perspective. Increasingly, edited texts incorporate a variety of perspectives when focusing on particular regions, offering the reader a broad view as well as detailed information on the topic. And then there are wonderfully crafted volumes, such as those produced by Travell & Simons, covering the spectrum of 'myofascial pain and dysfunction' and incorporating these authors' deeply researched and evolving model of care.

The authors of this text decided that the Travell & Simons view of the human body offered a valuable regional approach model on which to base our own perspectives. To this practical and intellectually satisfying model, we have added detailed anatomical and physiological descriptions, coupled with clinically practical 'bodywork' solutions to the problems located in each region. In this first volume of the text, the upper body is covered, and in volume 2, the region from the waist

down is surveyed in the same way. As authors, we have attempted to place in context the relative importance and significance of local conditions, pain and/or dysfunction, which are quite logically the main focus for the patient. However, we believe it is vital that local problems should be commonly seen by the practitioner to form part of a larger picture of compensation, adaptation and/or decompensation and that the background causes (of local myofascial pain, for example) be sought and, where possible, removed or at least modified.

We also take the position that it is the practitioner's role to take account of biochemical (nutritional and hormonal influences, allergy, etc.), biomechanical (posture, breathing patterns, habits of use, etc.) and/or psychosocial (anxiety, depression, stress factors, etc.) influences which might be involved, as far as this is possible. If appropriate, suitable advice or treatment can then be offered; if the practitioner is not trained and licensed to do so, however, professional referral becomes the obvious choice. In this way, the focus of health care goes beyond treatment of local conditions and moves toward holism, to the benefit of the patient.

In this volume, the person applying the techniques is referred to as the 'practitioner' so as to include all therapists, physicians, nurses or others who apply manual techniques. To ease confusion, the practitioner is depicted as male and the recipient of the treatment modalities (the patient) is depicted as female so that gender references (he, his, she, hers) used within the text are not ambiguous. In volume 2, the roles are reversed with the female practitioner treating the male patient.

The methods described in this text fall largely within the biomechanical arena, with the main emphasis being the first comprehensive, detailed description of the clinical application of NMT (neuromuscular *therapy* in the USA, neuromuscular *technique* in Europe). The descriptions of NMT are mainly of the modern American version, as described by Judith DeLany, whose many years of involvement with NMT, both clinically and academically, make her a leading authority on the subject.

Additional therapeutic choices, including nutritional and hydrotherapeutic, as well as complementary body-work methods, such as muscle energy, positional release and variations of myofascial release techniques, and the European version of NMT, are largely the contribution of Leon Chaitow, as are, to a large extent, the opening chapters regarding the physiology of pain and dysfunction.

By combining our clinical experience, we believe we have offered an expanded perspective which readers can use as a safe guide to the application of the methods described, especially if they have had previous training in soft tissue palpation and treatment. The text of this book is therefore intended as a framework for the clinical application of NMT for those already qualified (and, where appropriate, licensed to practice), as well as being a learning tool for those in training. It is definitely not meant to be a substitute for hands-on training with skilled instructors.

In addition to the practical application sections of the book, a number of chapters offer a wide-ranging overview of current thinking and research into the background of the dysfunctional states for which solutions and suggestions are provided in later chapters. The overview, 'big picture' chapters cover the latest research findings and information relevant to understanding fascia, muscles, neurological factors, patterns of dysfunction, pain and inflammation, myofascial trigger points, emotional and nutritional influences and much more. It is our assertion that the combination of the 'big picture', together with the detailed NMT protocols, offers a foundation on which to build the exceptional palpation and treatment skills necessary for finding effective, practical solutions to chronic pain conditions.

London 2000   LC
Florida 2000   JD

Acknowledgements

Books are written by the efforts of numerous people, although most of the support team is invisible to the reader. We humbly express our appreciation to our friends and colleagues who assisted in this project and who enrich our lives simply by being themselves.

From the long list of staff members and practitioners who dedicated time and effort to read and comment on this text, we are especially grateful to Jamie Alagna, Paula Bergs, Bruno Chikly, Renée Evers, Jose Fernandez, Gretchen Fiery, Barbara Ingram-Rice, Donald Kelley, Leslie Lynch, Aaron Mattes, Charna Rosenholtz, Cindy Scifres, Alex Spassoff, Bonnie Thompson and Paul Witt for reviewing pages of material, often at a moment's notice. And to those whose work has inspired segments of this text, such as John Hannon, Tom Myers, David Simons, Janet Travell and others, we offer our heartfelt appreciation for their many contributions to myofascial therapies.

John and Lois Ermatinger spent many hours as models for the photographs in the book, some of which eventually became line art while Mary Beth Wagner dedicated her time coordinating each photo session. The enthusiastic attitudes and tremendous patience shown by each of them turned what could have been tedious tasks into pleasant events.

Many people offered personal support so that quality time to write was available, including Lois Allison, Jan Carter, Linda Condon, Andrew DeLany, Valerie Fox, Patricia Guillote, Alissa Miller, and Trish Solito. Special appreciation is given to Mary Beth Wagner and Andrea Conley for juggling many, many ongoing tasks which serve to enhance and fortify this work.

Jane Shanks, Katrina Mather, and Valerie Dearing each put forth exceptional dedication to find clarity, organization and balance within this text, which was exceeded only by their patience. The illustration team as well as the many authors, artists and publishers who loaned artwork from other books have added visual impact to help the material come alive.

To Mary Law, we express our deepest appreciation for her vision and commitment to complementary medicine worldwide. Mary's ability to foster organization amidst chaos, to find solutions to enormous challenges and to simply provide a listening ear when one is needed has endeared her to our hearts.

And finally, to each of our families, we offer our deepest gratitude for their inspiration, patience, and ever present understanding. Their supporting love made this project possible.

1

Connective tissue and the fascial system

Connective tissue forms the single largest tissue component of the body. The material we know as fascia is one of the many forms of connective tissue. In this chapter we will examine some of the key features and functions of fascia in particular, and connective tissue in general, with specific focus on the ways in which:

- these tissues influence myofascial pain and dysfunction
- their unique characteristics determine how they respond to therapeutic interventions, as well as to adaptive stresses imposed on them.

In order to understand myofascial dysfunction, it is important to have a clear picture of that single network which enfolds and embraces all other soft tissues and organs of the body, the fascial web. In the treatment focus in subsequent chapters, a great deal of reductionist thinking will be called for as we identify focal points of dysfunction, local trigger points, individual muscular stresses and attachment problems, with appropriate local and general treatment descriptions flowing from these

---

Box 1.1   Definitions

Stedman's medical dictionary (1998) says fascia is:

A sheet of fibrous tissue that envelops the body beneath the skin; it also encloses muscles and groups of muscles, and separates their several layers or groups

and that connective tissue is

The supporting or framework tissue of the ... body, formed of fibrous and ground substance with more or less numerous cells of various kinds; it is derived from the mesenchyme, and this in turn from the mesoderm; the varieties of connective tissue are: areolar or loose; adipose; dense, regular or irregular, white fibrous; elastic; mucous; and lymphoid tissue; cartilage; and bone; the blood and lymph may be regarded as connective tissues, the ground substance of which is a liquid.

Fascia, therefore, is one form of connective tissue.

identified areas and structures. The truth, of course, is that no tissue exists in isolation but acts – is bound and is interwoven – with other structures, to the extent that a fallen arch can directly be shown to influence TMJ dysfunction (Janda 1986). When we work on a local area, we need to keep a constant awareness of the fact that we are influencing the whole body.

THE FASCIAL NETWORK

Fascia comprises one integrated and totally connected network, from the attachments on the inner aspects of the skull to the fascia in the soles of the feet. If any part of this network becomes deformed or distorted, there may be negative stresses imposed on distant aspects and on the structures which it divides, envelopes, enmeshes, supports and with which it connects. There is ample evidence that Wolff's law (see Box 1.3) applies, in that fascia accommodates to chronic stress patterns and

---

Box 1.2 Biomechanical terms relating to fascia

Creep Continued deformation (increasing strain) of a viscoelastic material with time under constant load (traction, compression, twist)
Hysteresis Process of energy loss due to friction when tissues are loaded and unloaded
Load The degree of force (stress) applied to an area
Strain Change in shape as a result of stress
Stress Force (load) normalized over the area on which it acts (All tissues exhibit stress–strain responses)
Thixotropy A quality of colloids in which the more rapidly force is applied (load), the more rigid the tissue response
Viscoelastic The potential to deform elastically when load is applied and to return to the original non-deformed state when load is removed
Viscoplastic A permanent deformation resulting from the elastic potential having been exceeded or pressure forces sustained

---

Box 1.3 Biomechanical laws

Mechanical principles influencing the body neurologically and anatomically are governed by basic laws.

- Wolff's law states that biological systems (including soft and hard tissues) deform in relation to the lines of force imposed on them.
- Hooke's law states that deformation (resulting from strain) imposed on an elastic body is in proportion to the stress (force/load) placed on it.
- Newton's third law states that when two bodies interact, the force exerted by the first on the second is equal in magnitude and opposite in direction to the force exerted by the second on the first.
- Ardnt–Schultz's law states that weak stimuli excite physiologic activity, moderately strong ones favor it, strong ones retard it and very strong ones arrest it.
- Hilton's law states that the nerve supplying a joint also supplies the muscles which move the joint and the skin covering the articular insertion of those muscles.

deforms itself, something which often precedes deformity of osseous and cartilaginous structures in chronic diseases.

Visualize a complex, interrelated, symbiotically functioning assortment of tissues comprising skin, muscles, ligaments, tendons, bones as well as the neural structures, blood and lymph channels and vessels which bisect and invest these tissues – all given shape, cohesion and functional ability by the fascia. Now imagine removing from this all that is not connective tissue. What remains would still demonstrate the total form of the body, from the shape of the eyeball to the hollow voids for organ placement.

FASCIA AND PROPRIOCEPTION

Research has shown that:

- muscle and fascia are anatomically inseparable
- fascia moves in response to complex muscular activities acting on bone, joints, ligaments, tendons and fascia
- fascia, according to Bonica (1990), is critically involved in proprioception, which is, of course, essential for postural integrity (see Chapter 3)
- research by Professor J Staubesand (using electron microscope studies) shows that 'numerous' myelinated sensory neural structures exist in fascia, relating to both proprioception and pain reception (Staubesand 1996)
- after joint and muscle spindle input is taken into account, the majority of remaining proprioception occurs in fascial sheaths (Earl 1965, Wilson 1966).

FASCIA: COLLAGENOUS CONTINUITY

Fascia is one form of connective tissue, formed from collagen, which is ubiquitous. The human framework depends upon fascia to provide form, cohesion, separation and support and to allow movement between neighboring structures without irritation. Since fascia comprises a single structure, from the soles of the feet (plantar fascia) to the inside of the cranium (dura and meninges), the implications for bodywide repercussions of distortions in that structure are clear. An example is to be found in the fascial divisions within the cranium, the tentorium cerebelli and falx cerebri, which are commonly warped during birthing difficulties (too long or too short a time in the birth canal, forceps delivery, etc.) and which are noted in craniosacral therapy as affecting total body mechanics via their influence on fascia (and therefore the musculature) throughout the body (Brookes 1984).

Dr Leon Page (1952) discusses the cranial continuity of fascia:

The cervical fascia extends from the base of the skull to the mediastinum and forms compartments enclosing esophagus, trachea and carotid vessels and provides support for the pharynx, larynx and thyroid gland. There is direct continuity of fascia from the apex of the diaphragm to the base of the skull. Extending through the fibrous pericardium upward through the deep cervical fascia and the continuity extends not only to the outer surface of the sphenoid, occipital and temporal bones but proceeds further through the foramina in the base of the skull around the vessels and nerves to join the dura.

FURTHER FASCIAL CONSIDERATIONS

Fascia is colloidal, as is most of the soft tissue of the body (a colloid is defined as comprising particles of solid material suspended in fluid – for example, wall paper paste or, indeed, much of the human body). Scariati (1991) points out that colloids are not rigid – they conform to the shape of their container and respond to pressure even though they are not compressible. The amount of resistance colloids offer increases proportionally to the

velocity of force applied to them. This makes a gentle touch a fundamental requirement if viscous drag and resistance are to be avoided when attempting to produce a change in, or release of, restricted fascial structures, which are all colloidal in their behavior.

ELASTICITY

Soft tissues, and other biological structures, have an innate, variable degree of elasticity, springiness, resilience or 'give' which allows them to withstand deformation when force or pressure is applied. This provides the potential for subsequent recovery of tissue to which force has been applied, so that it returns to its starting shape and size. This quality of elasticity derives from these tissues' (soft or osseous) ability to store some of the mechanical energy applied to them and to utilize this in their movement back to their original status. This is a process known as hysteresis (see below).

Box 1.4   Connective tissue

Connective tissue is composed of cells (including fibroblasts and chondrocytes) and an extracellular matrix of collagen and elastic fibers surrounded by a ground substance made primarily of acid glycosaminoglycans (AGAGs) and water (*Gray's anatomy* 1995, Lederman 1997). Its patterns of deposition change from location to location, depending upon its role and the stresses applied to it.

The collagen component is composed of three polypeptide chains wound around each other to form triple helixes. These microfilaments are arranged in parallel manner and bound together by crosslinking hydrogen bonds, which 'glue' the elements together to provide strength and stability when mechanical stress is applied. Movement encourages the collagen fibers to align themselves along the lines of structural stress as well as improves the balance of glycosaminoglycans and water, therefore lubricating and hydrating the connective tissue (Lederman 1997).

While these bonding crossbridges do provide structural support, injury, chronic stress and immobility cause excessive bonding, leading to the formation of scars and adhesions which limit the movement of these usually resilient tissues (Juhan 1987). The loss of tissue lengthening potential would then not be due to the *volume* of collagen but to the random pattern in which it is laid down and the abnormal crossbridges which prevent normal movement. Following tissue injury, it is important that activity be introduced as soon as the healing process will allow in order to prevent maturation of the scar tissue and development of adhesive crosslinks (Lederman 1997).

Lederman (1997) tells us:

The pattern of collagen deposition varies in different types of connective tissue. It is an adaptive process related to the direction of forces imposed on the tissue. In tendon, collagen fibers are organized in parallel arrangement; this gives the tendon stiffness and strength under unidirectional loads. In ligaments, the organization of the fibers is looser, groups of fibers lying in different directions. This reflects the multidirectional forces that ligaments are subjected to, for example during complex movements of a joint such as flexion combined with rotation and shearing ... Elastin has an arrangement similar to that of collagen in the extracellular matrix,

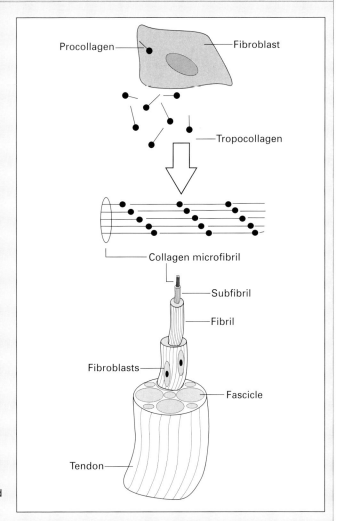

Figure 1.1   Collagen is produced locally for repair of damaged connective tissue (after Lederman 1997).

Box 1.4   (cont'd)

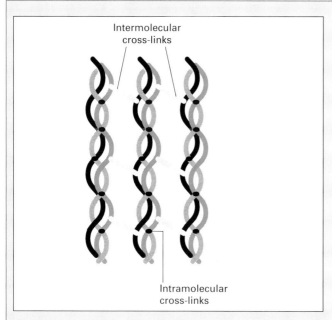

Figure 1.2 Collagen's triple helices are bound together by inter- and intramolecular crosslinking bonds.

and its deposition is also dependent on the mechanical stresses imposed on the tissue.

Elastin provides an elastic-like quality which allows the connective tissue to stretch to the limit of the collagen fiber's length, while absorbing tensile force. If this elastic quality is stretched over time, it may lose its ability to recoil (as seen in the stretch marks of pregnancy). When stress is applied, the tissue can be stretched to the limit of the collagen fiber length with flexibility being dependent upon elastic quality (and quantity) as well as the extent of crossbridging which has occurred between the collagen fibers. Additionally, if heavy pressure is suddenly applied, the connective tissue may respond as brittle and may more easily tear (Kurz 1986).

  Surrounding the collagen and elastic fibers is a viscous, gel-like ground substance, composed of proteoglycans and hyaluronan (formerly called hyaluronic acid), which lubricates these fibers and allows them to slide over one another (Barnes 1990, *Gray's anatomy* 1995).

- Ground substances provides the immediate environment for every cell in the body.
- The protein component is hydrophilic (draws water into the tissue), producing a cushion effect as well as maintaining space between the collagen fibers.
- Ground substance provides the medium through which other elements are exchanged, such as gases, nutrients, hormones, cellular waste, antibodies and white blood cells (Juhan 1987).
- The condition of the ground substance can then affect the rate of diffusion and therefore the health of the cells it surrounds.

Juhan (1987) notes:

Where we find mostly fluid and few fibers, we have a watery intercellular medium that is ideal for metabolic activities; with less fluid and more fibers, we have a soft, flexible lattice that can hold skin cells or liver cells or nerve cells into place; with little fluid and many fibers, we have the tough, stringy material of muscle sacs, tendons, and ligaments. If chondroblasts (cartilage-producing cells) and their hyaline secretions are added to this matrix, we obtain more solidity, and in the bones this cartilaginous secretion is replaced by mineral salts to achieve a rock-like hardness.

Unless irreversible fibrotic changes have occurred or other pathologies exist, connective tissue's state can be changed from a gelatinous-like substance to a more solute (watery) state by the introduction of energy through muscular activity (active or passive movement provided by activity or stretching), soft tissue manipulation (as provided by massage) or heat (as in hydrotherapies). This characteristic, called *thixotropy*, is 'a property of certain gels of becoming less viscous when shaken or subjected to shearing forces and returning to the original viscosity upon standing' (Stedman's 1998). Without thixotropic properties, movement would eventually cease due to solidification of synovium and connective tissue.
  Oschman states (1997):

If stress, disuse and lack of movement cause the gel to dehydrate, contract and harden (an idea that is supported both by scientific evidence and by the experiences of many somato-therapists) the application of pressure seems to bring about a rapid solation and rehydration. Removal of the pressure allows the system to rapidly re-gel, but in the process the tissue is transformed, both in its water content and in its ability to conduct energy and movement. The ground substance becomes more porous, a better medium for the diffusion of nutrients, oxygen, waste products of metabolism and the enzymes and building blocks involved in the 'metabolic regeneration' process...

Plastic and elastic features

Greenman (1989) describes how fascia responds to loads and stresses in both a plastic and an elastic manner, its response depending, among other factors, upon the type, duration and amount of the load. When stressful forces (undesirable or therapeutic) are gradually applied to fascia (or other biological material), there is at first an elastic reaction in which a degree of slack is allowed to be taken up, followed, if the force persists, by what is colloquially referred to as *creep* – a variable degree of resistance (depending upon the state of the tissues). This gradual change in shape results from the viscoelastic property of tissue.

Creep, then, is a term which accurately describes the slow, delayed, yet continuous deformation which occurs in response to a sustained, slowly applied load, as long as this is gentle enough not to provoke the resistance of colloidal 'drag'. During creep, tissues lengthen or distort ('deflect') until a point of balance is achieved. An example often used of creep is that which occurs in intervertebral discs as they gradually compress during periods of upright stance.

Stiffness of any tissue relates to its viscoelastic properties and, therefore, to the thixotropic colloidal nature of collagen/fascia. Thixotropy relates to the quality of colloids in which the more rapidly force is applied (load), the more rigid the tissue response will be – hence the

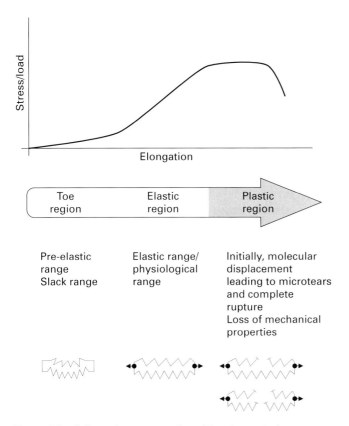

Figure 1.3 Schematic representation of the stress–strain curve.

likelihood of fracture when rapid force meets the resistance of bone. If force is gradually applied, 'energy' is absorbed by and stored in the tissues. The usefulness of this in tendon function is obvious and its implications in therapeutic terms profound (Binkley 1989).

Hysteresis is the term used to describe the process of energy loss due to friction and to minute structural damage which occurs when tissues are loaded and unloaded. Heat will be produced during such a sequence, which can be illustrated by the way intervertebral discs absorb force transmitted through them as a person jumps up and down. During treatment (tensing and relaxing of tissues, for example, or on-and-off pressure application), hysteresis induction reduces stiffness and improves the way the tissue will respond to subsequent demands. The properties of hysteresis and creep provide much of the rationale for myofascial release techniques and aspects of neuromuscular therapy and need to be taken into account during technique applications. Especially important are the facts that:

- rapidly applied force to collagen structures leads to defensive tightening
- slowly applied load is accepted by collagen structures and allows for lengthening or distortion processes to commence.

When tissues (cartilage, for example) which are behaving

viscoelastically are loaded for any length of time, they first deform elastically. Subsequently, there is an actual volume change as water is forced from the tissue as they become less *sol*-like and more *gel*-like. Ultimately, when the applied force ceases, there should be a return to the original non-deformed state. However, if the elastic potential has been exceeded or pressure forces are sustained, a *viscoplastic* response develops and deformation can become permanent. The time taken for tissues to return to normal, via elastic recoil, when the application of force ceases depends upon the uptake of water by the tissues and this relates directly to osmotic pressure and to whether the viscoelastic potential of the tissues has been exceeded, resulting in a viscoplastic (permanent deformation) response.

Cantu & Grodin (1992) describe what they see as the 'unique' feature of connective tissue as its 'deformation characteristics'. This refers to the combined viscous (permanent, plastic) deformation characteristic, as well as an elastic (temporary) deformation status discussed above. The fact that connective tissues respond to applied mechanical force by first changing in length, followed by some of the change being lost while some remains, has implications in the application of stretching techniques to such tissues, as well as helping us to understand how and why soft tissues respond as they do to postural and other repetitive insults which exert load on them, often over long periods.

It is worth emphasizing that although viscoplastic changes are described as 'permanent', this is a relative term. Such changes are not necessarily absolutely permanent since collagen (the raw material of fascia/connective tissue) has a limited (300–500 day) half-life and, just as bone adapts to stresses imposed upon it, so will fascia. If negative stresses (such as poor posture, use, etc.) are modified for the better and/or positive (therapeutic) 'stresses' are imposed by means of appropriate manipulation and/or exercise, apparently 'permanent' changes can modify for the better. Dysfunctional connective tissue changes can usually be improved, if not quickly then certainly over time (Neuberger 1953).

Important features of the response of tissue to load include:

- the degree of the load
- the amount of surface area to which force is applied
- the rate, uniformity and speed at which it is applied
- how long load is maintained
- the configuration of the collagen fibers (i.e. are they parallel to or differently oriented to the direction of force, offering greater or lesser degrees of resistance?)
- the permeability of the tissues (to water)

- the relative degree of hydration or dehydration of the individual and of the tissues involved
- the status and age of the individual, since elastic and plastic qualities diminish with age
- another factor (apart from the nature of the stress load) which influences the way fascia responds to application of a stress load, and what the individual feels regarding the process, relates to the number of collagen and elastic fibers contained in any given region.

TRIGGER POINTS, FASCIA AND THE NERVOUS SYSTEM

Changes which occur in connective tissue, and which result in alterations such as thickening, shortening, calcification and erosion, may be a painful result of sudden or sustained tension or traction. Cathie (1974) points out that many trigger points (he calls them trigger 'spots') correspond to points where nerves pierce fascial investments. Hence, sustained tension or traction on the fascia may lead to varying degrees of fascial entrapment of neural structures and consequently a wide range of symptoms and dysfunctions. Neural receptors within the fascia report to the central nervous system as part of any adaptation process, with the pacinian corpuscles being particularly important (these inform the CNS about the rate of acceleration of movement taking place in the area) in terms of their involvement in reflex responses. Other neural input into the pool of activity and responses to biomechanical stress involve fascial structures, such as tendons and ligaments, which contain highly specialized and sensitive mechanoreceptors and proprioceptive reporting stations (see reporting stations, Chapter 3).

Additionally:

- German research has shown that fascia is 'regularly' penetrated (via 'perforations') by a triad of venous, arterial and neural structures (Staubesand 1996)
- these seem to correspond with fascial perforations previously identified by Heine which have been correlated (82% correlation) with known acupuncture points (Heine 1995)
- many of these fascial neural structures are sensory and capable of being involved in pain syndromes.

Staubesand states:

The receptors we found in the lower leg fascia in humans could be responsible for several types of myofascial pain sensations ... Another and more specific aspect is the innervation and direct connection of fascia with the autonomic nervous system. It now appears that the fascial tonus might be influenced and regulated by the state of the autonomic nervous system ... intervention in the fascial system might have an effect on the autonomic nervous system, in general, and upon the organs which are directly effected from it. (Schleip 1998)

SUMMARY OF FASCIAL AND CONNECTIVE TISSUE FUNCTION

Fascia is involved in numerous complex biochemical activities.

- Connective tissue provides a supporting matrix for more highly organized structures and attaches extensively to and invests into muscles.
- Individual muscle fibers are enveloped by endomysium which is connected to the stronger perimysium which surrounds the fasciculi.
- The perimysium's fibers attach to the even stronger epimysium which surrounds the muscle as a whole and which attaches to fascial tissues nearby.
- Because it contains mesenchymal cells of an embryonic type, connective tissue provides a generalized tissue capable of giving rise, under certain circumstances, to more specialized elements.
- It provides (by its fascial planes) pathways for nerves, blood and lymphatic vessels and structures.
- Many of the neural structures in fascia are sensory in nature.
- Fascia supplies restraining mechanisms by the differentiation of retention bands, fibrous pulleys and check ligaments as well as assisting in the harmonious production and control of movement.
- Where connective tissue is loose in texture it allows movement between adjacent structures and, by the formation of bursal sacs, it reduces the effects of pressure and friction.
- Deep fascia ensheaths and preserves the characteristic contour of the limbs and promotes the circulation in the veins and lymphatic vessels.
- The superficial fascia, which forms the panniculus adiposis, allows for the storage of fat and also provides a surface covering which aids in the conservation of body heat.
- By virtue of its fibroblastic activity, connective tissue aids in the repair of injuries by the deposition of collagenous fibers (scar tissue).
- The ensheathing layer of deep fascia, as well as intermuscular septa and interosseous membranes, provides vast surface areas used for muscular attachment.
- The meshes of loose connective tissue contain the 'tissue fluid' and provide an essential medium through which the cellular elements of other tissues are brought into functional relation with blood and lymph.
- This occurs partly by diffusion and partly by means of hydrokinetic transportation encouraged by alterations in pressure gradients – for example, between the thorax and the abdominal cavity during inhalation and exhalation.
- Connective tissue has a nutritive function and houses nearly a quarter of all body fluids.

Box 1.5 Myers' fascial trains (Myers 1997)

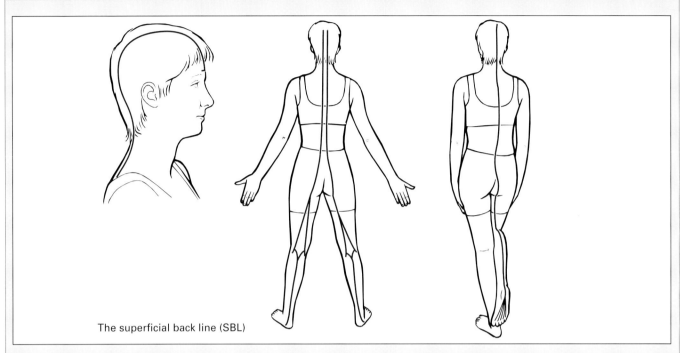

The superficial back line (SBL)

Figure 1.4 Myers' superficial fascial back line (reproduced, with permission, from the *Journal of Bodywork and Movement Therapies* 1997; **1**(2):95).

Tom Myers, a distinguished teacher of structural integration, has described a number of clinically useful sets of myofascial chains. The connections between different structures ('long functional continuities') which these insights allow will be drawn on and referred to when treatment protocols are discussed in this text. They are of particular importance in helping draw attention to (for example) dysfunctional patterns in the lower limb which impact directly (via these chains) on structures in the upper body.

The five major fascial chains

The superficial back line **(Fig. 1.4)** involves a chain which starts with:

- the plantar fascia, linking the plantar surface of the toes to the calcaneus
- gastrocnemius, linking calcaneus to the femoral condyles
- hamstrings, linking the femoral condyles to the ischial tuberosities
- subcutaneous ligament, linking the ischial tuberosities to sacrum
- lumbosacral fascia, erector spinae and nuchal ligament, linking the sacrum to the occiput
- scalp fascia, linking the occiput to the brow ridge.

The superficial front line **(Fig. 1.5)** involves a chain which starts with:

- the anterior compartment and the periostium of the tibia, linking the dorsal surface of the toes to the tibial tuberosity
- rectus femoris, linking the tibial tuberosity to the anterior inferior iliac spine and pubic tubercle
- rectus abdominis as well as pectoralis and sternalis fascia, linking the pubic tubercle and the anterior inferior iliac spine with the manubrium
- sternocleidomastoid, linking the manubrium with the mastoid process of the temporal bone.

The lateral line involves a chain which starts with:

- peroneal muscles, linking the 1st and 5th metatarsal bases with the fibular head
- iliotibial tract, tensor fascia latae and gluteus maximus, linking the fibular head with the iliac crest
- external obliques, internal obliques and (deeper) quadratus lumborum, linking the iliac crest with the lower ribs

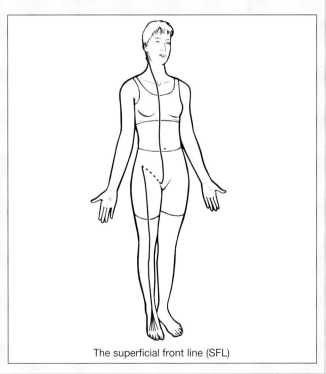

The superficial front line (SFL)

Figure 1.5 Myers' superficial fascial front line (reproduced, with permission, from the *Journal of Bodywork and Movement Therapies* 1997; **1**(2):97).

Box 1.5 *(cont'd)*

- external intercostals and internal intercostals, linking the lower ribs with the remaining ribs
- splenius cervicis, iliocostalis cervicis, sternocleidomastoid and (deeper) scalenes, linking the ribs with the mastoid process of the temporal bone.

The spiral line involves a chain which starts with:

- splenius capitis, which wraps across from one side to the other, linking the occipital ridge (say, on the right) with the spinous processes of the lower cervical and upper thoracic spine on the left
- continuing in this direction, the rhomboids (on the left) link via the medial border of the scapula with serratus anterior and the ribs (still on the left), wrapping around the trunk via the external obliques and the abdominal aponeurosis on the left, to connect with the internal obliques on the right and then to a strong anchor point on the anterior superior iliac spine (right side)
- from the ASIS, the tensor fascia latae and the iliotibial tract link to the lateral tibial condyle
- tibialis anterior links the lateral tibial condyle with the 1st metatarsal and cuneiform
- from this apparent endpoint of the chain (1st metatarsal and cuneiform), peroneus longus rises to link with the fibular head
- biceps femoris connects the fibular head to the ischial tuberosity
- the sacrotuberous ligament links the ischial tuberosity to the sacrum
- the sacral fascia and the erector spinae link the sacrum to the occipital ridge.

The deep front line describes several alternative chains involving the structures anterior to the spine (internally, for example):

- the anterior longitudinal ligament, diaphragm, pericardium, mediastinum, parietal pleura, fascia prevertebralis and the scalene fascia, which connect the lumbar spine (bodies and transverse processes) to the cervical transverse processes and via longus capitis to the basilar portion of the occiput
- other links in this chain might involve a connection between the posterior manubrium and the hyoid bone via the subhyoid muscles and
- the fascia pretrachealis between the hyoid and the cranium/mandible, involving suprahyoid muscles
- the muscles of the jaw linking the mandible to the face and cranium.

Myers includes in his chain description structures of the lower limbs which connect the tarsum of the foot to the lower lumbar spine, making the linkage complete. Additional smaller chains involving the arms are described as follows.

Back of the arm lines

- The broad sweep of trapezius links the occipital ridge and the cervical spinous processes to the spine of the scapula and the clavicle.
- The deltoid, together with the lateral intermuscular septum, connects the scapula and clavicle with the lateral epicondyle.
- The lateral epicondyle is joined to the hand and fingers by the common extensor tendon.
- Another track on the back of the arm can arise from the rhomboids, which link the thoracic transverse processes to the medial border of the scapula.
- The scapula in turn is linked to the olecranon of the ulna by infraspinatus and the triceps.
- The olecranon of the ulna connects of the small finger via the periostium of the ulna.
- A 'stabilization' feature in the back of the arm involves latissimus dorsi and the thoracolumbar fascia, which connects the arm with the spinous processes, the contralateral sacral fascia and gluteus maximus, which in turn attaches to the shaft of the femur.
- Vastus lateralis connects the femur shaft to the tibial tuberosity and (via this) to the periostium of the tibia.

Front of the arm line

- Latissimus dorsi, teres major and pectoralis major attach to the humerus close to the medial intramuscular septum, connecting it to the back of the trunk.
- The medial intramuscular septum connects the humerus to the medial epicondyle which connects with the palmar hand and fingers by means of the common flexor tendon.
- An additional line on the front of the arm involves pectoralis minor, the costocoracoid ligament, the brachial neurovascular bundle and the fascia clavipectoralis, which attach to the coracoid process.
- The coracoid process also provides the attachment for biceps brachii (and coracobrachialis) linking this to the radius and the thumb via the flexor compartment of the forearm.
- A 'stabilization' line on the front of the arm involves pectoralis major attaching to the ribs, as do the external obliques, which then run to the pubic tubercle, where a connection is made to the contralateral adductor longus, gracilis, pes anserinus, and the tibial periostium.

In the following chapters' discussions of local dysfunctional patterns involving the cervical, thoracic, shoulder and arm regions, it will be useful to hold in mind the direct muscular and fascial connections which Myers highlights, so that the possibility of distant influences is never forgotten.

- Fascia is a major arena of inflammatory processes (Cathie 1974) (see Chapter 7).
- Fluids and infectious processes often travel along fascial planes (Cathie 1974).
- Chemical (nutritional) factors influence fascial behavior directly. Pauling (1976) showed that, 'Many of the results of deprivation of ascorbic acid [vitamin C] involve a deficiency in connective tissue which is largely responsible for the strength of bones, teeth, and skin of the body and which consists of the fibrous protein collagen'.
- The histiocytes of connective tissue comprise part of

an important defense mechanism against bacterial invasion by their phagocytic activity.
- They also play a part as scavengers in removing cell debris and foreign material.
- Connective tissue represents an important 'neutralizer' or detoxicator to both endogenous toxins (those produced under physiological conditions) and exogenous toxins.
- The mechanical barrier presented by fascia has important defensive functions in cases of infection and toxemia.
- Fascia, then, is not just a background structure with little function apart from its obvious supporting role,

but is an ubiquitous, tenacious, living tissue which is deeply involved in almost all of the fundamental processes of the body's structure, function and metabolism.

- In therapeutic terms, there can be little logic in trying to consider muscle as a separate structure from fascia since they are so intimately related.

- Remove connective tissue from the scene and any muscle left would be a jelly-like structure without form or functional ability.

Box 1.6 Tensegrity

Tensegrity, a term coined by architect/engineer Buckminster Fuller, represents a system characterized by a discontinuous set of compressional elements (struts) which are held together, uprighted and/or moved by a continuous tensional network (Myers 1999, Oschman 1997). Fuller, one of the most original thinkers of the 20th century, developed a system of geometry based on tetrahedral (four-sided) shapes found in nature which maximize strength while occupying minimal space (maximum stability with a minimum of materials) (Juhan 1987). From these concepts he designed the geodesic dome, including the US Pavilion at Expo '67 in Montreal.

Tensegrity structures actually become stronger when they are stressed as the load applied is distributed not only to the area being directly loaded but throughout the structure (Barnes 1990). They employ both compressional and tensional elements. When applying the principles of tensegrity to the human body, one can readily see the bones and intervertebral discs as the discontinuous compressional units and the myofascial tissues (muscles, tendons, ligament, fascia and to some degree the discs) as the tensional elements. When load is applied (as in lifting) both the osseous and myofascial tissues distribute the stress incurred.

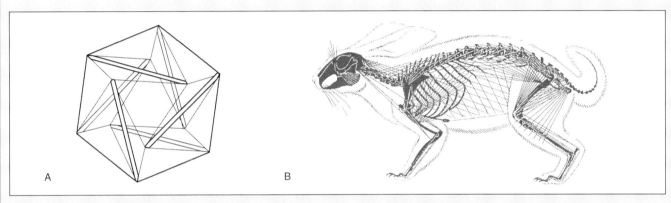

A   B

Figure 1.6 A&B: Tensegrity-based structures (reproduced, with permission, from the *Journal of Bodywork and Movement Therapies* 1997; **1**(5):300–302).

Of tensegrity, Juhan tells us:

Besides this hydrostatic pressure (which is exerted by every fascial compartment, not just the outer wrapping), the connective tissue framework – in conjunction with active muscles – provides another kind of tensional force that is crucial to the upright structure of the skeleton. We are not made up of stacks of building blocks resting securely upon one another, but rather of poles and guy-wires, whose stability relies not upon flat stacked surfaces, but upon proper angles of the poles and balanced tensions on the wires … There is not a single horizontal surface anywhere in the skeleton that provides a stable base for anything to be stacked upon it. Our design was not conceived by a stone-mason. Weight applied to any bone would cause it to slide right off its joints if it were not for the tensional balances that hold it in place and control its pivoting. Like the beams in a simple tensegrity structure, our bones act more as spacers than as compressional members; more weight is actually borne by the connective system of cables than by the bony beams.

Oschman (1997) concurs, adding another element:

Robbie (1977) reaches the remarkable conclusion that the soft tissues around the spine, when under appropriate tension, can actually lift each vertebra off the one below it. He views the spine as a tensegrity mast. The various ligaments form 'slings' that are capable of supporting the weight of the body without applying compressive forces to the vertebrae and intervertebral discs. In other words, the vertebral column is not, as it is usually portrayed, a simple stack of blocks, each cushioned by an intervertebral disc.

Later Oschman continues:

Cells and nuclei are tensegrity systems (Coffey 1985, Ingber & Folkman 1989, Ingber & Jamieson 1985). Elegant research has documented how the gravity system connects, via a family of molecules known as integrins, to the cytoskeletons of cells throughout the body. Integrins 'glue' every cell in the body to neighbouring cells and to the surrounding connective tissue matrix. An important study by Wang et al (1993) documents that integrin molecules carry tension from the extracellular matrix, across the cell surface, to the cytoskeleton, which behaves as a tensegrity matrix. Ingber (1993a,b) has shown how cell shape and function are regulated by an interacting tension and compression system within the cytoskeleton.

Levin (1997) informs us that once spherical shapes involving tensegrity structures occur (as in the cells of the body), a many-sided framework evolves which has 20 triangular faces. This is the hierarchically constructed tensegrity icosahedron (*icosa* is 20 in Greek) which are stacked together to form an infinite number of tissues.

Levin (1997) further explains architectural aspects of tensegrity, as it relates to the human body. He discusses the work of White & Panjabi (1978) who have shown that any part of the body which is free to move in any direction has 12 degrees of freedom: the ability to rotate around three axes, in each direction (six degrees of freedom) as well as the ability to translate on three planes in either direction (a further six degrees of freedom). He then asks, how is this stabilized?

Box 1.6 (cont'd)

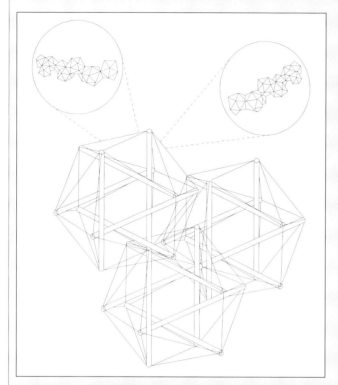

Figure 1.7 Tensegrity-based structures.

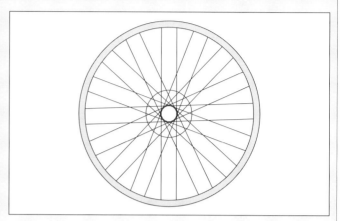

Figure 1.8 Cycle wheel structure allows compressive load to be distributed to rim through tension network.

To fix in space a body that has 12 degrees of freedom it seems logical that there need to be 12 restraints. Fuller (1975) proves this ... This principle is demonstrated in a wire-spoked bicycle wheel. A minimum of 12 tension spokes rigidly fixes the hub in space (anything more than 12 is a fail safe mechanism).

Levin points out that the tension-loaded spokes transmit compressive loads from the frame to the ground while the hub remains suspended in its tensegrity network of spokes: 'the load distributes evenly around the rim and the bicycle frame and its load hangs from the hubs like a hammock between trees'.

Other examples of tensegrity in common use include a tennis racket and the children's toy, a Jacob's ladder. In the body this architectural principle is seen in many tissues, most specifically in the way the sacrum is suspended between the ilia. This is detailed in Volume 2 of this text.

FASCIAL DYSFUNCTION

Mark Barnes (1997) states:

Fascial restrictions can create abnormal strain patterns that can crowd, or pull the osseous structures out of proper alignment, resulting in compression of joints, producing pain and/or dysfunction. Neural and vascular structures can also become entrapped in these restrictions, causing neurological or ischemic conditions. Shortening of the myofascial fascicle can limit its functional length – reducing its strength, contractile potential and deceleration capacity. Facilitating positive change in this system [by therapeutic intervention] would be a clinically relevant event.

Cantu & Grodin (1992) have stated that 'The response of normal connective tissue [fascia] to immobilization provides a basis for understanding traumatized conditions'.

A sequence of dysfunction has been demonstrated as follows (Akeson & Amiel 1977, Amiel & Akeson 1983, Evans 1960).

- The longer the immobilization, the greater the amount of infiltrate there will be.
- If immobilization continues beyond about 12 weeks

collagen loss is noted; however, in the early days of any restriction, a significant degree of ground substance loss occurs, particularly glycosaminoglycans and water.
- Since one of the primary purposes of ground substance is the lubrication of the tissues it separates (collagen fibers), its loss leads inevitably to the distance between these fibers being reduced.
- Loss of interfiber distance impedes the ability of collagen to glide smoothly, encouraging adhesion development
- This allows crosslinkage between collagen fibers and newly formed connective tissue, which reduces the degree of fascial extensibility as adjacent fibers become more and more closely bound.
- Because of immobility, these new fiber connections will not have a stress load to guide them into a directional format and they will be laid down randomly.
- Similar responses are observed in ligamentous as well as periarticular connective tissues.
- Mobilization of the restricted tissues can reverse the

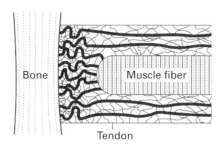 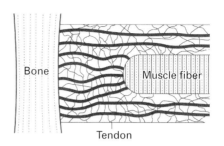

Figure 1.9 A: Dehydration of ground substance may cause kinking of collagen fibers. B: Sustained pressure may result in temporary solation of ground substance, allowing kinked collagen fibers to lengthen, thereby reducing muscular strain (reproduced, with permission, from the *Journal of Bodywork and Movement Therapies* 1997; **1**(5):309).

effects of immobilization as long as this has not been for an excessive period.

- If, due to injury, inflammatory processes occur as well as immobilization, a more serious evolution occurs, as inflammatory exudate triggers the process of contracture, resulting in shortening of connective tissue.
- This means that following injury, two separate processes may be occurring simultaneously: there may be a process of scar tissue development in the traumatized tissues and also fibrosis in the surrounding tissues (as a result of the presence of inflammatory exudate).
- Cantu & Grodin (1992) give an example: 'A shoulder may be frozen due to macroscopic scar adhesion in the folds of the inferior capsule … a frozen shoulder may also be caused by capsulitis, where the entire capsule shrinks'.
- Capsulitis could therefore be the result of fibrosis involving the entire fabric of the capsule, rather than a localized scar formation at the site of injury.

RESTORING GEL TO SOL

Mark Barnes (1997) insists that therapeutic methods which try to deal with this sort of fascial, connective tissue change (summarized above in relation to trauma or immobilization) would be to 'elongate and soften the connective tissue, creating permanent three-dimensional depth and width'.

To achieve this, he says:

Most important is the change in the ground substance from a gel to a sol. This occurs with a state phase realignment of crystals exposed to electromagnetic fields. This may occur as a piezoelectric event (changing a mechanical force to electric

energy) which changes the electrical charge of collagen and proteoglycans within the extracellular matrix.

In offering this opinion Barnes is basing his comments on the research evidence relating to connective tissue behavior which takes the properties of fascia into an area of study involving liquid crystal and piezoelectric events (Athenstaedt 1974, Pischinger 1991). Appropriately applied manual therapy can, Barnes suggests, often achieve such changes, whether this involves stretching, direct pressure, myofascial release or other approaches. All these elements form part of neuromuscular therapy interventions.

THERAPEUTIC SEQUENCING

Cantu & Grodin (1992), in their evaluation of the myofascial complex, conclude that therapeutic approaches which sequence their treatment protocols to involve the superficial tissues (involving autonomic responses) as well as deeper tissues (influencing the mechanical components of the musculoskeletal system) and which also address the factor of mobility (movement) meet with the requirements of the body when dysfunctional problems are being treated. NMT, as presented in this text, adopts this comprehensive approach and achieves at least some of its beneficial effects because of its influence on fascia.

In the upcoming chapters we will see how influences from the nervous system, inflammatory processes and patterns of use affect (and are affected by) the fascial network. In the second volume of this text, the principles of tensegrity, thixotropy and postural balance will be seen to form an intricate part of the foundations of whole-body structural integrity.

Box 1.7 Postural (fascial) patterns (Zink & Lawson 1979)

Zink & Lawson have described patterns of postural patterning determined by fascial compensation and decompensation.

- Fascial compensation is seen as a useful, beneficial and, above all, functional adaptation (i.e. no obvious symptoms) on the part of the musculoskeletal system, for example, in response to anomalies such as a short leg, or to overuse.
- Decompensation describes the same phenomenon but only in relation to a situation in which adaptive changes are seen to be dysfunctional, to produce symptoms, evidencing a failure of homeostatic adaptation.

By testing the tissue 'preferences' in different areas it is possible to classify patterns in clinically useful ways:

- *ideal* (minimal adaptive load transferred to other regions)
- *compensated* patterns which alternate in direction from area to area (e.g. atlantooccipital, cervicothoracic, thoracolumbar, lumbosacral) and which are commonly adaptive in nature
- *uncompensated* patterns which do not alternate and which are commonly the result of trauma.

Functional evaluation of fascial postural patterns

Zink & Lawson (1979) have described methods for testing tissue preference.

- There are four crossover sites where fascial tensions can be noted: occipitoatlantal (OA), cervicothoracic (CT), thoracolumbar (TL) and lumbosacral (LS).
- These sites are tested for their rotation and side-bending preferences.
- Zink & Lawson's research showed that most people display alternating patterns of rotatory preference with about 80% of people showing a common pattern of left-right-left-right (termed the common compensatory pattern or CCP) 'reading' from the occipitoatlantal region downwards.

- Zink & Lawson observed that the 20% of people whose compensatory pattern did not alternate had poor health histories.
- Treatment of either CCP or uncompensated fascial patterns has the objective of trying as far as is possible to create a symmetrical degree of rotatory motion at the key crossover sites.
- The treatment methods used to achieve this range from direct muscle energy approaches to indirect positional release techniques.

Assessment of tissue preference

Occipitoatlantal area (Fig. 1.10)

- Patient is supine.
- Practitioner sits at head, and cradles upper cervical region.
- The neck is fully flexed.
- The occiput is rotated on the atlas to evaluate tissue preference as the head is slowly rotated left and then right.

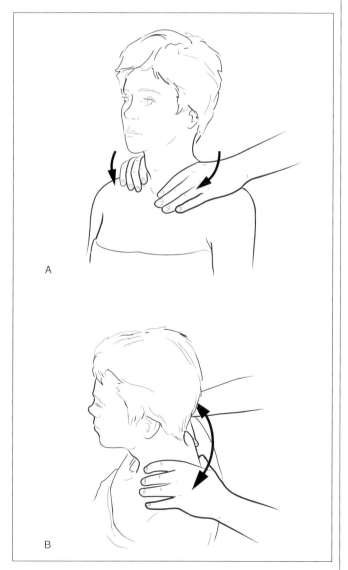

A

B

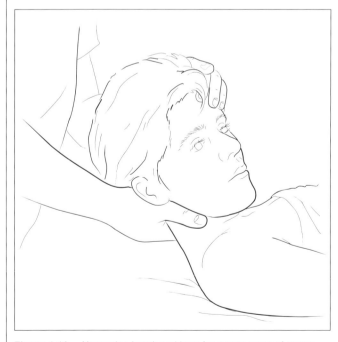

Figure 1.10 Alternative hand positions for assessment of upper cervical region tissue direction preference.

Figure 1.11 A&B: Hand positions for assessment of upper cervicothoracic region tissue direction preference.

Box 1.7 (cont'd)

Cervicothoracic area (Fig. 1.11)

- Patient is seated in relaxed posture with practitioner behind, with hands placed to cover medial aspects of upper trapezius so that fingers rest over the clavicles.
- The hands assess the area being palpated for its 'tightness/looseness' preferences as a slight degree of rotation left and then right is introduced at the level of the cervicothoracic junction.

Thoracolumbar area

- Patient is supine, practitioner stands at waist level facing cephalad and places hands over lower thoracic structures, fingers along lower rib shafts laterally.
- Treating the structure being palpated as a cylinder, the hands test the preference the lower thorax has to rotate around its central axis, one way and then the other.

Lumbosacral area

- Patient is supine, practitioner stands below waist level facing cephalad and places hands on anterior pelvic structures, using

the contact as a 'steering wheel' to evaluate tissue preference as the pelvis is rotated around its central axis while seeking information as to its 'tightness/looseness' preferences.

NOTE: By holding tissues in their 'loose' or ease positions, by holding tissues in their 'tight' or bind positions and introducing an isometric contraction or by just holding tissues at their barrier, waiting for a release, changes can be encouraged. The latter approach would be inducing the myofascial release in response to light, sustained load.

Questions following assessment exercise:

1. Was there an 'alternating' pattern to the tissue preferences?
2. Or was there a tendency for the tissue preference to be the same in all or most of the four areas assessed?
3. If the latter was the case, was this in an individual whose health is more compromised than average – in line with Zink & Lawson's suggestion?
4. By means of any of the methods suggested in the 'Note' above, are you able to produce a more balanced degree of tissue preference?

REFERENCES

Akeson W, Amiel D 1977 Collagen cross linking alterations in joint contractures. Connective Tissue Research 5:15–19

Amiel D, Akeson W 1983 Stress deprivation effect on metabolic turnover of medial collateral ligament collagen. Clinical Orthopedics 172:265–270

Athenstaedt H 1974 Pyroelectric and piezoelectric properties of vertebrates. Annals of New York Academy of Sciences 238:68–110

Barnes J F 1990 Myofascial release: the search for excellence. Myofascial Release Seminars, Paoli, PA

Barnes M 1997 The basic science of myofascial release. Journal of Bodywork and Movement Therapies 1(4):231–238

Binkley J 1989 Overview of ligaments and tendon structure and mechanics. Physiotherapy Canada 41(1):24–30

Bonica J 1990 The management of pain, 2nd edn. Lea and Febiger, Philadelphia

Brookes D 1984 Cranial osteopathy. Thorsons, London

Cantu R, Grodin A 1992 Myofascial manipulation. Aspen Publications, Maryland

Cathie A 1974 Selected writings. Academy of Applied Osteopathy Yearbook, Maidstone, England

Coffey D 1985 See Levine J The man who says YES. Johns Hopkins Magazine February / April:34–44

Earl E 1965 The dual sensory role of the muscle spindles. Physical Therapy Journal 45:4

Evans E 1960 Experimental immobilization and mobilization. Journal of Bone and Joint Surgery 42A:737–758

Fuller B 1975 Synergetics. Macmillan, New York

Gray's anatomy, 1995 (38th edn). Churchill Livingstone, Edinburgh

Greenman P 1989 Principles of manual medicine. Williams and Wilkins, Philadelphia

Heine H 1995 Functional anatomy of traditional Chinese acupuncture points. Acta Anatomica 152:293

Ingber D E, Folkman J 1989 Tension and compression as basic determinants of cell form and function: utilization of a cellular tensegrity mechanism. In: Stein W, Bronner F (eds) Cell shape: determinants, regulation and regulatory role. Academic Press, San Diego, pp 1–32

Ingber D E, Jamieson J 1985 Cells as tensegrity structures. In: Andersson L L, Gahmberg C G, Ekblom P E (eds) Gene expression during normal and malignant differentiation. Academic Press,

New York, pp 13–32

Ingber D E 1993a Cellular tensegrity: defining new rules of biological design that govern the cytoskeleton. Journal of Cell Science 104:613–627

Ingber D E 1993b The riddle of morphogenesis: a question of solution chemistry or molecular cell engineering. Cell 75:1249–1252

Janda V 1986 Extracranial causes of facial pain. Journal of Prosthetic Dentistry 56(4):484–487

Juhan D 1987 Job's body: a handbook for bodywork. Station Hill Press, Barrytown NY

Kurz I 1986 Textbook of Dr Vodder's manual lymph drainage, vol 2: Therapy, 2nd edn. Karl F Haug, Heidelberg

Lederman E 1997 Fundamentals of manual therapy. Physiology, neurology and psychology. Churchill Livingstone, Edinburgh

Levin S 1997 Tensegrity. In: Vleeming A, Mooney V, Dorman T, Snijders C, Stoeckart R (eds) Movement, stability and low back pain. Churchill Livingstone, Edinburgh

Myers T 1997 Anatomy trains. Journal of Bodywork and Movement Therapies 1(2):91–101 and 1(3):134–145

Myers T 1999 Kinesthetic dystonia parts 1 and 2. Journal of Bodywork and Movement Therapies 3(1):36–43 and 3(2):107–117

Neuberger A 1953 Metabolism of collagen. Journal of Biochemistry 53:47–52

Oschman J L 1997 What is healing energy? Pt 5: gravity, structure, and emotions. Journal of Bodywork and Movement Therapies 1(5): p 307–308

Page L 1952 Academy of Applied Osteopathy Yearbook

Pauling L 1976 The common cold and flu. W H Freeman, New York

Pischinger A 1991 Matrix and matrix regulation. Haug International, Brussels

Robbie D L 1977 Tensional forces in the human body. Orthopaedic Review 6:45–48

Scariati P 1991 Myofascial release concepts. In: DiGiovanna E (ed) An osteopathic approach to diagnosis and treatment. Lippincott, London

Schleip R 1998 Interview with Prof.Dr.med. J Staubesand in Rolf Lines. Rolf Institute, Boulder, Colorado

Staubesand J 1996 Zum Feinbau der fascia cruris mit Berucksichtigung epi-und intrafaszialar Nerven. Manuella Medezin 34:196–200

Stedman's Electronic Medical Dictionary 1998 version 4.0.

Wang J Y, Butler J P, Ingber D E 1993 Mechanotransduction across the cell surface and through the cytoskeleton. Science 260:1124–1127

White A, Panjabi M 1978 Clinical biomechanics of the spine. J B Lippincott, Philadelphia

Wilson V 1966 Inhibition in the CNS. Scientific American 5:102–106

Zink G, Lawson W 1979 An osteopathic structural examination and functional interpretation of the soma. Osteopathic Annals 12(7):433–440

2

Muscles

In this chapter we will focus attention on the prime movers and stabilizers of the body, the muscles. It is necessary to understand those aspects of their structure, function and dysfunction which can help to make selection and application of therapeutic interventions as suitable and effective as possible.

The skeleton provides the body with an appropriately rigid framework which has facility for movement at its junctions and joints. However, it is the muscular system

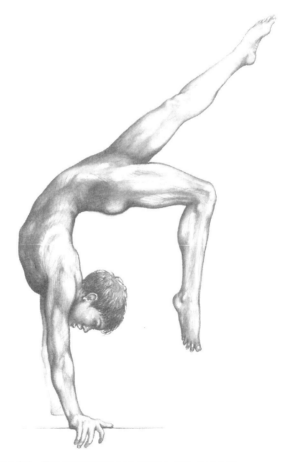

Figure 2.1   The miraculous possibilities of human balance (reproduced, with permission, from *Gray's anatomy* (1995)).

(given cohesion by the fascia, see Chapter 1) which both supports and propels this framework, providing us with the ability to express ourselves through movement, in activities ranging from chopping wood to brain surgery, climbing mountains to giving a massage. Almost everything, from facial expression to the beating of the heart, is dependent on muscular function.

Healthy, well-coordinated muscles receive and respond to a multitude of signals from the nervous system, providing the opportunity for coherent movement. When, through overuse, misuse, abuse, disuse, disease or trauma, the smooth interaction between the nervous, circulatory and the musculoskeletal systems is disturbed, movement becomes difficult, restricted, commonly painful and sometimes impossible. Dysfunctional patterns affecting the musculoskeletal system (see Chapter 5), which emerge from such a background, lead to compensatory adaptations and a need for therapeutic, rehabilitation and/or educational interventions. This chapter will highlight some of the unique qualities of the muscular system. On this foundation it will be possible to commence exploration of the many dysfunctional patterns which can interfere with the quality of life and create painful modifications of the framework, which leads to degenerative changes.

Because the anatomy and physiology of muscles are adequately covered elsewhere (see further reading list at the end of this chapter), the information in this chapter will be presented largely in summary form, with some specific topics (muscle type, for example) receiving a fuller discussion due to the significance they have in regard to neuromuscular therapy.

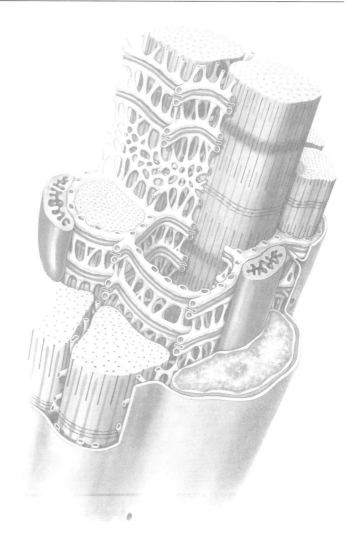

Figure 2.2 Details of the intricate organization of skeletal muscle (reproduced, with permission, from *Gray's anatomy* (1995)).

ESSENTIAL INFORMATION ABOUT MUSCLES (Fritz 1998, Jacob & Falls 1997, Lederman 1998, Liebenson 1996, Schafer 1987)

- Skeletal muscles are derived embryologically from mesenchyme and possess a particular ability to contract when neurologically stimulated.
- Skeletal muscle fibers comprise a single cell with hundreds of nuclei.
- The fibers are arranged into bundles (*fasciculi*) with connective tissue filling the spaces between the fibers (the *endomysium*) as well as surrounding the fasciculi (the *perimysium*).
- Entire muscles are surrounded by denser connective tissue (fascia, see Chapter 1) where it is known as the *epimysium*.
- The epimysium is continuous with the connective tissue of surrounding structures.
- Individual muscle fibers can vary in length from a few millimeters to an amazing 30 cm (in sartorius, for example) and in diameter from 10 to 60 μm.

TYPES OF MUSCLE

Muscle fibers can be broadly grouped into those which are:

- *longitudinal* (or *strap* or *parallel*), which have lengthy fascicles, largely oriented with the longitudinal axis of the body or its parts. These fascicles favor speedy action and are usually involved in range of movement (sartorius, for example, or biceps brachii)
- *pennate*, which have fascicles running at an angle to the muscle's central tendon (its longitudinal axis). These fascicles favor strong movement and are divided into unipennate (flexor digitorum longus), bipennate, which has a feather-like appearance (rectus femoris, peroneus longus) and multipennate (deltoid) forms, depending on the configuration of their fibers in relation to their tendinous attachments
- *circular*, as in the sphincters

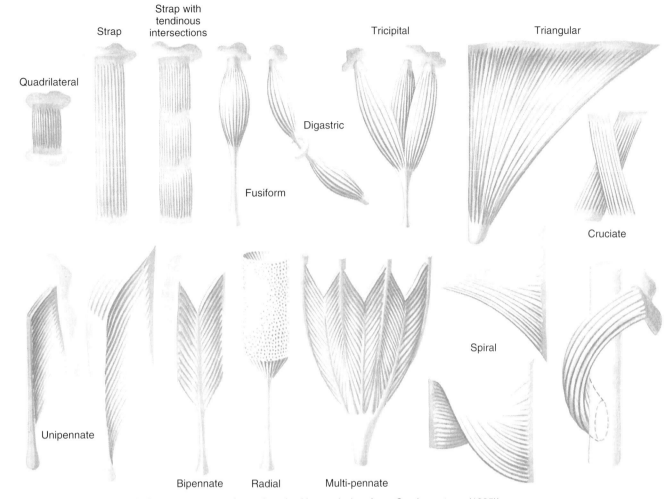

Figure 2.3 Types of muscle fiber arrangement (reproduced, with permission, from *Gray's anatomy* (1995)).

- *triangular* or *convergent*, where a broad origin ends with a narrow attachment, as in pectoralis major
- *spiral* or *twisted*, as in latissimus dorsi or levator scapulae.

MUSCLE ENERGY SOURCES

- Muscles are the body's force generators. In order to achieve this function, they require a source of power, which they derive from their ability to produce mechanical energy from chemically bound energy (in the form of adenosine triphosphate – ATP).
- Some of the energy so produced is stored in contractile tissues for subsequent use when activity occurs. The force which skeletal muscles generate is used to either produce or prevent movement, to induce motion or to ensure stability.
- Muscular contractions can be described in relation to what has been termed a *strength continuum*, varying from

a small degree of force, capable of lengthy maintenance, to a full-strength contraction, which can be sustained for very short periods.

- When a contraction involves more than 70% of available strength, blood flow is reduced and oxygen availability diminishes.

MUSCLES AND BLOOD SUPPLY

Gray's anatomy (1973, p. 483) explains the intricacy of blood supply to skeletal muscle as follows:

The blood supply of muscles is derived from the muscular branches of neighboring arteries. In many the branches of the principal artery and nerve enter together along a strip ... termed the neurovascular hilus. Subsidiary arteries are generally present and enter at the periphery or close to the ends of the muscle. These branch into smaller arteries and arterioles which ramify in the perimysial septa. These capillaries lie in the endomysium, mainly parallel with the muscle fibers, but they present frequent transverse anastomosis forming a three-dimensional lattice.

Gray's also tells us that the capillary bed of predominantly red muscle (type I postural, see below) is far denser than that of white (type II phasic) muscle.

Research has shown that there are two distinct circulations in skeletal muscle (Grant & Payling Wright 1968). *Nutritive circulation*:

derives from arteriolar branches of arteries entering by way of the neurovascular hilus. These penetrate to the endomysium where all the blood passes through to the capillary bed before collection into venules and veins to leave again through the hilus. Alternatively, some of the blood passes into the arterioles of the epi- and perimysium in which few capillaries are present. Arteriovenous anastomosis [a coupling of blood vessels] are abundant here, and most of the blood returns to the veins without passing through the capillaries; this circuit therefore constitutes a *non-nutritive* [collateral] pathway through which blood may pass when the flow in the endomysial capillary bed is impeded, e.g. during contraction.

In this way blood would keep moving but would not be nourishing the tissues it was destined for, if access to the capillary bed was blocked for any reason. This is particularly relevant to deep pressure techniques, designed to create 'ischemic compression', when treating myofascial trigger points, for example.

This means that if ischemic compression is applied, the blood destined for the tissues being obstructed by this pressure (the trigger point site) will diffuse elsewhere until pressure is released, at which time a 'flushing' of the previously ischemic tissues will occur.

Some areas of the body have relatively inefficient anastomosis and are termed *hypovascular*. These are particularly prone to injury and dysfunction. Examples include the supraspinatus tendon which, it is reported, corresponds with 'the most common site of rotator cuff tendinitis, calcification and spontaneous rupture' (Cailliet 1991, Tulos & Bennett 1984). Other hypovascular sites include the insertion of the infraspinatus tendon and the intrascapular aspect of the biceps tendon (Brewer 1979).

The lymphatic drainage of muscles occurs via lymphatic capillaries which lie in the epi- and perimysial sheaths. They converge into larger lymphatic vessels which travel close to the veins as they leave the muscle.

Box 2.1 Lymphatic system

Coming in contact with lymph is to connect with the liquid dimension of the organism. (Chikly 1996)

The lymphatic system serves as a collecting and filtering system for the body's interstitial fluids, while removing the body's cellular debris. It is able to process the waste materials from cellular metabolism and provide a strong line of defense against foreign invaders while recapturing the protein elements and water content for recycling by the body. Through 'immunological memory', lymphocyte cells, which reside in the lymph and blood and are part of the general immune system, recognize invaders (antigens) and rapidly act to neutralize these. This system of defending during invasion and then cleaning up the battleground makes the lymphatic system essential to the health of the organism.

Organization of the lymph system

The lymphatic system comprises an extensive network of lymphatic capillaries, a series of collecting vessels and lymph nodes. It is associated with the lymphoid system (lymph nodes, spleen, thymus, tonsils, appendix, mucosal-associated lymphoid tissue such as Peyer's patches and bone marrow), which is primarily responsible for the immune response (Braem 1994, Chikly 1996). The lymphatic system is:

- an essential defensive component of the immune system
- a carrier of (especially heavy and large) debris on behalf of the circulatory system
- a transporter of fat-soluble nutrients (and fat itself) from the digestive tract to the bloodstream.

Chikly (1996) notes:

The lymphatic system is a second pathway back to the heart, parallel to the venous system. The interstitial fluid is a very important fluid. It is the real interior milieu (Claude Bernard, 1813–1878) in which the cells are immersed, receive their nutritive substances and reject damaging by-products. [Interstitial fluid] *originates in the connective tissue spaces of the body. Once it is in the first lymph capillaries, the interstitial fluid is called lymph.*

Collection begins in the interstitial spaces as a portion of the circulating blood is picked up by the lymphatic system. This fluid is comprised primarily of large waste particles, debris and other material from which protein might need to be recovered or which may need to be disposed. Foreign particulate matter and pathogenic bacteria are screened out by the lymph nodes which are interposed along the course of the vessels. Nodes also produce lymphocytes, which makes their location at various points along the transportation pathway convenient should infectious material be encountered.

Lymph nodes (Chikly 1996):

- filter and purify
- capture and destroy toxins
- reabsorb about 40% of the lymphatic liquids, so concentrating the lymph while recycling the removed water
- produce mature lymphocytes – white blood cells which destroy bacteria, virus-infected cells, foreign matter and waste materials.

Production of lymphocytes increases (in nodes) when lymphatic flow is increased (for example, with lymphatic drainage techniques).

A lymphatic capillary network made of vessels slightly larger than blood capillaries drains tissue fluid from nearly all tissues and organs that have a blood vascularization. The blood circulatory system is a closed system, whereas the lymphatic system is an open-end system, beginning blind in the interstitial spaces. The moment the fluid enters a lymph capillary, a flap valve prevents it from returning into the interstitial spaces. The fluids, now called 'lymph', continue coursing through these 'precollector' vessels which empty into lymph collectors.

The collectors have valves every 6–20 mm which occur directly between two to three layers of spiral muscles, the unit being called a *lymphangion* (**Fig. 2.4**). The alternation of valves and muscles

Box 2.1 (*cont'd*)

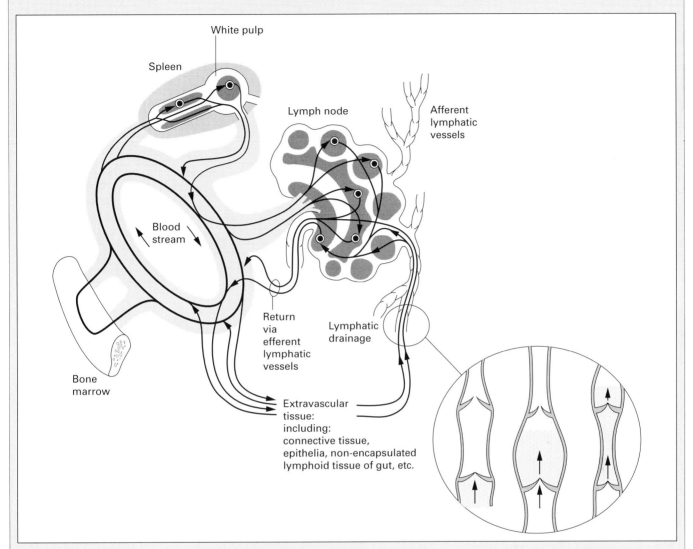

Figure 2.4 A lymphangion (shown in insert).

gives a characteristic 'moniliform' shape to these vessels, like pearls on a string. The lymphangions contract in a peristaltic manner which assists in pressing the fluids through the valved system. When stimulated, the muscles can substantially increase (up to 20 times) the capacity of the whole lymphatic system (Chikly 1996).

The largest of the lymphatic vessels is the thoracic duct, which begins at the cisterna chyli, a large sac-like structure within the abdominal cavity located at approximately the level of the 2nd lumbar vertebra. The thoracic duct, containing lymph fluids from both of the lower extremities and all abdominal viscera except part of the liver, runs posterior to the stomach and intestines. Lymph fluids from the left upper extremity, left thorax and the left side of cranium and neck may join it just before it empties into the left subclavian vein or may empty nearby into the internal jugular vein, brachiocephalic junction or directly into the subclavian vein. The right lymphatic duct drains the right upper extremity, right side of the head and neck and right side of the thorax and empties in a similar manner to that of the left side.

Stimulation of lymphangions (and therefore lymph movement) occurs as a result of automotoricity of the lymphangions (electrical potentials from the autonomic nervous system) (Kurz 1986). As the

spiral muscles of the vessels contract, they force the lymph through the flap valve, which prevents its return. Additionally, stretching of the muscle fibers of the next lymphangion (by increased fluid volume of the segment) leads to reflex muscle contraction (internally stimulated), thereby producing peristaltic waves along the lymphatic vessel. There are also external stretch receptors which may be activated by manual methods of lymph drainage which create a similar peristalsis.

Lymph movement is also augmented by respiration as the altering intrathoracic pressure produces a suction on the thoracic duct and cisterna chyli and thereby increases lymph movement in the duct and presses it toward the venous arch (Kurz 1986, 1987). Skeletal muscle contractions, movement of limbs, peristalsis of smooth muscles, the speed of blood movement in the veins into which the ducts empty and the pulsing of nearby arteries all contribute to lymph movement (Wittlinger & Wittlinger 1982). Exposure to cold, tight clothing, lack of exercise and excess protein consumption can hinder lymphatic flow (Kurz 1986, Wittlinger & Wittlinger 1982).

Contraction of neighboring muscles compresses lymph vessels, moving lymph in the directions determined by their valves;

Box 2.1 *(cont'd)*

extremely little lymph flows in an immobilized limb, whereas flow is increased by either active or passive movements. This fact has been used clinically to diminish dissemination of toxins from infected tissues by immobilization of the relevant regions. Conversely, massage aids the flow of lymph from oedematous regions (Gray's anatomy 1995).

By recovering up to 20% of the interstitial fluids, the lymphatic system relieves the venous system (and therefore the heart) of the responsibility of transporting the large molecules of protein and debris back to the general circulation. Additionally, the lymphocytes remove particulate matter by means of *phagocytosis*, that is, the process of ingestion and digestion by cells of solid substances (other cells, bacteria, bits of necrosed tissue, foreign particles). By the time the fluid has been returned to the veins, it is ultrafiltered, condensed and highly concentrated.

In effect, if the lymphatic system did not regain the 2–20% of the protein-rich liquid that escaped in the interstitium (a large part of which the venous system cannot recover), the body would probably develop major edemas and autointoxication and die within 24–48 hours (Chikly 1996, Guyton 1986).

Conversely, when applying lymph drainage techniques, care must be taken to avoid excessive increases in the volume of lymph flow in people who have heart conditions as the venous system must accommodate the load once the fluid has been delivered to the subclavian veins. Significantly increasing the load could place excessive strain on the heart.

Lymphatic circulation is separated into two layers. The superficial circulation, which constitutes approximately 60–70% of lymph circulation in the extremities (Chikly 1996), is located just under the dermoepidermic junction. The deep muscular and visceral circulation, below the fascia, is activated by muscular contraction; however, the superficial circulation is not directly stimulated by exercise. Additionally, lymph capillaries (lacteals) in the jejunum and ileum of the digestive tract absorb fat and fat-soluble nutrients which ultimately reach the liver through the blood circulation (Braem 1994).

Manual or mechanical lymphatic drainage techniques are effective ways to increase lymph removal from stagnant or edemic tissue. The manual techniques use extremely light pressure which significantly increases lymph movement by crosswise and lengthwise stretching of the anchoring filaments which open the lymph capillaries, thus allowing the interstitial fluid to enter the lymphatic system. However, shearing forces (like those created by deep pressure gliding techniques) can lead to temporary inhibition of lymph flow by inducing spasms of lymphatic muscles (Kurz 1986). Lymphatic movement can then be reactivated by use of manual techniques which stimulate the lymphangions.

While each case has to be considered individually, numerous conditions, ranging from postoperative edema to premenstrual fluid retention, may benefit from lymphatic drainage. There are, however, conditions for which lymphatic drainage would be contraindicated or precautions exercised. Some of the more serious of these conditions include:

- acute infections and acute inflammation (generalized and local)
- thrombosis
- circulatory problems
- cardiac conditions
- hemorrhage
- malignant cancers
- thyroid problems
- acute phlebitis.

Conditions which might benefit from lymphatic drainage but for which precautions are indicated include:

- certain edemas, depending upon their cause, such as cardiac insufficiency
- carotid stenosis
- bronchial asthma
- burns, scars, bruises, moles
- abdominal surgery, radiation or undetermined bleeding or pain
- removed spleen
- major kidney problems or insufficiency
- menstruation (drain prior to menses)
- gynecological infections, fibromas or cysts
- some pregnancies (especially in the first 3 months)
- chronic infections or inflammation
- low blood pressure.

MAJOR TYPES OF VOLUNTARY CONTRACTION

Muscle contractions can be:

- *isometric* (with no movement resulting)
- *isotonic concentric* (where shortening of the muscle produces approximation of its attachments and the structures to which the muscle attaches) or
- *isotonic eccentric* (in which the muscle lengthens during its contraction, therefore the attachments separate during contraction of the muscle).

TERMINOLOGY

- The terms *origin* and *insertion* are somewhat inaccurate, with *attachments* being more appropriate.
- In many instances, muscular attachments can adaptively reverse their roles, depending on what action is involved and therefore which attachment is fixed.
- As an example, psoas can flex the hip when its lumbar attachment is 'the origin' (fixed point) or it can flex the spine when the femoral attachment becomes 'the origin', i.e. the point towards which motion is taking place.

MUSCLE TONE AND CONTRACTION

Muscles display *excitability* – the ability to respond to stimuli and, by means of a stimulus, to be able to *actively contract*, *extend* (lengthen) or to *elastically recoil* from a distended position, as well as to be able to *passively relax* when stimulus ceases.

Lederman (1998) suggests that *muscle tone* in a resting muscle relates to biomechanical elements – a mix of fascial and connective tissue tension together with intramuscular fluid pressure, with no neurological input (therefore, not measurable by EMG). If a muscle has altered morphologically, due to chronic shortening, for example, or compartment syndrome, then muscle tone even at rest will be altered and palpable.

He differentiates this from *motor tone*, which is measurable by means of EMG and which is present in a resting muscle only under abnormal circumstances – for example, when psychological stress or protective activity is involved.

Motor tone is either *phasic* or *tonic*, depending upon the nature of the activity being demanded of the muscle – to move something (phasic) or to stabilize it (tonic). In normal muscles, both activities vanish when gravitational and activity demands are absent.

Contraction occurs in response to a motor nerve impulse acting on muscle fibers.

A motor nerve fiber will always activate more than one muscle fiber and the collection of fibers it innervates is called a *motor unit*. The greater the degree of fine control a muscle is required to produce, the fewer muscle fibers a nerve fiber will innervate in that muscle. This can range from between six and 12 muscle fibers being innervated by a single motor neuron in the extrinsic eye muscles to one motor neuron innervating 2000 fibers in major limb muscles (*Gray's anatomy* 1973).

Because there is a diffuse spread of influence from a single motor neuron throughout a muscle (i.e. neural influence does not necessarily correspond to fascicular divisions) only a few need to be active to influence the entire muscle.

The functional contractile unit of a muscle fiber is its *sarcomere*, which contains filaments of actin and myosin. These myofilaments (actin and myosin) interact in order to shorten the muscle fiber. *Gray's anatomy* (1973) describes the process as follows:

Two types of myofilament are distinguishable in each sarcomere, fine ones about 5 nm in diameter and thicker ones about 12 nm across – these have been characterized as actin and myosin respectively. The actin filaments are each attached at one end to a Z band and are free at the other to interdigitate with the myosin filaments ... In contracted muscle the actin filaments have slid in relation to the myosin towards the center of the sarcomere, so bringing the attached Z bands closer together with shortening of the whole contractile unit ... muscle contraction may be caused by the successive making and breaking of cross connections between the thick myosin and the thin actin filaments in a cyclical fashion, so pulling the thin ones between the thick ones towards the sarcomere center.

VULNERABLE AREAS

- In order to transfer force to its attachment site, contractile units merge with the collagen fibers of the tendon which attaches the muscle to bone.
- At the transition area, between muscle and tendon, these structures virtually 'fold' together, increasing strength while reducing the elastic quality.
- This increased ability to handle shear forces is achieved at the expense of the tissue's capacity to handle tensile forces.

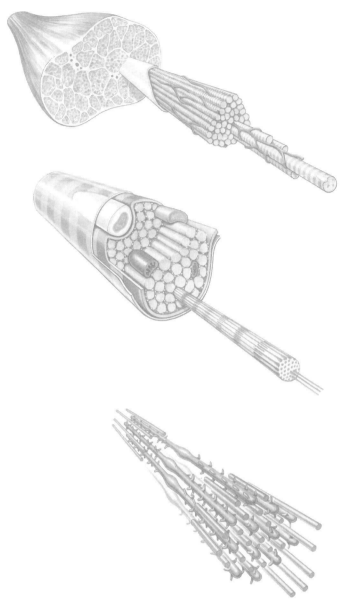

Figure 2.5 From whole muscle to the sarcomere's actin and myosin elements (reproduced, with permission, from *Gray's anatomy* (1995)).

- The chance of injury increases at those locations where elastic muscle tissue transitions to less elastic tendon and finally to non-elastic bone – the attachment sites of the body.

MUSCLE TYPES

Muscle fibers exist in various motor unit types – basically type I slow red tonic and type II fast white phasic (see below). Type I are fatigue resistant while type II are more easily fatigued.

All muscles have a mixture of fiber types (both I and II), although in most there is a predominance of one or the other, depending on the primary tasks of the muscle (postural stabilizer or phasic mover).

Those which contract slowly (slow-twitch fibers) are classified as *type I* (Engel 1986, Woo 1987). These have very low stores of energy-supplying glycogen, but carry high concentrations of myoglobulin and mitochondria. These fibers fatigue slowly and are mainly involved in postural and stabilizing tasks. The effect of overuse, misuse, abuse or disuse on postural muscles (see Chapters 4 and 5) is that, over time, they will shorten. This tendency to shorten is a clinically important distinction between the response to 'stress' of type I and type II muscle fibers (see below).

There are also several phasic (*type II*) fiber forms, notably:

- type IIa (fast-twitch fibers) which contract more speedily than type I and are moderately resistant to fatigue with relatively high concentrations of mitochondria and myoglobulin
- type IIb (fast-twitch glycolytic fibers) which are less fatigue resistant and depend more on glycolytic sources of energy, with low levels of mitochondria and myoglobulin
- type IIm (superfast fibers) which depend upon a unique myosin structure which, along with a high glycogen content, differentiates them from the other type II fibers (Rowlerson 1981). These are found mainly in the jaw muscles.

As mentioned above, long-term stress involving type I muscle fibers leads to them shortening, whereas type II fibers, undergoing similar stress, will weaken without shortening over their whole length (they may, however, develop localized areas of sarcomere contracture, for example where trigger points evolve without shortening overall).

Shortness/tightness of a postural muscle does not necessarily imply strength. Such muscles may test as strong or weak. However, a weak phasic muscle will not shorten overall and will always test as weak.

Fiber type is not totally fixed, in that evidence exists as to the potential for adaptability of muscles, so that committed muscle fibers can be transformed from slow twitch to fast twitch and vice versa (Lin 1994).

An example of this potential, which has profound clinical significance, involves the scalene muscles. Lewit (1985) confirms that they can be classified as either a postural or a phasic muscle. If the scalenes, which are largely phasic and dedicated to movement, have postural functions thrust upon them (for example, where there is an inappropriate degree of upper chest breathing involving the upper ribs being regularly elevated to provide inhalation) and are therefore regularly stressed, their fiber type will alter and they will shorten, as would any postural muscles when chronically stressed.

Among the more important postural muscles which become hypertonic in response to dysfunction are:

- trapezius (upper), sternocleidomastoid, levator scapula and upper aspects of pectoralis major in the upper trunk and the flexors of the arms
- quadratus lumborum, erector spinae, oblique abdominals and iliopsoas, in the lower trunk
- tensor fascia latae, rectus femoris, biceps femoris, adductors (longus, brevis and magnus), piriformis, hamstrings and semitendinosus in the pelvic and lower extremity region.

Phasic muscles, which weaken in response to dysfunction (i.e. are inhibited), include the paravertebral muscles (not erector spinae), scalenii and deep neck flexors, deltoid, the abdominal (or lower) aspects of pectoralis major, middle and inferior aspects of trapezius, the rhomboids, serratus anterior, rectus abdominis, gluteals, the peroneal muscles, vasti and the extensors of the arms.

Muscle groups, such as the scalenii, are equivocal. Although commonly listed as phasic muscles, this is how they start life but they can end up as postural ones if sufficient demands are made on them (see above).

COOPERATIVE MUSCLE ACTIVITY

Few, if any, muscles work in isolation, with most movements involving the combined effort of two or more, with one or more acting as the 'prime mover' or *agonist*.

Almost every skeletal muscle has an *antagonist* which performs the opposite action, with one of the most obvious examples being the elbow flexors (biceps brachii) and extensors (triceps brachii).

Prime movers usually have *synergistic* muscles which assist them and which contract at almost the same time. An example of these roles would be hip abduction, in which gluteus medius is the prime mover, with tensor fascia latae acting synergistically and the hip adductors acting as antagonists, being *reciprocally inhibited* (RI) by the action of the agonists. RI is the physiological phenomenon in which there is an automatic inhibition of a muscle when its antagonist contracts, also known as Sherrington's law.

Movement can only take place normally if there is co-ordination of all the interacting muscular elements. With many habitual complex movements, such as how to rise from a sitting position, a great number of involuntary, largely unconscious reflex activities are involved. This means that altering such patterns has to involve a relearning or repatterning process.

The most important action of an antagonist occurs at the outset of a movement, where its function is to facilitate a smooth, controlled initiation of movement by the agonist and its *synergists*, those muscles which share in and support the movement. When agonist and antagonist

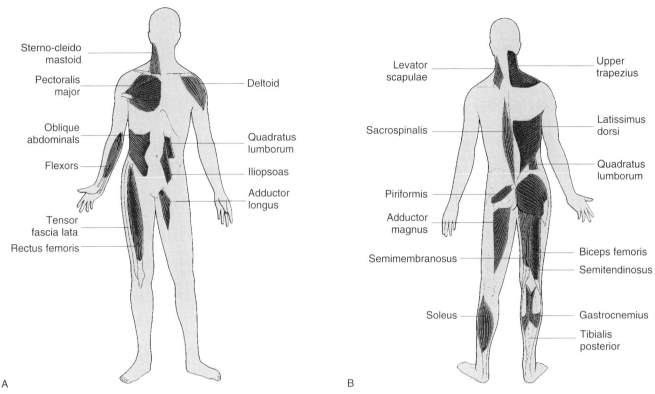

Figure 2.6 Major postural muscles. A: Anterior. B: Posterior (reproduced, with permission, from *Chaitow* (1996)).

Box 2.2 An alternative categorization of muscles

Because of overuse, misuse or disuse, muscular imbalance occurs in which certain muscles tend towards shortening, while others tend to become weak (i.e. inhibited). Norris (1995a,b,c,d,e, 1998) designates muscles according to their major functions, i.e. as 'stabilizers' or 'mobilizers'.

According to Norris' research (1995a,b,c,d,e, 1998) inhibited/weak muscles lengthen, adding to the instability of the region in which they operate, and it is the 'stabilizers' which have this tendency, i.e. if they are inhibited because of deconditioning they become unable to adequately perform the role of stabilizing joints in their 'neutral posture'.

'Stabilizer' muscles which fall into this category (i.e. they are more deeply situated, are slow twitch and have a tendency to weaken and lengthen if deconditioned) include transverse abdominis, multifidus, internal obliques, medial fibers of external oblique, quadratus lumborum, deep neck flexors, serratus anterior, lower trapezius, gluteus maximus and medius. These muscles can

be correlated, to a large extent (apart from quadratus lumborum) with muscles designated by Lewit (1999) and Janda (1983) as 'phasic'.

The more superficial, fast-twitch muscles which have a tendency to shortening (i.e. 'mobilizers' in Norris terminology) include the suboccipital group, sternocleidomastoid, upper trapezius, levator scapulae, iliopsoas and hamstrings. These fall into the category of 'postural' muscles as described by Lewit, Janda and Liebenson. Norris calls these mobilizers because they cross more than one joint. This redefining of 'postural' as 'mobilizer' appears to be confusing, and many (Liebenson 1999) prefer to simply refer to these muscles as 'having a tendency to shortening'.

Examples of patterns of imbalance which emerge as some muscles weaken and lengthen and their synergists become overworked, while their antagonists shorten, can be summarized as follows.

Lengthened or underactive stabilizer	*Overactive synergist*	*Shortened antagonist*
1. Gluteus medius	TFL., QL., piriformis	Thigh adductors
2. Gluteus maximus	Iliocostalis lumborum & hamstrings	Iliopsoas, rectus femoris
3. Transversus abdominis	Rectus abdominis	Iliocostalis lumborum
4. Lower trapezius	Lev. scapulae/U.trapezius	Pectoralis major
5. Deep neck flexors	SCM	Suboccipitals
6. Serratus anterior	Pectoralis major/minor	Rhomboids
7. Diaphragm		Scalenes, pectoralis major

Observation

Observation can often provide evidence of an imbalance involving cross patterns of weakness/lengthening and shortness. A number

of tests can be used to assess muscle imbalance: postural inspection, muscle length tests, movement patterns and inner holding endurance times. Posture is valuable because it provides a quick screen.

Box 2.2 (cont'd)

Muscle inhibition/weakness/lengthening	Observable sign
Transversus abdominis	Protruding umbilicus
Serratus anterior	Winged scapula
Lower trapezius	Elevated shoulder girdle ('gothic' shoulders)
Deep neck flexors	Chin 'poking'
Gluteus medius	Unlevel pelvis on one-legged standing
Gluteus maximus	Sagging buttock

Inner range endurance tests

'Inner holding isometric endurance' tests can be performed for muscles which have a tendency to lengthen, in order to assess their ability to maintain joint alignment in a neutral zone. Usually a lengthened muscle will demonstrate a loss of endurance, when tested in a shortened position. This can be tested by the practitioner passively prepositioning the muscle in a shortened position and assessing the duration of time that the patient can hold the muscle in this position. There are various methods used, including 10 repetitions of the holding position for 10 seconds at a time. Alternatively, a single 30-second hold can be requested. If the patient cannot hold the position actively from the moment of passive prepositioning, this is a sign of inappropriate antagonist muscle shortening.

Norris (1999) describes an example of inner range holding tests.

- *Iliopsoas*: patient is seated. Practitioner lifts one leg into greater hip flexion so that foot is well clear of floor and the patient is asked to hold this position.
- *Gluteus maximus*: Patient is prone and practitioner lifts one leg into extension at the hip (knee flexed to 90°) and the patient is asked to hold the leg in this position.
- *Posterior fibers of gluteus medius*: Patient is sidelying with lower leg straight and uppermost leg flexed at hip and knee so that both the knee and foot are resting on the floor/surface. The practitioner places the flexed leg into a position of maximal unforced external rotation at the hip, foot still resting on the floor, and the patient is asked to maintain this position.

Norris states

Optimal endurance is indicated when the full inner range position can be held for 10 to 20 seconds. Muscle lengthening is present if the limb falls away from the inner range position immediately.

---

muscles contract simultaneously they act in a stabilizing *fixator* role.

Sometimes a muscle has the ability to have one part acting as an antagonist to other parts of the same muscle, a phenomenon seen in the deltoid.

The ways in which skeletal muscles produce movement in the body, or in part of it, can be classified as:

- *postural*, where stability is induced. If this relates to standing still, it is worth noting that the maintenance of the body's center of gravity over its base of support requires constant fine tuning of a multitude of muscles, with continuous tiny shifts back and forth and from side to side
- *ballistic*, in which the momentum of an action carries on beyond the activation produced by muscular activity (the act of throwing, for example)
- *tension movement*, where fine control requires constant muscular activity (playing a musical instrument such as the violin, for example, or giving a massage).

MUSCLE SPASM, TENSION, ATROPHY
(Liebenson 1996, Walsh 1992)

Muscles are often said to be short, tight, tense or in spasm; however, these terms are used very loosely.

Muscles experience either neuromuscular, viscoelastic or connective tissue alterations or combinations of these. A tight muscle could have either increased neuro-

muscular tension or connective tissue modification (for example, fibrosis).

Spasm (tension with EMG elevation)

- Muscle spasm is a neuromuscular phenomenon relating either to an upper motor neuron disease or an acute reaction to pain or tissue injury.
- Electromyographic (EMG) activity is increased in these cases.
- Examples include spinal cord injury, reflex spasm (such as in a case of appendicitis) or acute lumbar antalgia with loss of flexion relaxation response (Triano & Schultz 1987).
- Long-lasting noxious (pain) stimulation has been shown to activate the flexion withdrawal reflex (Dahl et al 1992).
- Using electromyographic evidence Simons (1994) has shown that myofascial trigger points can 'cause reflex spasm and reflex inhibition in other muscles, and can cause motor incoordination in the muscle with the trigger point'.

Contracture (tension of muscles without EMG elevation)

- Increased muscle tension can occur without a consistently elevated EMG.
- An example is trigger points, in which muscle fibers fail to relax properly.

• Muscle fibers housing trigger points have been shown to have different levels of EMG activity within the same functional muscle unit.

• Hyperexcitability, as shown by EMG readings, has been demonstrated in the nidus of the trigger point, which is situated in a taut band (which shows no increased EMG activity) and has a characteristic pattern of reproducible referred pain (Hubbard & Berkoff 1993, Simons et al 1998).

• When pressure is applied to an active trigger point EMG activity is found to increase in the muscles to which sensations are being referred ('target area') (Simons 1994).

Increased stretch sensitivity

• Increased sensitivity to stretch can lead to increased muscle tension.

• This can occur under conditions of local ischemia, which have also been demonstrated in the nidus of trigger points, as part of the 'energy crisis' which, it is hypothesized (see Chapter 6), produces them (Mense 1993, Simons 1994).

• Liebenson confirms that *'Local ischemia is a key factor involved in increased muscle tone. Under conditions of ischemia groups III and IV muscle afferents become more sensitive to stretch'* (Liebenson 1996).

• These same afferents also become sensitized in response to a build-up of metabolites when sustained mild contractions occur, such as occurs in prolonged slumped sitting (Johansson 1991).

• Mense suggests that a range of dysfunctional events emerge from the production of local ischemia which can occur as a result of venous congestion, local contracture and tonic activation of muscles by descending motor pathways.

• Sensitization (which is in all but name the same phenomenon as facilitation, which is discussed more fully in Chapter 6) involves a change in the stimulus–response profile of neurons leading to a decreased threshold as well as increased spontaneous activity of types III and IV primary afferents.

• Schiable & Grubb (1993) have implicated reflex discharges from (dysfunctional) joints in the production of such neuromuscular tension.

• According to Janda (1991), neuromuscular tension can also be increased by central influences due to limbic dysfunction.

Viscoelastic influence

• Muscle stiffness is a viscoelastic phenomenon which has to do with fluid mechanics and viscosity (so-called sol or gel) of tissue, which was explained more fully in Chapter 1 (Walsh 1992).

• Fibrosis occurs in muscle or fascia gradually and is typically related to post trauma adhesion formation (see notes on fibrotic change in Chapter 1, p. 11).

• Fibroblasts proliferate in injured tissue during the inflammatory phase (Lehto et al 1986).

• If the inflammatory phase is prolonged then a connective tissue scar will form as the fibrosis is not absorbed.

Atrophy and chronic back pain

• In chronic back pain patients, generalized atrophy has been observed and to a greater extent on the symptomatic side (Stokes 1992).

• Type I (postural or aerobic) fibers *hypertrophy* on the symptomatic side and type II (phasic or anaerobic) fibers *atrophy* bilaterally in chronic back pain patients (Fitzmaurice et al 1992).

Box 2.3 Muscle strength testing

For efficient muscle strength testing it is necessary to ensure that:

• the patient builds force slowly after engaging the barrier of resistance offered by the practitioner
• the patient uses maximum controlled effort to move in the prescribed direction
• the practitioner ensures that the point of muscle origin is efficiently stabilized
• care is taken to avoid use by the patient of 'tricks' in which synergists are recruited.

Muscle strength is most usually graded as follows.

• Grade 5 is normal, demonstrating a complete (100%) range of movement against gravity, with firm resistance offered by the practitioner.
• Grade 4 is 75% efficiency in achieving range of motion against gravity with slight resistance.
• Grade 3 is 50% efficiency in achieving range of motion against gravity without resistance.
• Grade 2 is 25% efficiency in achieving range of motion with gravity eliminated.
• Grade 1 shows slight contractility without joint motion.
• Grade 0 shows no evidence of contractility.

Box 2.4 Two-joint muscle testing

As a rule when testing a two-joint muscle good fixation is essential. The same applies to all muscles in children and in adults whose cooperation is poor and whose movements are incoordinated and weak. The better the extremity is steadied, the less the stabilizers are activated and the better and more accurate are the results of the muscle function test. (Janda 1983)

WHAT IS WEAKNESS?

True muscle weakness is a result of lower motor neuron disease (i.e. nerve root compression or myofascial entrapment) or disuse atrophy. In chronic back pain patients, generalized atrophy has been demonstrated. This atrophy is selective in the type II (phasic) muscle fibers bilaterally.

Muscle weakness is another term that is used loosely. A muscle may simply be inhibited, meaning that it has not suffered disuse atrophy but is weak due to a reflex phenomenon. Inhibited muscles are capable of spontaneous strengthening when the inhibitory reflex is identified and remedied (commonly achieved through soft tissue or joint manipulation).

A typical example is reflex inhibition from an antagonist muscle due to Sherrington's law of reciprocal inhibition, which declares that a muscle will be inhibited when its antagonist contracts.

- Reflex inhibition of the vastus medialis oblique (VMO) muscle after knee inflammation/injury has been repeatedly demonstrated (DeAndrade et al 1965, Spencer et al 1984).
- Hides has found unilateral, segmental wasting of the multifidus in acute back pain patients (Hides et al 1994). This occurred rapidly and thus was not considered to be a disuse atrophy.
- In 1994, Hallgren et al found that some individuals with chronic neck pain exhibited fatty degeneration and atrophy of the rectus capitis posterior major and minor muscles as visualized by MRI. Atrophy of these small suboccipital muscles obliterates their important proprioceptive output which may destabilize postural balance (McPartland 1997) (see Chapter 3 for more detail on these muscles).

Various pathologic situations have been listed, which can affect either the flexibility or strength of muscles. The result is muscular imbalance involving increased tension or tightness in postural muscles, coincidental with inhibition or weakness of phasic muscles.

TRICK PATTERNS

Altered muscular movement patterns were first recognized clinically by Janda when it was noticed that classic muscle-testing methods did not differentiate between normal recruitment of muscles and 'trick' patterns of substitution during an action. So-called trick movements (see below) are uneconomical and place unusual strain on joints. They involve muscles in uncoordinated ways and are related to poor endurance.

In a traditional test of prone hip extension it is difficult to identify overactivity of the lumbar erector spinae or hamstrings as substitutes for an inhibited gluteus maximus. Tests developed by Janda are far more sensitive and allow us to identify muscle imbalances, faulty (trick) movement patterns and joint overstrain by observing or palpating abnormal substitution during muscle-testing protocols. For example, in a prone position, hip extension should be initiated by gluteus maximus. If the hamstrings

undertake the role of prime mover and gluteus maximus is inhibited, this is easily noted by palpating activity within each of them as movement is initiated.

Similar imbalances can be palpated and observed in the shoulder region where the upper fixators dominate the lower fixators by inhibiting them, which results in major neck and shoulder stress. These patterns have major repercussions, as will become clear when crossed syndromes, and Janda's functional assessment methods, are outlined in Chapter 5 (Janda 1978).

Joint implications

When a movement pattern is altered, the activation sequence, or firing order of different muscles involved in a specific movement, is disturbed. The prime mover may be slow to activate while synergists or stabilizers substitute and become overactive. When this is the case, new joint stresses will be encountered. Sometimes the timing sequence is normal yet the overall range may be limited due to joint stiffness or antagonist muscle shortening. Pain may well be a feature of such dysfunctional patterns.

WHEN SHOULD PAIN AND DYSFUNCTION BE LEFT ALONE?

Splinting (spasm) can occur as a defensive, protective, involuntary phenomenon associated with trauma (fracture) or pathology (osteoporosis, secondary bone tumors, neurogenic influences, etc.). Splinting-type spasm commonly differs from more common forms of contraction and hypertonicity because it releases when the tissues which it is protecting, or immobilizing, are placed at rest.

When splinting remains long term, secondary problems may arise as a result, in associated joints (e.g. contractures) and bone (e.g. osteoporosis). Travell & Simons (1983) note that 'Muscle-splinting pain is usually part of a complex process. Hemiplegic and brain-injured patients do identify pain that depends on muscle spasm'. They also note 'a degree of masseteric spasm which may develop to relieve strain in trigger points in its parallel muscle, the temporalis'.

Travell & Simons (1983) note a similar phenomenon in the lower back:

In patients with low back pain and with tenderness to palpation of the paraspinal muscles, the superficial layer tended to show less than a normal amount of EMG activity until the test movement became painful. Then these muscles showed increased motor unit activity or 'splinting' ... This observation fits the concept of normal muscles 'taking over' (protective spasm) to unload and protect a parallel muscle that is the site of significant trigger point activity.

Recognition of this degree of spasm in soft tissues is a matter of training and intuition. Whether attempts should be made to release, or relieve, what appears to be protective spasm depends on understanding the reasons for its existence. If splinting is the result of a cooperative attempt to unload a painful but not pathologically compromised structure, in an injured knee or shoulder for example, then treatment is obviously appropriate to ease the cause of the original need to protect and support. If, on the other hand, spasm or splinting is indeed protecting the structure it surrounds (or supports) from movement and further (possibly) serious damage, as in a case of advanced osteoporosis, for example, then it should clearly be left alone.

Beneficially overactive muscles

Van Wingerden et al (1997) report that both intrinsic and extrinsic support for the sacroiliac joint (SIJ) derives, in part, from hamstring (biceps femoris) status. Intrinsically, the influence is via the close anatomical and physiological relationship between biceps femoris and the sacrotuberous ligament (they frequently attach via a strong tendinous link). They state: *'Force from the biceps femoris muscle can lead to increased tension of the sacrotuberous ligament in various ways. Since increased tension of the sacrotuberous ligament diminishes the range of sacroiliac joint motion, the biceps femoris can play a role in stabilization of the SIJ'* (Van Wingerden et al 1997; see also Vleeming 1989).

Van Wingerden (1997) also notes that in low back patients forward flexion is often painful as the load on the spine increases. This happens whether flexion occurs in the spine or via the hip joints (tilting of the pelvis). If the hamstrings are tight and short, they effectively prevent pelvic tilting. *'In this respect, an increase in hamstring tension might well be part of a defensive arthrokinematic reflex mechanism of the body to diminish spinal load.'*

If such a state of affairs is long standing, the hamstrings (biceps femoris) will shorten (see discussion of the effects of stress on postural muscles, p. 22), possibly influencing sacroiliac and lumbar spine dysfunction. The decision to treat a tight hamstring should therefore take account of why it is tight and consider that, in some circumstances, it is offering beneficial support to the SIJ or that it is reducing low back stress. It is possible to conceive similar supportive responses in a variety of settings, including the shoulder joint when lower scapular fixators have weakened, thus throwing the load onto other muscles (see discussion of upper crossed syndrome in Chapter 5).

SOMATIZATION – MIND AND MUSCLES

It is entirely possible for musculoskeletal symptoms to represent an unconscious attempt by the patient to entomb their emotional distress. As most cogently expressed by Philip Latey (1996), pain and dysfunction may have psychological distress as their root cause. The patient may be somatizing the distress and presenting with apparently somatic problems (see Chapter 4).

But how is one to know?

Karel Lewit (1992) suggests that, *'In doubtful cases, the physical and psychological components will be distinguished during the treatment, when repeated comparison of (changing) physical signs and the patient's own assessment of them will provide objective criteria'.* In the main, he suggests, if the patient is able to give a fairly precise description and localization of his pain, we should be reluctant to regard it as 'merely psychological'.

In masked depression, Lewit suggests, the reported symptoms may well be of vertebral pain, particularly involving the cervical region, with associated muscle tension and 'cramped' posture. As well as being alerted by abnormal responses during the course of treatment to the fact that there may be something other than biomechanical causes of the problem, the history should provide clues. If the masked depression is treated appropriately the vertebrogenic pain will clear up rapidly, he states.

In particular, Lewit notes, *'The most important symptom is disturbed sleep. Characteristically, the patient falls asleep normally but wakes within a few hours and cannot get back to sleep'.* Pain and dysfunction can be masking major psychological distress and awareness of it, how and when to cross-refer should be part of the responsible practitioner's skills base.

Muscles cannot be separated, in reality or intellectually, from the fascia which envelopes and supports them. Whenever it appears we have done so in this book, it is meant to highlight and reinforce particular characteristics of each. When it comes to clinical applications, these structures have to be considered as integrated units. As muscular dysfunction is being modified and corrected it is almost impossible to conceive that fascial structures are not also being remodeled. Some of the quite amazingly varied functions of fascia were detailed in Chapter 1. In this chapter we have reviewed some of the important features of muscles themselves, their structure, function and at least some of the influences which cause them to become dysfunctional, in unique ways, depending in part on their fiber type.

In the next chapter, as we review the myriad reporting stations embedded in the soft tissues in general and the muscles in particular, it will become clear that muscles are as much an organ of sense as they are agents of movement and stability.

REFERENCES

Braem T 1994 The organs of the human anatomy – the lymphatic system. Bryan Edwards, Anaheim

Brewer B 1979 Aging and the rotator cuff. American Journal of Sports Medicine 7:102–110

Cailliet R 1991 Shoulder pain. F A Davis, Philadelphia

Chaitow L 1999 Muscle energy techniques. Churchill Livingstone, Edinburgh

Chikly B 1996 Lymph drainage therapy study guide, level 1. U I Publishing, Palm Beach Gardens

Dahl J B, Erichsen C J, Fuglsang-Frederiksen A, Kehlet H 1992 Pain sensation and nociceptive reflex excitability in surgical patients and human volunteers. British Journal of Anaesthesia 69:117–121

DeAndrade J R, Grant C, Dixon A St J 1965 Joint distension and reflex muscle inhibition in the knee. Journal of Bone and Joint Surgery 47:313–322

Engel A 1986 Skeletal muscle types in myology. McGraw-Hill, New York

Fitzmaurice R, Cooper R G, Freemont A J 1992 A histo-morphometric comparison of muscle biopsies from normal subjects and patients with ankylosing spondylitis and severe mechanical low back pain. Journal of Pathology 163:182

Fritz S 1998 Mosby's basic science for soft tissue and movement therapies. Mosby, St Louis

Grant T, Payling Wright H 1968 Further observations on the blood vessels of skeletal muscle. Journal of Anatomy 103:553–565

Gray's anatomy 1973 (35th edn). Churchill Livingstone, Edinburgh, p 483

Gray's anatomy 1995 (38th edn). Churchill Livingstone, New York

Guyton A 1986 Textbook of medical physiology, 7th edn. W B Saunders, Philadelphia

Hallgren R C, Greenman P E, Rechtien J J 1994 Atrophy of suboccipital muscles in patients with chronic pain: a pilot study. Journal of the American Osteopathic Association 94:1032–1038

Hides J A, Stokes M J, Saide M 1994 Evidence of lumbar multifidus muscle wasting ipsilateral to symptoms in patients with acute/subacute low back pain. Spine 19:165–172

Hubbard D R, Berkoff G M 1993 Myofascial trigger points show spontaneous needle EMG activity. Spine 18:1803–1807

Jacob A, Falls W 1997 Anatomy. In: Ward R (ed) Foundations for osteopathic medicine. Williams and Wilkins, Baltimore

Janda V 1978 Muscles, central nervous motor regulation, and back problems. In: Korr I M (ed) Neurobiologic mechanisms in manipulative therapy. Plenum, New York

Janda V 1983 Muscle function testing. Butterworths, London

Janda V 1991 Muscle spasm – a proposed procedure for differential diagnosis. Manual Medicine 1001:6136–6139

Johansson H 1991 Pathophysiological mechanisms involved in genesis and spread of muscular tension. A hypothesis. Medical Hypotheses 35:196

Kurz I 1986 Textbook of Dr. Vodder's manual lymph drainage, vol 2: therapy, 2nd edn. Karl F Haug, Heidelberg

Kurz I 1987 Introduction to Dr. Vodder's manual lymph drainage, vol 3: therapy II (treatment manual). Karl F Haug, Heidelberg

Latey P 1996 Feelings, muscles and movement. Journal of Bodywork and Movement Therapies 1(1):44–52

Lederman E 1998 Fundamentals of manual therapy. Churchill Livingstone, Edinburgh

Lehto M, Jarvinen M, Nelimarkka O 1986 Scar formation after skeletal muscle injury. Archives of Orthopaedic Trauma Surgery 104:366–370

Lewit K 1985 Manipulative therapy in rehabilitation of the locomotor system. Butterworths, London

Lewit K 1992 Manipulative therapy in rehabilitation of the locomotor system, 2nd edn. Butterworths, London

Lewit K 1999 Manipulation in rehabilitation of the motor system, 3rd edn. Butterworths, London

Liebenson C 1996 Rehabilitation of the spine. Williams and Wilkins, Baltimore

Liebenson C 1999 Muscular imbalance – an update. Dynamic Chiropractic Online <http//www.chiroweb.com/dynamic>

Lin J-P 1994 Physiological maturation of muscles in childhood. Lancet June 4: 1386–1389

McPartland J M 1997 Chronic neck pain, standing balance, and suboccipital muscle atrophy. Journal of Manipulative and Physiological Therapeutics 21(1):24–29

Mense S 1993 Nociception from skeletal muscle in relation to clinical muscle pain. Pain 54:241–290

Norris C M 1995a Spinal stabilisation. 1. Active lumbar stabilisation – concepts. Physiotherapy 81(2):61–64

Norris C M 1995b Spinal stabilisation. 2. Limiting factors to end-range motion in the lumbar spine. Physiotherapy 81(2):64–72

Norris C M 1995c Spinal stabilisation. 3. Stabilisation mechanisms of the lumbar spine. Physiotherapy 81(2):72–79

Norris C M 1995d, Spinal stabilisation. 4. Muscle imbalance and the low back. Physiotherapy 81(3):127–138

Norris C M 1995e Spinal stabilisation. 5. An exercise program to enhance lumbar stabilisation. Physiotherapy 81(3):138–146

Norris C M 1998 Sports injuries, diagnosis and management, 2nd edn. Butterworths, London

Norris C M 1999 Functional load abdominal training. Journal of Bodywork and Movement Therapies 3(3):150–158

Rowlerson A 1981 A novel myosin. Journal of Muscle Research 2:415–438

Schafer R 1987 Clinical biomechanics, 2nd edn. Williams and Wilkins, Baltimore

Schiable H G, Grubb B D 1993 Afferent and spinal mechanisms of joint pain. Pain 55:5–54

Simons D 1994 In: Vecchiet L, Albe-Fessard D, Lindblom U, Giamberardino M (eds) New trends in referred pain and hyperalgesia. Pain research and clinical management, vol 7. Elsevier Science Publishers, Amsterdam

Simons D, Travell J, Simons L 1998 Myofascial pain and dysfunction: the trigger point manual, vol 1, upper half of body, 2nd edn. Williams and Wilkins, Baltimore

Spencer J D, Hayes K C, Alexander I J 1984 Knee joint effusion and quadriceps reflex inhibition in man. Archives of Physical Medicine and Rehabilitation 65:171–177

Stokes M J, Cooper R G, Jayson M I V 1992 Selective changes in multifidus dimensions in patients with chronic low back pain. European Spine Journal 1:38–42

Travell J, Simons D 1983 Myofascial pain and dysfunction: the trigger point manual, vol. 1, upper half of body, 1st edn. Williams and Wilkins, Baltimore

Tulos H, Bennett J 1984 The shoulder in sports. In: Scott W (ed) Principles of sports medicine. Williams and Willkins, Baltimore

Triano J, Schultz A B 1987 Correlation of objective measure of trunk motion and muscle function with low-back disability ratings. Spine 12:561

Van Wingerden J-P, Vleeming A, Kleinvensink G, Stoekart R 1997 The role of the hamstrings in pelvic and spinal function. In: Vleeming A et al (eds) Movement, stability and low back pain. Churchill Livingstone, Edinburgh

Vleeming A 1989 Load application to the sacrotuberous ligament: influences on sacroiliac joint mechanics. Clinical Biomechanics 4:204–209

Walsh E G 1992 Muscles, masses and motion. The physiology of normality, hypotonicity, spasticity, and rigidity. MacKeith Press, Blackwell Scientific, Oxford

Wittlinger H, Wittlinger G 1982 Textbook of Dr. Vodder's manual lymph drainage, vol 1: basic course, 3rd edn. Karl F Haug, Heidelberg

Woo S L-Y 1987 Injury and repair of musculoskeletal soft tissues. American Academy of Orthopedic Surgeons Symposium, Savannah GA

3

Reporting stations and the brain

Irwin Korr (1970), osteopathy's premier researcher into the physiology of the musculoskeletal system, described it as 'the primary machinery of life'.

The musculoskeletal system (not our digestive or our immune system) is the largest energy consumer in the body. It allows us to perform tasks, play games and musical instruments, make love, give treatment, paint and, in a multitude of other ways, engage in life. Korr stated that the parts of the body act together 'to transmit and modify force and motion through which man acts out his life'. This coordinated integration takes place under the control of the central nervous system as it responds to a huge amount of sensory input from both the internal and the external environment.

Our journey through the structures which make up these communication pathways includes an overview of the ways in which information, most notably from the soft tissues, reaches the higher centers. The neural reporting stations represent 'the first line of contact between the environment and the human system' (Boucher 1996).

PROPRIOCEPTION

Information which is fed into the central control systems of the body relating to the external environment flows from exteroceptors (mainly involving data relating to things we see, hear and smell). A wide variety of internal reporting stations also transmit data on everything from the tone of muscles to the position and movement of every part of the body. The volume of information entering the central nervous system for processing almost defies comprehension and it is little wonder that, at times, the mechanisms providing the information or the way it is transmitted or received or the way it is processed and responded to become dysfunctional.

Proprioception can be described as the process of delivering information to the central nervous system, as to the position and motion of the internal parts of the body. The information is derived from neural reporting stations (afferent receptors) in the muscles, the skin, other soft tissues and joints. The term proprioception was first used by Sherrington in 1907 to describe the sense of position, posture and movement. Janda (1996) states that it is now used ('not quite correctly') in a broader way, 'to describe the function of the entire afferent system'.

Schafer (1987) describes proprioception as 'kinesthetic awareness' relating to 'body posture, position, movement, weight, pressure, tension, changes in equilibrium, resistance of external objects, and associated stereotyped response patterns'. In addition to the unconscious data being transmitted from the proprioceptors, Schafer lists the sensory receptors as:

- *mechanoreceptors*, which detect deformation of adjacent tissues. These are excited by mechanical pressures or distortions and so would respond to touch or to muscular movement. Mechanoreceptors can become sensitized following what is termed a 'nociceptive barrage' so that they start to behave as though they are pain receptors. This would lead to pain being sensed (reported) centrally in response to what would normally have been reported as movement or touch (Schaible & Grubb 1993, Willis 1993)
- *chemoreceptors*, which report on obvious information such as taste and smell, as well as local biochemical changes such as CO_2 and O_2 levels
- *thermoreceptors*, which detect modifications in temperature. These are used in palpation of tissue temperature variations and are most dense on the hands and forearms (and the tongue)
- *electromagnetic receptors*, which respond to light entering the retina
- *nociceptors*, which register pain. These receptors can become sensitized when chronically stimulated, leading to a drop in their threshold (see notes on facilitation, Chapter 6, p. 70). This is thought to be a process associated with trigger point evolution (Korr 1976).

Lewit has shown that altered function can produce increased pain perception and that this is a far more common occurrence than pain resulting from direct compression of neural structures (which produces radicular pain).

There is no need to explain pain by mechanical irritation of nervous structures, as is frequently suggested, under the obvious influence of the root-compression model. It would be a peculiar conception of the nervous system (a system dealing with information) that would have it reacting, as a rule, not to stimulation of its receptors but to mechanical damage to its own structures (Lewit 1985).

Lewit offers as examples of the reflex nature of much pain perception: referred pain from deeper structures (organs or ligaments) which produce radiating pain, altered skin sensitivity (hyperalgesia) and sometimes muscle spasm.

These reflex referrals are discussed later in this chapter in the context of somatosomatic and viscerosomatic reflexes. True radicular pain (for example, resulting from disc prolapse) mainly involves stimulation of nociceptors which are present in profusion in the dural sheaths and the dura and not direct compression which produces paresis and anesthesia (loss of motor power and numbness) *but not pain*. Pain derives from irritation of pain receptors and where this results from functional changes (such as inappropriate degrees of maintained tension in muscles), Lewit has offered the descriptive term 'functional pathology of the motor system'.

Fascia and proprioception

Bonica (1990) suggests that fascia is critically involved in proprioception and that, after joint and muscle spindle input is taken into account, the majority of remaining proprioception occurs in fascial sheaths (Earl 1965, Wilson 1966). Staubesand (1996) confirms this and has demonstrated that myelinated sensory neural structures exist in fascia, relating to both proprioception and pain reception.

The various neural reporting organs in the body provide a constant source of information feedback to the central nervous system, and higher centers, as to the current state of tone, tension, movement, etc. of the tissues housing them (Travell & Simons 1983, 1992, Wall & Melzack 1991). It is important to realize that the traffic between the center and the periphery in this dynamic mechanism operates in both directions along efferent and afferent pathways, so that any alteration in normal function at the periphery (such as a proprioceptive source of information) leads to adaptive mechanisms being initiated in the central nervous system – and vice versa (Freeman 1967).

It is also important to realize that it is not just neural impulses which are transmitted along nerve pathways, in both directions, but a host of important trophic substances. This process of the transmission of trophic substances, in a two-way traffic along neural pathways, is arguably at least as important as the passage of impulses with which we usually associate nerve function (see Box 3.1).

REFLEX MECHANISMS

The basis of reflex arcs which control much of the motion of the body can be summarized as follows (Sato 1992).

- A receptor (proprioceptor, mechanoreceptor, etc.) is stimulated.
- An afferent impulse travels, via the central nervous system, to a part of the brain which we can call an integrative center.
- This integrative center evaluates the message and,

Box 3.1 Neurotrophic influences

Irvin Korr (Korr 1967, 1986) spent half a century investigating the scientific background to osteopathic methodology and theory. Some of his most important work related to the role of neural structures in the delivery of trophic substances. The various patterns of stress which will be covered in the next chapter are capable of drastically affecting this axoplasmic transportation.

Korr states:

These 'trophic' proteins are thought to exert long-term influences on the developmental, morphologic, metabolic and functional qualities of the tissues – even on their viability. Biomechanical abnormalities in the musculoskeletal system can cause trophic disturbances in at least two ways: (1) by mechanical deformation (compression, stretching, angulation, torsion) of the nerves, which impedes axonal transport; and (2) by sustained hyperactivity of neurons in facilitated segments of the spinal cord [see discussion of this phenomenon in Chapter 6] which slows axonal transport and which, because of metabolic changes, may affect protein synthesis by the neurons. It appears that manipulative treatment would alleviate such impairments of neurotrophic function.

The manufacturing process of macromolecules for transportation takes place in nerve cells, is packaged by the Golgi apparatus and transported along the neural axon to the target neurons (Ochs & Ranish 1969). The speed of transportation along axons is sometimes remarkably swift at the rate of up to half a meter per day (although much slower than the 120 meters per second of actual neural transmission) (Ochs 1975).

Once the macromolecules reach their destination, where they influence the development and maintenance of the tissues being supplied, a return transportation of materials for reprocessing commences. When there is interference in axonal flow (because of compression, etc.) the tissues not receiving the trophic material degenerate and a build-up of axoplasm occurs, forming a swelling (Schwartz 1980).

Korr (1981) has shown that when a muscle is denervated by injury and atrophies, it is the interruption of trophic substances which causes this rather than loss of neural impulses (see notes on rectus capitis posterior minor denervation following whiplash, p. 34).

Research has shown that when the neural supply to a postural (predominantly red fiber) muscle is surgically altered, so that it receives neurotrophic material originally destined for a phasic (white fiber) muscle, there is a transformation in which the postural muscle can become a phasic muscle (and vice versa) based on the trophic material it receives. This suggests that genetic expression is neurally mediated. The axoplasm tells the muscle what its function is going to be (Guth 1968).

with influences from higher centers, sends an efferent response.

● This travels to an effector unit, perhaps a motor endplate, and a response occurs.

As Schafer (1987) points out, 'The human body exhibits an astonishingly complex array of neural circuitry'. It is possible to characterize the reflex mechanisms which operate as part of involuntary nervous system function as follows.

● *Somatosomatic reflexes* which may involve stimulus of sensory receptors in the skin, subcutaneous tissue, fascia, striated muscle, tendon, ligament or joint producing reflex responses in segmentally related somatic structures;

for example, from one such site on the body to another segmentally related site on the body. Such reflexes are commonly evoked in manual therapy techniques (compression, vibration, massage, manipulation, application of heat or cold, etc.).

● *Somatovisceral reflexes* which involve a localized somatic stimulation (from cutaneous, subcutaneous or musculoskeletal sites) producing a reflex response in a segmentally related visceral structure (internal organ or gland) (Simons et al 1998). Such reflexes are also commonly evoked in manual therapy techniques (compression, vibration, massage, manipulation, application of heat or cold, etc.).

● *Viscerosomatic reflex* in which a localized visceral (internal organ or gland) stimulus produces a reflex response in a segmentally related somatic structure (cutaneous, subcutaneous or musculoskeletal) (Fig. 3.1). It has been suggested that such reflexes feeding in to the superficial structures of the body can give rise to trigger points in the somatic tissues (De Sterno 1977, Simons et al 1998). Balduc (1983) reports that these reflexes are intensity oriented, which is to say that the degree of reflex response relates directly to the intensity of the visceral stimulus.

● *Viscerocutaneous reflex* in which organ dysfunction stimuli produce superficial effects involving the skin (including pain, tenderness, etc.). Obvious examples of this include right shoulder pain in gall bladder disease and cardiac ischemia producing the typical angina distribution of left arm and thoracic pain.

● *Viscerovisceral reflex* in which a stimulus in an internal organ or gland produces a reflex response in another segmentally related internal organ or gland.

Whether such reflexes have bidirectional potential is debated. Some research suggests that a visceral problem

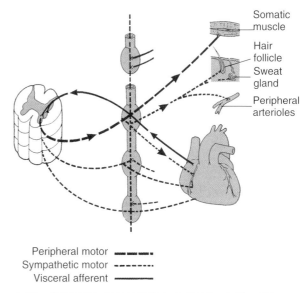

Peripheral motor ▬ ▬ ▬
Sympathetic motor - - - - - -
Visceral afferent ▬▬▬▬

Figure 3.1 Schematic representation of viscerosomatic reflex (reproduced, with permission, from Chaitow (1996a)).

can exhibit in a specific dermatomal segment via a viscerocutaneous reflex and that stimulation of the skin could have a distinct effect on related visceral area via a cutaneovisceral reflex. Schafer (1987) makes the very important observation that, 'The difference between somatovisceral and viscerosomatic reflexes appears to be only quantitative and to be accounted for by the lesser density of nociceptive receptors in the viscera'.

This can best be understood by means of Head's law, which states that when a painful stimulus is applied to a body part of low sensitivity (such as an organ) that is in close central connection (the same segmental supply) with an area of higher sensitivity (such as a part of the soma), pain will be felt at the point of higher sensitivity rather than where the stimulus was applied.

Local reflexes

A number of mechanisms exist in which reflexes are stimulated by sensory impulses from a muscle leading to a response being transmitted to the same muscle. Examples include the stretch reflexes, myotatic reflexes and the deep tendon reflexes. The stretch reflex is a protective mechanism in which a contraction is triggered when the annulospiral receptors in a muscle spindle are rapidly elongated. Concurrently there are inhibitory messages transmitted to the motor neurons of the antagonist muscles inducing reciprocal inhibition, with simultaneous facilitating impulses to the synergists. If enough fibers are involved the threshold of the Golgi tendon organs will be breached, leading to the muscle 'giving way'. This is a reflex process known as *autogenic inhibition* (Ng 1980).

Central influences

Sensory information received by the central nervous system can be modulated and modified both by the influence of the mind and changes in blood chemistry, to which the sympathetic nervous system is sensitive (see notes on carbon dioxide influences on neural sensitivity, Chapter 4, p. 51). Whatever local biochemical influences may be operating, the ultimate overriding control on the response to any neural input derives from the brain itself.

- Afferent messages are received centrally from somatic vestibular (ears) and visual sources, both reporting new data and providing feedback for requested information.
- If all or any of this information is excessive, noxious or inappropriately prolonged, sensitization (see notes on facilitation, Chapter 6, p. 70) can occur in aspects of the central control mechanisms, which results in dysfunctional and inappropriate output.
- The limbic system of the brain can also become dysfunctional and inappropriately process incoming data, leading to complex problems, such as fibromyalgia (Goldstein 1996) (see Box 3.4).

- The entire suprasegmental motor system, including the cortex, basal ganglia, cerebellum, etc., responds to the afferent data input with efferent motor instructions to the body parts, with skeletal activity receiving its input from alpha and gamma motor neurons, as well as the motor aspects of cranial nerves.

Schafer (1987) sums up the process:

Whether a person is awake or asleep, the brain is constantly bombarded by input from all skin and internal receptors. This barrage of incoming messages is examined, valued, and translated relative to a framework composed of instincts, experiences and psychic conditioning. In some yet to be discovered manner, an appropriate decision is arrived at that is transmitted to all pertinent muscles necessary for the response desired. By means of varying synaptic facilitation and restraints within the appropriate circuits, an almost limitless variety of neural integration and signal transmission is possible.

The sum of proprioceptive information results in specific responses.

- Motor activity is refined and reflex corrections of movement patterns occur almost instantly.
- A conscious awareness occurs of the position of the body and the part in space.
- Over time, learned processes can be modified in response to altered proprioceptive information and new movement patterns can be learned and stored.
- It is this latter aspect, the possibility of learning new patterns of use, which makes proprioceptive influence so important in rehabilitation.

NEUROMUSCULAR DYSFUNCTION FOLLOWING INJURY (Ryan 1994)

- Functional instability may result from altered proprioception following trauma, e.g. the ankle 'gives way' (functional instability) during walking when no apparent structural reason exists (Lederman 1997).
- Proprioceptive loss following injury has been demonstrated in spine, knee, ankle and TMJ (following trauma, surgery, etc.) (Spencer 1984).
- These changes contribute to progressive degenerative joint disease and muscular atrophy (Fitzmaurice 1992).
- The motor system will have lost feedback information for refinement of movement, leading to abnormal mechanical stresses of muscles/joints. Such effects of proprioceptive deficit may not be evident for many months after trauma.

MECHANISMS WHICH ALTER PROPRIOCEPTION (Lederman 1997)

- Ischemic or inflammatory events at receptor sites may produce diminished proprioceptive sensitivity due to the build-up of metabolic by-products which stimulate

---

Box 3.2 Reporting stations

Some important structures involved in this internal information highway, which may under given circumstances be involved in the production or maintenance of pain (LaMotte 1992), are listed below.

Ruffini end-organs. Found within the joint capsule, around the joints, so that each is responsible for describing what is happening over an angle of approximately 15°, with a degree of overlap between it and the adjacent end-organ. These organs are not easily fatigued and are progressively recruited as the joint moves, so that movement is smooth and not jerky. The prime concern of Ruffini end-organs is a steady position. They are also to some extent concerned with reporting the direction of movement.

Golgi end-organs. These, too, adapt slowly and continue to discharge over a lengthy period. They are found in the ligaments associated with the joint. Unlike the Ruffini end-organs, which respond to muscular contraction which alters tension in the joint capsule, Golgi end-organs can deliver information independently of the state of muscular contraction. This helps the body to know just where the joint is at any given moment, irrespective of muscular activity.

Slow-adapting joint receptors (above) have a powerful modulating influence on reflex responses (for example, in the sacroiliac joint) and seem to have the ability to produce long-lasting influences, either in maintaining dysfunction or in helping in its resolution (if pressure/stress on them can be normalized). Direct joint manipulation (Lefebvre et al 1993) can have just such an effect or, as Lewit has shown, so can normalization of joint function by less direct means. Lewit (1985) emphasizes this by saying:

The basic [soft tissue] techniques ... are very gentle and are also very effective for mobilization, using muscular facilitation and inhibition, i.e. the inherent forces of the patient. It is most unfortunate that in the minds of most people, physicians and laymen alike, manipulation is tantamount to thrusting techniques – techniques that should rather be the exception.

The pacinian corpuscle. This is found in periarticular connective tissue and adapts rapidly. It triggers discharges, and then ceases reporting in a very short space of time. These messages occur successively, during motion, and the CNS can, therefore, be aware of the rate of acceleration of movement taking place in the area. It is sometimes called an acceleration receptor.

Skin receptors are responsive to touch, pressure and pain and are involved in primitive responses such as withdrawal and grasp reflexes.

Cervical receptors, especially relative to the suboccipital

musculature (see notes on rectus capitis posterior minor on p. 34), interact with the *labyrinthine* (ear) *receptors* to maintain balance and an appropriate positioning of the head in space.

There are other end-organs, but those described above can be seen to provide information on the present status, position, direction and rate of movement of any muscle or joint and of the body as a whole.

Muscle spindle. This receptor is sensitive and complex.

- It detects, evaluates, reports and adjusts the length of the muscle in which it lies, setting its tone.
- Acting with the Golgi tendon organ, most of the information as to muscle tone and movement is reported.
- Spindles lie parallel to the muscle fibers and are attached to either skeletal muscle or the tendinous portion of the muscle.
- Inside the spindle are fibers which may be one of two types. One is described as a 'nuclear bag' fiber and the other as a chain fiber.
- In different muscles, the ratio of these internal spindle fibers differs.
- In the center of the spindle is a receptor called the annulospiral receptor (or primary ending) and on each side of this lies a 'flower spray receptor' (secondary ending).
- The primary ending discharges rapidly and this occurs in response to even small changes in muscle length.
- The secondary ending compensates for this, because it fires messages only when larger changes in muscle length have occurred.
- The spindle is a 'length comparator' (also called a 'stretch receptor') and it may discharge for long periods at a time.
- Within the spindle there are fine, intrafusal fibers which alter the sensitivity of the spindle. These can be altered without any actual change taking place in the length of the muscle itself, via an independent gamma efferent supply to the intrafusal fibers. This has implications in a variety of acute and chronic problems.
- The activities of the spindle appear to provide information as to length, velocity of contraction and changes in velocity. How long is the muscle, how quickly is it changing length and what is happening to this rate of change of length (*Gray's anatomy* 1973)?

Golgi tendon receptors. These structures indicate how hard the muscle is working (whether contracting or stretching) since they reflect the tension of the muscle, rather than its length. If the tendon organ detects excessive overload it may cause cessation of function of the muscle to prevent damage. This produces relaxation.

---

group III and IV, mainly pain afferents (this also occurs in muscle fatigue).

- Physical trauma can directly affect receptor axons (articular receptors, muscle spindles and their innervations).
  1. In direct trauma to muscle, spindle damage can lead to denervation (for example, following whiplash) (Hallgren et al 1993).
  2. Structural changes in parent tissue lead to atrophy and loss of sensitivity in detecting movement, plus altered firing rate (for example, during stretching).
- Loss of muscle force (and possibly wasting) may result when reduced afferent pattern leads to central reflexogenic inhibition of motor neurons supplying the affected muscle.
- Psychomotor influences (e.g. feeling of insecurity)

can alter patterns of muscle recruitment at local level and may result in disuse and muscle weakness.
- The combination of muscular inhibition, joint restriction and trigger point activity is, according to Liebenson (1996), 'the key peripheral component of the functional pathology of the motor system'.

AN EXAMPLE OF PROPRIOCEPTIVE DYSFUNCTION

In order to appreciate some of the profound influences which proprioceptive function offers and the devastating effect disturbance of this function can produce in terms of postural stability and pain, a particular example is summarized below involving rectus capitis posterior minor.

Rectus capitis posterior minor (RCPMin) research evidence

- In head extension, the posterior atlas arch maintains a mid-position between the occiput and the axis. In forward head translation, this space nearly vanishes (Penning 1989).
- Hack et al (1995) noted that a fascial bridge between the RCPMin and the dura is oriented perpendicularly, resisting movement of the dura towards the spinal cord with head translation.
- The attachment of the ligamentum nuchae into the dura between the atlas and axis serves a complementary function with the RCPMins (Mitchell et al 1998).
- Through the ligamentum nuchae, other posterior muscles may also be acting indirectly with the RCPMin to coordinate dural position with head movement.
- EMG studies suggest RCPMin does not fire during extension, but rather does so when the head translates forwards (Greenman 1997, personal communication).
- The high density of muscle spindles found in the RCPMs suggests the value of these muscles lies not in their motor function but in their role as 'proprioceptive monitors' of the cervical spine and head.
- Observations linking the suboccipital and cervical muscles with equilibrium are not new (Longet 1845).
- In 1955, the importance of proprioceptors in this region was recognized and the term 'cervical vertigo' was coined (Ryan & Cope 1955).
- Cervical proprioception currently is recognized as an essential component in maintaining balance. This is particularly true in the elderly, in whom there is a shift in emphasis from vestibular reflexes to cervical reflexes in maintaining balance (Wyke 1985).

Proprioception and pain

- Proprioceptive signals from these suboccipital

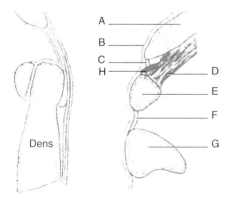

Figure 3.2 Main structures of the atlantooccipital region (sagittal section, showing bridge connecting RCPMin to dura. A: occiput; B: posterior dura; C: posterior atlantooccipital membrane; D: rectus capitis posterior minor muscle; E: atlas (posterior arch); F: posterior atlantoaxial ligament; G: axis; H: bridge to dura (reproduced, with permission, from the *Journal of Bodywork and Movement Therapies* 1999; **3**(1):31).

muscles may also serve as a 'gate' that blocks nociceptor (pain fiber) transmission into the spinal cord and higher centers of the central nervous system (Wall 1989).
- According to the gate theory of pain, large-diameter (A-beta) fibers from proprioceptors and mechanoreceptors enter the spinal cord and synapse on *interneurons* in the dorsal horn of the spinal cord.
- Interneurons inhibit nociceptor transmission, specifically nociceptors which synapse in lamina V of the dorsal horn.
- Chronic postural stress (slouching or 'chin poking') or trauma may lead to hypertonic suboccipital muscles.
- Hallgren et al (1994) found that some individuals with chronic neck pain exhibited fatty degeneration and atrophy of the RCPMin and RCPMaj, as visualized by MRI.
- Atrophy of the RCPMin reduces its proprioceptive output and this may destabilize postural balance (McPartland 1997).
- Subjects with chronic neck pain (and RCPMin atrophy as seen by MRI) showed a decrease in standing balance when compared to control subjects.
- Reduced proprioceptive input facilitates the transmission of impulses from a wide dynamic range of nociceptors, which can develop into a chronic pain syndrome.
- When muscle pain increases in intensity, referral of the pain sensation to remote sites occurs, such as to other muscles, fascia, tendons, joints and ligaments (Mense & Skeppar 1991).
- Noxious stimulation of the rectus capitis posterior muscles causes reflex EMG activity in distal muscles, including the trapezius and the masseter muscles (Hu et al 1993). Hu and colleagues (1995) showed that irritation of the dural vasculature in the upper cervical leads to reflexive EMG activity of the neck and jaw muscles.
- Injury or dysfunction of the RCPMin may irritate the C1 nerve which, if chronic, may lead to facilitation of sympathetic fibers associated with C1, resulting in a chronic pain syndrome.
- Alternatively, chronic C1 irritation may refer pain to the neck and face, via C1's connections with C2 and cranial nerve V.
- Conclusion: RCPMin dysfunction (atrophy) leads to increased pain perception, reduced proprioceptive input, reflexively affecting, for example, other cervical and jaw muscles (Hack et al 1995).

RCPMin evaluation and treatment

- McPartland (1997) palpated individuals with RCPMin atrophy and found they had twice as many cervical somatic dysfunctions as control subjects.
- Somatic dysfunctions were identified by tenderness of paraspinal muscles, asymmetry of joints, restriction in ROM and tissue texture abnormalities.

• Janda (1978) screened for proprioceptive dysfunction by testing standing balance with eyes closed. A normal individual should be able to stand on one leg with arms crossed and eyes closed for 30 seconds. Anything less than this is regarded as indicating degrees of proprioceptive dysfunction. Patients with proprioceptive dysfunction are treated with 'sensory motor retraining' – balance retraining with the eyes closed.

NEURAL INFLUENCES

Effect of contradictory proprioceptive information

Korr (1976) reminds us:

The spinal cord is the keyboard on which the brain plays when it calls for activity or for change in activity. But each 'key' in the console sounds, not an individual 'tone', such as the contraction of a particular group of muscle fibers, but a whole 'melody' of activity, even a 'symphony' of motion. In other words, built into the cord is a large repertoire of patterns of activity, each involving the complex, harmonious, delicately balanced orchestration of the contractions and relaxations of many muscles. The brain 'thinks' in terms of whole motions, not individual muscles. It calls selectively, for the preprogrammed patterns in the cord and brain stem, modifying them in countless ways and combining them in an infinite variety of still more complex patterns. Each activity is also subject to further modulation, refinement, and adjustment by the afferent feedback continually streaming in from the participating muscles, tendons, and joints.

This means that the pattern of information fed back to the CNS and brain reflects, at any given time, the steady state of joints, the direction as well as speed of alteration in position of joints, together with data on the length of muscle fibers, the degree of load that is being borne and the tension this involves. It is a totality of information which is received rather than individual pieces of information from particular reporting stations.

Should any of this mass of information be contradictory and actually conflict with other information being received, what then? If conflicting reports reach the cord from a variety of sources simultaneously, no discernible pattern may be recognized by the CNS (see Korr's discussion below and Box 3.3). In such a case no adequate response would be forthcoming and it is probable that activity would be stopped and a protective co-contraction ('freezing', splinting) spasm could be the result.

Neural overload, entrapment and crosstalk

Korr (1976) discusses a variety of insults which may result in increased neural excitability including the triggering of a barrage of supernumerary impulses to and from the cord and 'crosstalk', in which axons may overload and pass impulses to one another directly. Muscle contraction disturbances, vasomotion, pain impulses, reflex mecha-

nisms and disturbances in sympathetic activity may all result from such behavior, due to what might be relatively slight tissue changes (in the intervertebral foramina, for example), possibly involving neural compression or actual entrapment.

In addition, Korr states that normal patterned transmission from the periphery can be jammed when any tissue is disturbed, whether bone, joint, ligament or muscle. These factors, combined with any mechanical alterations in the tissues, are the background to much somatic dysfunction.

Korr summarizes the picture as follows:

These are the somatic insults, the sources of incoherent and meaningless feedback, that cause the spinal cord to halt normal operations and to freeze the status quo in the offending and offended tissues. It is these phenomena that are detectable at the body surface and are reflected in disorders of muscle tension, tissue texture, visceral and circulatory function, and even secretory function; the elements that are so much a part of osteopathic diagnosis.

Goldstein (1996) offers a more complex scenario in which the brain itself (or at least part of it, becomes hyperreactive and starts to misinterpret incoming information (Box 3.4).

Manipulating the reporting stations

There exist various ways of 'manipulating' the neural reporting stations to produce physiological modifications in soft tissues.

• *Muscle energy technique* (MET) – isometric contractions utilized in MET affect the Golgi tendon organs, although the degree of subsequent inhibition of muscle tone is strongly debated. Some take a position that this is a minimal effect (Lederman 1997), while others suggest a strong, if temporary, influence which allows for an easier stretch of previously shortened structures (Lewit 1985).

• *Positional release techniques* (PRT) – muscle spindles are influenced by methods which take them into an 'ease' state and which theoretically allow them an opportunity to 'reset' and reduce hypertonic status. Jones' (1995) Strain and counterstrain and other positional release methods use the slow and controlled return of distressed tissues to the position of strain as a means of offering spindles a chance to reset and so normalize function. This is particularly effective if they have inappropriately held an area in just such protective splinting.

• *Direct influences* can be achieved, for example, by means of pressure applied to the spindles or Golgi tendon organs (sometimes termed 'ischemic compression' or 'inhibitory pressure', equivalent to acupressure methodology) (Stiles 1984).

• *Proprioceptive manipulation* (applied kinesiology) is possible (Walther 1988). For example, kinesiological muscle tone correction utilizes two key receptors in muscles to achieve its effects. A muscle in spasm may

Box 3.3 Co-contraction and strain

The work of Laurence Jones DO (1995) in developing his treatment method of strain and counterstrain (see Chapter 9) led him to research the mechanisms which might occur under conditions of acute strain. His concept is based on the predictable physiological responses of muscles in given situations.

Jones describes how in a balanced state the proprioceptive functions of the various muscles supporting a joint will be feeding a flow of information derived from the neural receptors in those muscles and their tendons. For example, the Golgi tendon organs will be reporting on tone, while the various receptors in the spindles will be firing a constant stream of information (slowly or rapidly, depending upon the demands being placed on the tissues) regarding their resting length and any changes which might be occurring in that length (Korr 1947, 1974, Mathews 1981).

Jones (1964) first observed the phenomenon of spontaneous release when he 'accidentally' placed a patient who was in considerable pain and some degree of compensatory distortion into a position of comfort (ease) on a treatment table. Despite no other treatment being given, after just 20 minutes resting in a position of relative ease the patient was able to stand upright and was free of pain. The pain-free position of ease into which Jones had helped the patient was one which exaggerated the degree of distortion in which his body was being held. He had taken the patient into the direction of ease (rather than towards tension or 'bind') since any attempt to correct or straighten the body would have been met by both resistance and pain. In contrast, moving the body further into distortion was acceptable and easy and seemed to allow operation of the physiological processes involved in resolution of spasm.

The events which occur at the moment of strain provide the key to understanding the mechanisms of neurologically induced positional release. For example, consider an all too common example of someone bending forward. At this time the trunk flexors would be short of their resting length and their muscle spindles would be firing slowly, indicating little or no activity and no change of length taking place. At the same time the spinal erector group would be stretched, or stretching, and firing rapidly. Any stretch affecting a muscle (and therefore its spindles) will increase the rate of reporting which will reflexively induce further contraction (myotatic stretch reflex) and an increase in tone in that muscle. This produces an instant reciprocal inhibition of the functional antagonists to it (flexors), reducing even further the already limited degree of reporting from their muscle spindles.

This feedback link with the central nervous system is the *primary muscle spindle afferent response*, modulated by an additional muscle spindle function, *the gamma efferent system*, which is controlled from higher (brain) centers. In simple terms, the gamma efferent system influences the primary afferent system, for example when a muscle is in a quiescent state. When it is relaxed and short with little information coming from the primary receptors, the gamma efferent system might fine-tune and increase ('turn up') the sensitivity of the primary afferents to ensure a continued information flow (Mathews 1981).

Crisis

Now imagine an emergency situation in which immediate demands for stabilization are made on both sets of muscles (the short, relatively 'quiet' flexors and the stretched, relatively actively firing extensors) even though they are in quite different states of preparedness for action.

The flexors would be 'unloaded', relaxed and providing minimal feedback to the control centers, while the spinal extensors would be at stretch, providing a rapid outflow of spindle-derived information, some of which ensures that the relaxed flexor muscles remain even more relaxed due to inhibitory activity.

The central nervous system would at this time have minimal information as to the status of the relaxed flexors and, at the

moment when the crisis demand for stabilization occurred, these shortened and relaxed flexors would be obliged to stretch quickly to a length which would balance the already stretched extensors – which would be contracting rapidly to stabilize the area.

As this happened the annulospiral receptors in the short (flexor)

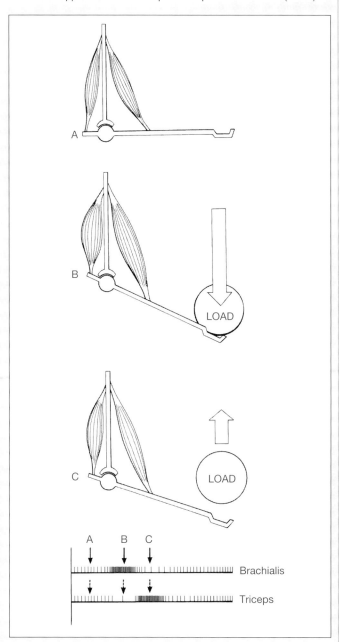

Figure 3.3 A: Arm flexor (brachialis) and extensor (triceps brachii) in easy normal relationship indicated by rate of firing on the scale for each muscle. B: When sudden force is applied, the flexors are stretched and the extensors protect the joint by rapidly shortening. C: Stretch receptors in the flexors continue to fire as though stretch continues. Firing of both flexors and extensors continues at inappropriately high rates, producing the effect noted in a strained joint where restriction exists within the joint's physiological range of motion (reproduced, with permission, from Chaitow (1996b)).

Box 3.3 (cont'd)

muscles would respond to the sudden stretch demand by contracting even more, as the stretch reflex was triggered. The neural reporting stations in these shortened muscles would be firing impulses as if the muscles were being stretched – *even when the muscle remained well short of its normal resting length*. At the same time the extensor muscles, which had been at stretch and which in the alarm situation were obliged to rapidly shorten, would remain longer than their normal resting length as they were attempting to stabilize the situation.

Korr has described what happens in the abdominal muscles (flexors) in such a situation. He says that, because of their relaxed status short of their resting length, a silencing of the spindles occurs. However, due to the sudden demand for information by the higher centers, gamma gain is increased so that, as the muscle contracts rapidly to stabilize the situation and demands for information are received from the central nervous system, the muscle reports back that it is being stretched when it is actually short of its normal resting length. This results in co-contraction of both sets of muscles, agonists and antagonists. In effect, the muscles would have adopted a restricted position as a result of inappropriate proprioceptive reporting (Korr 1976). The two opposing sets of muscles become locked into positions of imbalance in relation to their normal function. One would be shorter and one longer than its normal resting length.

At this time any attempt to extend the area/joint(s) would be strongly resisted by the tonically shortened flexor group. The individual would be locked into a forward-bending distortion, in this example. The joints involved would not have been taken beyond their normal physiological range and yet the normal range would be unavailable due to the shortened status of the flexor group (in this particular example). Going further into flexion, however, would present no problems or pain.

Walther (1988) summarizes the situation as follows.

When proprioceptors send conflicting information there may be simultaneous contraction of the antagonists ... without antagonist muscle inhibition joint and other strain results ... a reflex pattern develops which causes muscle or other tissue to maintain this continuing strain. It [strain dysfunction] often relates to the inappropriate signaling from muscle proprioceptors that have been strained from rapid change that does not allow proper adaptation.

This situation would be unlikely to resolve itself spontaneously and is the 'strain' position in Jones' Strain/counterstrain method. We can recognize it in an acute setting in torticollis as well as in acute 'lumbago'. It is also recognizable as a feature of many types of chronic somatic dysfunction in which joints remain restricted due to muscular imbalances of this type.

This is a time of intense neurological and proprioceptive confusion. This is the moment of 'strain'.

Box 3.4 Biochemistry, the mind and neurosomatic disorders

Goldstein (1996) has described many chronic health conditions, including chronic fatigue and fibromyalgia syndromes (CFS, FMS), as neurosomatic disorders, quoting Yunus (1994) who says they are '...the commonest group of illnesses for which patients consult physicians'.

Neurosomatic disorders are illnesses which Goldstein suggests are caused by 'a complex interaction of genetic, developmental and environmental factors', often involving the possibility of early physical, sexual or psychological abuse (Fry 1993). Symptoms emerge as a result of 'impaired sensory information processing' by the neural network (including the brain). Examples given are of light touch being painful, mild odours producing nausea, walking a short distance being exhausting, climbing stairs being like going up a mountain, reading something light causing cognitive impairment – all of which examples are true for many people with CFS/FMS.

Goldstein is critical of psychological approaches to treatment of such conditions, apart from cognitive behaviour therapy which he suggests '... may be more appropriate, since coping with the vicissitudes of these illnesses, which wax and wane unpredictably, is a major problem for most of those afflicted'. He claims that most major medical journals, concerned with psychosomatic medicine, rarely discuss neurobiology and 'apply the concept of somatization to virtually every topic between their covers' (Hudson 1992, Yunus 1994).

The four basic influences on neurosomatic illness are, he believes, as follows.

1. Genetic susceptibility, which can be strong or weak. If only a weak tendency exists other factors are needed to influence the trait.
2. If a child feels unsafe between birth and puberty, hypervigilance may develop and interpretation of sensory input will alter.
3. Genetically predetermined susceptibility to viral infection affecting the neurons and glia. 'Persistent CNS viral infections could alter production of transmitters as well as cellular mechanisms'.

4. Increased susceptibility to environmental stressors due to reduction in neural plasticity (resulting from all or any of causes listed in 1–3 above). This might include deficiency in glutamate or nitric oxide (NO) secretions which results in encoding new memory. 'Neural plasticity' capacity may be easily overtaxed in such individuals which, Goldstein suggests, is why neurosomatic patients often develop their problems after a degree of increased exposure to environmental stressors such as acute infection, sustained attention, exercise, immunization, emergence from anesthesia, trauma, etc.

Goldstein (1996) describes the limbic system and its dysregulation thus.

1. The limbic system acts as a regulator (integrative processing) in the brain with effects on fatigue, pain, sleep, memory, attention, weight, appetite, libido, respiration, temperature, blood pressure, mood, immune and endocrine function.
2. Limbic function dysregulation influences all or any of these functions and systems.
3. Regulation of autonomic control of respiration derives from the limbic system and major abnormalities (hyperventilation tendencies, irregularity in tidal volume, etc.) in breathing function are noted in people with chronic fatigue syndrome, along with abnormal responses to exercise (including failure to find expected levels of cortisol increase, catecholamines, growth hormone, somatostatin, increased core temperature, etc.) (Gerra 1993, Goldstein & Daly 1993, Griep 1993, Munschauer 1991).
4. Dysfunction of the limbic system can result from central or peripheral influences ('stress').
5. Sensory gating (the weight given to sensory inputs) has been shown to be less effectively inhibited in women than in men (Swerdlow 1993).
6. Many biochemical imbalances are involved in limbic dysfunction and no attempt will be made in this summary to detail them all.
7. The trigeminal nerve, states Goldstein, modulates limbic

Box 3.4 *(cont'd)*

regulation. 'The trigeminal nerve may produce expansion of the receptive field zones of wide dynamic-range neurons and nociceptive-specific neurons under certain conditions, perhaps involving increased secretion of substance P, so that a greater number of neurons will be activated by stimulation of a receptive zone, causing innocuous stimuli to be perceived as painful' (Dubner 1992).

8. Goldstein reports that nitrous oxide, which is a primary vasodilator in the brain, has profound influences on glutamate secretion and the neurotransmitters which influence short-term memory (Sandman 1993), anxiety (Jones 1994), dopamine release (Hanbauer 1992) (so affecting fatigue), descending pain inhibition processes, sleep induction and even menstrual problems: 'Female patients with CFS/FMS usually have premenstrual exacerbations of their symptoms. Most of the symptoms of late luteal phase dysphoric disorder are similar to those of CFS, and it is likely that this disorder has a limbic etiology similar to CFS/FMS' (Iadecola 1993).

Allostasis is a major feature of Goldstein's model. He reports the following.

• Approximately 40% of FMS/CFS patients screened have been shown to have been physically, psychologically or sexually abused in childhood. By testing for brain electricity imbalances, using brain electricity activity mapping (BEAM) techniques, Goldstein has been able to demonstrate abnormalities in the left temporal area, a feature of people who have been physically, psychologically or sexually abused in childhood (as compared with non-abused controls) (Teicher 1993).

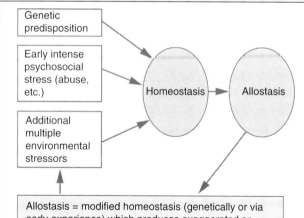

Allostasis = modified homeostasis (genetically or via early experience) which produces exaggerated or insufficient responses, for example:
• stress-hormone elevation
• behavioral and neuroimmunoendocrine disorders
• physiological regulation of abnormal states (out of balance)
• glucocorticoid elevation
• various key sites in the brain produce neurohumoral changes potentially influencing almost any part of the body or its functions.

Figure 3.4 Schematic representation of allostasis (reproduced, with permission, from Chaitow (1999)).

• Major childhood stress, he reports, increases cortisol levels which can affect hippocampal function and structure (McEwan 1994, Sapolsky 1990). It seems that early experience and environmental stimuli interacting with undeveloped biological systems lead to altered homeostatic responses: 'For example, exaggerated or insufficient HPA axis responses to defend a homeostatic state in a stressful situation could result in behavioural and neuro-immunoendocrine disorders in adulthood, particularly if stimuli that should be non-stressful were evaluated ... inappropriately by the prefrontal cortex ...' (Meaney 1994).

• Sapolsky (1990) has studied this area of 'allostasis' (regulation of internal milieu through dynamic change in a number of hormonal and physical variables that are not in a steady-state condition) and identifies as a primary feature a sense of lack of control. Sapolsky also identifies a sense of lack of predictability and various other stressors which influence the HPA axis and which are less balanced in individuals with CFS/FMS; all these stressors involve 'marked absence of control, predictability, or outlets for frustration'.

• In studies of this topic CFS/FMS patients are found to predominantly attribute their symptoms to external factors (virus, etc.) while control subjects (depressives) usually experience inward attribution (Powell 1990).

• Allostatic load, in contrast to homeostatic mechanisms which stabilize deviations in normal variables, is 'the price the body pays for containing the effects of arousing stimuli and the expectation of negative consequences' (Schulkin 1994).

• Chronic negative expectations and subsequent arousal seem to increase allostatic load. This is characterized by anxiety and anticipation of adversity leading to elevated stress hormone levels (Sterling & Eyer 1981).

• Goldstein attempts to explain the immensely complex biochemical and neural interactions which are involved in this scenario, embracing areas of the brain such as the amygdala, the prefrontal cortex, the lower brainstem and other sites, as well as myriad secretions including hormones (including glucocorticoids), neurotransmitters, substance P, dopamine and nitric oxide.

• Finally, he states, prefrontal cortex function can be altered by numerous triggering agents *in the predisposed individual* (possibly involving genetic features or early trauma) including:
1. viral infections that alter neuronal function
2. immunizations that deplete biogenic amines (Gardier 1994)
3. organophosphate or hydrocarbon exposure
4. head injury
5. childbirth
6. electromagnetic fields
7. sleep deprivation
8. general anesthesia
9. 'stress', e.g. physical, such as marathon running, or mental or emotional.

What Goldstein is reporting is an altered neurohumoral response in individuals whose defense and repair systems are predisposed to this happening, either because of inherited tendencies or because of early developmental (physical or psychological) insult(s), to which additional multiple stressors have been added. His solution is a biochemical (drug) modification of the imbalances he identifies as key features of this situation.

Alternative approaches might attempt to modify behavior or to alter other aspects of the complex disturbances, possibly using nutritional approaches. Goldstein has offered us insights and his own solutions. Not everyone will necessarily accept these solutions but the illumination of the highly complicated mechanisms involved, which he offers, is to be commended.

It is also worth reflecting on the possible effects, on predisposed mechanisms, of whiplash-type injuries, as discussed in this chapter.

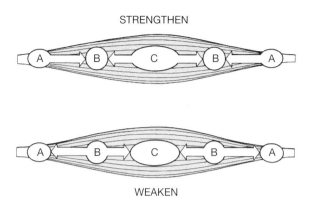

STRENGTHEN

WEAKEN

A = golgi tendon organs

B = belly of muscle

C = muscle spindle

Figure 3.5 Proprioceptive manipulation of muscles as described in the text (reproduced, with permission, from Chaitow (1996c)).

be helped to relax by the application of direct pressure (using approximately 2 lbs or 0.5 kilos of pressure) away from the belly of the muscle, in the area of the Golgi tendon organs, and/or by the application of the same amount of pressure towards the belly of the muscle, in the area of the muscle spindle cells (Fig. 3.5).

• The precise opposite effect (i.e. temporary toning or strengthening of the muscle) is achieved by applying pressure away from the belly, in the muscle spindle region, or towards the belly of the muscle in the tendon organ region.

• The mechanoreceptors in the skin are very responsive to stretching or pressure and are therefore easily influenced by methods which rub them (e.g. massage), apply pressure to them (NMT, reflexology, acupressure, shiatsu, etc.), stretch them or 'ease' them (as in osteopathic functional technique – see Chapter 9).

• The mechanoreceptors in the joints, tendons and ligaments are influenced to varying degrees by active or passive movement including articulation, mobilization, adjustment and exercise (Lederman 1997).

THERAPEUTIC REHABILITATION USING REFLEX SYSTEMS

Vladimir Janda has researched and developed ways in which reeducation of dysfunctional patterns of use can best be achieved, using our knowledge of neural reporting stations – a 'sensory motor' approach (Janda 1996). There are, he states, two stages to the process of learning new motor skills or relearning old ones.

1. The first is characterized by the learning of new ways of performing particular functions. This involves the cortex of the brain in conscious participation in the process of skill acquisition. As this process proceeds, Janda says, 'the brain tries to minimize the pathways and to simplify the regulatory circuits', speeding up this relatively slow means of rehabilitation. However, he warns, 'If such a motor program has become fixed once, it is difficult, if not impossible, to change it. This calls for other approaches'.

2. The speedier approach to motor learning involves balance exercises which attempt to assist the proprioceptive system and associated pathways relating to posture and equilibrium. Janda informs us that, 'From the point of view of afference, receptors in the sole of the foot, from the neck muscles, and in the sacroiliac area have the main proprioceptive influence' (Abrahams 1977, Freeman et al 1965, Hinoki & Ushio 1975).

Aids to stimulating the proprioceptors in these areas include wobble boards, rocker boards, balance shoes, mini trampolines and many others. The principles of this approach are based on the work of Bobath & Bobath (1964) who developed motor education programs for children with cerebral palsy. A program of reeducation of sensory motor function can apparently double the speed of muscle contraction, significantly improving general and postural function (Bullock-Saxton et al 1993).

CONCLUSION

An appreciation of the roles of the neural reporting stations helps us in our understanding of the ways in which dysfunctional adaptive responses progress, as they evolve out of patterns of overuse, misuse, abuse and disuse. Compensatory changes which emerge over time or as a result of adaptation to a single traumatic event are seen to have a logical progression. We will focus on these patterns in the next chapter. There we will take both a broad and local view of compensations and adaptations to the normal (gravity) and abnormal (use patterns or trauma) stresses of life and how these impact our remarkably resilient bodies.

REFERENCES

Abrahams V 1977 Physiology of neck muscles: their role in head movement and maintenance of posture. Canadian Journal of Physiology and Pharmacology 55:332

Balduc H 1983 Overview of contemporary chiropractic. Convention Notes, Northwestern College of Chiropractic, April 24

Bobath K, Bobath B 1964 Facilitation of normal postural reactions and movement in treatment of cerebral palsy. Physiotherapy 50:246

Bonica J 1990 The management of pain, 2nd edn. Lea and Febiger, Philadelphia

Boucher J 1996 Training and exercise science. In: Liebenson C (ed) Rehabilitation of the spine. Williams and Wilkins, Baltimore

Bullock-Saxton J, Janda V, Bullock M 1993 Reflex activation of gluteal muscles in walking. Spine 18:704

Chaitow L 1996a Muscle energy techniques. Churchill Livingstone, Edinburgh

Chaitow L 1996b Positional release techniques. Churchill Livingstone, Edinburgh

Chaitow L 1996c Modern Neuromuscular techniques. Churchill Livingstone, Edinburgh

Chaitow L 1999 Fibromyalgia Syndrome. Churchill Livingstone, Edinburgh

De Sterno C 1977 The pathophysiology of TMJ dysfunction. In: Gelb H (ed) Clinical management of head, neck and TMJ pain and dysfunction. W B Saunders, Philadelphia

Dubner R 1992 Hyperalgesia and expanded receptive fields. Pain 48:3–4

Earl E 1965 The dual sensory role of the muscle spindles. Physical Therapy Journal 45:4

Fitzmaurice R 1992 A histo-morphometric comparison of muscle biopsies from normal subjects and patients with ankylosing spondylitis and severe mechanical low back pain. Journal of Pathology 163:182

Freeman M 1967 Articular reflexes at the ankle joint. British Journal of Surgery 54:990

Freeman M, Dean M, Hanham I 1965 Etiology and prevention of functional instability of the foot. Journal of Bone and Joint Surgery (UK) 47:678

Fry R 1993 Adult physical illness and childhood sexual abuse. Journal of Psychosomatic Research 37(2):89–103

Gardier A 1994 Effects of a primary immune response to T-cell dependent antigen on serotonin metabolism in the frontal cortex [rat study]. Brain Research 645:1150–1156

Gerra G 1993 Noradrenergic and hormonal responses to physical exercise in adolescents. Neuropsychobiology 27(2):65–71

Goldstein J 1996 Betrayal by the brain. Haworth Medical Press, Binghampton, NY

Goldstein J, Daly J 1993 Neuroimmunoendocrine findings in CFS before and after exercise. Cited in Chronic fatigue syndrome: the limbic hypothesis. Haworth Press, Binghampton, NY

Gray's anatomy 1973 (35th edn). Longman, London

Griep E 1993 Altered reactivity of the hypothalamic-pituitary-adrenal axis in primary fibromyalgia syndrome. Journal of Rheumatology 20:469–474

Guth L 1968 Trophic influences of nerve on muscle. Physiology Review 48:177

Hack G D, Koritzer R T, Robinson W L et al 1995 Anatomic relation between the rectus capitis posterior minor muscle and the dura mater. Spine 20:2484–2486

Hallgren R, Greenman P, Rechtien J 1993 MRI of normal and atrophic muscles of the upper cervical spine. Journal of Clinical Engineering 18(5):433–439

Hallgren R, Greenman P, Rechtien J 1994 Atrophy of suboccipital muscles in patients with chronic pain: a pilot study. Journal of the American Osteopathic Association 94:1032–1038

Hanbauer I 1992 Role of nitric oxide in NMDA-evoked release of [³H]dopamine from striatal slices. NeuroReports 3(5):409–412

Hinoki M, Ushio N 1975 Lumbosacral proprioceptive reflexes in body equilibrium. Acta Otolaryngologia 330 (suppl):197

Hu J W, Yu X M, Vernon H, Sessle B J 1993 Excitatory effects on neck and jaw muscle activity of inflammatory irritant applied to cervical paraspinal tissues. Pain 55:243–250

Hu J W, Vernon H, Tatourian I 1995 Changes in neck electromyography associated with meningeal noxious stimulation. Journal of Manipulative Physiology and Therapeutics 18:577–581

Hudson J 1992 Comorbidity of fibromyalgia with medical and psychiatric disorders. American Journal of Medicine 92(4):363–367

Iadecola C 1993 Localization of NAPDH diaphorase in neurons in rostral ventral medulla: possible role of nitric oxide in central autonomic regulations and chemoreception. Brain Research 603:173–179

Janda V 1978 Muscles, central nervous motor regulation and back problems. In: Korr I M (ed) The neurobiologic mechanisms in manipulative therapy. Plenum Press, New York, pp 27–41

Janda V 1996 Sensory motor stimulation. In: Liebenson C (ed) Rehabilitation of the spine. Williams and Wilkins, Baltimore

Jones L 1964 Spontaneous release by positioning. The DO 4:109–116

Jones L 1995 Jones strain-counterstrain. JSCS Inc, Boise ID

Jones N 1994 Diverse roles for nitric oxide in synaptic signaling after activation of NMDA release-regularing receptors. Neuropharmacology 33:1351–1356

Korr I M 1947 The neural basis of the osteopathic lesion. Journal of the American Osteopathic Association 48:191–198

Korr I M 1967 Axonal delivery of neuroplasmic components to muscle cells. Science 155:342–345

Korr I M 1970 The physiological basis of osteopathic medicine. Postgraduate Institute of Osteopathic Medicine and Surgery, New York

Korr I M 1974 Proprioceptors and somatic dysfunction. Journal of the American Osteopathic Association 74:638–650

Korr I M 1976 Spinal cord as organiser of disease process. Academy of Applied Osteopathy Yearbook

Korr I M 1981 Spinal cord as organizer of disease processes. IV. Axonal transport and neurotrophic function. Journal of the American Osteopathic Association 80:451

Korr I M 1986 Somatic dysfunction, osteopathic manipulative treatment and the nervous system. Journal of the American Osteopathic Association 86(2):109–114

LaMotte R 1992 Subpopulations of 'nocisensor neurons' contributing to pain and allodynia, itch and allokinesis. APS Journal 2:115

Lederman E 1997 Fundamentals of manual therapy. Churchill Livingstone, Edinburgh

Lefebvre S et al 1993 Modulation of segmental spinal excitability by mechanical stress upon the sacroiliac joint. Proceedings of the International Conference on Spinal Manipulation, FCR, Arlington, pp 56–57

Lewit K 1985 Manipulative therapy in rehabilitation of the locomotor system. Butterworths, London

Liebenson C 1996 Rehabilitation of the spine. Williams and Wilkins, Baltimore

Longet F A 1845 Sur les troubles qui surviennent dans l'équilibration, la station et la locomotion des animaux, après la section des parties molles de la nuque. Gazette Medicale France 13:565–567

Mathews P 1981 Muscle spindles. In: Brooks V (ed) Handbook of physiology, section 1, the nervous system, vol 2. American Physiological Society, Bethesda, pp 189–228

McEwan B 1994 The plasticity of the hippocampus is the reason for its vulnerability. Seminal Neuroscience 6:239–246

McPartland J M 1997 Chronic neck pain, standing balance, and suboccipital muscle atrophy. Journal of Manipulative and Physiological Therapeutics 21(1):24–29

Meaney M 1994 Early environmental programming of hypothalamic-pituitary-adrenal responses to stress. Seminal Neuroscience 6:247–259

Mense S, Skeppar P 1991 Discharge behaviour of feline gamma-motoneurones following induction of an artificial myositis. Pain 46:201–210

Mitchell B S, Humphreys B K, O'Sullivan E 1998 Attachments of the ligamentum nuchae to cervical posterior spinal dura and the lateral part of the occipital bone. Journal of Manipulative and Physiological Therapeutics 21:145–148

Munschauer F 1991 Selective paralysis of voluntary but not limbically influenced autonomic respirations. Archives of Neurology 48:1190–1192

Ng S 1980 Skeletal muscle spasms. American Chiropractic Association Journal 14(23)

Ochs R, Ranish S 1969 Characteristics of fast transport in mammalian nerve fibers. Journal of Neurobiology 1:247

Ochs S 1975 Brief review of material transport in nerve fibers. In: Goldstein M (ed) Research status of spinal manipulative therapy. Monograph 15, HEW/NINCDS, Bethesda

Penning P 1989 Functional anatomy of joints and discs. In: Sherk H H (ed) The cervical spine, 2nd edn. J B Lippincott, Philadelphia, pp 33–56

Powell R 1990 Attributions and self-esteem in depression and chronic fatigue syndromes. Journal of Pyschosomatic Research 14(6):665–671

Ryan G M S, Cope S 1955 Cervical vertigo. Lancet 2:1355–1358

Ryan L 1994 Mechanical instability, muscle strength and proprioception in the functionally unstable ankle. Australian Journal of Physiotherapy 40:41–47

Sato A 1992 Spinal reflex physiology. In: Haldeman S (ed) Principles and practice of chiropractic. Appleton and Lange, East Norwalk

Sandman C 1993 Memory deficits associated with chronic fatigue immune dysfunction syndrome (CFIDS). Biological Psychiatry 33:618–623

Sapolsky R 1990 Hippocampal damage associated with prolonged glucocorticoid exposure in primates. Journal of Neuroscience 10:2897–2902

Schafer R 1987 Clinical biomechanics, 2nd edn. Williams and Wilkins, Baltimore

Schaible H, Grubb B 1993 Afferent and spinal mechanisms of joint pain. Pain 55:5

Schulkin J 1994 Allostasis, amygdala and anticipatory angst. Neuroscience Biobehavioural Review 18(3):385–396

Schwartz J 1980 The transport of substances in nerve cells. Scientific American 243:152

Sherrington C 1907 On reciprocal innervation of antagonistic muscles. Proceedings of Royal Society, London 79(B):337

Simons D, Travell J, Simons L 1998 Myofascial pain and dysfunction: the trigger point manual, vol 1: upper half of body, 2nd edn. Williams and Wilkins, Baltimore

Spencer J 1984 Knee joint effusion and quadriceps reflex inhibition in man. Archives of Physical Medicine and Rehabilitation 65:171

Staubesand J 1996 Zum Feinbau der fascia cruris mit Berucksichtigung epi- und intrafaszialar Nerven. Manuella Medezin 34:196–200

Sterling P, Eyer J 1981 Allostasis: a new paradigm to explain arousal pathology. In: Fisher S, Reason H (eds) Handbook of life stress, cognition and health. John Wiley, New York

Stiles E 1984 Patient care, May

Swerdlow N 1993 Men are more inhibited than women by weak prepulses. Biological Psychiatry 34:253–260

Teicher M 1993 Early childhood abuse and limbic system ratings in adult psychiatric outpatients. Journal of Neuropsychiatry and Clinical Neuroscience 5(3):301–306

Travell J, Simons D 1983 Myofascial pain and dysfunction: the trigger point manual, vol 1: upper half of body. Williams and Wilkins, Baltimore

Travell J, Simons D 1992 Myofascial pain and dysfunction: the trigger point manual, vol 2: the lower extremities. Williams and Wilkins, Baltimore

Wall P D 1989 The dorsal horn. In: Wall P D, Melzack R (eds) Textbook of pain, 2nd edn. Churchill Livingstone, Edinburgh, pp 102–111

Wall P D, Melzack R 1991 Textbook of pain, 3rd edn. Churchill Livingstone, Edinburgh

Walther D 1988 Applied kinesiology. SDC Systems, Pueblo

Willis W 1993 Mechanical allodynia – a role for sensitized nociceptive tract cells with convergent input from mechanoreceptors and nociceptors APS Journal 1:23

Wilson V 1966 Inhibition in the CNS. Scientific American 5:102–106

Wyke B D 1985 Articular neurology and manipulative therapy. In: Glasgow E F, Twomey L T, Scull E R, Kleynhans A M, Idczak R M (eds) Aspects of manipulative therapy. Churchill Livingstone, Edinburgh, pp 72–77

Yunus M 1994 Psychological aspects of fibromyalgia syndrome. In: Masi A (ed) Fibromyalgia and myofascial pain syndromes. Baillière Tindall, London

4

Causes of musculoskeletal dysfunction

The struggle with gravity is a lifelong battle, often complicated by the sheer range of adaptive stresses to which we subject our bodies throughout life. Adaptation and compensation are the processes by which our functions are gradually compromised as we respond to an endless series of demands, ranging from postural repositioning in our work and leisure activities to habitual patterns (such as how we choose to sit, walk, stand or breathe). There are local tissue changes as well as whole body compensations to short- and long-term insults imposed on the body. A summary discussion of the adaptive mechanisms involved, together with a deeper examination of key features in the evolution of musculoskeletal dysfunction, will support an understanding of how the body adapts, how it may be assisted and when it might be appropriate to leave the adaptation alone.

ADAPTATION – GAS AND LAS

When we examine musculoskeletal function and dysfunction we become aware of a system which can become compromised as a result of adaptive demands exceeding its capacity to absorb the load, while attempting to maintain something approaching normal function. Elastic limits may at times be exceeded, resulting in structural and functional modifications. Assessing these dysfunctional patterns – making sense of what can be observed, palpated, demonstrated – allows for detection of causes and guidance toward remedial action.

The demands which lead to dysfunction can either be violent, forceful, single events or they can be the cumulative influence of numerous minor events. Each such event is a form of stress and provides its own load demand on the local area as well as the body as a whole. In order to better understand these processes it is useful to refer back to the principal researcher of this phenomenon, Hans Selye.

Selye (1956) called stress the 'non-specific element' in disease production. He described the *general adaptation syndrome* (GAS) as being composed of three distinct stages:

- the alarm reaction when initial defense responses occur ('fight or flight')
- the resistance (adaptation) phase (which can last for many years, as long as homeostatic – self-regulating – mechanisms can maintain function)
- the exhaustion phase (when adaptation fails) where frank disease emerges.

GAS affects the organism as a whole, while the *local adaptation syndrome* (LAS) goes through the same stages but affects localized areas of the body. For example, imagine the tissue response to digging the garden, chopping wood or playing tennis after a period of relative inactivity – an 'acute adaptive response' would result with accompanying stiffness and aching, followed by resolution of the stress effects after a few days. Imagine the same activity repeated over and over again, in which adaptive ('training') responses would result, leading to chronic tissue responses involving hypertrophy, possible shortening, strengthening and so on. Anyone who regularly trains by running or lifting weights will recognize this sequence. The body, or part of the body, responds to the repetitive stress (running, lifting, etc.) by adapting to the needs imposed on it. It gets stronger or fitter, unless the adaptive demands are excessive, in which case it would ultimately break down or become dysfunctional.

Selye demonstrated that stress results in a pattern of adaptation, individual to each organism. He also showed that when an individual is acutely alarmed, stressed or aroused, homeostatic (self-normalizing) mechanisms are activated. However, if the alarm status is prolonged or if adaptive demands are excessive, long-term, chronic changes occur and these are almost always at the expense of optimal functional integrity.

When assessing or palpating a patient or a dysfunctional area, neuromusculoskeletal changes can often be seen to represent a record of the body's attempts to adapt and adjust to the multiple and varied stresses which have been imposed upon it over time. The results of repeated postural and traumatic insults over a lifetime, combined with the somatic effects of emotional and psychological origin, will often present a confusing pattern of tense, shortened, bunched, fatigued and, ultimately, fibrous tissue (Chaitow 1989).

POSTURE, RESPIRATORY FUNCTION AND THE ADAPTATION PHENOMENON

Some of the many forms of soft tissue stress responses which affect the body include the following (Barlow 1959, Basmajian 1974, Dvorak & Dvorak 1984, Janda 1982, 1983, Korr 1978, Lewit 1985, Travell & Simons 1983, 1992).

1. Congenital and inborn factors, such as short or long leg, small hemipelvis, fascial influences (e.g. cranial distortions involving the reciprocal tension membranes due to birthing difficulties, such as forceps delivery).
2. Overuse, misuse and abuse factors, such as injury or inappropriate or repetitive patterns of use involved in work, sport or regular activities.
3. Immobilization, disuse (irreversible changes can occur after just 8 weeks).
4. Postural stress patterns (see below).
5. Inappropriate breathing patterns (see below).
6. Chronic negative emotional states such as depression, anxiety, etc. (see below).
7. Reflexive influences (trigger points, facilitated spinal regions) (see Chapter 6).

As a result of these influences, which affect each and every one of us to some degree, acute and painful adaptive changes occur, thereby producing the dysfunctional patterns and events on which neuromuscular therapies focus.

When the musculoskeletal system is 'stressed', by these or other means, a sequence of events occurs as follows.

- 'Something' (see list above) occurs which leads to increased muscular tone.
- If this increased tone is anything but short term, retention of metabolic wastes occurs.
- Increased tone simultaneously results in a degree of localized oxygen deficiency (relative to the tissue needs) and the development of ischemia.
- Ischemia is itself not a producer of pain but an ischemic muscle which contracts rapidly does produce pain (Lewis 1942, Liebenson 1996).
- Increased tone might also lead to a degree of edema.
- These factors (retention of wastes/ischemia/edema) all contribute to discomfort or pain.
- Discomfort or pain reinforces hypertonicity.
- Inflammation or, at least, chronic irritation may result.
- Neurological reporting stations in these distressed hypertonic tissues will bombard the CNS with information regarding their status leading, in time, to a degree of sensitization of neural structures and the evolution of facilitation and its accompanying hyperreactivity.
- Macrophages are activated, as is increased vascularity and fibroblastic activity.
- Connective tissue production increases with crosslinkage, leading to shortened fascia.
- Chronic muscular stress (a combination of the load involved and the number of repetitions or the degree of sustained influence) results in the gradual development of hysteresis in which collagen fibers and proteoglycans are rearranged to produce an altered structural pattern.
- This results in tissues which are far more easily fatigued and prone to frank damage, if strained.

- Since all fascia and other connective tissue is continuous throughout the body, any distortions or contractions which develop in one region can potentially create fascial deformations elsewhere, resulting in negative influences on structures which are supported or attached to the fascia, including nerves, muscles, lymph structures and blood vessels.
- Hypertonicity in any muscle will produce inhibition of its antagonist(s) and aberrant behavior in its synergist(s).
- Chain reactions evolve in which some muscles (postural – type I) shorten while others (phasic – type II) weaken.
- Because of sustained increased muscle tension, ischemia in tendinous structures occurs, as it does in localized areas of muscles, leading to the development of periosteal pain.
- Compensatory adaptations evolve, leading to habitual, 'built-in' patterns of use emerging as the CNS learns to compensate for modifications in muscle strength, length and functional behavior (as a result of inhibition, for example).
- Abnormal biomechanics result, involving malcoordination of movement (with antagonistic muscle groups being either hypertonic or weak; for example, erector spinae tightens while rectus abdominis is inhibited and weakens).
- The normal firing sequence of muscles involved in particular movements alters, resulting in additional strain.
- Joint biomechanics are directly influenced by the accumulated influences of such soft tissue changes and can themselves become significant sources of referred and local pain, reinforcing soft tissue dysfunctional patterns (Schaible & Grubb 1993).
- Deconditioning of the soft tissues becomes progressive as a result of the combination of simultaneous events involved in soft tissue pain, 'spasm' (hypertonic guarding), joint stiffness, antagonist weakness, overactive synergists, etc.
- Progressive evolution of localized areas of hyperreactivity of neural structures occurs (facilitated areas) in paraspinal regions or within muscles (myofascial trigger points).
- In the region of these trigger points (see discussion of myofascial triggers on p. 65) a great deal of increased neurological activity occurs (for which there is EMG evidence) which is capable of influencing distant tissues adversely (Hubbard 1993, Simons 1993).
- Energy wastage due to unnecessarily sustained hypertonicity and excessively active musculature leads to generalized fatigue as well as to a local 'energy crisis' in the local tissues (see trigger point discussion on p. 65).
- More widespread functional changes develop – for example, affecting respiratory function and body posture – with repercussions on the total economy of the body.
- In the presence of a constant neurological feedback of impulses to the CNS/brain from neural reporting stations, indicating heightened arousal (a hypertonic muscle status is part of the alarm reaction of the flight/fight alarm response), there will be increased levels of psychological arousal and a reduction in the ability of the individual, or the local hypertonic tissues, to relax effectively, with consequent reinforcement of hypertonicity.
- Functional patterns of use of a biologically unsustainable nature will emerge, probably involving chronic musculoskeletal problems and pain.
- At this stage, restoration of normal function requires therapeutic input which addresses both the multiple changes which have occurred and the need for a reeducation of the individual as to how to use their body, to breathe and to carry themselves in more sustainable ways.
- The chronic adaptive changes which develop in such a scenario lead to the increased likelihood of future acute exacerbations as the increasingly chronic, less supple and resilient, biomechanical structures attempt to cope with additional stress factors resulting from the normal demands of modern living.

MAKING SENSE OF THE PICTURE

In the broader discussion below, attention will be given to three core elements – musculoskeletal stress resulting from postural, emotional and respiratory causes. These three factors interface with each other and reinforce any resulting dysfunctions. As will become clear in these descriptions, there is a constant merging and mixing of fundamental influences on health and ill health. In trying to make sense of a patient's problems, it is frequently clinically valuable to cluster etiological factors. One model which the authors find useful divides negative influences into:

- biomechanical (congenital, overuse, misuse, trauma, disuse, etc.)
- biochemical (toxicity, endocrine imbalance, nutritional deficiency, ischemia, inflammation)
- psychosocial (anxiety, depression, unresolved emotional states, somatization, etc.).

The usefulness of this approach is that it allows a focus to be brought to factors which are amenable to change via (for example):

- manual methods, rehabilitation, reeducation and exercise, which influence biomechanical factors

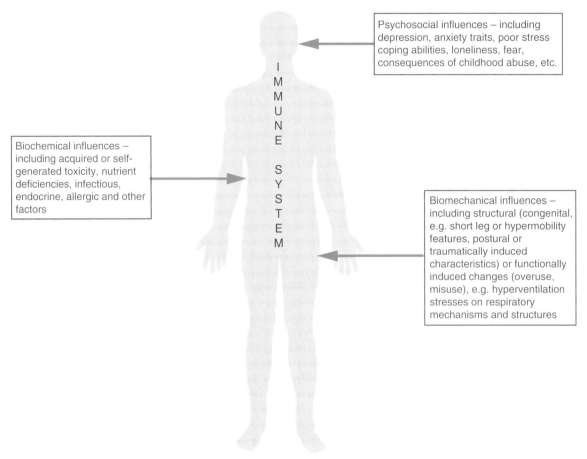

Psychosocial influences – including depression, anxiety traits, poor stress coping abilities, loneliness, fear, consequences of childhood abuse, etc.

Biochemical influences – including acquired or self-generated toxicity, nutrient deficiencies, infectious, endocrine, allergic and other factors

Biomechanical influences – including structural (congenital, e.g. short leg or hypermobility features, postural or traumatically induced characteristics) or functionally induced changes (overuse, misuse), e.g. hyperventilation stresses on respiratory mechanisms and structures

The interacting influences of a biochemical, biomechanical and psychosocial nature do not produce single changes. For example:
- a negative emotional state (e.g. depression) produces specific biochemical changes, impairs immune function and leads to altered muscle tone.
- hyperventilation modifies blood acidity, alters neural reporting (initially hyper and then hypo), creates feelings of anxiety/apprehension and directly impacts on the structural components of the thoracic and cervical region – muscles and joints.
- altered chemistry affects mood; altered mood changes blood chemistry; altered structure (posture for example) modifies function and therefore impacts on chemistry (e.g. liver function) and potentially on mood.

Within these categories – biochemical, biomechanical and psychosocial – are to be found most major influences on health.

Figure 4.1 Biochemical, biomechanical and psychosocial influences on health (reproduced, with permission, from Chaitow (1999)).

- nutritional or pharmaceutical tactics which modify biochemical influences, and
- psychological approaches which deal with psychosocial influences.

In truth, the overlap between these causative categories is so great that in many cases interventions can be randomly selected since, if effective, all will (to some degree) modify the adaptation demands or enhance self-regulatory functions sufficiently for benefit to be noted.

Example

Consider someone who is habitually breathing in an upper chest mode, the stress of which will place adaptive demands on the accessory breathing muscles, with consequent stiffness, pain, trigger point activity (particularly in the scalenes) and joint involvement. This individual will probably display evidence of anxiety (see below) as a direct result of the CO_2 imbalance caused by this breathing pattern or might possibly be breathing in this way because of a predisposing anxiety (Timmons 1994).

- Interventions which reduce anxiety will help all associated symptoms and these could involve biochemical modification (herbs, drugs), stress coping approaches or psychotherapy.
- Interventions which improve breathing function, probably involving easing of soft tissue distress (including deactivation of trigger points) and/or

joint restrictions, as well as breathing retraining should also help to reduce the symptoms.

The most appropriate approach will be the one which most closely deals with causes rather than effects and which allows for long-term changes which will reduce the likelihood of recurrence. Biochemistry, biomechanics and the mind are seen in this example to be inextricably melded to each other. In other examples, etiological influences may not always be seen to be as clearly defined; however, they will almost always impact on each other.

The theme of respiratory influence on musculoskeletal dysfunction will be explored further later in this chapter. Before that, a summary of postural and emotional influences will prepare us for a more comprehensive understanding of one of the most important body processes – respiration.

POSTURAL AND EMOTIONAL INFLUENCES ON MUSCULOSKELETAL DYSFUNCTION

An insightful Charlie Brown cartoon depicts him standing in a pronounced stooping posture, while he philosophizes to Lucy that it is only possible to get the most out of being depressed if you stand this way. Standing up straight, he asserts, removes all sense of being depressed.

Once again, as in the breathing dysfunction example above, we can see how emotions and biomechanics are closely linked. Anything which relieved the depressed state would almost certainly result in a change of body language and, if Charlie is correct, standing tall should impact (to some extent at least) on his state of mind.

Australian-based British osteopath Philip Latey (1996) has found a useful metaphor to describe observable and palpable patterns of distortion which coincide with particular clinical problems. He uses the analogy of 'clenched fists' because, he says, the unclenching of a fist correlates with physiological relaxation while the clenched fist indicates fixity, rigidity, overcontracted muscles, emotional turmoil, withdrawal from communication and so on.

Latey states:

The 'lower fist' is centered entirely on pelvic function. When I describe the 'upper fist' I will include the head, neck, shoulders and arms with the upper chest, throat and jaw. The 'middle fist' will be focused mainly on the lower chest and upper abdomen.

We find Latey's manner of describing the emotional background to physical responses a meaningful vehicle with which to accompany more mechanistic interpretations of what may be happening in any given dysfunctional pattern. Below is a brief discussion of his work insofar as this relates to the main theme of this book.

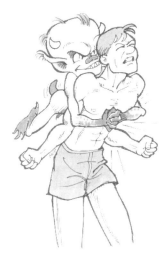

Figure 4.2 Cartoon showing Latey's 'middle fist' concept (reproduced, with permission, from the *Journal of Bodywork and Movement Therapies* 1996; **1**(1):50).

Postural interpretations

Latey describes the patient entering the consulting room as displaying an *image posture*, which is the impression the patient subconsciously wishes you to see.

If the patient is requested to relax as far as possible, the next image noted is that of *slump posture*, in which gravity acts on the body as it responds according to its unique attributes, tensions and weakness. Here it is common to observe overactive muscle groups coming into operation – hands, feet, jaw and facial muscle may writhe and clench or twitch.

Finally, when the patient lies down and relaxes we come to the deeper image, the *residual posture*. Here are to be found the tensions the patient cannot release. These are palpable and, says Latey, leaving aside sweat, skin and circulation, represent the deepest 'layer of the onion' available to examination.

Contraction patterns

What is seen varies from person to person according to their state of mind and well-being. Apparent is a record or psychophysical pattern of the patient's responses, actions, transactions and interactions with his or her environment. The patterns of contraction which are observed and palpated often have a direct relationship with the patient's unconscious and provide a reliable avenue for discovery and treatment.

One of Latey's concepts involves a mechanism which leads to muscular contraction as a means of disguising a sensory barrage resulting from an emotional state. Thus Latey describes:

- a sensation which might arise from the pit of the stomach being hidden, masked, by contraction of the muscles attached to the lower ribs, upper abdomen and the junction between the chest and lower spine

- genital and anal sensations which might be drowned out by contraction of hip, leg and low back musculature
- throat sensations which might be concealed with contraction of the shoulder girdle, neck, arms and hands.

Emotional contractions

A restrained expression of emotion itself results in suppression of activity and, ultimately, chronic contraction of the muscles which would be used were these emotions to be expressed (as rage, fear, anger, joy, frustration, sorrow or anything else). Latey points out that all areas of the body producing sensations which arouse emotional excitement may have their blood supply reduced by muscular contraction. Also sphincters and hollow organs can be held tight until numb. He gives as examples the muscles which surround the genitals and anus as well as the mouth, nose, throat, lungs, stomach and bowel.

When considering the 'middle fist', Latey concentrates his attention on respiratory and diaphragm function and the many emotional inputs which affect this region. He discounts as a popular misconception the idea that breathing is produced by contraction of the diaphragm and the muscles which raise the rib cage, with exhalation being but a relaxation of these muscles. He states: 'The even flow of easy breathing should be produced by dynamic interaction of … two sets of muscles'.

The active exhalation phase of breathing is instigated, he suggests, by the following muscles.

1. Transversus thoracis which lies inside the front of the chest and attaches to the back of the sternum, while fanning out inside the rib cage and then continuing to the lower ribs where the fibers separate. This forms an inverted 'V' below the chest. This muscle, Latey says, has direct intrinsic abilities to generate all manner of uniquely powerful sensations, with even light contact sometimes producing reflex contractions of the whole body or of the abdomen or chest. Feelings of nausea and choking and all types of anxiety, fear, anger, laughter, sadness, weeping and other emotions may be displayed. He discounts the idea that the muscle's sensitivity is related to the 'solar plexus', suggesting that its closeness to the internal thoracic artery is probably more significant since when it is contracted, it can exert direct pressure on the artery. He believes that physiological breathing has, as its central event, a rhythmical relaxation and contraction of this muscle. Rigidity is often seen in the patient with 'middle fist' problems, where 'control' dampens the emotions which relate to it.

2. The other main exhalation muscle is serratus posterior inferior which runs from the lower thoracic and upper lumbar spine and fans upwards and outwards over the lower ribs, which it grasps from behind to pull them down and inwards on exhalation. These two muscles mirror each other and work together. Latey states that it is common to find a static overcontracture of serratus posterior inferior, with the underlying back muscles in a state of fibrous shortening and degeneration, reflecting 'the fixity of the transversus, and the extent of the emotional blockage.'

'Middle fist' functions

Latey reports that laughing, weeping and vomiting are three emotional 'safety valve' functions of 'middle fist' function, used by the body to help resolve internal imbalance. Anything stored internally which cannot be contained emerges explosively via this route. In laughing and weeping, there is a definite rhythm of contraction/relaxation of transversus whereas, in vomiting, it remains in total contraction throughout each eliminative wave. Between waves of vomiting the breathing remains in the inspiratory phase, with upper chest panting. Transversus is slack in this phase. Latey suggests that often it is only muscle fatigue which breaks cycles of laughter/weeping/vomiting.

The clinical problems associated with 'middle fist' dysfunction relate to distortions of blood vessels, internal organs, autonomic nervous system involvement and alteration in the neuroendocrine balance. Diarrhea, constipation and colitis may be involved but more direct results relate to lung and stomach problems. Thus, bronchial asthma is an obvious example of 'middle fist' fixation.

There is a typical, associated posture with the shoulder girdle raised and expanded as if any letting go would precipitate a crisis. Compensatory changes usually include very taut, deep neck and shoulder muscles (see Janda's upper crossed syndrome description, discussed in Chapter 5) (Janda 1983).

In treating such a problem, Latey starts by encouraging function of the 'middle fist' itself, then extending into the neck and shoulder muscles, while encouraging them to relax and drop. He then goes back to the 'middle fist'. Dramatic expressions of alarm, unease and panic may be seen. The patient, on discussing what they feel, might report sensations of being smothered, drowned, choked, engulfed or crushed.

'Upper fist' functions

The 'upper fist' involves muscles which extend from the thorax to the back of the head, where the skull and spine join, and extends sideways to include the muscles of the shoulder girdle. These muscles therefore set the relative positions of the head, neck, jaw, shoulders and upper chest and, to a large extent, the rest of the body follows this lead (it was F.M. Alexander (1932) who showed that the head–neck relationship is the primary postural control mechanism). This region, says Latey, is 'the center, *par excellence*, of anxieties, tensions and other amorphous expressions of unease'.

In chronic states of disturbed 'upper fist' function, he asserts, the main physical impression is one of a restrained, overcontrolled, damped down expression. The feeling of the muscles is that they are controlling an 'explosion of affect'. Those experiences which are not allowed free play on the face are expressed in the muscles of the skull and the base of the skull. This is, he believes, of central importance in problems of headache, especially migraine. Says Latey, 'I have never seen a migraine sufferer who has not lost complete ranges of facial expression, at least temporarily'.

Effects of 'upper fist' patterns

The mechanical consequences of 'upper fist' fixations are many and varied, ranging from stiff neck to compression factors leading to disc degeneration and facet wear. Swallowing and speech difficulties are common, as are shoulder dysfunctions including brachial neuritis, Reynaud's syndrome and carpal tunnel problems. Latey states:

The medical significance of 'upper fist' contracture is mainly circulatory. Just as 'lower fist' contraction contributes to circulatory stasis in the legs, pelvis, perineum and lower abdomen, so may 'upper fist' contracture have an even more profound effect. The blood supply to the head, face, special senses, the mucosa of the nose, mouth, upper respiratory tract, the heart itself and the main blood vessels are controlled by the sympathetic nervous system and its main 'junction boxes' (ganglia) lie just to the front of the vertebrae at the base of the neck.

Thus, headaches, eye pain, ear problems, nose and throat as well as many cardiovascular troubles may contain strong mechanical elements relating to 'upper fist' muscle contractions. He reminds us that it is not uncommon for cardiovascular problems to manifest at the same time as chronic muscular shoulder pain (such as avascular necrosis of the rotator cuff tendons) and that the longus colli muscles are often centrally involved in such states.

He looks to the nose, mouth, lips, tongue, teeth, jaws and throat for evidence of functional change related to 'upper fist' dysfunction, with relatively simple psychosomatic disturbances underlying these. Sniffing, sucking, biting, chewing, tearing, swallowing, gulping, spitting, dribbling, burping, vomiting, sound making and so on are all significant functions which might be disturbed acutely or chronically. These patterns of use can all be approached via breathing function.

When all the components of the 'upper fist' are relaxed, the act of expiration produces a noticeable rhythmical movement. The neck lengthens, the jaw rises slightly (rocking the whole head), the face fills out, the upper chest drops. When the patient is in difficulty I may try to encourage these movements by manual work on the muscles and gentle direction to assist relaxed expiration. Again, by asking the patient to let go and let feelings happen, I encourage resolution. Specific elements often emerge quite readily, especially those mentioned with the 'middle fist', the need to vomit, cry, scream, etc.

Note: More detail of Latey's perspective regarding 'lower fist' function is presented in Volume 2 of this book which deals with the lower body.

Cautions and questions

There is (justifiably) intense debate regarding the question of the intentional induction of 'emotional release' in clinical settings in which the therapist is relatively untrained in psychotherapy.

- If the most appropriate response an individual can currently make to the turmoil of their life is the 'locking away' of the resulting emotions into their musculoskeletal system, what is the advisability of unlocking the emotions which the tensions and contractions hold?
- If there exists no current ability to mentally process the pain that these somatic areas are holding, are they not best left where they are until counseling or psychotherapy or self-awareness leads to the individual's ability to reflect, handle, deal with and eventually work through the issues and memories?
- What are the advantages of triggering a release of emotions, manifested by crying, laughing, vomiting or whatever – as described by Latey and others – if neither the individual nor the therapist can then take the process further?
- In the experience of one of the authors (LC) there are indeed patients whose musculoskeletal and other symptoms are patently linked to devastating life events (torture, abuse, witness to genocide, refugee status and so on) to the extent that extreme caution is called for in addressing their obvious symptoms for the reasons suggested above. What would emerge from a 'release'? How would they handle it? The truth is that there are many examples in modern times of people whose symptoms represent the end result of appalling social conditions and life experiences. Their healing may require a changed life (often impossible to envisage) or many years of work with psychological rehabilitation and not interventions which address apparent symptoms, which may be the merest tips of large icebergs.

The contradictory perspective to these questions suggests that there would not be a 'spontaneous' release of 'emotional baggage' unless the person was able to intellectually and emotionally handle whatever emerged from the process. This is indeed a debate without obvious resolution. The authors feel it worthy of exposure in this context but cannot offer definitive answers. These questions are intended to be thought provoking and it is suggested that each patient and each therapist/practitioner should reflect on these issues before removing (however gently and however temporarily) the defensive armoring that life may have obliged vulnerable individuals (almost all of us at one time or another) to erect and maintain. It may be that, in some circumstances, an individual's 'physical tensions' may be all that are preventing them from fragmenting emotionally.

At the very least we should all learn skills which allow the safe handling of 'emotional releases', which may occur with or without deliberate efforts to induce them. And we should have a referral process in place to direct the person for further professional help.

As a first-aid approach, should such an event occur during or following treatment, emphasis should be on initiating calm and this may best be achieved through slow breathing, focusing on the outbreath. The patient should be allowed to talk if they wish but, unless adequately trained, the therapist should avoid any attempt to advise or to try to 'sort out' the patient's problems. The focus should be on helping them through the crisis before offering an appropriate referral.

POSTURAL IMBALANCE AND THE DIAPHRAGM (Goldthwaite 1945)

Goldthwaite, in his classic 1930s discussion of posture, links a wide array of health problems with the absence of balanced posture. Clearly, some of what he hypothesized remains conjecture but we can see just how much impact postural stress can have on associated tissues, starting with diaphragmatic weakness.

The main factors which determine the maintenance of the abdominal viscera in position are the diaphragm and the abdominal muscles, both of which are relaxed and cease to support in faulty posture. The disturbances of circulation resulting from a low diaphragm and ptosis may give rise to chronic passive congestion in one or all of the organs of the abdomen and pelvis, since the local as well as general venous drainage may be impeded by the failure of the diaphragmatic pump to do its full work in the drooped body. Furthermore, the drag of these congested organs on their nerve supply, as well as the pressure on the sympathetic ganglia and plexuses, probably causes many irregularities in their function, varying from partial paralysis to overstimulation. All these organs receive fibers from both the vagus and sympathetic systems, either one of which may be disturbed. It is probable that one or all of these factors are active at various times in both the stocky and the slender anatomic types, and are responsible for many functional digestive disturbances. These disturbances, if continued long enough, may lead to diseases later in life. Faulty body mechanics in early life, then, becomes a vital factor in the production of the vicious cycle of chronic diseases and presents a chief point of attack in its prevention ... In this upright position, as one becomes older, the tendency is for the abdomen to relax and sag more and more,

allowing a ptosic condition of the abdominal and pelvic organs unless the supporting lower abdominal muscles are taught to contract properly. As the abdomen relaxes, there is a great tendency towards a drooped chest, with narrow rib angle, forward shoulders, prominent shoulder blades, a forward position of the head, and probably pronated feet. When the human machine is out of balance, physiological function cannot be perfect; muscles and ligaments are in an abnormal state of tension and strain. A well-poised body means a machine working perfectly, with the least amount of muscular effort, and therefore better health and strength for daily life.

Note how closely Goldthwaite mirrors the picture Janda paints in his upper and lower crossed syndrome and 'posture and facial pain' descriptions (see Chapter 5, p. 55).

RESPIRATORY INFLUENCES

In modern inner cities in particular and late 20th-century existence in general, there exists a vast expression of respiratory imbalance ('paradoxical breathing'). Breathing dysfunction is seen to be at least an associated factor in most chronically fatigued and anxious people and almost all people subject to panic attacks and phobic behavior, many of whom also display multiple musculoskeletal symptoms.

As a tendency towards upper chest breathing becomes more pronounced, biochemical imbalances occur when excessive amounts of carbon dioxide (CO_2) are exhaled leading to relative alkalosis, which automatically produces a sense of apprehension and anxiety. This condition frequently leads to panic attacks and phobic behavior, from which recovery is possible only when breathing is normalized (King 1988, Lum 1981).

Since carbon dioxide is one of the major regulators of cerebral vascular tone, any reduction due to hyperventilation patterns leads to vasoconstriction and cerebral oxygen deficiency. Whatever oxygen there is in the bloodstream then has a tendency to become more tightly bound to its hemoglobin carrier molecule, leading to decreased oxygenation of tissues. All this is accompanied by a decreased threshold of peripheral nerve firing.

Summary of effects of hyperventilation

- Reduction in PCO_2 (tension or partial pressure of carbon dioxide) causes respiratory alkalosis via reduction in arterial carbonic acid, which leads to abnormally decreased arterial carbon dioxide tension (hypocapnia) and major systemic repercussions (see Figs 4.2 and 4.3).
- The first and most direct response to hyperventilation is cerebral vascular constriction, reducing oxygen availability by about 50%.
- Of all body tissues, the cerebral cortex is the most vulnerable to hypoxia which depresses cortical activity

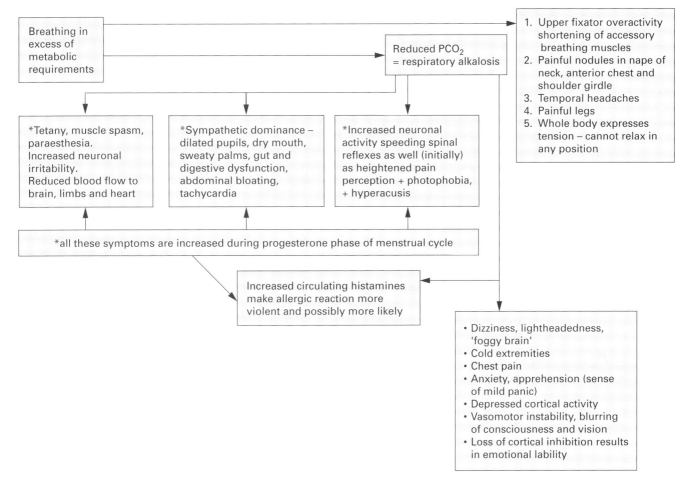

Figure 4.3 Negative health influences of a dysfunctional breathing pattern such as hyperventilation.

Box 4.1 Partial pressure symbols

Partial pressure was formerly symbolized by p, followed by the chemical symbol in capital letters (e.g. pCO$_2$, pO$_2$). Currently, in respiratory physiology, P, followed by subscripts, denotes location and/or chemical species (e.g. PCO$_2$, PO$_2$, PO$_2$, PACO$_2$).

PCO$_2$ = partial pressure of carbon dioxide
PO$_2$ = partial pressure of oxygen
PACO$_2$ = arterial carbon dioxide tension (where A = arterial)

Box 4.2 Hyperventilation in context

The simplest definition of hyperventilation is that it represents a pattern of (over)breathing which is in excess of metabolic requirements. It is normal to hyperventilate ('puffing and panting') in association with physical exertion such as running or if there exists a heightened degree of acid in the bloodstream (acidosis), possibly a result of kidney or liver disease. In these examples the rapid breathing pattern produces a reduction in acidity via exhalation of CO$_2$ and is therefore seen to be helping to restore normal acid – alkaline balance (pH 7.4).

It is when a pattern of overbreathing occurs without an associated acidosis that problems arise, as this leads to alkalosis and all the symptoms which flow from that state (see main text for details).

There are many individuals whose blood gas profile would not categorize them as having reached a state of true hyperventilation, but who are clearly progressing towards that state. It is such individuals who often display many of the early signs of chronic unwellness, ranging from fatigue to chronic muscular pains and loss of concentration. These individuals may well benefit from a combination of stress management, musculoskeletal normalization and breathing retraining approaches.

---

and causes dizziness, vasomotor instability, blurred consciousness ('foggy brain') and visual disturbances.

● Loss of cortical inhibition results in emotional lability.

Neural repercussions

● Loss of CO$_2$ ions from neurons during moderate hyperventilation stimulates neuronal activity, while producing muscular tension and spasm, speeding spinal reflexes as well as producing heightened perception (pain, photophobia, hyperacusis) – all of which are of major importance in chronic pain conditions.

● When hypocapnia is more severe or prolonged it depresses neural activity until the nerve cell becomes inert.

• What seems to occur in advanced or extreme hyperventilation is a change in neuronal metabolism; anaerobic glycolysis produces lactic acid in nerve cells, while lowering pH. Neuronal activity is then diminished so that in extreme hypocapnia (reduced levels of CO_2), neurons become inert. Thus, in the extremes of this clinical condition, initial hyperactivity gives way to exhaustion, stupor and coma (Lum 1981).

Tetany

According to *Stedman's medical dictionary* (1998) tetany is characterized by muscle twitches, cramps and cramping of the hands and feet and, if severe, may include laryngospasm and seizures. These findings reflect irritability of the central and peripheral nervous systems, which may result from low serum levels of ionized calcium or, rarely, magnesium. A reduced degree of CO_2 resulting in excessive alkalinity can also produce this effect.

In tetany which is secondary to alkalosis (excessive alkalinity), muscles which maintain 'attack-defense' mode (hunched shoulders, jutting head, clenched teeth, scowling) are those most likely to be affected and these are also common sites for active myofascial trigger points (Timmons 1994).

• Painful muscular contractions ('nodules') develop and are easily felt in the nape of the neck, anterior chest and shoulder girdle.
• Temporal headaches centered on painful nodules in the parietal region are common.
• Sympathetic dominance is evident by virtue of dilated pupils, dry mouth, sweaty palms, gut and digestive dysfunction, abdominal bloating and tachycardia.
• Allergies and food intolerances are common due to increased circulating histamines.

Biomechanical changes in response to upper chest breathing

Whereas Goldthwaite (1945), Janda (1982) and others point to the collapse of normal posture leading inevitably to changes which preclude normal breathing function, Garland (1994) presents the picture in reverse, suggesting that it is the functional change of inappropriate breathing (e.g. hyperventilation or upper chest patterns of breathing) which ultimately modifies structure. It was Garland who coined the memorable phrase 'where psychology overwhelms physiology' to describe the changes which occur.

Garland describes the somatic changes which follow from a pattern of hyperventilation and upper chest breathing.

• A degree of visceral stasis and pelvic floor weakness will develop, as will an imbalance between increasingly weak abdominal muscles and increasingly tight erector spinae muscles.
• Fascial restriction from the central tendon via the pericardial fascia, all the way up to the basiocciput, will be noted.
• The upper ribs will be elevated and there will be sensitive costal cartilage tension.
• The thoracic spine will be disturbed by virtue of the lack of normal motion of the articulation with the ribs and sympathetic outflow from this area may be affected.
• Accessory muscle hypertonia, notably affecting the scalenes, upper trapezius and levator scapulae, will be palpable and observable.
• Fibrosis will develop in these muscles as will myofascial trigger points (see p. 65).
• The cervical spine will become progressively more rigid with a fixed lordosis being a common feature in the lower cervical spine.
• A reduction in the mobility of the 2nd cervical segment and disturbance of vagal outflow from this region are likely.
• Although not noted in Garland's list of dysfunctions, the other changes which Janda has listed in his upper crossed syndrome (see p. 55) are likely consequences, including the potentially devastating effects on shoulder function of the altered position of the scapulae and glenoid fossae as this pattern evolves.
• Also worth noting in relation to breathing function and dysfunction are the likely effects on two important muscles, not included in Garland's description of the dysfunctions resulting from inappropriate breathing patterns, quadratus lumborum and iliopsoas, both of which merge fibers with the diaphragm.
• Since these are both postural muscles, with a propensity to shortening when stressed, the impact of such shortening, uni- or bilaterally, can be seen to have major implications for respiratory function, whether the primary feature of such a dysfunction lies in diaphragmatic or muscular distress.
• Among possible stress factors which will result in shortening of postural muscles is disuse. When upper chest breathing has replaced diaphragmatic breathing as the norm, reduced diaphragmatic excursion results and consequent reduction in activity for those aspects of quadratus lumborum and psoas which are integral with it. Shortening (of any of these) would likely be a result of this disuse pattern.

Garland concludes his listing of somatic changes associated with hyperventilation: 'Physically and physiologically [all of] this runs against a biologically sustainable pattern, and in a vicious cycle, abnormal function (use) alters normal structure, which disallows return to normal function'.

Garland also suggests that counseling (for associated

anxiety or depression, perhaps) and breathing retraining are far more likely to be successfully initiated if the biomechanical component(s), as outlined, are appropriately treated.

Pioneer osteopathic physician Carl McConnell (1962) reminds us of wider implications of respiratory dysfunction.

Remember that the functional status of the diaphragm is probably the most powerful mechanism of the whole body. It not only mechanically engages the tissues of the pharynx to the perineum, several times per minute, but is physiologically indispensable to the activity of every cell in the body. A working knowledge of the crura, tendon, and the extensive ramification of the diaphragmatic tissues, graphically depicts the significance of structural continuity and functional unity. The wealth of soft tissue work centering in the powerful mechanism is beyond compute, and clinically it is very practical'.

ADDITIONAL EMOTIONAL FACTORS AND MUSCULOSKELETAL DYSFUNCTION

• Use of electromyographic techniques has shown a statistical correlation between unconscious hostility and arm tension as well as leg muscle tension and sexual disturbances (Malmo 1949).

• Sainsbury (1954) showed that when 'neurotic' patients complained of feeling tension in the scalp muscles, there was electromyographic evidence of scalp muscle tension.

• Wolff (1948) proved that the majority of patients with headache showed 'marked contraction in the muscles of the neck … most commonly due to sustained contractions associated with emotional strain, dissatisfaction, apprehension and anxiety'.

• Barlow (1959) sums up the emotion/muscle connection thus: *'muscle is not only the vehicle of speech and expressive gesture, but has at least a finger in a number of other emotional pies – for example, breathing regulation, control of excretion, sexual functioning and, above all, an influence on the body schema through proprioception. Not only are emotional attitudes, say, of fear and aggression, mirrored immediately in the muscle, but also such moods as depression, excitement and evasion have their characteristic muscular patterns and postures'.*

SELECTIVE MOTOR UNIT INVOLVEMENT
(Waersted et al 1992, 1993)

The effect of psychogenic influences on muscles may be more complex than a simplistic 'whole' muscle or regional involvement. Researchers at the National Institute of Occupational Health in Oslo, Norway, have demonstrated that a small number of motor units in particular muscles may display almost constant, or repeated, activity when influenced psychogenically. In their study normal individuals performing reaction time tasks were evaluated, creating a 'time pressure' anxiety. Using the trapezius muscle as the focus of attention, the researchers were able to demonstrate low-amplitude levels of activity (using surface EMG) even when the muscle was not being employed. They explain this phenomenon as follows.

In spite of low total activity level of the muscle, a small pool of low-threshold motor units may be under considerable load for prolonged periods of time. Such a recruitment pattern would be in agreement with the 'size principle' first proposed by Henneman (1957), saying that motor units are recruited according to their size. Motor units with type I [postural] fibers are predominant among the small, low-threshold units. If tension-provoking factors [anxiety, for example] are frequently present and the subject, as a result, repeatedly recruits the same motor units, the hypothesized overload may follow, possibly resulting in a metabolic crisis and the appearance of type I fibers with abnormally large diameters, or 'ragged-red' fibers, which are interpreted as a sign of mitochondrial overload. (Edwards 1988, Larsson et al 1990)

The researchers report that similar observations have been noted in a pilot study (Waersted et al 1992).

The implications of this information are profound since they suggest that emotional stress can selectively involve postural fibers of muscles, which shorten over time when stressed (Janda 1983). The possible 'metabolic crisis' suggested by this research has strong parallels with the evolution of myofascial trigger points as suggested by Simons, a topic which will be discussed in greater detail in later chapters (Wolfe & Simons 1992).

CONCLUSION

We have observed in this chapter evidence of the negative influence on the biomechanical components of the body, the muscles, joints, etc. of overuse, misuse, abuse and disuse, whether of a mechanical (posture) or psychological (depression, anxiety, etc.) nature. We have also seen the interaction of biomechanics and biochemistry in such processes, with breathing dysfunction as a key example of this. In the next chapter we will explore some of the patterns which emerge as dysfunction progresses.

REFERENCES

Alexander F M 1932 The use of the self. E P Dutton, London
Barlow W 1959 Anxiety and muscle tension pain. British Journal of Clinical Practice 13(5):
Basmajian J 1974 Muscles alive. Williams and Wilkins, Baltimore

Brostoff J 1992 Complete guide to food allergy. Bloomsbury, London
Chaitow L 1989 Soft tissue manipulation. Thorsons, London
Chaitow L 1999 Fibromalgia Syndrome. Churchill Livingstone, Edinburgh

Dvorak J, Dvorak V 1984 Manual medicine – diagnostics. Georg Thieme Verlag, Stuttgart

Edwards R 1988 Hypotheses of peripheral and central mechanisms underlying occupational muscle pain and injury. European Journal of Applied Physiology 57:275–281

Garland W 1994 Somatic changes in the hyperventilating subject. Presentation to the Respiratory Function Congress, Paris

Goldthwaite J 1945 Essentials of body mechanics. Lippincott, Philadelphia

Henneman E 1957 Relation between size of neurons and their susceptibility to discharge. Science 126:1345–1347

Hubbard D 1993 Myofascial trigger points show spontaneous EMG activity. Spine 18:1803

Janda V 1982 Introduction to functional pathology of the motor system. Proceedings of the VII Commonwealth and International Conference on Sport. Physiotherapy in Sport 3:39

Janda V 1983 Muscle function testing. Butterworths, London

King J 1988 Hyperventilation – a therapist's point of view. Journal of the Royal Society of Medicine 81:532–536

Korr I M 1978 Neurologic mechanisms in manipulative therapy. Plenum Press, New York, p 27

Larsson S-E et al 1990 Chronic trapezius myalgia – morphology and blood flow studied in 17 patients. Acta Orthopaedica Scandinavica 61:394–398

Latey P 1996 Feelings, muscles and movement. Journal of Bodywork and Movement Therapies 1(1):44–52

Lewis T 1942 Pain. Macmillan, New York

Lewit K 1985 Manipulation in rehabilitation of the locomotor system. Butterworths, London

Liebenson C 1996 Rehabilitation of the spine. Williams and Wilkins, Baltimore

Lum L 1981 Hyperventilation – an anxiety state. Journal of the Royal Society of Medicine 74:1–4

Malmo R 1949 Psychosomatic Medicine 2:9

McConnell C 1962 Yearbook. Osteopathic Institute of Applied Technique, Boulder, Colorado, pp 75–78

Sainsbury 1954 Journal of Neurology, Neurosurgery and Psychiatry 17:3

Schiable H, Grubb B 1993 Afferent and spinal mechanisms of joint pain. Pain 55:5

Selye H 1956 The stress of life. McGraw Hill, New York

Simons D 1993 Referred phenomena of myofascial trigger points. In: Vecchiet L (ed) New trends in referred pain and hyperalgesia. Elsevier, Amsterdam

Stedman's Electronic Dictionary 1998, version 4.0. Williams and Wilkins, Baltimore

Timmons B 1994 Behavioral and psychological approaches to breathing disorders. Plenum Press, New York

Travell J, Simons D 1983 Myofascial pain and dysfunction: the trigger point manual, vol 1: upper half of body. Williams and Wilkins, Baltimore

Travell J, Simons D 1992 Myofascial pain and dysfunction: the trigger point manual, vol 2: the lower extremities. Williams and Wilkins, Baltimore

Waersted M, Eken T, Westgaard R 1992 Single motor unit activity in psychogenic trapezius muscle tension. Arbete och Halsa 17:319–321

Waersted M, Eken T, Westgaard R 1993 Psychogenic motor unit activity – a possible muscle injury mechanism studied in a healthy subject. Journal of Musculoskeletal Pain 1(3/4): 185–190

Wolfe F, Simons D 1992 Fibromyalgia and myofascial pain syndromes. Journal of Rheumatology 19(6): 944–951

Wolff H G 1948 Headache and other head pain. Oxford University Press, Oxford

5

Patterns of dysfunction

We have seen something of the interconnectedness of the structures of the body in Myers' fascial network model. As a consequence of the imposition of sustained or acute stresses, adaptation takes place in the musculoskeletal system and chain reactions of dysfunction emerge. These can be extremely useful indicators of the way adaptation has occurred and can often be 'read' by the clinician in order to help establish a therapeutic plan of action.

When a chain reaction develops, in which some muscles shorten (postural type 1) and others weaken (phasic type 2), predictable patterns involving imbalances emerge. Czech researcher Vladimir Janda MD (1982, 1983) describes two of these, *the upper and lower crossed syndromes*, as follows.

UPPER CROSSED SYNDROME (Fig. 5.1)

The upper crossed syndrome involves the following basic imbalance.

Pectoralis major and minor
Upper trapezius   which all tighten and
Levator scapulae   shorten
Sternomastoid
while
Lower and middle trapezius   } all weaken
Serratus anterior and rhomboids

As these changes take place they alter the relative positions of the head, neck and shoulders as follows.

1. The occiput and C1 and C2 will hyperextend, with the head being translated anteriorly. There will be weakness of the deep neck flexors and increased tone in the suboccipital musculature.
2. The lower cervicals down to the 4th thoracic vertebrae will be posturally stressed as a result.
3. Rotation and abduction of the scapulae occur as the increased tone in the upper fixators of the shoulder (upper trapezius and levator scapulae, for example) causes then to become stressed and shorten,

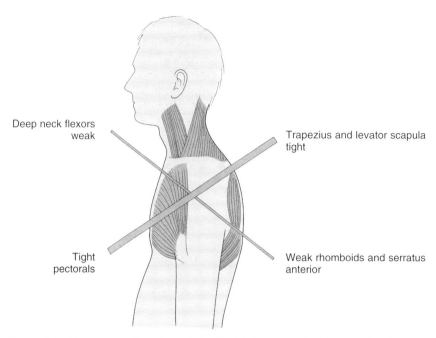

Figure 5.1 Upper crossed syndrome (after Janda) (reproduced, with permission, from Chaitow (1996)).

inhibiting the lower fixators, such as serratus anterior and the lower trapezius.

4. As a result the scapula loses its stability and an altered direction of the axis of the glenoid fossa evolves, resulting in humeral instability which involves additional levator scapulae, upper trapezius and supraspinatus activity to maintain functional efficiency.

These changes lead to cervical segment strain, the evolution of trigger points in the stressed structures and referred pain to the chest, shoulders and arms. Pain mimicking angina may be noted, plus a decline in respiratory efficiency.

The solution, according to Janda, is to be able to identify the shortened structures and to release (stretch and relax) these, followed by reeducation toward more appropriate function. This key underlying pattern of dysfunction will be found to relate to a great many of the painful conditions of the neck, shoulder and arm, all of which will be considered in later chapters. Whatever other local treatment these receive, consideration and reform of patterns, such as the upper crossed syndrome, must form a basis for long-term rehabilitation.

LOWER CROSSED SYNDROME (Fig. 5.2)

The lower crossed syndrome involves the following basic imbalance.

Iliopsoas, rectus femoris
TFL, short adductors   } which all tighten and shorten
Erector spinae group of the trunk

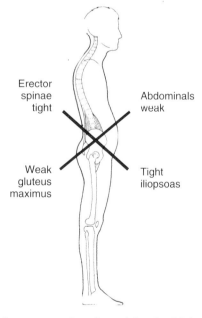

Figure 5.2 Lower crossed syndrome (after Janda) (reproduced, with permission, from Chaitow (1996)).

while
Abdominal and gluteal muscles } all weaken

The result of this chain reaction is to tilt the pelvis forward on the frontal plane, while flexing the hip joints and exaggerating lumbar lordosis. L5–S1 will have increased likelihood of soft tissue and joint distress, accompanied by pain and irritation. An additional stress feature commonly appears in the sagittal plane in which:

Quadratus lumborum   shortens
while
Gluteus maximus and medius   weaken

When this 'lateral corset' becomes unstable the pelvis is held in increased elevation and is accentuated when walking. This instability results in L5–S1 stress in the sagittal plane, which leads to lower back pain. The combined stresses described produce instability at the lumbodorsal junction, an unstable transition point at best.

The piriformis muscles are also commonly involved. In 10–20% of individuals, the right piriformis is penetrated by either the peroneal portion of the sciatic nerve or, rarely, by the whole nerve (the incidence of this is greatly increased in individuals of Asian descent) (Kuchera & Goodridge 1997). Piriformis syndrome can therefore produce direct sciatic pressure and pain (but not beyond the knee) (Heinking et al 1997).

Arterial involvement of piriformis shortness can produce ischemia of the lower extremity and, through a relative fixation of the sacrum, sacroiliac dysfunction and pain in the hip. Dural dysfunction is also possible when sacral mechanics are distorted in this way as the deformations place tension and torsion on the dural tube.

An almost inevitable consequence of a lower crossed syndrome pattern is that stresses will translate superiorly, thereby triggering or aggravating the upper crossed syndrome pattern outlined above. We can once again see how the upper and lower body interact with each other, not only functionally but dysfunctionally as well.

The solution for these common patterns is to identify both the shortened and the weakened structures and to set about normalizing their dysfunctional status. This might involve:

- deactivating trigger points within them or which might be influencing them
- normalizing the short and weak muscles, with the objective of restoring balance. This may involve purely soft tissue approaches or be combined with osseous adjustment/mobilization
- such approaches should coincide with reeducation of posture and body usage, if results are to be other than short term.

CHAIN REACTION LEADING TO FACIAL AND JAW PAIN: AN EXAMPLE

In case it is thought that such imbalances are of merely academic interest, a practical example of the negative effects of the chain reactions described above is given by Janda (1986). His premise is that TMJ problems and facial pain can be analyzed in relation to the person's whole posture.

Janda has hypothesized that the muscular pattern associated with TMJ problems may be considered as locally involving hyperactivity and tension in the temporal and masseter muscles while, because of this hypertonicity, reciprocal inhibition occurs in the suprahyoid, digastric and mylohyoid muscles. The external pterygoid, in particular, often develops spasm.

This imbalance between 'jaw adductors' (mandibular elevators) and 'jaw openers' (mandibular depressors) alters the ideal position of the condyle and leads to a consequent redistribution of stress on the joint while contributing to degenerative changes.

Janda describes a typical pattern of muscular dysfunction of an individual with TMJ problems as involving upper trapezius, levator scapulae, scalenii, sternocleidomastoid, suprahyoid, lateral and medial pterygoid, masseter and temporalis muscles, all of which show a tendency to tighten and to develop spasm. He notes that while the scalenes are unpredictable, commonly when overloaded they will become atrophied and weak and may also develop spasm, tenderness and trigger points.

The postural pattern associated with TMJ dysfunction might therefore involve:

1. hyperextension of the knee joints
2. increased anterior tilt of the pelvis
3. pronounced flexion of the hip joints
4. hyperlordosis of the lumbar spine
5. rounded shoulders and winged (rotated and abducted) scapulae
6. cervical hyperlordosis
7. forward thrust of the head
8. compensatory overactivity of the upper trapezius and levator scapulae muscles
9. forward thrust of the head results in opening of the mouth and retraction of the mandible.

This series of changes provokes increased activity of the jaw adductor (mandibular elevator) and protractor muscles, creating a vicious cycle of dysfunctional activity. Intervertebral joint stress in the cervical spine follows.

The message which can be drawn from this example is that patterns first need to be identified before they can be assessed for the role they might be playing in the person's pain and restriction conditions and certainly before these can be successfully and appropriately treated. Various protocols will be outlined in later chapters which can assist in this form of functional assessment.

PATTERNS AS HABITS OF USE

Lederman (1997) separates the patterns of dysfunction which emerge from habitual use (poor posture and hunched shoulders when typing, for example) and those which result from injury. Following structural damage tissue repair may lead to compensating patterns of use, with reduction in muscle force and possible wasting, often observed in backache and trauma patients. If uncorrected, such patterns of use inevitably lead to the development of habitual motor patterns and eventually to structural modifications.

Lederman lists the possible sequelae to trauma as follows.

- Modified proprioceptive function due to alteration in mechanoreceptor behavior (see notes on suboccipital injury as an example of this: Chapter 3, p. 34).
- If joint damage is part of the picture there may be inhibition of joint afferents influencing local muscular function. This may involve the build-up of metabolic by-products (Johansson 1993).
- Altered motor patterns resulting from higher center responses to injury. These psychomotor changes may involve a sense of insecurity and the development of protective behavior patterns, resulting eventually in actual structural modification such as muscle wasting.
- Reflexogenic responses to pain and also to injury which is not painful (Hurley 1991).

Treatment of patterns of imbalance which result from trauma, or from habitually stressful patterns of use, needs to address the causes of residual pain, as well as aiming to improve these patterns of voluntary use, with a focus on rehabilitation towards normal proprioceptive function. Active, dynamic rehabilitation processes which reeducate the individual and which enhance neurological organization may usefully be assisted by passive manual methods, including basic massage methodology and soft tissue approaches as outlined in this text.

THE BIG PICTURE AND THE LOCAL EVENT

As adaptive changes take place in the musculoskeletal system and as decompensation progresses toward an inevitably more compromised degree of function, structural modifications become evident. Whole-body, regional and local postural changes, such as those described by Janda (crossed syndromes) and epitomized in the case of facial pain outlined above, commonly result.

Simultaneously, with gross compensatory changes manifesting as structural distortion, local influences are noted in the soft tissues and the neural reporting stations situated within them, most notably in the proprioceptors and the nociceptors. These adaptive modifications include the phenomenon of facilitation and the evolution of re-flexogenically active structures in the myofascia (detailed in Chapter 6, p. 70).

JANDA'S 'PRIMARY AND SECONDARY' RESPONSES

It has become a truism that we need to consider the body as a whole; however, local focus still seems to be the dominant clinical approach. Janda (1988) gives various additional examples of why this is extremely shortsighted. He discusses the events which follow on from the presence of a short leg, which might well include:

- altered pelvic position
- scoliosis
- probable joint dysfunction, particularly at the cervicocranial junction
- compensatory activity of the small cervicooccipital muscles
- modified head position
- later compensation of neck musculature
- increased muscle tone
- muscle spasm
- and a sequence of events which would then include compensation and adaptation responses in many muscles, followed by the evolution of a variety of possible syndromes involving head/neck, TMJ, shoulder/arm or others.

Janda's point is that after all the adaptation that has taken place, treatment of the most obvious cervical restrictions, where the person might be aware of pain and restriction, would offer limited benefit. He points to the existence of oculopelvic and pelviocular reflexes, which indicate that any change in pelvic orientation alters the position of the eyes and vice versa, and to the fact that eye position modifies muscle tone, particularly the suboccipital muscles (look up and extensors tighten, look down and flexors prepare for activity, etc.). The implications of modified eye position due to altered pelvic position therefore become yet another factor to be considered when unraveling chain reactions of interacting elements (Komendatov 1945). 'These examples,' Janda says, 'serve to emphasize that one should not limit consideration to local clinical symptomatology … but [that we] should always maintain a general view'.

Grieve (1986) echoes this viewpoint. He explains how a patient presenting with pain, loss of functional movement or altered patterns of strength, power or endurance will probably either have suffered a major trauma, which has overwhelmed the physiological limits of relatively healthy tissues, or will be displaying 'gradual decompensation demonstrating slow exhaustion of the tissue's adaptive potential, with or without trauma'. As this process of decompensation occurs, progressive postural adaptation, influenced by time factors and possibly by trauma, leads to exhaustion of the body's adaptive potential and results in dysfunction and, ultimately, symptoms.

Grieve reminds us of Hooke's law, which states that within the elastic limits of any substance, the ratio of the stress applied to the strain produced is constant (Bennet 1952).

In simple terms, this means that tissue capable of deformation will absorb or adapt to forces applied to it

Box 5.1 Hooke's law

The stress applied to stretch or compress a body is proportional to the strain or change in length thus produced, so long as the limit of elasticity of the body is not exceeded.

within its elastic limits, beyond which it will break down or fail to compensate (leading to decompensation). Grieve rightly reminds us that while attention to specific tissues incriminated in producing symptoms often gives excellent short-term results, 'Unless treatment is also focused towards restoring function in asymptomatic tissues responsible for the original postural adaptation and subsequent decompensation, the symptoms will recur'.

RECOGNIZING DYSFUNCTIONAL PATTERNS

Vasilyeva & Lewit (1996) have cataloged observable changes in muscle, elevating the art of inspection to a higher level. They state:

Because muscular imbalances manifest in individual muscles and therefore (primarily) in certain regions, but are followed by compensatory reactions in other areas that restore balance, it is most important to determine which muscle(s) and which region are primarily affected and where compensation is taking place.

Among the main criteria examined when assessing for patterns of imbalance, for example in an extremity joint, are the following.

- Can the movement be carried out in the desired direction?
- Is the movement smooth and of constant speed?
- Does the movement follow the shortest path?
- Does the movement involve the full range?

The decision as to which muscles are probably implicated when abnormal responses are noted is based on the following.

- Dysfunction of agonists and synergists when the direction of movement is abnormal.
- Neutralizer muscles are implicated if precise motion is missing.
- If movement is other than smooth, antagonists are implicated.

What happens if the main culprits in disturbed motor patterns are short muscles?

The shortened muscle is also hyperactive as a rule. Its irritation threshold is lowered and therefore it contracts sooner than normal, i.e. the order in which muscles contract in the normal pattern is altered. If, therefore, the agonist is shortened, the relationship to the synergists, neutralizers, fixators and antagonists is out of balance and the local pattern, i.e. the direction, smoothness, speed and range of motion, is disturbed in a characteristic way. (Vasilyeva & Lewit 1996)

What happens if the main culprits in disturbed motor patterns are weak muscles?

The threshold of irritation in the weakened muscle is raised and therefore, as a rule, the muscle contracts later than normal or, in some cases, not at all. Hence the order in which muscles contract is altered, as is coordination. The most characteristic feature, however, is substitution, altering the entire pattern. This change is particularly evident if the weak muscle is the agonist. If, however, the neutralizers and/or fixators are weak, the basic pattern persists but there is accessory motion; if the antagonists are weak, the range of motion is increased. (Vasilyeva & Lewit 1996)

An example of Vasilyeva & Lewit's findings, relating specifically to a shortened upper trapezius, includes the following observations.

With a short upper trapezius muscle the attachments will deviate as follows, causing the listed changes.

- The occipital bone will be pulled caudoventrally and slightly laterally, causing the head to deviate forward and to the side with rotation to the opposite side leading to craniocervical lordosis.
- There will be pull on the spinous processes adding to side bending and rotation to the opposite side. In compensation, scoliosis will develop at the cervicothoracic junction, to the ipsilateral side, with increased kyphosis.
- There will be relative fixation of the cervical and upper thoracic spine with increased mobility at the craniocervical and cervicothoracic junctions.
- The acromion will be pulled craniomedially leading to the clavicle and acromion deviating craniomedially, producing compression of the clavicle at the sternal articulation, with compensation involving side bending at the shoulder girdle towards the opposite side, with rotation to the ipsilateral side.

The motor patterns during shoulder abduction which will be disturbed with a shortened upper trapezius include the following.

- There will be a shearing between the clavicle and scapula at the acromioclavicular joint.
- The head and cervical spine will move into extension, ipsilateral flexion and contralateral rotation.
- The shoulder girdle will displace superiorly.

Observation may also alert the practitioner to the presence of a crossed syndrome – pelvis tilted anteriorly, protruding abdomen, increased thoracic kyphosis, head thrust forward, rounded shoulders, etc. But which muscles, specifically, among the many involved are demonstrating relative shortness or weakness or both? Testing is needed and this can involve functional tests (below), as well as assessment of length and strength. A number of these tests will be detailed in the text associated with particular regions and joints later in the book.

Janda has developed a series of assessments – functional tests – which can be used to show changes which suggest imbalance, via evidence of over- or underactivity. Some of these are outlined below.

FUNCTIONAL SCREENING SEQUENCE
(Janda 1996)

Altered movement patterns can be tested as part of a screening examination for locomotor dysfunction. In general, observation alone is all that is needed to determine the altered movement pattern. However, light palpation may also be used if observation is difficult due to poor lighting, a visual problem or if the person is not sufficiently disrobed.

Although some of these tests relate directly to the lower back and limb, their relevance to the upper regions of the body should be clear, based on the interconnectedness of body mechanics which has been previously discussed.

Prone hip extension test (Fig. 5.3)

- The person lies prone and the practitioner stands to the side at waist level with the cephalad hand spanning the lower lumbar musculature and assessing erector spinae activity.
- The caudad hand is placed so that the heel lies on the gluteal muscle mass with the fingertips on the hamstrings.
- The person is asked to raise the leg into extension as the practitioner assesses the firing sequence.
- The normal activation sequence is (1) gluteus maximus, (2) hamstrings, followed by (3) erector spinae contralateral, then (4) ipsilateral. (*Note*: not all clinicians agree with this sequence definition; some believe hamstrings fire first or that there should be a simultaneous contraction of hamstrings and gluteus maximus.)

- If the hamstrings and/or erectors take on the role of gluteus as the prime mover, they will become shortened (see notes on postural and phasic muscle response to stress and overuse in Chapter 2).
- Janda says, 'The poorest pattern occurs when the erector spinae on the ipsilateral side, or even the shoulder girdle muscles, initiate the movement and activation of gluteus maximus is weak and substantially delayed … the leg lift is achieved by pelvic forward tilt and hyperlordosis of the lumbar spine, which undoubtedly stresses this region'.

Variation

- When the hip extension movement is performed there should be a sense of the lower limb 'hinging' from the hip joint.
- If, instead, the hinge seems to exist in the lumbar spine, the indication is that the lumbar spinal extensors have adopted much of the role of gluteus maximus and that these extensors (and probably hamstrings) will have shortened.

Trunk flexion test (Fig. 5.4)

- The person is supine with arms folded, hands placed on opposite shoulders, knees flexed and feet flat on table.

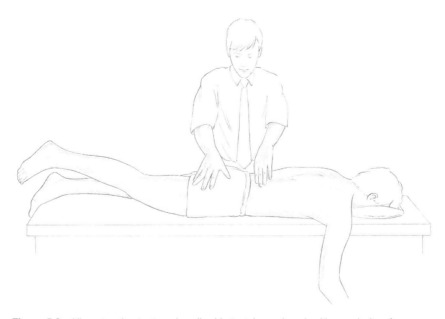

Figure 5.3 Hip extension test as described in text (reproduced, with permission, from Chaitow (1996)).

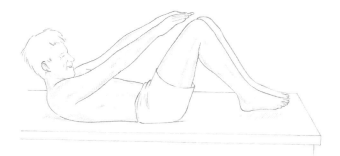

Figure 5.4 Trunk flexion test. If feet leave the surface or back arches, psoas shortness is indicated (reproduced, with permission, from Chaitow (1996)).

- The person is asked to maintain the lumbar spine against the table and to slowly lift the head, then the shoulders and then the shoulder blades from the table.
- Normal function is represented by the ability to raise the trunk until the scapulae are clear of the table without the feet lifting *or* the lower back arching.
- Abnormal function is indicated when the feet (or a foot) lift from the table *or* the low back arches, before the scapulae are raised from the table. This indicates psoas overactivity and weakness of the abdominals.

Hip abduction test

- The person lies on the side, ideally with head on a cushion, with the upper leg straight and the lower leg flexed at hip and knee, for balance.
- The practitioner, who is observing not palpating, stands in front of the person and toward the head end of the table.
- The person is asked to slowly raise the leg into abduction.
- Normal is represented by pure hip abduction to 45°.

- Abnormal is represented by:
  1. hip flexion during abduction, indicating tensor fascia lata (TFL) shortness, and/or
  2. the leg externally rotating during abduction, indicating piriformis shortness, and/or
  3. 'hip hiking', indicating quadratus lumborum shortness (and probable gluteus medius weakness), and/or
  4. posterior pelvic rotation, suggesting short antagonistic hip adductors.

Variation 1

- Before the test is performed the practitioner (standing behind the sidelying patient) lightly places the fingertips of the cephalad hand onto the lateral margin of quadratus lumborum while also placing the caudad hand so that the heel is on gluteus medius and the fingertips on TFL.
- If quadratus lumborum is overactive (and, by definition, shortened – see p. 57), it will fire before gluteus and possibly before TFL.
- The indication would be that quadratus (and possibly TFL) had shortened and that gluteus medius was inhibited and weak.

Variation 2

- When observing the abduction of the hip, there should be a sense of 'hinging' occurring at the hip and not at waist level.
- If there is a definite sense of the hinge being in the low back/waist area the implication is the same as in variation 1 – that quadratus is overactive and shortened, while gluteus medius is inhibited and weak.

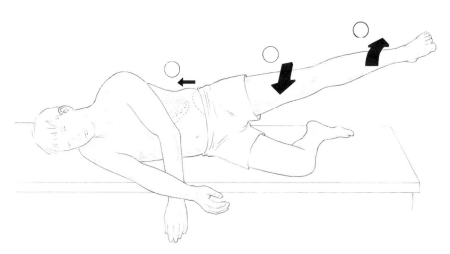

Figure 5.5 Hip abduction test which, if normal, occurs without 'hip hike', hip flexion or external rotation (reproduced, with permission, from Chaitow (1996)).

Scapulohumeral rhythm test

- This test has direct implications for neck and shoulder dysfunction.
- The person is seated and the practitioner stands behind to observe.
- The person is asked to let the arm being tested hang down and to flex the elbow to 90° with the thumb pointing upward.
- The person is asked to slowly abduct the arm toward the horizontal.
- A normal abduction will include elevation of the shoulder and/or rotation or superior movement of the scapula only after 60° of abduction.
- Abnormal performance of this test occurs if elevation of the shoulder, rotation, superior movement or winging of the scapula occurs within the first 60° of shoulder abduction, indicating levator and/or upper trapezius as being overactive and shortened, while lower and middle trapezius and serratus anterior are inhibited and are therefore weak.

Variation 1

- The person performs the abduction of the arm as described above and the practitioner observes from behind.
- A 'hinging' should be seen to take place at the shoulder joint, if upper trapezius and levator are normal.
- If 'hinging' appears to be occurring at the base of the neck, this is an indication of excessive activity in the upper fixators of the shoulder and shortness of upper trapezius and/or levator scapulae is suggested.

Variation 2

- The person is seated or standing with the practitioner standing behind with a finger tip resting on the mid-portion of the upper trapezius muscle of the side to be tested.
- The person is asked to take the arm into extension (a movement which should not involve upper trapezius).
- If there is discernible firing of upper trapezius during this movement of the arm, upper trapezius is overactive and, by implication, shortened.

Neck flexion test

- The person is supine without a pillow.
- The person is asked to lift the head and place the

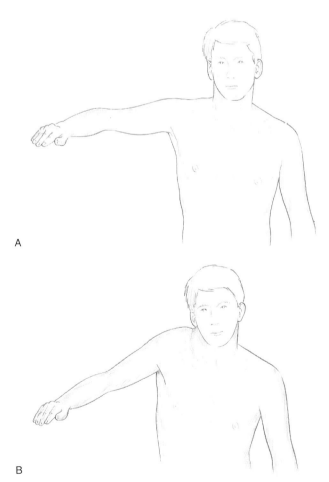

A

B

Figure 5.6 Scapulohumeral rhythm test. A: Normal. B: Imbalance due to elevation of the shoulder within first 60° of abduction (reproduced, with permission, from Chaitow (1996)).

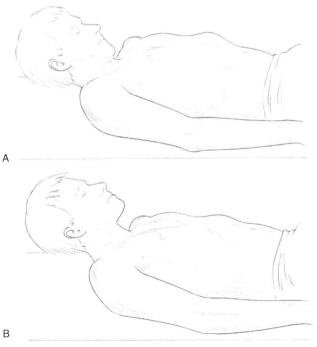

A

B

Figure 5.7 Neck flexion test. A: Normal flexion. B: Abnormal flexion ('chin poking'), suggesting shortness of SCM (reproduced, with permission, from Chaitow (1996)).

chin on the chest while raising the head no more than 2 centimeters from the table.

- A normal result occurs if there is an ability to hold the chin tucked in while flexing the head/neck.
- Abnormal is represented by the chin poking forward during this movement, which indicates sternocleidomastoid shortness and weak deep neck flexors.

Push-up test

- The person is asked to perform a push-up and/or to lower themselves from a push-up position, as the practitioner observes scapulae behavior.
- A normal result will be evidenced by the scapulae protracting (moving toward the spine) without winging or shifting superiorly as the trunk is lowered.
- If the scapulae wing, shift superiorly or rotate, the indication is that the lower stabilizers of the scapulae are weak (serratus anterior, upper and middle trapezius).

In addition to these 'snapshot' pictures of functional imbalance, which offer strong indications of which muscles might individually be short and/or weak, a range of tests exists for individual muscles. Some of these will be detailed in the appropriate sections of the therapeutic applications section of the book.

TRIGGER POINT CHAINS (Mense 1993, Patterson 1976, Travell & Simons 1983, 1992)

As compensatory postural patterns emerge, such as Janda's crossed syndromes, which involve distinctive and (usually) easily identifiable rearrangements of fascia, muscle and joints, it is inevitable that local, discrete changes should also evolve within these distressed tissues. Such changes include areas which, because of the particular stresses imposed on them, have become irritated and sensitized.

If particular local conditions apply (see Chapter 6), these irritable spots may eventually become hyperreactive, even reflexogenically active, and mature into major sources of pain and dysfunction. This form of dysfunctional adaptation can occur segmentally (often involving several adjacent spinal segments) or in soft tissues anywhere in the body (as myofascial trigger points). The activation and perpetuation of myofascial trigger points now becomes a focal point of even more adaptational changes.

Clinical experience has shown that trigger point 'chains' emerge over time, often contributing to predictable patterns of pain and dysfunction. Hong (1994), for example, has shown in his research that deactivation of particular trigger points (by means of injection) effectively inactivates remote triggers (see Box 5.2). In the next chapter the trigger point phenomenon will be examined in some detail.

Box 5.2 Trigger point chains (Hong 1994)	
When key trigger points were deactivated, Hong noted that trigger points in distant areas, which had previously tested as active, became inactive.	
Deactivated trigger	Inactivated associated triggers
Sternocleidomastoid	Temporalis, masseter, digastric
Upper trapezius	Temporalis, masseter, splenius, semispinalis, levator scapulae, rhomboid minor
Scalenii	Deltoid, extensor carpi radialis, extensor digitorum communis
Splenius capitis	Temporalis, semispinalis
Supraspinatus	Deltoid, extensor carpi radialis
Infraspinatus	Biceps brachii
Pectoralis minor	Flexor carpi radialis, flexor carpi ulnaris, first dorsal interosseous
Latissimus dorsi	Triceps, flexor carpi ulnaris
Serratus posterior superior	Triceps, latissimus dorsi, extensor digitorum communis, extensor carpi ulnaris, flexor carpi ulnaris
Deep paraspinal muscles (L5–S1)	Gluteus maximus, medius, minimus; piriformis, hamstrings, tibialis, peroneus longus, soleus, gastrocnemius
Quadratus lumborum	Gluteus maximus, medius, minimus; piriformis
Piriformis	Hamstrings
Hamstrings	Peroneus longus, gastrocnemius, soleus

REFERENCES

Bennet C 1952 Physics. Barnes and Noble, New York
Chaitow L 1996 Muscle Energy Techniques. Churchill Livingstone, Edinburgh
Grieve G 1986 Modern manual therapy. Churchill Livingstone, London
Heinking K, Jones III J M, Kappler R 1997 Pelvis and sacrum. In: Ward R (ed) American Osteopathic Association: foundations for osteopathic medicine. Williams and Wilkins, Baltimore
Hong C-Z 1994 Considerations and recommendations regarding myofascial trigger point injection. Journal of Musculoskeletal Pain 2(1):29–59
Hurley M 1991 Isokinetic and isometric muscle strength and inhibition after elbow arthroplasty. Journal of Orthopedic Rheumatology 4:83–95
Janda V 1982 Introduction to functional pathology of the motor system. Proceedings of the VII Commonwealth and International Conference on Sport. Physiotherapy in Sport 3:39
Janda V 1983 Muscle function testing. Butterworths, London
Janda V 1986 Extracranial causes of facial pain. Journal of Prosthetic Dentistry 56(4):484–487

Janda V 1988 In: Grant R (ed) Physical therapy in the cervical and thoracic spine. Churchill Livingstone, New York

Janda V 1996 Evaluation of muscular balance. In: Liebenson C (ed) Rehabilitation of the spine. Williams and Wilkins, Baltimore

Johansson H 1993 Influence on gamma-muscle spindle system from muscle afferents stimulated by KCL and lactic acid. Neuroscience Research 16(1):49–57

Komendatov G 1945 Proprioceptivnije reflexi glaza i golovy u krolikov. Fiziologiceskij Zurnal 31:62

Kuchera M, Goodridge J 1997 Lower extremity. In: Ward R (ed) American Osteopathic Association: foundations for osteopathic medicine. Williams and Wilkins, Baltimore

Lederman E 1997 Fundamentals of manual therapy. Churchill Livingstone, Edinburgh

Mense S 1993 Peripheral mechanisms of muscle nociception and local muscle pain. Journal of Musculoskeletal Pain 1(1):133–170

Patterson M 1976 Model mechanism for spinal segmental facilitation. Academy of Applied Osteopathy Yearbook, Colorado Springs, Colorado

Travell J, Simons D 1983 Myofascial pain and dysfunction, vol 1. Williams and Wilkins, Baltimore

Travell J, Simons D 1992 Myofascial pain and dysfunction, vol 2. Williams and Wilkins, Baltimore

Vasilyeva L, Lewit K 1996 Diagnosis of muscular dysfunction by inspection. In: Liebenson C (ed) Rehabilitation of the spine. Williams and Wilkins, Baltimore

6

Trigger points

NMT has among its key aims the removal of sources of pain and dysfunction. Modern pain research has demonstrated that a feature of all chronic pain is the presence, as part of etiology (often the major part), of localized areas of soft tissue dysfunction which promote pain and distress in distant structures (Melzack & Wall 1988). These are the loci which are known as trigger points, the focus of enormous research effort and clinical treatment. This chapter has as its primary objective the task of summarizing current knowledge and thinking on this topic.

A great deal of research into the trigger point phenomenon – much of it outlined in this chapter – has been conducted worldwide since the first edition of Travell & Simons' (1983a) *Myofascial pain and dysfunction: the trigger point manual, volume 1: upper half of the body* was released by Williams and Wilkins. That book rapidly became the preeminent resource relative to myofascial trigger points and their treatment. Its companion volume for the lower extremities was published in 1992.

In the second edition of volume 1 of the *Trigger point manual*, published in 1998, Simons et al have built on more recent research to modify not only the concepts around the theoretical basis of trigger point formation but also the most useful treatment protocols. Changes in technique application, including emphasis on massage and trigger point pressure release methods, accompany discussion of injection techniques, so that appropriate manual methods are now far more clearly defined. Suggested new terminology assists in clarifying differences and relationships between central (CTrP) and attachment (ATrP) trigger points, key and satellite trigger points, active and latent trigger points, and contractures which often result in enthesitis. Many of these definitions have been incorporated in this text to encourage the development of a common language among practitioners regarding these mechanisms.

In the new edition, Simons et al (1998) present an explanation as to the way they believe myofascial trigger points form and why they form where they do. Combining information from electrophysical and histopathological sources, their integrated trigger point hypothesis is seen to be based solidly on current understanding of physiology and function. Additionally, the authors have:

- validated their theories using research evidence
- cited older research (some dating back over 100 years) as referring to these same mechanisms (see Box 6.1 for a brief historical summary)

- analyzed and in some instances refuted previous research into the area of myofascial trigger points, some of which they assert was poorly designed
- suggested future research direction and design.

Simons et al (1998) present evidence which suggests that what they term 'central' trigger points (those forming in the belly of the muscle) develop almost directly in the

---

Box 6.1 Historical research into chronic referred muscle pain (Baldry 1993, Cohen & Gibbons 1998, Simons 1988, Straus 1991, Van Why 1994)

- F Valleix 1841 *Treatise on neuralgia*. Paris
  Noted that when certain painful points were palpated they produced shooting pain to other regions (*neuralgia*). He also reported that diet was a precipitating factor in the development of the painful aching symptoms of the back and cervical region.

- Johan Mezger, mid-19th century (Haberling W 1932 *Johan Georg Mezger of Amsterdam. Founder of modern scientific massage*. Medical Life)
  Dutch physician, developed massage techniques for treating 'nodules' and taut cord-like bands associated with this condition.

- T Inman 1858 *Remarks on myalgia or muscular pain*. British Medical Journal 407–408:866–868
  Was able to clearly state that radiating pain in these conditions (*myalgia*) was independent of nerve routes.

- Uno Helleday 1876 Nordiskt Medecinkst Arkiv 6 & 8 (8)
  Swedish physician described nodules as part of 'chronic myitis'.

- H Strauss 1898 Klinische Wochenschrift 35:89–91
  German physician distinguished between palpable nodules and 'bands'.

- A Cornelius 1903 *Narben und Nerven*. Deutsche Militartzlische Zeitschrift 32:657–673
  German physician who demonstrated the pain influencing features of tender points and nodules, insisting that the radiating pathway was not determined by the course of nerves. He also showed that external influences, including climatic, emotional or physical exertion, could exacerbate the already hyperreactive neural structures associated with these conditions. Cornelius also discussed these pain phenomena as being due to *reflex mechanisms*.

- A Muller 1912 *Untersuchbefund am rheumatish erkranten musckel*. Zeitschrift Klinische Medizine 74:34–73
  German physician who noted that to identify nodules and bands required refined palpation skills, aided, he suggested, by lubricating the skin.

- Sir William Gowers 1904 *Lumbago: its lessons and analogues*. British Medical Journal 1:117–121
  Suggested that the word *fibrositis* be used, believing erroneously that inflammation was a key feature of 'muscular rheumatism'. Lecture, National Hospital of Nervous Diseases, London.

- Ralph Stockman 1904 *Causes, pathology and treatment of chronic rheumatism*. Edinburgh Medical Journal 15:107–116, 223–225
  Offered support for Gowers' suggestion by reporting finding evidence of inflammation in connective tissue in such cases (never substantiated) and suggested that pain sensations emanating from nodules could be due to nerve pressure (now discounted).

- Sir William Osler 1909 *Principles and practice of medicine*. Appleton, New York
  Considered the painful aspects of muscular rheumatism (*myalgia*) to involve '*neuralgia of the sensory nerves* of the muscles'.

- W Telling 1911 *Nodular fibromyositis – an everyday affliction and its identity with so-called muscular rheumatism*. Lancet 1:154–158
  Called the condition '*nodular fibromyositis*'.

- L Llewellyn 1915 *Fibrositis*. Rebman New York
  Broadened the use of the word '*fibrositis*' to include other conditions including gout.

- F Albee 1927 *Myofascitis – a pathological explanation of any apparently dissimilar conditions*. American Journal of Surgery 3:523–533
  Called the condition '*myofascitis*'.

- F Gudzent 1927 *Testunt und heilbehandlung von rheumatismus und gicht mid specifischen allergen*. Deutsche Medizinsche Wochenschrift
  German physician noted that chronic '*muscular rheumatism*' may at times be allergic in origin and that removal of certain foods from the diet resulted in clinical improvement.

- C Hunter 1933 *Myalgia of the abdominal wall*. Canadian Medical Association Journal 28:157–161
  Described referred pain (*myalgia*) resulting from tender points situated in the abdominal musculature.

- J Edeiken, C Wolferth 1936 *Persistent pain in the shoulder region following myocardial infarction*. American Journal of Medical Science 191:201–210
  Showed that pressure applied to tender points in scapula region muscles could reproduce shoulder pain already being experienced. This work influenced Janet Travell – see below.

- Sir Thomas Lewis 1938 *Suggestions relating to the study of somatic pain*. British Medical Journal 1:321–325
  A major researcher into the phenomenon of pain in general, charted several patterns of pain referral and suggested that Kellgren (see below), who assisted him in these studies, continue the research.

- J Kellgren 1938 *Observations on referred pain arising from muscle*. Clinical Science 3:175–190
  Identified (in patients with '*fibrositis*' and '*myalgia*') many of the features of our current understanding of the trigger point phenomenon, including consistent patterns of pain referral – to distant muscles and other structures (teeth, bone, etc.) from pain points ('spots') in muscle, ligament, tendon, joint and periosteal tissue – which could be obliterated by use of novocaine injections.

- A Reichart 1938 *Reflexschmerzen auf grund von myoglosen*. Deutsche Medizinische Wochenschrift 64:823–824
  Czech physician who identified and charted patterns of distribution of *reflex pain* from tender points (nodules) in particular muscles.

- M Gutstein 1938 *Diagnosis and treatment of muscular rheumatism*. British Journal of Physical Medicine 1:302–321
  Refugee Polish physician working in Britain who identified that in treating *muscular rheumatism*, manual pressure applied to tender (later called 'trigger') points produced both local and referred symptoms and that these referral patterns were consistent in

Box 6.1 *(cont'd)*

everyone, if the original point was in the same location. He deactivated these by means of injection.

- A Steindler 1940 *The interpretation of sciatic radiation and the syndrome of low back pain.* Journal of Bone and Joint Surgery 22:28–34
  American orthopedic surgeon who demonstrated that novocaine injections into tender points located in the low back and gluteal regions could relieve sciatic pain. He called these points 'trigger points'. Janet Travell (see below) was influenced by his work and popularized the term 'trigger points'.

- M Gutstein-Good 1940 (same person as M Gutstein above) *Idiopathic myalgia simulating visceral and other diseases.* Lancet 2:326–328
  Called the condition '*idiopathic myalgia*'.

- M Good 1941 (same person as M Gutstein and M Gutstein-Good above) *Rheumatic myalgias.* The Practitioner 146:167–174
  Called the condition '*rheumatic myalgia*'.

- James Cyriax 1948 *Fibrositis.* British Medical Journal 2:251–255
  Believed that chronic muscle pain derived from nerve impingement due to disc degeneration. 'It [pressure on dura mater] has misled clinicians for decades and has given rise to endless misdiagnosis; for these areas of "*fibrositis*", "trigger points", or "myalgic spots", have been regarded as the primary lesion – not the result of pressure on the dura mater' (Cyriax J 1962 Textbook of orthopaedic medicine, vol. 1, 4th edn. Cassell, London).

- P Ellman, D Shaw 1950 *The chronic 'rheumatic' and his pains. Psychosomatic aspects of chronic non-articular rheumatism.* Annals of Rheumatic Disease 9:341–357
  Suggested that because there were few physical manifestations to support the pain claimed by patients with chronic muscle pain, their condition was essentially psychosomatic (*psychogenic rheumatism*): 'the patient aches in his limbs because he aches in his mind'.

- Theron Randolph 1951 *Allergic myalgia.* Journal of Michigan State Medical Society 50:487
  This leading American clinical ecologist described the condition as *allergic myalgia* and demonstrated that widespread and severe muscle pain (particularly of the neck region) could be reproduced 'at will under experimental circumstances' following trial ingestion of allergenic foods or inhalation of house dust extract or particular hydrocarbons, with relief of symptoms often being achieved by avoidance of allergens. Randolph reports that several of his patients who achieved relief by these means had previously been diagnosed as having '*psychosomatic rheumatism*'.

- James Mennell 1952 *The science and art of joint manipulation, vol. 1.* Churchill, London
  British physician described 'sensitive areas' which referred pain. Recommended treatment was a choice between manipulation, heat, pressure and deep friction. He also emphasized the importance of diet, fluid intake, rest, the possible use of cold and procaine injections as well as suggesting cupping, skin rolling, massage and stretching in normalization of '*fibrositic deposits*'.

- Janet Travell (and S Rinzler) 1952 *The myofascial genesis of pain.* Postgraduate Medicine 11:425–434
  Building on previous research and following her own detailed

studies of the tissues involved, coined the word 'myofascial', adding it to Steindler's term to produce 'myofascial trigger points' and finally '*myofascial pain syndrome*'.

- I Neufeld 1952 *Pathogenetic concepts of 'fibrositis' – fibropathic syndromes.* Archives of Physical Medicine 33:363–369
  Suggested that the pain of '*fibrositis-fibropathic syndromes*' was due to the brain misinterpreting sensations.

- F Speer 1954 *The allergic-tension-fatigue syndrome.* Pediatric Clinics of North America 1:1029
  Called the condition the '*Allergic-tension-fatigue syndrome*' and added to the pain, fatigue and general symptoms previously recognized (see Randolph above) the observation that edema was a feature, especially involving the eyes.

- R Gutstein 1955 *Review of myodysneuria (fibrositis).* American Practitioner 6:570–577
  Called the condition '*myodysneuria*'.

- R Nimmo 1957 *Receptors, effectors and tonus: a new approach.* Journal of the National Chiropractic Association 27(11):21
  After many years of research, which paralleled chronologically that of Travell, he described his concept of 'receptor-tonus technique', involving virtually the same mechanisms as those described by Travell & Simons but with a more manual emphasis. 'I have found that a proper degree of pressure, sequentially applied, causes the nervous system to release hypertonic muscle.'

- M Kelly 1962 *Local injections for rheumatism.* Medical Journal of Australia 1:45–50
  Australian physician who carried on Kellgren's concepts from the early 1940s, diagnosing and treating pain (*rheumatism*) by means of identification of pain points and deactivating these using injections.

- M Yunus et al 1981 *Primary fibromyalgia (fibrositis) clinical study of 50 patients with matched controls.* Seminars in Arthritis and Rheumatism 11:151–171
  First popularized the word '*fibromyalgia*'.

- Janet Travell, David Simons 1983 *Myofascial pain and dysfunction: the trigger point manual volume 1*
  The definitive work (with volume 2, 1992) on the subject of *myofascial pain syndrome* (MPS)

- David Simons 1986 *Fibrositis/fibromyalgia: a form of myofascial trigger points?* American Journal of Medicine 81 (suppl 3A):93–98
  American physician who collaborated with Travell in joint study of MPS and who also conducted his own studies into the connection between *myofascial pain syndrome* and *fibromyalgia syndrome*, finding a good deal of overlap.

- M Margoles 1989 *The concept of fibromyalgia.* Pain 36:391
  States that most patients with *fibromyalgia* demonstrate numerous active myofascial trigger points.

- R Bennett 1990 *Myofascial pain syndromes and the fibromyalgia syndrome.* In: Fricton R Awad E (eds) Advances in pain research and therapy. Raven Press, New York
  Showed that many 'tender points' in *fibromyalgia* are in reality latent trigger points. He believes that MPS and FMS are distinctive syndromes but are 'closely related'. States that many people with MPS progress on to develop fibromyalgia.

center of the muscle's fibers, where the motor endplate innervates it at the neuromuscular junction (Fig. 6.1). They postulate the following.

- Dysfunctional endplate activity occurs (commonly associated with a strain), which causes acetylcholine

(ACh) to be excessively released at the synapse, often associated with excess calcium.

- The presence of high calcium levels apparently keeps the calcium-charged gates open and the ACh continues to be released, resulting in ischemia.

- The consequent ischemia involves an oxygen/nutrient

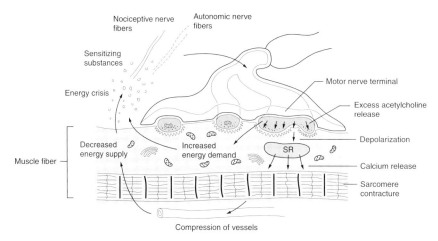

Figure 6.1 Integrated hypothesis of endplate dysfunction associated with trigger point formation (SR = sarcoplasmic reticulum).

deficit which, in turn, leads to a local energy crisis and inadequate adenosine triphosphate (ATP) production.

- Without available ATP the local tissue is unable to remove the calcium ions which are 'keeping the gates open' for ACh to continue releasing.
- Removing the superfluous calcium requires more energy than sustaining a contracture, so the contracture remains.
- The resulting muscle fiber contracture (involuntary, without motor potentials) needs to be distinguished from a contraction (voluntary, with motor potentials) and spasm (involuntary, with motor potentials).
- The contracture is sustained by the chemistry at the innervation site, not by action potentials from the spinal cord.
- As the endplate keeps producing ACh flow, the actin/myosin filaments slide to a fully shortened position (a weakened state) in the immediate area around the motor endplate (at the center of the fiber).
- As the sarcomeres shorten, they begin to bunch and a contracture 'knot' forms.
- This knot is the 'nodule' which is a palpable characteristic of a trigger point (Fig. 6.2).
- As this process occurs, the remainder of the sarcomeres of that fiber (those not bunching) are stretched, thereby creating the usually palpable taut band which is also a common trigger point characteristic.
- Attachment trigger points may develop at the attachment sites of these shortened tissues (periosteal, myotendinous) where muscular tension provokes inflammation, fibrosis and, eventually, deposition of calcium.

This model is explored in greater depth later in this chapter, since it represents the most widely held understanding as to the etiology of myofascial trigger points. Other models exist which attempt to explain the trigger point phenomenon, including the facilitation concept

Trigger point complex

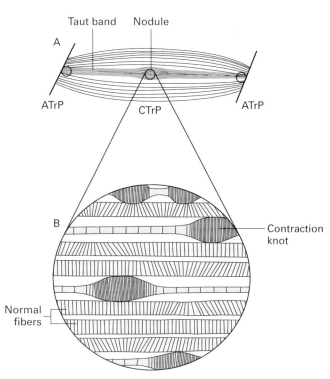

Figure 6.2 Tension produced by central trigger point can result in localized inflammatory response (attachment trigger point). Adapted from Simons et al (1998).

(below) and the ideas and methods developed by Raymond Nimmo DC (1981) (discussed below). Before examining these, it will be useful to investigate a key element of myofascial trigger point development and dysfunction – ischemia.

ISCHEMIA AND MUSCLE PAIN (Lewis 1942, Lewis et al 1931, Rodbard 1975, Uchida et al 1969)

Ischemia can be simply described as a state in which the current oxygen supply is inadequate for the current physiological needs of tissue. The causes of ischemia can be pathological, as in a narrowed artery or thrombus, or anatomical, as in particular hypovascular areas of the body, such as the region of the supraspinatus tendon 'between the anastomosis of the vascular supply from the humeral tuberosity and the longitudinally directed vessels arriving from the muscle's belly' (Tullos & Bennet 1984), or as occurs in trigger points as a result of the sequence of events outlined above involving excess calcium and decreased ATP production.

When the blood supply to a muscle is inhibited, pain is not usually noted until that muscle is asked to contract, at which time pain is likely to be noted within 60 seconds. This is the phenomenon which occurs in intermittent claudication. The precise mechanisms are open to debate but are thought to involve one or more of a number of processes, including lactate accumulation and potassium ion build-up.

Pain receptors are sensitized when under ischemic conditions, it is thought, due to bradykinin (a chemical mediator of inflammation) influence. This is confirmed by the use of drugs which inhibit bradykinin release, allowing an active ischemic muscle to remain relatively painless for longer periods of activity (Digiesi et al 1975). When ischemia ceases, pain receptor activation persists for a time and, conceivably, indeed probably, contributes to sensitization (facilitation) of such structures, a phenomenon noted in the evolution of myofascial trigger points (discussed further below). Research also shows that when pain receptors are stressed (mechanically or via ischemia) and are simultaneously exposed to elevated levels of adrenaline, their discharge rate increases, i.e. a greater volume of pain messages is sent to the brain (Kieschke et al 1988).

Trigger point activity itself may also induce relative ischemia in 'target' tissues (Baldry 1993). The mechanisms by which this occurs remain hypothetical but may involve a neurologically mediated increase in tone in the trigger point's reference zone (target tissues). According to Simons these target zones are usually peripheral to the trigger point, sometimes central to the trigger point and, more rarely (27%), the trigger point is located within the target zone of referral (Simons et al 1998). This translates to: If you are treating only the area of pain and the cause is myofascial trigger points, you are 'in the wrong spot' nearly 75% of the time!

The term 'essential pain zone' describes a referral pattern that is present in almost every person when a particular trigger point is active. Some trigger points may also produce a 'spillover pain zone' beyond the essential zone, or in place of it, where the referral pattern is usually less intense (Simons et al 1998). These target zones should be examined, and ideally palpated, for changes in tissue 'density', temperature, hydrosis and other characteristics associated with satellite trigger point formation (as discussed later in this chapter).

Any appropriate manual treatment, movement or exercise program which encourages normal circulatory function is likely to modulate these negative effects and reduce trigger point activity. A degree of normal function may return when the soft tissue's circulatory environment is improved and the stress-producing elements, whether of biomechanical, biochemical and/or psychosocial origin, are reduced or removed.

Increased lymphatic flow, which is enhanced by light gliding strokes and other forms of tugging on the skin surface, such as that created by lymphatic drainage therapy (Wittlinger & Wittlinger 1982), will assist in draining the waste materials which accumulate within the ischemic tissues, while altering the local cellular chemistry and reducing neuroexcitation. Many massage techniques drain lymphatic wastes and some are designed to dynamically induce lymph movement and drainage (Chikly 1996, Wittlinger & Wittlinger 1982). Use of these specialized techniques may greatly enhance the conditions of the interstitial fluids surrounding the cells. Such movement may also increase the flow of nutrients to the area, thus improving the cells' physiological status.

ISCHEMIA AND TRIGGER POINT EVOLUTION

Hypoxia (apoxia) involves tissues being deprived of adequate oxygen. This can occur in a number of ways, such as in ischemic tissues where circulation is impaired, possibly due to a sustained hypertonic state resulting from overuse or overstrain. The anatomy of a particular region may also predispose it to potential ischemia, as described above in relation to the supraspinatus tendon. Additional sites of relative hypovascularity include the insertion of the infraspinatus tendon and the intercapsular aspect of the biceps tendon. Prolonged compression crowding, such as is noted in side-lying sleeping posture, may lead to relative ischemia under the acromion process (Brewer 1979). These are precisely the sites most associated with rotator cuff tendinitis, calcification and spontaneous rupture, as well as trigger point activity (Cailliet 1991).

Additionally, a number of shoulder and neck muscles, including levator scapulae, scalenus anterior and medius, triceps brachii and trapezius, target the supraspinatus area as their referred zone and can produce not only pain but also autonomic and motor effects, including spasm, vasoconstriction, weakness, loss of coordination and loss of work tolerance (Simons et al 1998). Due to weakness and loss of coordination, the person may adapt by improperly using these and other muscles with resultant damage to the tissues (see patterns of dysfunction, Chapter 5, p. 55).

Trigger point connection

Mense (1993) describes the hypothesized evolution of a trigger point, clearly based on the Simons et al (1998) model.

A muscle lesion leads to the rupture of the sarcoplasmic reticulum and releases calcium from the intracellular stores. The increased calcium concentration causes sliding of the myosin and actin filaments; the result is a local contracture (myofilament activation without electrical activity) that has high oxygen consumption and causes hypoxia. An additional factor may be the traumatic release of vasoneuroactive substances (for example bradykinin) which produce local edema that in turn compresses venules and enhances the ischemia and hypoxia. Because of the hypoxia-induced drop in ATP concentrations, the function of the calcium pump in the muscle cell is impaired, and the sarcoplasmic calcium concentration remains elevated. This perpetuates the contracture.

The presence of oxygen deficit at the heart of the trigger point has been confirmed, according to Mense. *'Measurements of the tissue PO_2 with microprobes show that oxygen tension ... is extremely low. Thus, the pain and tenderness of a trigger point could be due to ischemia-induced release of bradykinin and other vasoneuroactive substances which activate and/or sensitize nociceptors'* (Bruckle et al 1990).

The original 'lesion' could have been the result of any of the multiple etiological and maintaining factors (overuse, misuse, abuse, disuse) outlined in the overview of stress and the musculoskeletal system in Chapter 4. It could be the result of a gross trauma, such as a blow, sudden elongation (as in whiplash) or laceration, occurring recently or even years before. It could also be the result of sustained emotional distress, with its influence on somatic structures, or of the effects of hormonal imbalance, specific nutritional deficiencies, allergic reactions or increased levels of toxic material in the tissues (see Chapter 4).

Simons describes the trigger point evolution as follows.

Visualize a spindle like a strand of yarn in a knitted sweater ... a metabolic crisis takes place which increases the temperature locally in the trigger point, shortens a minute part of the muscle (sarcomere) – like a snag in a sweater – and reduces the supply of oxygen and nutrients into the trigger point. During this disturbed episode an influx of calcium occurs and the muscle spindle does not have enough energy to pump the calcium outside the cell where it belongs. Thus a vicious cycle is maintained; the muscle spindle can't seem to loosen up and the affected muscle can't relax. (Wolfe & Simons 1992)

FACILITATION – SEGMENTAL AND LOCAL
(Korr 1976, Patterson 1976)

Neural sensitization can occur by means of a process known as facilitation. There are two forms of facilitation: segmental (spinal) and local (e.g. trigger point). If we are to make sense of soft tissue dysfunction, we should have an understanding of facilitation.

Facilitation occurs when a pool of neurons (premotor neurons, motoneurons or, in spinal regions, preganglionic sympathetic neurons) are in a state of partial or sub-threshold excitation. In this state, a lesser degree of afferent stimulation is required to trigger the discharge of impulses. Facilitation may be due to sustained increase in afferent input, aberrant patterns of afferent input or changes within the affected neurons themselves *or their chemical environment*. Once established, facilitation can be sustained by normal central nervous system activity. It is the example of neurons maintained in a hyperirritable state, due to an altered biochemical status in their local environment, that appears to come closest to the situation occurring in trigger point behavior. On a spinal segmental level the cause of facilitation may be the result of organ dysfunction as explained below (Ward 1997).

Organ dysfunction will result in sensitization and, ultimately, facilitation of the paraspinal structures at the level of the nerve supply to that organ. If, for example, there is any form of cardiac disease, there will be a 'feedback' toward the spine of impulses along the same nerves that supply the heart, so that the muscles alongside the spine in the upper thoracic level (T2,3,4 as a rule) will become hypertonic. If the cardiac problem continues, the area will become facilitated, with the nerves of the area, including those passing to the heart, becoming sensitized and hyperirritable. Electromyographic readings of the muscles alongside the spine at this upper thoracic level would show this region to be more active than the tissues above and below it. The muscles alongside the spine, at the facilitated level, would be hypertonic and almost certainly painful to pressure. The skin overlying this facilitated segmental area will alter in tone and function (increased levels of hydrosis as a rule) and will display a reduced threshold to electrical stimuli.

Once facilitation of the neural structures of an area has occurred, any additional stress *of any sort* which impacts the individual, whether emotional, physical, chemical, climatic, mechanical – indeed, absolutely anything which imposes adaptive demands on the person as a whole and not just this particular part of their body – leads to a marked increase in neural activity in the facilitated segments and not to the rest of the normal, 'unfacilitated' spinal structures.

Korr (1976) has called such an area a 'neurological lens' since it concentrates neural activity to the facilitated area, so creating more activity and also a local increase in muscle tone at that level of the spine. Similar segmental (spinal) facilitation occurs in response to any organ problem, affecting only the part of the spine from which the nerves supplying that organ emerge. Other causes of segmental (spinal) facilitation can include stress imposed on a part of the spine through injury, overactivity, repetitive patterns of use, poor posture or structural imbalance (short leg, for example).

Korr (1978) tells us that when subjects who have had facilitated segments identified were exposed to physical, environmental and psychological stimuli similar to those encountered in daily life, the sympathetic responses in those segments were exaggerated and prolonged. The disturbed segments behaved as though they were continually in, or bordering on, a state of 'physiologic alarm'.

In assessing and treating somatic dysfunction, the phenomenon of segmental facilitation needs to be borne in mind, since the causes and treatment of these facilitated segments may lie outside the scope of practice of many practitioners. In many instances, appropriate manipulative treatment can help to 'destress' facilitated areas. However, when a somatic dysfunction consistently returns after appropriate therapy has been given, the possibility of organ disease or dysfunction is a valid consideration and should be ruled out or confirmed by a physician.

How to recognize a facilitated spinal area

A number of observable and palpable signs indicate an area of segmental (spinal) facilitation.

- Beal (1983) tells us that such an area will usually involve two or more segments unless traumatically induced, in which case single segments are possible.
- The paraspinal tissues will palpate as rigid or board-like.
- With the person supine and the palpating hands under the paraspinal area to be tested (practitioner standing at the head of the table, for example, and reaching under the shoulders for the upper thoracic area), any ceiling-ward 'springing' attempt on these tissues will result in a distinct lack of elasticity, unlike more normal tissues above or below the facilitated area (Beal 1983).

Grieve (1986), Gunn & Milbrandt (1978) and Korr (1948) have all helped to define the palpable and visual signs which accompany facilitated dysfunction.

- A gooseflesh appearance is observable in facilitated areas when the skin is exposed to cool air, as a result of a facilitated pilomotor response.
- A palpable sense of 'drag' is noticeable as a light touch contact is made across such areas, due to increased sweat production resulting from facilitation of the sudomotor reflexes.
- There is likely to be cutaneous hyperesthesia in

the related dermatome, as the sensitivity is increased (facilitated).

- An 'orange peel' appearance is noticeable in the subcutaneous tissues when the skin is rolled over the affected segment, because of subcutaneous trophedema.
- There is commonly localized spasm of the muscles in a facilitated area, which is palpable segmentally as well as peripherally in the related myotome. This is likely to be accompanied by an enhanced myotatic reflex due to the process of facilitation.

Local facilitation in muscles

Baldry (1993) explains:

Palpable myofascial bands are electrically silent at rest. However, when such a band is 'plucked' with a finger … a transient burst of electrical activity with the same configuration as a motor unit's action potentials may be recorded (Dexter & Simons 1981). It is undoubtedly this electrical hyperactivity of motor and sensory nerve fibers at myofascial trigger points that is responsible for the so-called local twitch response, a transient contraction of muscle fibers which may be seen or felt … It is also neural hyperirritability which causes both myofascial and non-myofascial trigger points to be exquisitely tender to touch … The amount of pressure required to produce this is a measure of the degree of irritability present.

A similar process of facilitation occurs when particularly vulnerable sites of muscles (attachments, for example) are overused, abused, misused or disused in any of the many ways discussed in Chapter 4. Localized areas of hypertonicity may develop, sometimes accompanied by edema, sometimes with a stringy feel but always with a sensitivity to pressure.

Many of these tender, sensitive, localized, facilitated areas contain myofascial trigger points, which are not only painful themselves when palpated but will also transmit or activate pain (and other) sensations some distance away in 'target' tissues. Leading researchers into pain Melzack & Wall (1988) have stated that there are few, if any, chronic pain problems which do not have trigger point activity as a major part of the picture, perhaps not always as a prime cause but almost always as a maintaining feature. Similar to the facilitated areas alongside the spine, these trigger points will become more active when stress, of whatever type, makes adaptive demands on the body as a whole, not just on the area in which they lie.

When a trigger point is mechanically stimulated by compression, needling, stretch or other means, it will refer or intensify a referral pattern (usually of pain) to a target zone. An active trigger point refers a pattern that the person recognizes as being a part of their current symptom picture. When a latent trigger point is stimulated, it refers a pattern that may be unfamiliar to the person or an old pattern they used to have and have not had for a while (previously active, reverted to latent) (Simons et al 1998). All the same characteristics which denote an active trigger point (as detailed in this chapter) may be present in the latent trigger point, with the exception of the person's recognition of their active pain pattern. The same signs as described for segmental facilitation, such as increased hydrosis, a sense of 'drag' on the skin, loss of elasticity, etc., can be observed and palpated in these localized areas as well.

Lowering the neural threshold

There is another way of viewing facilitation processes. One of Selye's (1974) most important findings is commonly overlooked when the concurrent impact of multiple stressors on the system is being considered. Shealy (1984) summarizes as follows.

Selye has emphasized the fact that any systemic stress elicits an essentially generalized reaction, with release of adrenaline and glucocorticoids, in addition to any specific damage such stressor may cause. During the stage of resistance (adaptation), a given stressor may trigger less of an alarm; however, Selye insists that adaptation to one agent is acquired at the expense of resistance to other agents. That is, as one accommodates to a given stressor, other stressors may require lower thresholds for eliciting the alarm reaction. Of considerable importance is Selye's observation that concomitant exposure to several stressors elicits an alarm reaction at stress levels which individually are subthreshold. That is, one-third the dose of histamine, one-third the dose of cold, one-third the dose of formaldehyde, elicit an alarm reaction equal to a full dose of any one agent.

In short, therefore, as adaptation to life's stresses and stressors continues, thresholds drop and a lesser load is required to produce responses (pain, etc.) from facilitated structures, whether paraspinal or myofascial.

DIFFERENT MODELS FOR THE EVOLUTION OF TRIGGER POINTS
Awad's analysis of trigger points

In 1973, Awad examined dissected muscle fascicles (approximately 1 cm wide and 2 cm long) from muscle 'nodules'. Under a light microscope, in eight of the 10 specimens (different people), large amounts of 'amorphous material' were noted between muscle fascicles. This was shown to comprise acid mucopolysaccharides (with high water-binding properties) usually minimally present in muscle extracellular tissue. Electron microscopy showed clusters of platelets and mast cells discharging mucopolysaccharide-containing granules; also shown was increased connective tissue in five cases.

The space-occupying water-retaining substances stretch surrounding tissue, impair oxygen flow, increase acidity and sensitize nociceptors, converting the area into a pain-producing trigger point.

Baldry (1993) refers to questions raised by Awad (1990): 'Does the accumulation of mucopolysaccharides in … these nodules occur as a result of an increased production of this normally occurring substance, or a decrease in degradation, or a change in its quality?'

Awad therefore identifies edema as a part of the etiology of the trigger point, based on his analysis of the content of the tissue. Non-traumatic reduction of fluid levels and acidity, perhaps involving lymphatic drainage or traditional massage techniques, as well as improved oxygenation should therefore decrease nociceptive sensitization, something neuromuscular therapy has as a primary objective.

Improved oxygenation and reduced trigger point pain – an example

New Zealand physiotherapist Dinah Bradley (1999), an expert in breathing rehabilitation, identifies key trigger points in her patients, in the intercostals and upper trapezius as a rule, at the outset of their course of breathing rehabilitation. She asks patients to ascribe a value, out of 10, to the trigger point when under digital pressure, before they commence their exercise and treatment program (during which no direct treatment is given to the trigger points themselves) and periodically during their course, as well as at the time of discharge.

Bradley states:

I use trigger point testing as an objective measurement. Part of [the patient's] recovery is a reduction in musculoskeletal pain in these overused muscles. I use a numeric scale to quantify this. Patients themselves feel the reduction in tension and pain, a useful subjective marker for them, and an excellent motivator.

This use of trigger points, in which they are not directly deactivated but are used as monitors of improved breathing function, highlights several key points.

1. As oxygenation improves trigger points become less reactive and painful.
2. Enhanced breathing function also represents a reduction in overall stress, reinforcing the concepts associated with facilitation – that as stress of whatever kind reduces, trigger points react less violently.
3. Direct deactivation tactics are not the only way to handle trigger points.
4. Trigger points can be seen to be acting as 'alarm' signals, virtually quantifying the current levels of adaptive demand being imposed on the individual.

Nimmo's receptor-tonus techniques

Raymond Nimmo DC (1904–1986) developed an understanding of musculoskeletal pain syndromes which paralleled that of Janet Travell (1901–1997), whose work he admired (Cohen & Gibbons 1998). Nimmo arrived at a different (from Travell) understanding of the way in which trigger points (he called these 'noxious generative' points) evolve and of how to treat them. He held to a model in which increased muscle tone was the major feature initiating the triggers via the effect they had on neural receptors. He saw the trigger as an abnormal reflex arc.

- Excessive levels of muscle tone could result from repetitive or prolonged influence of stressors ('insults') such as cold, trauma, postural strain, etc., acting on them and causing projection of impulses through the posterior root to the gray matter of the cord.
- Here the highly excitatory internuncial neurons produce a prolonged motor discharge, increasing muscle tone.
- If there were a 'malfunction' in this feedback system (resulting, Nimmo suggested, from insults such as 'accidents, exposure to cold drafts or from occupations requiring prolonged periods of postural strain'), hypermyotonia could result, leading to even greater afferent input to the cord and amplification of additional efferent impulses to the muscles.
- This state of abnormally increased tone could become part of a self-perpetuating cycle, involving involuntary sympathetic activity, with reflex 'spillover' causing vasoconstriction, retention of metabolic wastes and pain.

Nimmo's treatment approach was based on releasing the hypertonic status of the muscles ('I found that a proper degree of pressure sequentially applied causes the nervous system to release a hypertonic muscle') (Nimmo 1981). He called his approach 'receptor-tonus' technique (Nimmo 1957) and it has had a major influence on modern neuromuscular therapy (DeLany 1999). A 1993 review of current chiropractic adjustive techniques found that just over 40% of chiropractors currently utilize Nimmo's approach on a regular basis (NBCE 1993).

Simons' current perspective

Simons et al (1998) see the strong need to differentiate 'central' from 'attachment' trigger points, both in their nature and in treatment requirements. The following highlights critical points to consider when applying therapy to trigger points. Much of this information is discussed at length in *Myofascial pain and dysfunction: the trigger point manual, vol. 1*, 2nd edn.

- Central trigger points are usually directly in the center of a fiber's belly.
- Motor points are consistently located (with a few exceptions) in the center of the muscle fiber's belly.
- The practitioner who knows fiber arrangement (fusiform, pennate, bipennate, multipennate, etc.), as well as attachment sites of each tissue being examined, will find it easy to locate the triggers since their sites

---

Box 6.2 Fibromyalgia and myofascial pain

Among the research into the connection between myofascial trigger point activity and fibromyalgia are the following.

1. Yunus (1993) suggests that 'Fibromyalgia and myofascial pain syndrome (MPS) [trigger point-derived pain] share several common features [and] it is possible that MPS represents an incomplete, regional or early form of fibromyalgia syndrome since many fibromyalgia patients give a clear history of localized pain before developing generalised pain.'
2. Granges & Littlejohn (1993) in Australia have researched the overlap between trigger points and the tender points in fibromyalgia and come to several conclusions, including:
   'Tender points in FMS represent a diffusely diminished pain threshold to pressure while trigger points are the expression of a local musculoskeletal abnormality.'
   'It is likely that trigger points in diffuse chronic pain states such as FMS … contribute only in a limited and localized way to decreasing the pain threshold to pressure in these patients.'
   'Taken individually the trigger points are an important clinical finding in some patients with FMS with nearly 70% of the FMS patients tested having at least one active trigger point.'
   Of those FMS patients with active trigger points, around 60% reported that pressure on the trigger 'reproduced a localized and familiar [FMS] pain'.
3. Researchers at Oregon Health Sciences University studied the history of patients with FMS and found that over 80% reported that prior to the onset of their generalized symptoms they suffered from regional pain problems (which almost always involve trigger points). Physical trauma was cited as the major cause of their pre-FMS regional pain. Only 18% had FMS which started without prior regional pain (Burckhardt 1993).
4. Research at UCLA has shown that injecting active trigger points with the pain-killing agent xylocaine produced marked benefits in FMS patients in terms of pain relief and reduction of stiffness but that this is not really significantly apparent for at least a week after the injections. FMS patients reported more local soreness following the injections than patients with only myofascial pain but improved after this settled down. This reinforces the opinion of many practitioners that myofascial trigger points contribute a large degree of the pain being experienced in FMS (Hong 1996).
5. Travell & Simons (1993) are clearly of this opinion, stating 'Most of these [fibromyalgia] patients would be likely to have specific myofascial pain syndromes that would respond to myofascial therapy.'

---

are moderately predictable (see pp. 16–17 in Chapter 2).
- Attachment trigger points are located where fibers merge into tendons or at periosteal insertions.
- Tension from taut bands on periosteal, connective or tendinous tissues can lead to enthesopathy or enthesitis (disease process where recurring concentrations of muscular stress provoke inflammation with a strong tendency toward the evolution of fibrosis and the deposition of calcium).
- Both central and attachment trigger points can have the same end result – referred pain. However, the local processes, according to Simons, are very different and should be addressed differently.
- Until they are thoroughly examined and tissue reaction noted, attachment trigger points should be treated with their tendency toward inflammation in

mind. For example, ice applications would be more appropriate than heat in areas where enthesitis has developed.

- Central trigger points would be treated with their contracted central sarcomeres and local ischemia in mind.
- Since the end of the taut band is likely to create enthesopathy, stretching the muscle before releasing its central trigger point might further inflame the attachments.
- Therefore, it is suggested, the attachment trigger points should first be addressed by releasing the associated central trigger point.
- Stretches, particularly involving active ranges of motion, will then further elongate the fibers but should be applied mildly until reaction is noted so as to avoid further tissue insult.
- When passive stretching is applied, care should be taken to assess for tendinous or periosteal inflammation, avoiding increased tension on already distressed connective tissue attachments.
- Gliding techniques may usefully be applied from the center of the fibers out toward the attachments, unless contraindicated (as in extremities where vein valves exist). By elongating the tissue toward the attachment, sarcomeres which are shortened at the center of the fiber will be lengthened and those which are overstretched near the attachment sites will have the tension released.
- Central trigger points often respond well to heat as warmth may encourage the gel of the fascia to turn more solute (Kurz 1986). Heat draws fresh blood to the area, bringing with it oxygenation and nutrients. Subsequent application of cold (see below and Chapter 10) or massage is required to prevent stasis and congestion following application of heat.
- Short (20–30 seconds) cold applications, once removed, produce a strong flushing of the tissues (Boyle & Saine 1988). Cold applications are likely to penetrate to deeper tissue than heat does, although prolonged, continuous applications of ice may decrease the pliability of connective tissue so that they are less easily stretched (Lowe 1995).
- Oxygen, ATP and nutrients offered by the incoming blood could reduce the local environmental deficits and encourage normalization of the dysfunctional tissues.
- When compression techniques are used, local chemistry can change due to blanching of the nodules followed by a flush of blood to the tissues when the compression is released.
- The effects of thermal or other neuro-altering applications (skin irritants, moxibustion, dry or wet needling, etc.) will usually induce the contracture to release more readily.

KEY AND SATELLITE TRIGGER POINTS

Clinical experience and research evidence suggest that 'key' triggers exist which, if deactivated, relieve activity in satellite trigger points (usually located within the target area of the key trigger). If these key trigger points are not relieved but the satellites are treated, the referral pattern usually returns.

Box 6.3 Trigger point activating factors

Primary activating factors include:

- persistent muscular contraction, strain or overuse (emotional or physical cause)
- trauma (local inflammatory reaction)
- adverse environmental conditions (cold, heat, damp, draughts, etc.)
- prolonged immobility
- febrile illness
- systemic biochemical imbalance (e.g. hormonal, nutritional).

Secondary activating factors include (Baldry 1993):

- compensating synergist and antagonist muscles to those housing primary triggers may develop triggers
- satellite triggers evolve in referral zone (from primary triggers or visceral disease referral, e.g. myocardial infarct).

Hong & Simons (1992) have reported on over 100 sites involving 75 patients in whom remote trigger points were inactivated by means of injection of key triggers. The details of the key and satellite triggers, as observed in this study, are listed below.

Key trigger	Satellite triggers
Sternocleidomastoid	Temporalis, masseter, digastric
Upper trapezius	Temporalis, masseter, splenius, semispinalis, levator scapulae, rhomboid major
Scalenii	Deltoid, extensor carpi radialis, extensor digitorum communis, extensor carpi ulnaris
Splenius capitis	Temporalis, semispinalis
Supraspinatus	Deltoid, extensor carpi radialis
Infraspinatus	Biceps brachii
Pectoralis minor	Flexor carpi radialis, flexor carpi ulnaris, first dorsal interosseous
Latissimus dorsi	Triceps, flexor carpi ulnaris
Serratus post. sup.	Triceps, latissimus dorsi, extensor digitorum communis, extensor carpi ulnaris, flexor carpi ulnaris
Deep paraspinals (L5–S1)	Gluteus maximus, medius and minimus, piriformis, hamstrings, tibialis, peroneus longus, gastrocnemius, soleus
Quadratus lumborum	Gluteus maximus, medius and minimus, piriformis
Piriformis	Hamstrings
Hamstrings	Peroneus longus, gastrocnemius, soleus

TRIGGER POINTS AND JOINT RESTRICTION (Kuchera & McPartland 1997)

Since trigger points influence associated muscles and are associated with loss of range of motion of the tissue housing them, the muscles associated with a joint suffering a restriction of movement should be examined for trigger point involvement in the restriction. Though this may occur at any joint, the following example is given for the shoulder region, as noted by Kuchera.

Trigger points associated with shoulder restriction (Kuchera & McPartland 1997)

Restricted motion	Muscle housing trigger point
Flexion	Triceps
Abduction	Subscapularis
	Infraspinatus
	Supraspinatus
	Teres major
	Levator scapulae
Internal rotation	Teres major
	Infraspinatus
External rotation	Subscapularis
	Pectoralis minor

Other trigger point sites

Trigger points may form in numerous body tissues; however, only those occurring in myofascial structures are named 'myofascial trigger points'. Trigger points may also occur in skin, fascia, ligaments, joints, capsules and periostium.

Trigger points often develop in scar tissue (Simons et al 1998) and may perpetuate the original pain pattern, even after the original cause of the pain has been removed. Additionally, the scar tissue might block normal lymphatic drainage (Chikly 1996), which results in a build-up of waste products in surrounding tissue and may encourage trigger point formation or recurrence.

Viscerosomatic referrals, such as the arm pain often experienced with a myocardial infarction, are commonly noted for most organs. Somatovisceral referrals could be silent as organs do not always report pain; however, recurrent viscerosomatic referrals (low back pain) could be an organ's painful cry for help (kidney stone, infection or disease) (see Chapter 4 and Fig. 6.3).

TESTING AND MEASURING TRIGGER POINTS

As the trigger point phenomenon continues to attract high levels of research interest, it becomes increasingly important for standardized criteria to be established relating to the skills required to identify and treat myofascial dysfunction.

Basic skill requirements

When designing and conducting clinical studies relating to soft tissue dysfunction, it is important that the examiners be experienced and well trained in those palpation skills and protocols required to accurately assess the tissues. Those who are inexperienced (recent graduates or students, for example) or experienced practitioners with insufficient training in the specific techniques required may well fall short of the skills needed to apply technique-sensitive strategies. This is especially true of those applying manual techniques, since palpation skills take time and practice to perfect. Experienced practitioners who are trained to palpate for, and identify, specific characteristics which form part of research criteria (see below) will offer the most useful and valid findings (Simons et al 1998).

Practitioners should be able to identify:

- bony structures
- individual muscles (where possible)
- palpable thickenings, bands and nodules within the myofascial tissues.

Additionally, knowledge of fiber arrangement and the shortened and stretched positions for each section of each muscle will allow the practitioner to apply the techniques in such a way as to obtain accurate and reliable results. Knowledge of (or accessible charts showing) trigger point reference zones will offer greater accuracy.

Simons et al (1998) discuss diagnostic criteria for identifying a trigger point:

- taut palpable band
- exquisite spot tenderness of a nodule in the taut band
- recognizable referral pattern (usually pain) by pressure on a tender nodule (active with familiar referral or latent with unfamiliar referral)
- painful limit to full stretch range of motion.

Additional observations:

- local twitch responses identified visually, tactilely or by needle penetration
- altered sensations in reference zones
- electromyographic verification of spontaneous electrical activity (SEA) found in active loci of trigger point.

Identification of a local twitch response is the most difficult; however, when it is present, it supports a strong confirmation that a trigger point has been located, especially when elicited by needle penetration. Additionally, pain upon contraction and weakness in the muscle may be observed.

Given the above criteria and the fact that no particular laboratory test or imaging technique has been officially established to identify trigger points (Simons et al 1998),

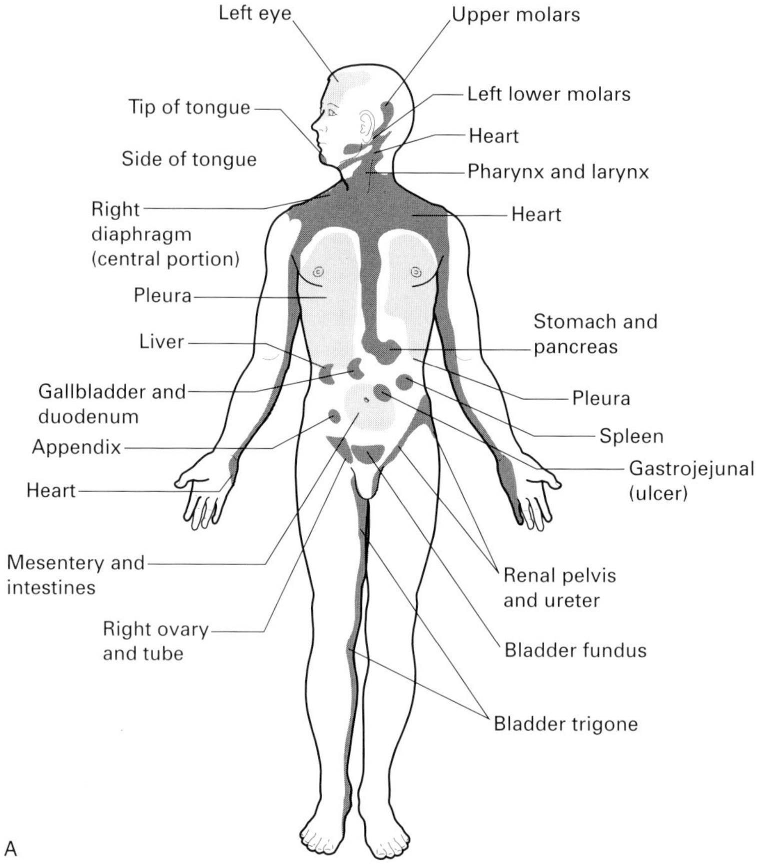

Left eye
Upper molars
Tip of tongue
Left lower molars
Side of tongue
Heart
Right diaphragm (central portion)
Pharynx and larynx
Heart
Pleura
Liver
Stomach and pancreas
Gallbladder and duodenum
Pleura
Appendix
Spleen
Heart
Gastrojejunal (ulcer)
Mesentery and intestines
Renal pelvis and ureter
Right ovary and tube
Bladder fundus
Bladder trigone

A

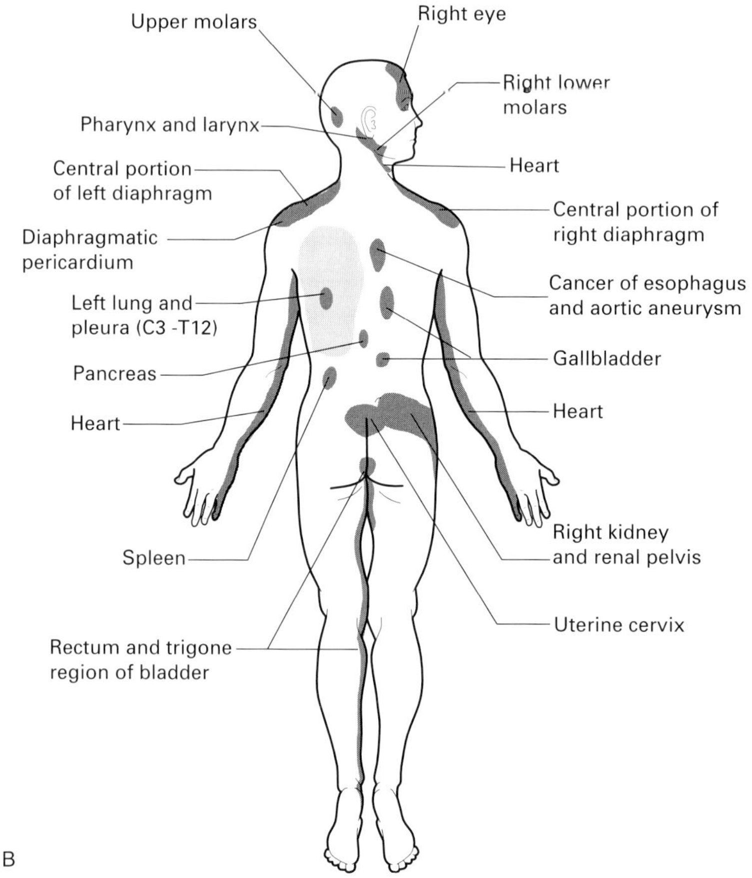

Upper molars
Right eye
Pharynx and larynx
Right lower molars
Central portion of left diaphragm
Heart
Diaphragmatic pericardium
Central portion of right diaphragm
Left lung and pleura (C3 -T12)
Cancer of esophagus and aortic aneurysm
Pancreas
Gallbladder
Heart
Heart
Spleen
Right kidney and renal pelvis
Rectum and trigone region of bladder
Uterine cervix

B

Figure 6.3 Pain referred from viscera.
A: Anterior view. B: Posterior view.
(Adapted from Rothstein et al (1991).

the development of palpation skills is even more important. Additionally, several testing procedures may be used as confirmatory evidence of the presence of a trigger point when coupled with the above minimal criteria.

Needle electromyography

While this method of testing would not be practical in most practice settings, the obvious value in clinical research is high. Though a thorough discussion of this material is beyond the scope of this text, the reader is referred to Simons et al (1998) who have extensively discussed spontaneous electrical activity, needle penetration methodology, abnormal endplate noise and other associated information which has only been briefly discussed here.

The above-mentioned text offers evidence of the importance of several factors when using EMG needling for trigger point diagnosis. They include:

- the type and size of needle used to penetrate the trigger point
- the speed and manner in which the needle is inserted
- the sweep speed used for recording
- the recording of both high-amplitude spike potentials and low-amplitude noise-like components
- the belief system of the operator as to what 'normal endplate noise' represents.

Simons et al (1998) state:

The issue of whether the endplate potentials now recognized by electromyographers as endplate noise arise from normal or abnormal endplates is critical and questions conventional belief. ... Since publication of the paper by Weiderholt in 1970, electromyographers have accepted his apparently mistaken conclusion that potentials similar to what we now identify as SEA [spontaneous electrical activity] represent *normal* miniature endplate potentials.

Electromyographers commonly identify the low-amplitude potentials as 'seashell' noise. Wiederholt was correct in concluding that the low-amplitude potentials arose from endplates, and illustrated one recording of a few discrete monophasic potentials having the configuration of normal miniature endplate potentials as described by physiologists. However, the continuous noise-like endplate potentials that he also illustrated and that we observe from active loci have an entirely different configuration and have an abnormal origin.

Advancing the penetrating needle very slowly and with gentle rotation is a key factor in arriving at the active loci without provoking an insertion-induced potential which could distort the noise produced by the dysfunctional endplate. Simons et al (1998) note:

As the needle advances through the TrP region in this electronically quiet background, the examiner occasionally hears a distant rumble of noise that swells to full SEA dimensions as the needle continues to advance. ... Sometimes the SEA can be increased or decreased by simply applying gentle side pressure to the hub of the EMG needle. The distance of the needle from the discrete source of the electrical activity can be that critical.

Ultrasound

Visual imaging of the local twitch response (LTR) provides objective evidence that an LTR has been provoked. While it may be clinically practical to use ultrasound, the practitioner would still need to provoke the LTR. This would involve needle penetration or the development of snapping palpation skills. Snapping palpation is a difficult technique to master and is not applicable to many of the muscles. However, when it is possible to do so, this method provides non-invasive supporting evidence that a trigger point has been found.

Surface electromyography

Surface EMG offers a promising possibility of studying the effects trigger points have on referred inhibition and referred spasm to other muscles. With well-designed studies, this may provide evidence that trigger points increase responsiveness and fatiguability and delay recovery of the muscle.

Algometer use for research and clinical training

When applying digital pressure to a tender point in order to ascertain its status (Does it hurt? Does it refer? etc.), it is important to have some way of knowing that pressure being applied is uniform. The term 'pressure threshold' is used to describe the least amount of pressure required to produce a report of pain and/or referred symptoms. It is obviously useful to know whether pain and/or referral symptoms occur with 1,2,3 or however many pounds of pressure and whether this degree of pressure changes before and after treatment or at a subsequent clinical encounter.

In diagnosing fibromyalgia, the criteria for a diagnosis depends upon 11 of 18 specific test sites testing as positive (hurting severely) on application of 4 kilograms of pressure (American College of Rheumatologists 1990). If it takes more than 4 kg of pressure to produce pain, the point does not count in the tally. Without a measuring device, such as an algometer, there would be no means of standardizing pressure application. An algometer is also a useful tool for training a practitioner to apply a standardized degree of pressure when treating and to 'know' how hard they are pressing.

Use of an algometer is not really practical in everyday clinical work but this becomes an important tool if research is being carried out, as an objective measurement of a change in the degree of pressure required to produce symptoms. The research by Hong and colleagues as to 'which treatment method is most successful in treating trigger points' reported on later in this chapter, utilized algometer readings before and after treatment and could not usefully have been carried out without such an instrument.

Belgian researchers Jonkheere & Pattyn (1998) explain how they have used algometers to identify what they term the 'myofascial pain index' (MPI). They also use it to define the nature of trigger points under investigation, with a slight variation on the way Travell & Simons use the terms 'active', 'latent', etc. 'The purpose of algometrics is to define whether a trigger point is active, latent, falsely positive or absent.' In order to achieve this objective, various standard locations are tested (for example, the 18 test sites used for fibromyalgia diagnosis). Based on the results of this, an MPI is calculated.

The purpose of this exercise is to create an objective base (the MPI), which emerges initially from the patient's subjective pain reports, when pressure is applied to test points. The calculation of the MPI determines the degree of pressure required to evoke pain in a trigger point and helps to sift 'false-positive' from 'active' points, with the latter receiving treatment and the former not.

The Belgian researchers acknowledge that they have based their approach on earlier work by Hong et al (1996), who investigated pressure thresholds of trigger points and the surrounding soft tissues.

Jonkheere & Pattyn define the various states of trigger points as follows.

1. An active trigger point, they say, is sensitive to palpation and produces an identifiable pain which corresponds, completely or partially, with the known pattern of a trigger point located at that particular site.
2. A latent trigger point is one which only produces localized pain on palpation.

3. A 'false-positive' trigger point is one which is sensitive to palpation and which refers pain:
   - but which does not correspond with known patterns, or
   - which produces a referral pattern which does correspond, completely or partially, with the known pattern of a trigger point located at that particular site, but only when the pressure required to evoke this response is greater than the MPI. This 'false-positive' point is, in Travell & Simons' terminology, also a latent point.

The 18 points tested are located in nine bilateral sites as defined by the American College of Rheumatology in 1990, as part of the diagnostic protocol for fibromyalgia syndrome (FMS) (Fig. 6.4). They are:

- at the suboccipital muscle insertions (close to where rectus capitis posterior minor inserts)
- at the anterolateral aspect of the intertransverse spaces between C5 and C7
- at the midpoint of the upper border of the upper trapezius muscle
- at the origin of the supraspinatus muscle above the scapula spine
- at the second costochondral junctions, on the upper surface, just lateral to the junctions
- 2 centimeters distal to the lateral epicondyles of the elbows
- in the upper outer quadrant of the buttocks in the anterior fold of gluteus medius
- posterior to the prominence of the greater trochanter (piriformis attachment)
- on the medial aspect of the knees, on the fatty pad, proximal to the joint line.

Using an algometer (the Belgians used an Algoprobe®) pressure is applied to each of the points at a precise 90° angle to the skin, sufficient to produce pain, with the measurement being taken when this is reported. The 18 values

---

Box 6.5 Trigger point incidence and location

1. 200 asymptomatic Air Force recruits aged 17–35 demonstrated trigger points in 54% of 100 females and 45% of 100 males tested (Sola 1951).
2. Triggers can occur in any myofascial tissue but the most commonly identified trigger points are found in the upper trapezius and quadratus lumborum (Travell & Simons 1983b). (A latent trigger point in the third finger extensor may be more common' Simons et al 1998.)
3. Incidence of primary myofascial syndromes noted in 85% of 283 consecutive chronic pain patients and 55% of 164 chronic head/neck pain patients (Fishbain et al 1986, Fricton et al 1985).
4. Most common trigger point sites are:
   - belly of muscle, close to motor point
   - close to attachments
   - free borders of muscle.

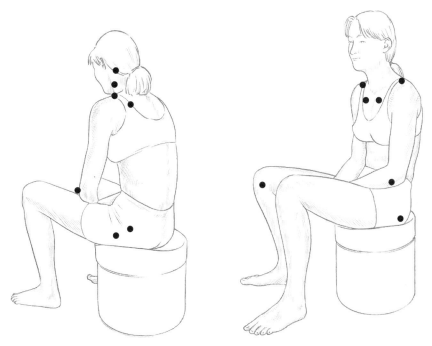

Figure 6.4 Nine pairs of points used in testing for fibromyalgia (reproduced, with permission, from Chaitow (1996)).

are recorded and then averaged, leaving a number which is the MPI.

Once established, this amount of pressure is used to judge the nature (active, 'false positive', etc.) of all other potential trigger point sites. A label of 'active' is assigned to any point where the referral pattern matches known referral distribution from that site and which requires less than the MPI degree of pressure to produce this response. Those triggers which meet the definition of 'active trigger point' are therefore noted and treated. If a greater degree of pressure than the MPI is required to evoke a pain response, the trigger point is not regarded as 'active'.

Jonkheere & Pattyn, utilizing the basic research of Simons et al (1998), have also identified 'chains' of trigger points which seem to be functionally or structurally related to the patient's reported pain symptoms. Before treatment, these are methodically tested using an algometer in the manner described above.

Baldry (1993) (referring to research by Fischer (1988) discusses algometer use (he calls it a 'pressure threshold meter') and suggests it should be used to measure the

degree of pressure needed to produce symptoms, 'before and after deactivation of a trigger point, for when this is successful, the pressure threshold over the trigger point increases by about 4 kg'.

Thermography and trigger points

Various forms of thermography are being used to identify trigger point activity, including infrared, electrical and liquid crystal (Baldry 1993). Swerdlow & Dieter (1992) found, after examining 365 patients with demonstrable trigger points in the upper back, that 'Although thermographic "hot-spots" are present in the majority, the sites are not necessarily where the trigger points are located'.

Simons suggests that while hot-spots may commonly represent trigger point sites, some triggers may exist in 'normal' temperature regions and hot-spots can exist for reasons other than the presence of trigger points.

Thermal examination of the reference zone (target area) usually shows skin temperature raised but not always. Simons (1987) attributes this anomaly to the different effects trigger points have on the autonomic nervous system. Simons (1993a) explains:

Depending upon the degree and manner in which the trigger point is modulating sympathetic control of skin circulation, the reference zone initially may be warmer, isothermic or cooler than unaffected skin. Painful pressure on the trigger point consistently and significantly reduced the temperature in the region of the referred pain and beyond.

Barrell (1996) has shown that manual-thermal diagnosis is only accurate regarding what the hand perceives as

---

Box 6.6 Trigger points and referred inhibition

- Various studies have demonstrated that trigger points in one muscle are related to inhibition of another functionally related muscle (Simons 1993b).
- In particular, it was shown by Simons that the deltoid muscle can be inhibited when there are infraspinatus trigger points present.
- Headley (1993) has shown that lower trapezius inhibition is related to trigger points in the upper trapezius.

'heat' 70% of the time. Apparently when scanning manually for heat, any area which is markedly different from surrounding tissues in temperature terms is considered 'hot' by the brain. Manual scanning for heat is therefore an accurate way of assessing 'difference' between tissues but not their actual thermal status.

CLINICAL FEATURES OF MYOFASCIAL TRIGGER POINTS (Kuchera & McPartland 1997)

Simons et al (1998) have detailed a recommended criteria for identifying a latent or active trigger point. They note all trigger points as having four essential characteristics and a number of possible confirmatory observations, which may or may not be present. 'Clearly, there is no one diagnostic examination that alone is a satisfactory criterion for routine clinical identification of a trigger point … The minimum acceptable criteria is the combination of spot tenderness in a palpable band and subject recognition of the pain.'

The four essential characteristics of active and latent trigger points are:

- taut, palpable band
- small nodular or spindle-shaped thickening in the fiber's center which is exquisitely tender when pressed (also called 'nidus' or 'active loci')
- person's recognition of current pain complaint (active TrP) or of an unfamiliar one (latent TrP) when the trigger point is mechanically stimulated
- painful limit of stretch range of motion.

Other common characteristics of active trigger points include:

- local twitch response (LTR) is seen (visually or by ultrasound) or felt as taut band is snapped or nodule is penetrated by a needle (both techniques are difficult to perform and require a high level of skill)
- compression of tender nodule produces pain or altered sensation in the target zone
- EMG evidence of SEA in active loci
- painful upon contraction
- muscle weakness.

Box 6.7 Trigger point perpetuating factors

Travell & Simons (1983a, 1992) confirm that the following stressors help to maintain and enhance trigger point activity:

- nutritional deficiency (especially vitamins C, B-complex and iron)
- hormonal imbalances (thyroid in particular)
- infections
- allergies (wheat and dairy, in particular)
- low oxygenation of tissues (aggravated by tension, stress, inactivity, poor respiration).

Box 6.8 'What trigger points are not'

Simons suggests that taut bands in which trigger points are found (Baldry 1993):

- are not areas of 'spasm' (no EMG activity)
- are not fibrositic change (tautness vanishes within seconds of stretching or acupuncture needle insertion)
- are not edematous (although local areas of the tissues around the trigger hold more fluid – see Awad's research above)
- do not involve colloidal gelling (myogelosis).

Other palpable signs have been observed by the authors of this text and others. These include:

- altered cutaneous temperature (increased or decreased)
- altered cutaneous humidity (usually increased)
- altered cutaneous texture (sandpaper-like quality, roughness)
- a 'jump' sign (or exclamation!) may accompany palpation due to extreme sensitivity
- local trophic changes or 'gooseflesh' may be evident overlying trigger site or in target zone.

Developing skills for TrP palpation

The following suggestions will help develop or refine palpation skills which are needed to locate and deactivate trigger points. While these points are generalized, advice regarding specific examination of individual muscles is offered in the second half of this text dealing with clinical applications of NMT.

- Central trigger points are usually palpable either with flat palpation (against underlying structures) or with pincer compression (tissue held more precisely between thumb and fingers like a C-clamp or held more broadly, with fingers extended like a clothes pin) (see hand positions, Chapter 9, Fig. 9.4).
- Compressions may be applied wherever the tissue may be lifted without compressing neurovascular bundles.

Box 6.9 What are taut bands?

Taut bands seem to represent areas in which:

- muscle fibers in circumscribed areas seem to be undergoing physiological contracture
- sarcoplasmic reticulum may have been 'damaged', releasing calcium ions and activating actin-myosin contractile mechanisms in contiguous muscle fiber sarcomeres
- there is evolution of ischemia and accumulation of metabolites, which leads to persistent vasoconstriction reflex response
- depletion of ATP prevents calcium from being returned to repository, so maintaining sarcomere shortening
- there are other factors yet to be identified which maintain calcium concentrations.

• A general thickening in the central portion of the muscle's belly will usually soften when a broad general pressure is applied by using a broad pincer compression (finger pads).

• A more specific compression of individual fibers is possible by using the more precise pincer compression using the tips of the digits or by using flat palpation against underlying structures, both of which methods entrap specific bands of tissue.

• The presence of underlying structures, including neurovascular courses which might be impinged or compressed and sharp surfaces such as foraminal gutters, will determine whether pincer compression or flat palpation is appropriate. Sometimes either can be used.

• Compression techniques between fingers and thumb have the advantage of offering information from two or more of the examiner's digits simultaneously, whereas flat palpation against underlying tissues offers a more solid and stable background against which to assess the tissue.

• Additionally, the tissue can be rolled between fingers and thumb to assess quality, density, fluidity and other characteristics which may offer information to the discerning touch.

• Tendons should be disregarded when looking for central trigger points with the fiber's actual length being considered. For example, the tendon of either biceps brachii head is not included when assessing for central trigger points in this muscle. Only the length of the belly of the muscle is considered, which places the predictable zone of central trigger point location much further distally on the upper arm than it would be if the tendon's length were included.

• Muscles with tendinous inscriptions (tendinous bands traversing muscles which divide them into sections, such as occurs in rectus abdominis) will have an endplate zone within each section.

• The fiber arrangement of all underlying and overlying tissues should be considered when approaching layers of muscles with manual assessment so as to include all of them.

Additional palpation skills may be used to discover the presence of trigger points, facilitated tissue and myofascial restrictions. These skills require practice before accuracy is reliable; however, once developed, they are clinically valuable. They include (Chaitow 1996a):

• off-body scan (manual thermal diagnosis), which offers evidence of variations in local circulation, probably resulting from variations in tone, as well as factors such as inflammation and ischemia. Trigger point activity is likely in areas of greatest 'difference'
• movement of skin on fascia – resistance to easy gliding of skin on fascia indicates general locality of reflexogenic activity, i.e. possible trigger point (Lewit

1992) and can indicate lymphatic congestion which may be contributing to the etiology
• local loss of skin elasticity – can refine localization of site of trigger points, as can
• extremely light single-digit stroking, which seeks to locate a 'drag' sensation (evidence of increased hydrosis in and under the skin), which offers pinpoint accuracy of location
• digital pressure (angled rather than perpendicular) into the suspected tissues seeks confirmation of active trigger or latent trigger points (Kuchera & McPartland 1997).

Trigger point deactivation possibilities, which will be examined in later sections of this book, include (Chaitow 1996b, Kuchera & McPartland 1997):

• inhibitory soft tissue techniques (also called ischemic compression or trigger point pressure release) including neuromuscular therapy/massage
• chilling techniques (cryospray, ice)
• acupuncture, injection, etc. (dry or wet needling)
• positional release methods
• muscle energy (stretch) techniques
• myofascial release methods
• combination sequences such as integrated neuromuscular inhibition technique (INIT; Chapter 9)
• correction of associated somatic dysfunction possibly involving high-velocity thrust (HVT) adjustments and/or osteopathic or chiropractic mobilization methods
• education and correction of contributory and perpetuating factors (posture, diet, stress, habits, etc.)

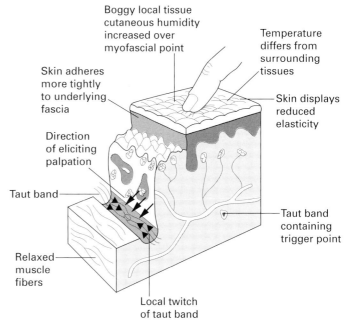

Figure 6.5 Altered physiology of tissues in region of myofascial trigger point.

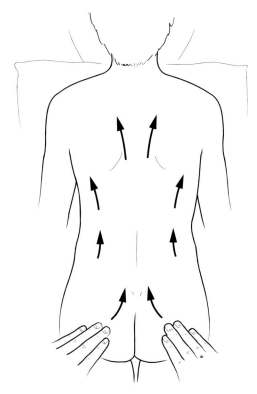

Figure 6.6 Testing skin and fascial mobility bilaterally as local tissues are taken towards the elastic end of range.

- self-help strategies (stretching, hydrotherapy methods, etc.).

Which method is more effective?

Researchers at the Department of Physical Medicine and Rehabilitation, University of California, Irvine, evaluated the immediate benefits of treating an active trigger point in the upper trapezius muscle by comparing four commonly used approaches as well as a placebo treatment (Hong et al 1993). The methods included:

1. ice spray and stretch (Travell & Simons approach)
2. superficial heat applied by a hydrocolator pack (20–30 minutes)
3. deep heat applied by ultrasound (1.2–1.5 watt/cm^2 for 5 minutes)
4. dummy ultrasound (0.0 watt/cm^2)
5. deep inhibitory pressure soft tissue massage (10–15 minutes of modified connective tissue massage and shiatsu/ischemic compression).

Twenty-four patients were selected who had active triggers in the upper trapezius which had been present for not less than 3 months and who had had no previous treatment for these for at least 1 month prior to the study (as well as no cervical radiculopathy or myelopathy, disc or degenerative disease).

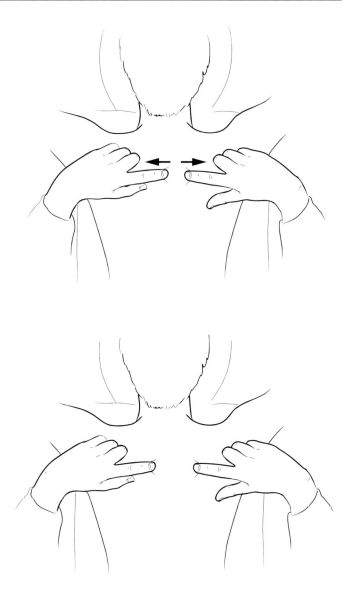

Figure 6.7 Skin elasticity is evaluated by stretching apart to the elastic barrier and comparing with the range of the surrounding skin.

- The pain threshold of the trigger point area was measured using a pressure algometer three times pretreatment and within 2 minutes of treatment.
- The average was recorded on each occasion.
- A control group were similarly measured twice (30 minutes apart) who received no treatment until after the second measurement.
- The results showed that all methods (but not the placebo ultrasound) produced a significant increase in pain threshold following treatment, with the greatest change being demonstrated by those receiving deep pressure treatment (which equates with the methods advocated in neuromuscular therapy).
- The spray and stretch method was the next most efficient in achieving increase in pain threshold.

Box 6.10 Clinical symptoms other than pain as result of trigger point activity (usually in same region as pain appearance) (Kuchera & McPartland 1997)

- Diarrhea, dysmenorrhea
- Diminished gastric motility
- Vasoconstriction and headache
- Dermatographia
- Proprioceptive disturbance, dizziness
- Excessive maxillary sinus secretion
- Localized sweating
- Cardiac arrhythmias (especially pectoralis major triggers)
- Gooseflesh
- Ptosis, excessive lacrimation
- Conjunctival reddening

Box 6.11 Lymphatic dysfunction and trigger point activity

Travell & Simons (1983a) have identified triggers which impede lymphatic function.

- The scalenes (anticus, in particular) can entrap structures passing through the thoracic inlet.
- This is aggravated by 1st rib (and clavicular) restriction (which can be caused by triggers in anterior and middle scalenes).
- Scalene trigger points have been shown to reflexively suppress lymphatic duct peristaltic contractions in the affected extremity.
- Triggers in the posterior axillary folds (subscapularis, teres major, latissimus dorsi) influence lymphatic drainage affecting upper extremities and breasts (Travell & Simons 1992). Similarly, triggers in the anterior axillary fold (pectoralis minor) can be implicated in lymphatic dysfunction affecting the breasts (Zink 1981).

The researchers suggest that:

Perhaps deep pressure massage, if done appropriately, can offer better stretching of the taut bands of muscle fibers than manual stretching because it applies stronger pressure to a relatively small area compared to the gross stretching of the whole muscle. Deep pressure may also offer ischemic compression which [has been shown to be] effective for myofascial pain therapy. (Simons 1989)

When precise palpation and release techniques are combined with elongation of the tissues (stretching), the combination can powerfully release the contractures and teach the person new skills for maintaining the release. Little long-term benefit is derived from the mechanical release alone. At-home stretching, changes in usage and attention to other perpetuating factors will alter the conditions which have helped build the trigger points and help prevent them from recurring.

REFERENCES

American College of Rheumatologists 1990 Criteria for the classification of fibromyalgia. Arthritis and Rheumatism 33:160–172

Awad E 1973 Interstitial myofibrositis. Archives of Physical Medicine 54:440–453

Awad E 1990 Histopathological changes in fibrositis. In: Fricton J, Awad E (eds) Advances in pain research and therapy, vol 17. Raven Press, New York, pp 248–258

Baldry P 1993 Acupuncture, trigger points and musculoskeletal pain. Churchill Livingstone, Edinburgh

Barrell J-P 1996 Manual-thermal diagnosis. Eastland Press, Seattle

Beal M 1983 Palpatory testing of somatic dysfunction in patients with cardiovascular disease. Journal of the American Osteopathic Association 82(11):73–82

Boyle W, Saine A 1988 Naturopathic hydrotherapy. Buckeye Naturopathic Press, East Palestine, Ohio

Bradley D 1999 In: Gilbert C (ed) Breathing retraining advice from three therapists. Journal of Bodywork and Movement Therapies 3(3):159–167

Brewer B 1979 Aging and the rotator cuff. American Journal of Sports Medicine 7:102–110

Bruckle W et al 1990 Gewebe-pO2-Messung in der verspannten Ruckenmuskulatur (erector spinae). Zeitschrift fur Rheumatologie 49:208–216

Burckhardt R 1995 Quoted in Fibromyalgia Network October: p 10

Cailliet R 1991 Shoulder pain. F A Davis, Philadelphia

Chaitow L 1996a Palpation skills. Churchill Livingstone, Edinburgh

Chaitow L 1996b Modern neuromuscular techniques. Churchill Livingstone, Edinburgh

Chaitow L 1999 Fibromyalgia syndrome. Churchill Livingstone, Edinburgh

Chikly B 1996 Lymph drainage therapy study guide level I. UI Publishing, Palm Beach Gardens, FL

Cohen J, Gibbons R 1998 Raymond Nimmo and the evolution of trigger point therapy. Journal of Manipulation and Physiological Therapeutics 21(3):167–172

DeLany J 1999 Stop the cycle of chronic pain with neuromuscular therapy's 6-point system. Massage Magazine 79:54–66

Dexter J, Simons D 1981 Local twitch response in human muscle evoked by palpation and needle penetration of a trigger point. Archives of Physical Medicine and Rehabilitation 62:521–522

Digiesi V et al 1975 Effect of proteinase inhibitor on intermittent claudication. Pain 1:385–389

Fischer A 1988 Documentation of muscle pain and soft tissue pathology. In: Kraus H (ed) Diagnosis and treatment of muscle pain. Quintessence, Chicago

Fishbain D et al 1986 Male and female chronic pain patients categorized. Pain 26:181–197

Fricton J et al 1985 Myofascial pain syndrome of the head and neck. Oral Surgery 6:615–663

Granges G, Littlejohn G 1993 Prevalence of myofascial pain syndrome in fibromyalgia syndrome and regional pain syndrome. Journal of Musculoskeletal Pain 1(2):19–34

Grieve G (ed) 1986 Modern manual therapy. Churchill Livingstone, Edinburgh

Gunn C, Milbrandt W 1978 Early and subtle signs in low back sprain. Spine 3:267–281

Headley B J 1993 Muscle inhibition. Physical Therapy Forum 24 November: 1

Hong C 1996 Difference in pain relief after trigger point injections in myofascial pain patients with and without fibromyalgia. Archives of Physical Medicine and Rehabilitation 77(11):1161–1166

Hong C-Z, Simons D 1992 Remote inactivation of myofascial trigger points by injection of trigger points in another muscle. Scandinavian Journal of Rheumatology 94(suppl):25

Hong C-Z, Chen Y-C, Pon C, Yu J 1993 Immediate effects of various physical medicine modalities on pain threshold of an active myofascial trigger point. Journal of Musculoskeletal Pain 1(2)

Hong C-Z, Chen Y-N, Twehouse D, Hong D 1996 Pressure threshold for referred pain by compression on trigger point and adjacent area. Journal of Musculoskeletal Pain 4(3):61–79

Jonkheere P, Pattyn J 1998 Myofascial muscle chains. Trigger vzw, Brugge, Belgium

Kieschke J et al 1988 Influences of adrenaline and hypoxia on rat muscle receptors. In: Hamman W (ed) Progress in brain research, volume 74. Elsevier, Amsterdam

Korr I 1948 The emerging concept of the osteopathic lesion. Journal of the American Osteopathic Association 48:127–138

Korr I 1976 Spinal cord as organizer of disease process. Academy of Applied Osteopathy Yearbook, Carmel, California

Korr I (ed) 1978 Sustained sympatheticotonia as a factor in disease. In: The neurobiological mechanisms in manipulative therapy. Plenum Press, New York

Kuchera M, McPartland J 1997 Myofascial trigger points. In: Ward R (ed) Foundations of osteopathic medicine. Williams and Wilkins, Baltimore

Kurz I 1986 Textbook of Dr. Vodder's manual lymph drainage, vol 2: therapy, 2nd edn. Karl F Haug, Heidelberg

Lewit K 1992 Manipulative therapy in rehabilitation of the locomotor system. Butterworths, London

Lewis T 1942 Pain. Macmillan, London

Lewis T et al 1931 Observations upon muscular pain in intermittent claudication. Heart 15:359–383

Lowe W W 1995 Orthopedic and sports massage reviews. Orthopedic Massage Education and Research Institute, Bend, Oregon

Melzack R, Wall P 1988 The challenge of pain. Penguin, London

Mense S 1993 Peripheral mechanisms of muscle nociception and local muscle pain. Journal of Musculoskeletal Pain 1(1):133–170

National Board of Chiropractic Economics 1993 Chiropractic treatment procedures, in job analysis of chiropractic (Table 9–11). Greeley, Colorado

Nimmo R 1957 Receptors, effectors and tonus. Journal of the National Chiropractic Association 27(11):21

Nimmo R 1981 Some remarks on the development of receptor–tonus technique. Privately circulated notes

Patterson M 1976 Model mechanism for spinal segmental facilitation. Academy of Applied Osteopathy Yearbook, Carmel, California

Rodbard S 1975 Pain associated with muscular activity. American Heart Journal 90:84–92

Rothstein J et al 1991 Rehabilitation specialists handbook. FA Davis, Philadelphia

Selye H 1974 Stress without distress. Lippincott, Philadelphia

Shealy C N 1984 Total life stress and symptomatology. Journal of Holistic Medicine 6(2):112–129

Simons D 1987 Myofascial pain due to trigger points. Monograph 1, International Rehabilitation Medicine Association, Houston, Texas

Simons D 1988 Myofascial pain syndromes: where are we? Where are we going? Archives of Physical Medicine and Rehabilitation 69:207–211

Simons D 1989 Myofascial pain syndromes. Current Therapy of Pain B.C. Decker Inc pp 251–266

Simons D 1993a Myofascial pain and dysfunction review. Journal of Musculoskeletal Pain 1(2):131

Simons D 1993b Referred phenomena of myofascial trigger points. In: Vecchiet L, Albe-Fessard D, Lindlom U (eds) New trends in referred pain and hyperalgesia. Elsevier, Amsterdam

Simons D, Travell J, Simons L 1998 Myofascial pain and dysfunction: the trigger point manual, vol 1: upper half of body, 2nd edn. Williams and Wilkins, Baltimore

Sola A et al 1951 Incidence of hypersensitive areas in posterior shoulder muscles. American Journal of Physical Medicine 34:585–590

Straus S 1991 History of chronic fatigue syndrome. Review of Infectious Diseases 13:S2–S7

Swerdlow B, Dieter N 1992 Evaluation of thermography. Pain 48:205–213

Travell J, Simons D 1983a Myofascial pain and dysfunction: the trigger point manual, vol 1: upper half of body. Williams and Wilkins, Baltimore

Travell J, Simons D 1983b Low back pain (pt 2). Postgraduate Medicine 73(2):81–92

Travell J, Simons D 1992 Myofascial pain and dysfunction, vol 2. Williams and Wilkins, Baltimore

Tullos H, Bennet J 1984 The shoulder in sports In: Scott W (ed) Principles of sports medicine. Williams and Wilkins, Baltimore

Uchida Y et al 1969 Kininogen and kinin activity during local ischemia in man. Japanese Heart Journal 10:503–508

Van Why R 1994 FMS and massage therapy. Self published

Ward R (ed) 1997 Foundations of osteopathic medicine. Williams and Wilkins, Baltimore

Wiederholt W C 1970 'End-plate noise' in electromyography. Neurology 20:214–224

Wittlinger H, Wittlinger G 1982 Textbook of Dr Vodder's manual lym.ph drainage, vol 1: basic course, 3rd edn. Karl F Haug, Heidelberg

Wolfe F, Simons D 1992 Fibromyalgia and myofascial pain syndromes. Journal of Rheumatology 19(6):944–951

Yunus M 1993 Research in fibromyalgia and myofascial pain syndromes. Journal of Musculoskeletal Pain 1(1):23–41

Zink J 1981 The posterior axillary folds: a gateway for osteopathic treatment of the upper extremities. Osteopathic Annals 9 (3):81–88

7

Inflammation and pain

This chapter focuses on the body's self-regulatory processes which are involved in repair and healing, with particular focus on the role of pain. As practitioners, we are faced with the apparent paradox of recognizing the importance in the healing process of inflammation, and of pain as an alarm signal, and yet being confronted with patients who demand the removal of these (to them) undesirable processes. This calls for an ability to explain and educate the patient as to the 'meaning' of symptoms and being able to modulate these, without suppressing the important roles they often play.

THE INFLAMMATORY RESPONSE

In response to trauma and other abuses, defensive repair processes commence with a primary focus on reorganization and repair of damaged tissues. The coordinated achievement of these processes, influenced by a plethora of biochemical mediators, occurs under the general heading of 'inflammation'.

These homeostatic adaptations usually take place in an orderly manner, although the stages involved can vary quite considerably in temporal terms, depending on the status of the individual and associated conditions (hygiene, for example). The stages of inflammation are known as *acute response (lag) phase*, *regeneration phase* and finally, if all is going well, *remodeling phase*.

The healing process needs to involve capillary repair and new growth, proliferation of fibroblasts, deposition of collagen and scar tissue formation. It is always worth reminding ourselves that inflammatory processes are usually beneficial and have a great healing potential.

Acute (lag) phase of the inflammatory response

The initial acute inflammation response results from tissue injury, which can be on a microscopic cellular level or could involve gross damage. This stage is characterized by initial vasodilation, increased local vascular permeability, tenderness, heat and edema. The way the organism reacts to trauma involves both local and systemic (neuroendocrine) responses. Numerous chemical mediators are involved in these processes, including bradykinin, prostaglandins, leukotrienes, cytokines, oxygen metabolites and enzymes.

During this phase the early repair of injured tissues commences, with damaged or dead cells being replaced. Various cytokines are thought to be intimately involved at this early inflammatory stage, primarily interleukin 1 (IL-1).

In the earliest stages, highly unstable fibrin structures are laid down to secure the damaged tissues (Barlow & Willoughby 1992) and anything which stresses these further (pressure, stretching, etc.) would, in all probability, aggravate and delay the healing process (Wahl 1989). Treatment in the early stages – which can last up to a week – should therefore involve standard rest, ice, compression (bandaging or taping for example) and elevation (RICE), with minimal stress to the tissues being allowed and certainly no active treatment. During the early stages following tissue injury, tensile strength is reduced and, therapeutically speaking, a primary task is to encourage the adaptive healing process by methods which promote early return of adequate tensile strength.

Regeneration phase

Under the influence of biological mediators such as IL-1, collagen synthesis occurs and new collagen fibers are laid down. Hunter (1998) suggests that this is a key time for initiating constructive treatment: 'The tendency for the formation of randomly oriented collagen fibers that restore structure but not function can be reduced by

careful tensioning of the healing tissue during the regeneration phase'. The key objective during this stage is the encouragement of enhanced tensile strength and stability, involving improved functional alignment of collagen fibers.

Remodeling phase

As collagen crosslinkage increases, stability returns but often at the expense of mobility. In order to prevent undue loss of pliability during this phase, treatment which carefully encourages full range of movement is helpful.

An understanding of the properties of connective tissue and fascia allows for the selection of appropriate treatment strategies (see notes on fascia in Chapter 1). Slow deliberate movements which localize tension to the injury site, as precisely as possible, are considered useful at this stage.

Difference between degenerative and inflammatory processes

Hunter, quoted above, makes a clear distinction between many conditions previously labeled as inflammatory which are, in fact, degenerative. In such conditions there may be scant evidence of the beneficial influences of inflammation. This 'mistaken identity' may occur, he notes, in Achilles tendinitis and patella tendinitis, a view which is evidence based (Kannus 1997).

'Evidence … suggests that degenerative tendon changes are evident in one third of the healthy urban population aged 35 or more.' Hunter reports that, at biopsy, degenerative changes (e.g. calcifying tendinopathy) may be found and that, without inflammation, there will be no stimulus to healing.

Treatment which deliberately mildly inflames the structure may, in such cases, be seen to offer a therapeutic stimulus. Controlled friction carefully applied to such structures could induce a mild inflammatory response and assist in achieving this. Methods such as crossfiber friction, as advocated by Cyriax (1962), would be selectively useful in such settings.

MUSCLES AND PAIN

Where pain exists in tense musculature (in the absence of other pathology), Barlow (1959) suggests that it results from:

- the muscle itself through some noxious metabolic product ('factor P') (Lewis 1942) or an interference in blood circulation due to spasm, resulting in relative ischemia
- the muscular insertion into the periosteum, such as that caused by an actual lifting of the periosteal tissue as a result of marked or repetitive muscular

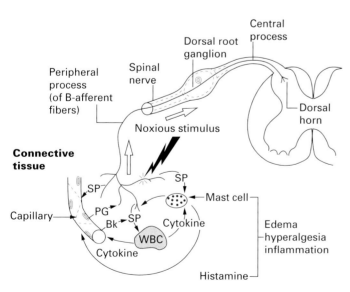

Figure 7.1 Schematic representation of neurogenic inflammation cascade. Key: SP=substance P; PG=prostaglandins; Bk=bradykinin.

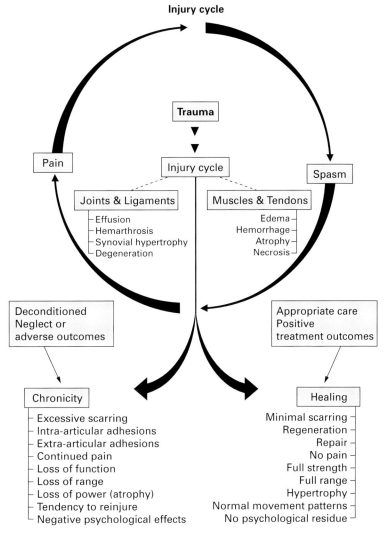

Figure 7.2 Schematic representation of the injury cycle.

tension dragging on the attachment and causing periosteal pain points (Lewit 1992)

- the joint, which can become restricted and overapproximated, to the extent that osteoarthritic changes can result from the repeated microtrauma of shortened and unbalanced soft tissue structures
- overapproximation of joint surfaces due to soft tissue shortening can also lead to uneven wear and tear, as for example when the tensor fascia lata structure shortens and crowds both the hip and lateral knee joint structures
- neural irritation, which can be produced spinally or along the course of the nerve, as a result of chronic muscular contractions. These can involve disc and general spinal mechanical faults (Korr 1976)
- variations in pain threshold (possibly to do with perception (Melzack 1983)), which can make all these factors more or less significant and obvious.

Baldry (1993) describes the progression of normal muscle to one which is in painful, chronic distress as commonly involving:

- initial or repetitive trauma (strain or excessive use) leading to
- release of chemical substances such as bradykinin, prostaglandins, histamine, serotonin and potassium ions
- subsequent sensitization of A-delta and C (Group IV) sensory nerve fibers with involvement of the brain (limbic system and the frontal lobe).

Liebenson (1996) has outlined the current understanding of pain in the spectrum of musculoskeletal dysfunction. He notes: 'The literature shows that prolonged or intense pain can lead to both psychological (abnormal illness behavior) and neurological (dorsal horn sensitization) consequences'.

We can see in this example a manifestation of an adaptive response by the nervous system, as well as the mind of the individual, to a long-standing stressor, pain. In the sequence that follows, Liebenson is describing pain associated with a spinal strain but the model holds true elsewhere. These features are, he believes, at 'the heart of the transition from an acute to a chronic pain syndrome'.

- Adaptation occurs to a painful event involving altered biomechanics.
- The demands on local functional capacity may be exceeded by such changes, leading to tissue fatigue, as the processes of hysteresis and creep evolve (see Chapter 1 on fascia, for details of these phenomena).
- In order to maintain accurate proprioception, type I and type II afferents are stimulated.
- The firing from muscle spindle, joint mechano-receptor and Golgi tendon organ afferents helps the adapting tissues avoid failure.
- These receptors are adaptive and therefore cease to discharge if the adaptation process continues for a lengthy period.
- Ultimately, however, as in all stress situations, adaptive capacity is exhausted and a painful, chronic, situation slowly emerges.
- At this stage, inflammatory processes commence (see more detail on inflammation later in this chapter) as does stimulation of non-adaptive types III and IV nociceptive afferents leading to protective mechanisms which immobilize the area.
- Immobilization is appropriate in acute injury situations but can become memorized and influence the evolution towards chronic behavior.

Liebenson (1996) summarizes:

Acute pain involves biomechanical insult (injury, repetitive strain), biochemical mediation (inflammation), facilitation of algesic pathways, and, finally, neuromuscular adaptation. If repetitive biomechanical insult is not avoided, abnormal illness behavior is present, or deconditioning occurs, resulting in inadequate neuromuscular adaptation, then chronic pain with central nervous system involvement (corticalization) can be expected.

Rehabilitation from the adverse effects of such a pain cycle requires the individual to be actively involved in understanding and modifying the processes involved, which might include:

- altering sources of external biomechanical overload (posture, habits of use in daily life including work and leisure activities, etc.)
- cognition and modification of abnormal illness behavior
- improvement of normal function via self-applied strengthening, stretching, fitness training, balance and coordination-enhancing strategies.

As these patterns are appropriately being addressed, functional rehabilitation of the motor system, through appropriate treatment and exercise, should be ongoing. When reading the sections of this book which focus most on the treatment aspects of neuromuscular pain and dysfunction, the reader should bear in mind the essential need for the person's active participation in the recovery process.

Reflex effects of muscular pain

Liebenson (1996) highlights the fact that muscular pain produces not just increased stiffness and tension but inhibition as well. He quotes from research that has demonstrated:

- in acute back pain, localized areas of the multifidus muscle show signs of unilateral wasting in association with a single dysfunctional vertebral segment (Hides 1994)
- as a result of chronic back pain, type I multifidus fibers (postural) hypertrophy on the symptomatic side, while type II fibers (phasic) atrophy bilaterally (Stokes 1992)
- reciprocal inhibition occurs in the abdominal muscles when erector spinae are excessively 'stiff' and they become spontaneously stronger again (without rehabilitation exercises) when the overactive erector spinae are stretched (Janda 1978).
- Myofascial trigger points in upper trapezius inhibit the functional activity of the lower trapezius muscle (Headley 1993)
- deltoid inhibition occurs as a result of myofascial trigger point activity in the supraspinatus muscle (Simons 1993).

SOURCE OF PAIN

Is it reflex or local?

Palpation of an area that the person reports to be painful will produce increased sensitivity or tenderness if the pain is originating from that area. If, however, palpation produces no such increase in sensitivity, then the chances are strong that the pain is being referred from elsewhere.

But where is it coming from? If the pain is indeed coming from a myofascial trigger point, knowledge of the distribution patterns of probable trigger point target zones (see Chapter 6) can allow for a swift focusing on suitable sites to search for an offending trigger. Unless the pattern is a result of combinations of several trigger point referrals, the patterns distributed by trigger points are fairly predictable and well documented by research (Simons et al 1998).

Radicular pain

The discomfort could, however, be a radicular symptom

coming from the spine. 'When pain is being referred into a limb due to a spinal problem, the greater the pain distally from the source, the greater the index of difficulty in applying quickly successful treatment', suggests Grieve (1984).

Dvorak & Dvorak (1984) state: 'For patients with acute radicular syndrome there is little diagnostic difficulty, which is not the case for patients with chronic back pain. Some differentiation for further therapy is especially important, although not always simple'. Noting that a mixed clinical picture is common, they then say: 'when testing for the radicular syndrome, particular attention is to be paid to the motor disturbances and the deep tendon reflexes. When examining sensory radicular disorders, the attention should be towards the algesias'.

Dvorak & Dvorak have charted a multitude of what they term 'spondylogenic reflexes' which derive primarily from intervertebral joints. The palpated changes are characterized as:

Painful swellings, tender upon pressure and detachable with palpation, located in the musculofascial tissue in topographically well-defined sites. The average size varies from 0.5 cm to 1 cm and the main characteristic is the absolutely timed and qualitative linkage to the extent of the functionally abnormal position (segmental dysfunction). As long as a disturbance exists, the zones of irritation can be identified, yet disappear immediately after the removal of the disturbance.

In this form of dysfunction, the joint (segment of the spine) is seen to be the maintaining factor in a soft tissue manifestation of pain. However, Dvorak & Dvorak also see altered mechanics in a vertebral unit as causing 're-flexogenic pathological change of the soft tissue, the most important being the "myotendinoses", which can be identified by palpation'. Many experts, including Lewit, cited above, would argue that soft tissue changes frequently precede the altered vertebral states, as a result perhaps of poor posture and patterns of overuse. 'It is in chronic pain patients that mobility of fascia is frequently impaired; in such cases, joint (spinal) mobility is as a rule restored by moving the fascia. It also follows that unless we restore normal mobility of the fascia, muscle and joint dysfunction will recur' (Lewit 1996).

The reader may reflect on the fact that, in these examples, the same phenomena are being observed (pain and joint dysfunction) and quite different interpretations as to cause and effect are being ascribed. Do the soft tissues determine and maintain the joint restriction and the pain that follows? Or does the joint restriction produce and maintain the soft tissue changes and the pain that follows? Or are both elements (joint and soft tissue) so intermeshed in their functional roles that this separation is artificial? The authors of this text take the view, based on clinical experience, that the soft tissues hold the primary role most of the time, but not always.

Are the reflexes normal? What is the source of the pain?

The referred pain may not be from either a trigger or the spine itself. Kellgren (1938, 1939) showed that: 'The superficial fascia of the back, the spinous processes and the supraspinous ligaments induce local pain upon stimulation, while stimulation of the superficial portions of the interspinous ligaments and the superficial muscles results in a diffused (more widespread) type of pain'.

Clearly ligaments and fascia must therefore also be considered as sources of referred pain and this is made clearer by Brugger (1960), who describes a number of syndromes in which altered arthromuscular components produce reflexogenic pain. These syndromes are attributed to painfully stimulated tissues (origins of tendons, joint capsules and so on) producing pain in muscles, tendons and overlying skin.

As an example, irritation and increased sensitivity in the region of the sternum, clavicles and rib attachments to the sternum, through occupational or postural strain, will cause pain in the intercostal muscles, scalenes, sternocleidomastoid, pectoralis major and cervical muscles. The increased tone in these muscles and the resultant stresses that they produce may lead to spondylogenic problems in the cervical region, with further spread of symptoms. Overall, this syndrome can produce chronic pain in the neck, head, chest wall, arm and hand (even mimicking heart disease) (Brugger 1960).

Neuropathic pain (Corderre 1993, Merskey 1988, Nachemson 1992)

The concept of sensitization and facilitation has been discussed in Chapter 6. A similar but more complex mechanism is proposed by those researchers and clinicians who advocate the view that neuropathic pain plays a major part in many chronic pain syndromes. This involves increased sensitization of nerve cells as a cause of persistent regional pain and associated symptoms and is seen to explain the pain of many people who have previously had a psychological etiology ascribed to their conditions (Corderre 1993, Merskey 1988, Nachemson 1992). Most manual therapists must have been consulted by patients whose symptoms have been labeled 'psychosomatic' in orgin and who have noted and successfully treated musculoskeletal (i.e. structural or functional) dysfunction. The ascribing of a psychological etiology to a biomechanical problem is not necessarily inaccurate, but it may be, and the neuropathic hypothesis offers a different view on chronic pain which could, in a different setting, attract a psychological diagnosis.

It is believed, by the proponents of this perspective, that following biomechanical stress (overuse, etc.) a *sustained* degree of normal neurological input (from types III and

IV mechanoreceptors, for example) to the dorsal horn neurons can sensitize the nerve cells and decrease their threshold to pain. Once sensitized, a situation of allodynia evolves, in which the pain threshold is lowered so that stimuli which would previously not be perceived as painful, such as normal physiological movement or light touch, become painful. If this occurs the affected areas will have become hyperalgesic.

As part of this process, which involves central mis-processing of received information, there may be a degree of cutaneous hypoasthesia in which, for example, pinprick sensations will be noted as reduced. The neuropathic pain pattern will usually also include poor motor control, malcoordination and balance control ('Can you stand on one leg with eyes closed for 10 seconds?'). There is also a strong likelihood of referred pain from associated myofascial trigger points. In such a situation palpation of superficial tissues will demonstrate the classic increase in sympathetic activity described in Chapter 6, including greater superficial hydrosis, reduced skin elasticity and tighter adherence of skin to underlying fascia. The reader may reflect on the degree of similarity and overlap between this neuropathic view of chronic pain etiology and the osteopathic facilitation concept, discussed in Chapter 6. There is also a degree of similarity with Nimmo's (Cohen & Gibbons 1998) and Travell & Rinzler's (1952) views on the way myofascial trigger points evolve, as well as chiropractic subluxation ideas and research evidence relating to zygapophyseal pain sources (Bogduk & Twomey 1991).

Differentiating between soft tissue and joint pain

Several simple screening tests have been proposed by Kaltenborn (1980).

1. Does passive stretching (traction) of the painful area increase the level of pain? If so, it is probably of soft tissue origin (extraarticular).

2. Does compression of the painful area increase the pain? If so, it is probably of joint origin (intraarticular) involving tissues belonging to that anatomical joint.

3. If active (controlled by the person) movement in one direction produces pain (and/or is restricted), while passive (controlled by the operator) movement in the opposite direction also produces pain (and/or is restricted), the contractile tissues (muscle, ligament, etc.) are implicated. Resisted movement tests, the principles of which are described below, can confirm the accuracy of this proposal.

4. If active movement and passive movement in the same direction produce pain (and/or restriction), joint dysfunction is probable. This can be confirmed by use of traction and compression (and gliding) of the joint.

Resisted tests are used to assess both strength of, and painful responses to, muscle contraction. These tests involve producing a *maximal* contraction of the suspected muscle while the joint is kept immobile, somewhere near the middle of its range. No joint motion should be allowed to occur during the contraction. If it is painful, contractile tissues are implicated in the painful problem.

These resisted tests are done after test 3 (described above) to confirm a soft tissue dysfunction rather than a joint involvement. Before performing the resisted test, it is wise to perform the compression test (2 above) to clear any suspicion of joint involvement.

Cyriax (1962) adds to this the following thoughts.

- If, on resisted testing, the muscle seems strong and is also painful, there is no more than a minor lesion/dysfunction of the muscle or its tendon.
- If it is weak and painful, there is a more serious lesion/dysfunction of the muscle or tendon.
- If it is weak and painless, there may be a neurological lesion or the tendon has ruptured.
- A normal muscle tests strong and pain free.

It is suggested that all these statements be tested on conditions of known etiology.

In many instances soft tissue dysfunction accompanies (precedes or follows) joint dysfunction. Joint involvement is less likely in the early stages of soft tissue dysfunction than (for example) in the chronic stages of muscle shortening. It is hard to conceive of joint conditions, acute or chronic, without accompanying soft tissue involvement. The tests described above will offer a strong indication as to whether the major involvement in such a situation is of soft tissue or osseous in nature.

Examples of a joint assessment involving compression are described by Blower & Griffin (1984) for sacroiliac dysfunction. They showed that pressure applied over the lower half of the sacrum or over the anterior superior iliac spines were diagnostic of sacroiliac problems (possibly indicating ankylosing spondylitis) if pain was produced in the sacrum and buttocks. Soft tissue dysfunction would not produce painful responses with this type of compression test.

Note: Lumbar pain is not significant if it occurs on sacral pressure, as this action causes movement of the lumbosacral joint, as well as some motion throughout the whole lumbar spine.

WHEN SHOULD PAIN AND DYSFUNCTION BE LEFT ALONE?

Splinting (spasm) can occur as a defensive, protective, involuntary phenomenon associated with trauma (fracture, for instance) or pathology (osteoporosis, secondary bone tumors, neurogenic influences, etc.)(Simons et al 1998). Splinting-type spasm commonly differs from more common forms of spasm because it releases when the tissues it is protecting or immobilizing are placed at rest. When splinting is long term, secondary problems may arise in associated joints as a result (e.g. contractures) and bone (e.g. osteoporosis). Travell & Simons (1983) note that, 'Muscle-splinting pain is usually part of a complex process. Hemiplegic and brain-injured patients do identify pain that depends on muscle spasm'. They also note 'a degree of masseteric spasm which may develop to relieve strain in trigger points in its parallel muscle, the temporalis', which suggests that spasm is sometimes a way of relieving overload elsewhere.

Travell & Simons (1983) also note a similar phenomenon in low back pain.

In patients with low back pain and with tenderness to palpation of the paraspinal muscles, the superficial layer tended to show less than a normal amount of EMG activity until the test movement became painful. Then these muscles showed increased motor unit activity or 'splinting' … This observation fits the concept of normal muscles 'taking over' (protective spasm) to unload and protect a parallel muscle that is the site of significant trigger point activity.

Recognition of this sort of spasm in soft tissues is a matter of training and intuition. Whether attempts should be made to release, or relieve, what appears to be protective spasm depends on understanding the reasons for its existence. If splinting is the result of a cooperative attempt to unload a painful but not pathologically compromised structure, then treatment is obviously appropriate to ease the cause of the original need to protect and support. If, on the other hand, spasm or splinting is indeed protecting the structure it surrounds (or supports) from movement and further (possibly) serious damage, then it should clearly be left alone. Experience alone can assist in differentiating between this sort of cooperative spasm and the board-like rigidity of spasm associated with, say, osteoporosis. It is safe to caution that if any doubt exists, the spasm should be left intact.

Somatization

It is entirely possible for musculoskeletal symptoms to represent an unconscious attempt by the person to entomb their emotional distress. As noted in the segment on emotion and musculoskeletal distress (see Chapter 4) and most cogently expressed by Philip Latey (1996), pain and dysfunction may have psychological distress as its root cause. The person may be somatizing this distress and presenting with apparently somatic problems. The earlier discussion relating to neuropathic pain suggested that sometimes a misattribution occurs as to the cause of pain being 'psychosomatic'. This should not lead the practitioner to ignore the fact that some very real and intense somatic pain involves roots in the psyche of the individual.

How is one to know?

Karel Lewit (1992) suggests that, 'In doubtful cases the physical and psychological components will be distinguished during the treatment, when repeated comparison of (changing) physical signs and the patient's own assessment of them will provide objective criteria'. In the main, he suggests, if the patient is able to give a fairly precise description and localization of his pain, we should be reluctant to regard it as 'merely psychological'.

In masked depression, Lewit suggests, the reported symptoms may be of vertebral pain, particularly involving the cervical region, with associated muscle tension and 'cramped' posture. The practitioner may be alerted by abnormal responses during the course of treatment to the fact that there may be something other than biomechanical causes of the problem. The history should also provide clues, especially if this is a 'thick file' individual, someone who has consulted many people before yourself. In particular, Lewit notes that, 'The most important symptom [associated with psychological distress] is disturbed sleep. Characteristically, the patient falls asleep normally but wakes within a few hours and cannot get back to sleep'.

If a masked depression is treated appropriately the vertebrogenic pain will clear up rapidly, he states. Pain and dysfunction can be masking major psychological distress. Awareness of if, how and when to crossrefer should be part of the responsible practitioner's skills base.

Becker (1996) informs us that somatizers may go years without an adequate diagnosis, with misdiagnosis being:

the inevitable precursor to prolonged and ineffective treatment, and frequently to multiple and inappropriate chemical, electrical and imaging studies; inappropriate medications, including narcotics (which frequently compound the problem); or, worse yet, to invasive procedures, including surgical intervention.

He reports that, 'Depressed and otherwise psychologically unwell persons frequently do not recognize the psychological nature of their problem. In fact they usually deny vehemently any psychological or emotional dimension to their clinical picture … [this] makes them particularly difficult to treat'.

Becker adds the important clue to recognizing somatizers, who need a special degree of help, not necessarily relating directly to their musculoskeletal symptoms: 'Certain individuals, emotionally shortchanged or scarred during their formative years, evidence a proclivity to somatize in the face of stressful untoward events and circumstances of adult life, especially ones that awaken untoward feelings buried in the unconscious and rooted in the past' (Becker 1991).

How are you to recognize such a patient? An abbreviated list of Becker's suggested 'red flags' is as follows.

In the history look for:

- vague and implausible history

- symptoms which proliferate and link different body areas
- highly emotionally charged descriptors (searing, blinding, cruel, etc.)
- hyperbole ('I couldn't move')
- discrepancies (patient reports 'cannot sit' but sits for duration of interview)
- passivity (e.g. acceptance of disabled status)
- evidence of deconditioning, weight gain and/or increased use of narcotic medication.

Psychosocial issues:

- apportioning of blame for financial or employment or personal problems to external sources
- feelings kept internally
- tearfulness during interview
- denial of link between symptoms and emotional status.

Mood disturbances:

- anger directed at employer or doctors may be displaced anger at parents
- failure of reasonable treatments – patient may report worsening symptoms to bewilderment of practitioner
- practitioner may start feeling anger towards patient (countertransference)
- 'emotional hunger' may be masked by increased weight gain and use of pain-relieving medication.

Examination findings:

- theatrical presentation (excessive limp, unnecessary use of walking stick, often in wrong hand, etc.)
- non-anatomic sensory findings (accentuating the need for careful testing)
- non-anatomic motor findings such as suboptimal grip attempts (accentuating the need for careful testing)
- inappropriate response to tests such as palpation and percussion, especially if practitioner's hand is pushed away in an exaggerated manner.

But, despite the importance of the warnings suggested by Becker and others, it is as well to remember that a great many people with bodywide pain and virtual disability do indeed have musculoskeletal (or associated) conditions and that their psychological distress derives directly from the pain and disability they suffer. The truth is that we should not make a hard demarcation between 'mind' and 'body' as origins of pain. This has been the folly of much medical practice in the past, although ever more apparent is a recognition of the need to deal with the whole person. If, as we know, psychological factors can influence the body (soma) then the reverse is patently true and it may well be that as part of the rehabilitation of someone with chronic pain and psychological distress,

appropriate bodywork can contribute towards recovery. What is needed, though, is a recognition that the emotional side needs skillful expert attention, just as much as do the somatic manifestations of dysfunction.

PAIN MANAGEMENT
Gunn's view

Pain expert Dr C Chan Gunn (1983) observes that pain management is simplified when it is realized that following injury, three sequential stages may be noted.

1. Immediate – a perception of noxious input which is transient unless tissue damage is sufficient to cause the next stage.
2. Inflammation – during which time algesic substances are released which sensitize higher threshold receptors, followed by
3. Chronic phase – where there may be persistent nociception (or prolonged inflammation). Hyperalgesia may exist where normally non-noxious stimuli are rendered excessive due to hypersensitive receptors.

Close similarities can be observed between facilitation concepts as outlined in Chapter 6, the neuropathic concept outlined above and the sequence described by Gunn.

Questions

During palpation and evaluation, questions need to be asked.

- Which of this person's symptoms, whether of pain or other forms of dysfunction, are the result of reflexogenic activity such as trigger points or possibly of spondylogenic or neuropathic origin?
- What palpable, measurable, identifiable evidence connects what we can observe, test and palpate to the symptoms (pain, restriction, fatigue, etc.) of this person?
- Is there evidence of a psychogenic influence to the person's complaint?
- And what, if anything, can be done to remedy or modify the situation, safely and effectively?

Pain control

Elimination of myofascial trigger points and inhibition of pain transmission is possible via a number of approaches, some pharmaceutical, some surgical, some electrical, some hydrotherapeutic and some manual (Jerome 1997).

- Local anesthetics (nerve blocks such as procaine, etc.).
- Neurolytic blocks which destroy small-fiber afferent

Box 7.1 Placebo power

If someone believes a form of treatment will relieve pain, it will do so far more effectively than if the belief is that the treatment cannot help. In trials involving over 1000 people suffering from chronic pain, dummy medication reduced the levels of the pain by at least 50% of that achieved by *any* form of pain-killing drug, including aspirin and morphine (Melzack & Wall 1989).

Melzack & Wall (1989) explain, 'This shows clearly that the psychological context – particularly the physician's and patient's expectations – contains powerful therapeutic value in its own right in addition to the effect of the drug itself'.

Placebo facts

- Placebos are far more effective against severe pain than mild pain.
- Placebos are more effective in people who are severely anxious and stressed than in people who are not, suggesting that the 'antianxiety' effect of placebos accounts for at least part of the reason for their usefulness.
- Placebos work best against headache-type pain (over 50% effectiveness).
- In about a third of all people, most pains are relieved by placebo.
- A placebo works more effectively if injected, rather than if taken by mouth.
- Placebos work more powerfully if accompanied by the suggestion that they are indeed powerful and that they will rapidly produce results.
- Placebos which are in capsule or tablet form work better if two are taken rather than one.
- Large capsules work as placebos more effectively than do small ones.
- Red placebos are most effective of all in helping pain problems.
- Green placebos help anxiety best.
- Blue placebos are the most sedative and calming.
- Yellow placebos are best for depression and pink are the most stimulating.
- Placebos have been shown to be effective in a wide variety of conditions including anorexia, depression, skin diseases, diarrhea and palpitation.
- Placebo effects do not only occur when taking something by mouth or injection; for example, any form of treatment from manipulation to acupuncture to surgery carries with it a degree of placebo effect.

Recognition of the placebo effect allows us to realize the importance of the power of suggestion on all of us, with some people being more influenced than others. It is essential that we should not think that because a placebo 'works' in an individual that the person is not genuinely suffering pain or that the reported relief is false (Millenson 1995).

A person's attitudes and emotions can be seen to be powerful aids (or hindrances) to recovery. The feelings of hope and expectation of improvement, coupled with a relationship with caring helpers, professional or otherwise, assist in recovery and coping.

tissue and therefore interfere with pain transmission (e.g. facet rhizotomy – thermocauterization which eliminates small-fiber afferent activity).

- Dry needling which inhibits ascending pain pathway transmission.
- Hot packs which increase blood flow (at least temporarily; hot followed by cold would be more effective), reducing nociceptive metabolites and decreasing segmental reflexes and sympathetic tone.
- Ice or cold sprays (ethyl chloride) which increase small-fiber activity, flooding afferent pathways and causing brainstem inhibition of nociceptive input from trigger area.
- TENS, which is thought to achieve its pain-reducing effects via:
  1. preferential activation of large myelinated fibers interfering with pain perception and increasing tolerance
  2. local axonal fatigue reducing small-fiber activity and therefore pain input
  3. activating descending inhibitory influences including opioid release.
- Vibration which differentially stimulates large proprioceptive afferent fibers interfering with pain perception.
- Direct inhibitory pressure (as used in neuromuscular therapy) which offers a combination of influences including:
  1. mechanical (stretching shortened myofascial fibers)
  2. circulatory enhancement when ischemic compression is released
  3. neurological influence via mechanoreceptors inhibiting pain transmission
  4. endorphin and enkephalin release
  5. and, possibly, energetic influences.
- Restoration of normal physiological (using manual methods) and psychological function, including:
  1. reeducation (e.g. cognitive behavior modification – see Chapter 8)
  2. comprehensive management of associated musculoskeletal dysfunction patterns (including HVT, mobilization/articulation together with trigger point deactivation, soft tissue stretching and/or strengthening, using NMT, MET, PRT, MFR and massage)
  3. rehabilitation and self-care – breathing, posture, etc.

In the next chapter, the focus turns to treatment methods and how selection of the most appropriate therapeutic approaches demands the systematic use of sound observation and assessment protocols.

REFERENCES

Baldry P 1993 Acupuncture, trigger points and musculoskeletal pain. Churchill Livingstone, London

Barlow T, Willoughby J 1992 Pathophysiology of soft tissue repair. British Medical Bulletin 48(3):698–711

Barlow W 1959 Anxiety and muscle tension pain. British Journal of Clinical Practice 13(5)

Becker G 1991 Chronic pain. Depression and the injured worker. Psychiatric Annals 21(1):391–404

Becker G 1996 Psychosocial factors in chronic pain. In: Liebenson C (ed) Rehabilitation of the spine. Williams and Wilkins, Baltimore

Blower A, Griffin B 1984 Annals of Rheumatic Disease 43:192–195

Bogduk N, Twomey L 1991 Clinical anatomy of the lumbar spine, 2nd edn. Churchill Livingstone, Edinburgh

Brugger A 1960 Pseudoradikulare syndrome. Acta Rheumatologica 18:1

Cohen J, Gibbons R 1998 Raymond Nimmo and the evolution of trigger point therapy. Journal of Manipulation and Physiological Therapeutics 21(3):167–172

Corderre T 1993 Contribution of central neuroplasticity to pathological pain. Pain 52:259

Cyriax J 1962 Textbook of orthopaedic medicine, vol 1: soft tissue lesions. Cassell, London

Dvorak J, Dvorak V 1984 Manual medicine: diagnostics. Georg Thieme. Verlag, New York

Grieve G 1984 Mobilisation of the spine. Churchill Livingstone, Edinburgh

Gunn C C 1983 Three phases of pain. Acupuncture and Electro Therapeutics 8(3/4):334

Headley B 1993 Muscle inhibition. Physical Therapy Forum, November 1: 24–26

Hides J 1994 Evidence of lumbar multifidus muscles wasting ipsilateral to symptoms in patients with acute/subacute back pain. Spine 19:165

Hunter G 1998 Specific soft tissue mobilization in management of soft tissue dysfunction. Manual Therapy 3(1):2–11

Janda V 1978 Muscles, central nervous motor regulation and back problems. In: Korr I (ed) Neurobiological mechanisms in manipulative therapy. Plenum Press, New York

Jerome J 1997 Pain management. In: Ward R (ed) Foundations of osteopathic medicine. Williams and Wilkins, Baltimore

Kaltenborn F 1980 Mobilization of the extremity joints. Olaf Novlis Bokhandel, Oslo

Kannus O 1997 Tendon pathology: basic science and clinical applications. Sports Exercise and Injury 3:62–75

Kellgren J 1938 Observation of referred pain arising from muscles. Clinical Science 3:175

Kellgren J 1939 On the distribution of pain arising from deep somatic structures. Clinical Science 4:35

Korr I 1976 Spinal cord as organiser of the disease process. Academy of Applied Osteopathy Yearbook, Carmel, California

Latey P 1996 Feelings, muscles and movement. Journal of Bodywork and Movement Therapies 1(1):44–52

Lewis T 1942 Pain. Macmillan, New York

Lewit K 1992 Manipulative therapy in rehabilitation of the locomotor system. Butterworths, London

Lewit K 1996 Role of manipulation in spinal rehabilitation. In: Liebenson C (ed) Rehabilitation of the spine. Williams and Wilkins, Baltimore

Liebenson C 1996 Integrating rehabilitation into chiropractic practice. In: Liebenson C (ed) Rehabilitation of the spine. Williams and Wilkins, Baltimore

Melzack R 1983 The challenge of pain. Penguin, London

Melzack R, Wall P 1989 Textbook of pain, 2nd edn. Churchill Livingstone, London

Merskey H 1988 Regional pain is rarely hysterical. Archives of Neurology 45:915

Millenson J 1995 Mind matters – psychological medicine in holistic practice. Eastland Press, Seattle

Nachemson A 1992 Newest knowledge of low back pain. Clinical Orthopedics 279:8

Simons D 1993 Referred phenomena of myofascial trigger points. In: Vecchiet L (ed) New trends in referred pain and hyperalgesia. Elsevier, Amsterdam

Simons D, Travell J, Simons L 1998 Myofascial pain and dysfunction: the trigger point manual, vol 1, 2nd edn. Williams and Wilkins, Baltimore

Stokes M 1992 Selective changes in multifidus dimensions in patients with chronic low back pain. European Spine Journal 1:38

Travell J, Rinzler S 1952 The myofascial genesis of pain. Postgraduate Medicine 11:425

Travell J, Simons D 1983 Myofascial pain and dysfunction: the trigger point manual, vol 1: upper half of body. Williams and Wilkins, Baltimore

Wahl S 1989 Role of growth factors in inflammation and repair. Journal of Cell Biochemistry 40:343–351

8

Assessment, treatment and rehabilitation

In this chapter several interacting influences on health in general, and musculoskeletal dysfunction in particular, will be considered, including biomechanical, biochemical and psychosocial factors. Awareness of the need to consider the range of health influences impacting an individual forms the foundation for sound complementary health care.

As will be noted later in this chapter, this calls for not only attention to the structural and functional patterns associated with pain or dysfunction but also to how well or poorly nourished the individual is; whether or not there may be food intolerances associated with their symptoms; how their beliefs and attitudes impact on their condition and their willingness and ability to undertake a rehabilitation program. It is not within the scope of practice, or skills base, of many practitioners and therapists to handle all such health influences but this should not prevent them being aware of their potential to affect recovery. At the least, advice can be offered regarding sources of information and appropriate professional care. In chronic pain conditions a team approach is often ideal, as will be explained in the notes on cognitive behavior therapy, later in this chapter.

Making sense of what is happening in a body which is adapting to the stresses of life requires a framework (or several frameworks) of evaluation and grids of (relative) normality, against which the person's current status can be measured. This might involve all or any of the following.

- Assessing muscles for strength or weakness.
- Evaluation of relative 'shortness' of muscles.
- Testing range of motion of soft tissues and joints.
- Evaluating for presence, absence or overactivity of neurological reflexes.
- Evaluating for presence of localized, reflexogenically active structures, such as myofascial trigger points or spinal (segmental facilitation) hyperreactivity.
- Assessment of postural (a)symmetry.
- Gait function assessment.

- Evaluating respiratory function.
- Consideration of nutritional and lifestyle influences.
- Awareness of psychosocial influences.

A BIOMECHANICAL EXAMPLE

In the earlier discussion of the upper crossed syndrome (p. 55) we saw an example of a number of these elements of assessment interacting. This particular (upper crossed syndrome) dysfunctional postural pattern included:

- observable postural imbalance, with the head forward of its center of gravity, chin poked forwards, increased cervical lordosis and dorsal kyphosis and rounded shoulder stance
- identifiable shortness in postural muscles of the region, using assessments described in a later chapter
- demonstrable malcoordination between muscles as those which have become hypertonic will be inhibiting their antagonists (e.g. levator scapula tight, serratus anterior weak), as demonstrated by Janda's (1982) functional assessment methods as described in Chapter 5
- the presence of active myofascial trigger points in key predictable sites (for example, upper trapezius, sternocleidomastoid) which can be identified by means of palpation, as described in Chapter 6, and utilizing neuromuscular evaluation palpation methods (modern American and European approaches) described in the clinical applications section of the book
- probable rotator cuff dysfunction due to altered position of glenoid fossa in relation to humerus
- upper thoracic, cervical, atlantooccipital, temporomandibular restrictions or imbalances, which can be evaluated by normal palpation and assessment methods
- altered respiratory function, which can be evaluated using methods described in Chapter 14
- in addition, there may be evidence of emotional or psychosocial factors which might be directly or indirectly linked with the presenting symptoms.

The person's history, as well as the presenting symptoms, should be laid against this accumulation of dysfunctional patterns. When this is done a picture should emerge which suggests a line of action designed to minimize present symptoms, as well as to rehabilitate towards a more normal status. This should also prevent or reduce the likelihood of recurrence.

Unless the cause of the person's problems relates to a specific trauma, the present dysfunctional patterns are likely to represent the body's attempts to adapt to whatever overuse, misuse, abuse and disuse stresses it has been subjected to. Treatment needs to deal with these adaptive changes, as far as is possible, as well as assist

in regaining an awareness of normal function while also evaluating ways of preventing a return to the very patterns which produced the symptoms. If all these elements are not incorporated into treatment, results will be short term at best.

In order to be truly successful, such a program would include:

- attention to soft tissue changes (abnormal tension, fibrosis, etc.) – possibly involving massage, NMT, MET, MFR, PRT and/or articulation/mobilization
- deactivation of myofascial trigger points – possibly involving massage, NMT, MET, MFR, PRT and/or articulation/mobilization
- releasing and stretching the shortened soft tissues – utilizing MFR, MET or other stretching procedures, including yoga
- strengthening weakened structures – involving exercise and rehabilitation methods, such as Pilates
- proprioceptive reeducation – utilizing physical therapy methods (e.g. wobble board) as well as methods such as those devised by Trager (1987), Feldenkrais (1972), Pilates (Knaster 1996), Hanna (1988) and others
- postural and breathing reeducation – using physical therapy approaches as well as Alexander, yoga, tai chi and other similar systems
- ergonomic, nutritional and stress management strategies, as appropriate
- attention to any psychosocial elements which may be factoring into the etiology or maintenance of symptoms
- occupational therapy which specializes in activating healthy coping mechanisms, determining functional capacity, increasing activity that will produce greater 'concordance' than rote exercise and developing adaptive strategies to return the individual to a greater level of self-reliance and quality of life (Lewthwaite 1990).

In evaluating for musculoskeletal imbalances, specific tests and assessments are necessary (see Chapters 9 and 10). Broader views are also useful, such as that previously described in which Tom Myers (1997) suggests 'chains' of soft tissue connections in which the fascial structures are key (see Chapter 1).

'LOOSENESS AND TIGHTNESS' AS PART OF THE BIOMECHANICAL MODEL

A different conceptual model is offered by Robert Ward DO (1997). Ward discusses the 'loose–tight' concept as an image required to appreciate three-dimensionality as the body, or part of it, is palpated/assessed. This can involve large or small areas in which interactive asymmetry produces areas, or structures, which are 'tight and loose', relative to each other. Ward illustrates this with the following examples:

- a 'tight' sacroiliac/hip on one side and 'loose' on the other
- a 'tight' SCM and 'loose' scalenes on the same side
- one shoulder area 'tight' and the other 'loose'.

In positional release methodology (strain/counterstrain, functional technique, etc., see Chapters 9 and 10), the terms 'ease' and 'bind' describe similar phenomena. Assessment of 'tethering' of tissues and of the subtle qualities of 'end-feel' in soft tissues and joints is a prerequisite for appropriate treatment being applied, whether this is of a direct or indirect nature or whether it is active or passive. Indeed, the awareness of these features (end-feel, tight/loose, ease/bind) may be the deciding factor as to which therapeutic approaches are introduced and in what sequence.

Ward (1997) states, 'Tightness suggests tethering, while looseness suggests joint and/or soft tissue laxity, with or without neural inhibition'. These barriers (tight and loose) can also be seen to refer to the obstacles which are sought in preparation for direct (toward bind, tightness) and indirect (towards ease, looseness) techniques.

Clinically it is always worth considering whether restriction barriers ought to be released, in case they are offering some protective benefit. As an example, Van Wingerden (1997) reports that both intrinsic and extrinsic support for the sacroiliac joint derives in part from hamstring (biceps femoris) status. Intrinsically, the influence is via the close anatomical and physiological relationship between biceps femoris and the sacrotuberous ligament (they frequently attach via a strong tendinous link). He states, 'Force from the biceps femoris muscle can lead to increased tension of the sacrotuberous ligament in various ways. Since increased tension of the sacrotuberous ligament diminishes the range of sacroiliac joint motion, the biceps femoris can play a role in stabilization of the SIJ' (Van Wingerden 1997; see also Vleeming et al 1989). He also notes that in low back patients forward flexion is often painful as the load on the spine increases. This happens whether flexion occurs in the spine or via the hip joints (tilting of the pelvis). If the hamstrings are tight and short they effectively prevent pelvic tilting. 'In this respect, an increase in hamstring tension might well be part of a defensive arthrokinematic reflex mechanism of the body to diminish spinal load.' If such a state of affairs is long standing the hamstrings (biceps femoris) will shorten (see discussion of the effects of stress on postural muscles in Chapters 4 and 5), possibly influencing sacroiliac and lumbar spine dysfunction. The decision to treat a tight ('tethered') hamstring should therefore take account of why it is tight and consider that in some circumstances it is offering beneficial support to the SIJ or that it is reducing low back stress.

Lewit (1996) and 'loose–tight' thinking

Lewit notes that pain is often noted on the 'loose' side when there is an imbalance in which a joint or muscle (group) on one side of the body differs from the other.

A 'tight and loose complex', i.e. one side is restricted and the other side is hypotonic, is frequently noted. Shifting [Lewit is referring to stretching of fascial structures] is examined and treated in a craniocaudal or caudocranial direction on the back, but it should be assessed and treated in a circular manner around the axis of the neck and the extremities.

Soft tissue treatment and barriers

- MET methods can be utilized to identify the tight bind barrier and, using isometric contractions of agonist or antagonist, attempt directly to push this barrier back or to pass through it.
- Myofascial release (in its direct usage) also addresses its directions of force directly towards the barrier of restriction.
- In contrast, positional release methods seek the indirect, 'ease' or 'loose' barriers. This concept will be made explicit when positional release methods are described in Chapter 10.

Pain and the tight–loose concept

Pain is more commonly associated with tight and bound/tethered structures, which may be due to local overuse/misuse/abuse factors, scar tissue, reflexively induced influences or centrally mediated neural control. When a tight tissue is then asked to either fully contract or fully lengthen, pain is often experienced. Paradoxically, as pointed out by Lewit above, pain is also often noted in the 'loose' rather than the 'tight' areas of the body, which may involve hypermobility and ligamentous laxity at the 'loose' joint or site. These (lax, loose) areas are vulnerable to injury and prone to recurrent dysfunctional episodes (SI joint, TMJ, etc.).

Box 8.1 Tight–loose palpation exercise (Ward 1997)

- Person is supine.
- Practitioner grasps person's wrists.
- A slow movement is made of both arms to full overhead extension as particular focused attention is paid to symmetry of freedom of movement and any sense of restriction commencing at the wrist contact but possibly involving the body as a whole.
- Attention needs to be paid to both *quality* and *amplitude* of the passive movement.
- The same exercise should be performed on each arm independently, as well as simultaneously, while attention is paid to any sensations of restriction and the end-feel associated with it.
- Ward states, 'With practice, variable tension and loads are readily sensed from the hands and wrists into the lumbodorsal fascia and pelvis'.

Myofascial trigger points may develop in either 'tight' or 'loose' structures but usually appear more frequently, and are more stressed, in those which are tethered, restricted or tight. Myofascial trigger points will continue to evolve if the etiological factors which created and/or sustained them are not corrected and, unless the trigger points are deactivated, they will help to sustain the dysfunctional postural patterns which subsequently emerge.

THREE-DIMENSIONAL PATTERNS

Areas of dysfunction will usually involve vertical, horizontal and 'encircling' (also described as crossover, spiral, or 'wrap-around') patterns of involvement. Ward offers a 'typical' wrap-around pattern associated with a tight left low back area (which ends up involving the entire trunk and cervical area) as 'tight' areas evolve to compensate for loose, inhibited areas (or vice versa).

- 'Tightness' in the posterior left hip, SI joint, lumbar erector spinae and lower rib cage.
- 'Looseness' on the right low back.
- Tight lateral and anterior rib cage on the right.
- Tight left thoracic inlet, posteriorly.
- Tight left craniocervical attachments (involving jaw mechanics).

At any given treatment session, as tight areas are freed or loosened, even if only to a degree, inhibiting influences on 'loose' weak areas diminish and allow a return of tone. It is at this time that rehabilitation, proprioceptive and educational patterns of use need to be introduced and practiced by the person, so that what initially 'feels wrong' in terms of posture and usage (proper position and movement) becomes comfortable and starts to feel 'right'.

Methods for restoration of 'three-dimensionally patterned functional symmetry'

1. Identification of patterns of ease/bind–loose/tight in a given body area or the body as a whole. This can emerge from sequential assessment of muscle shortness and restriction or palpation methods, such as those described by Ward (above), or any other comprehensive evaluation of the status of the soft tissues of the body as a whole (Ward 1997).

2. Appropriate methods for release of areas identified as tight, restricted, tethered (possibly involving myofascial release, MET, NMT, PRT, singly or in combination, plus other manual approaches).

3. If joints fail to respond adequately to soft tissue mobilization, the use of articulation/mobilization or high-velocity thrust methods may be incorporated into this sequence as appropriate to the status (age, structural

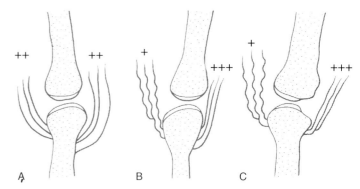

Figure 8.1 Muscular imbalance altering joint mechanics. A: Symmetrical muscle tone. B: Unbalanced muscle tone. C: Joint surface degeneration (reproduced, with permission, from the *Journal of Bodywork and Movement Therapies* 1999; **3**(3):154).

integrity, inflammatory status, pain levels, etc.) of the individual and the scope of practice of the practitioner.

4. Identification and appropriate deactivation (using NMT or other appropriate means) of myofascial trigger points contained within these structures. Whether step 2 precedes step 4 or vice versa is a matter of clinical judgment (and debate). They may happen simultaneously.

5. Trigger points always require stretching of the affected tissues towards the end of treatment applied to their deactivation.

6. Reeducation and rehabilitation (including homework) of posture, breathing, patterns of use, in order to restore functional integrity and prevent recurrence, as far as is possible.

7. Exercise (homework) has to be focused, time efficient and within the person's easy comprehension and capabilities, if cooperation is to be achieved.

MANAGING SOFT TISSUE DYSFUNCTION

There are many ways of usefully applying manual methods to the musculoskeletal system. Treatment approaches can be categorized as direct and indirect, active and passive, gentle or mechanically invasive and all have value in their appropriate settings.

A great many of the methods of manual treatment can cluster under a heading of 'neuromuscular' inasmuch as they focus on the soft tissues, including musculature, and they incorporate into their methodology influences on neural function. Methods which are seen to be natural allies of neuromuscular therapy (NMT), as applied in Europe and the USA, include:

- muscle energy techniques (MET) (and other forms of induced stretching or release)
- positional release techniques (PRT) (including strain/counterstrain (SCS), functional technique, craniosacral techniques, etc.)
- myofascial release (MFR) (varying from dynamic to extremely gentle)

- direct manual pressure (also called ischemic compression, trigger point pressure release, inhibition technique, acupressure)
- direct manual variations (such as crossfiber friction, specific soft tissue mobilization, etc.)
- rhythmically applied release methods (including percussion and harmonic technique)
- mobilization of associated joints (including articulation, rhythmic pulsating approaches, e.g. Ruddy's technique (Ruddy 1962), high-velocity thrust (HVT))
- variations on these basic themes.

Manipulating tissues

Lederman (1997) points out that in effect there are only a limited number of ways of treating tissues ('modes of loading') and most of the various direct 'techniques' employed by manual therapists are variations of these (Carlstedt & Nordin 1989). Indirect approaches which 'unload' tissues (i.e. they move away from any perceived restriction barrier), such as osteopathic functional technique and strain/counterstrain, are not included in this summary of direct approaches. Lederman's perspective on variations of possible application of direct treatment forces (with additions from the authors) includes the following.

1. *Tension loading* in which factors such as traction, stretching, extension and elongation are involved. The objective is to lengthen tissue. The effect, if sustained, is to encourage an increase in collagen aggregation and therefore denser and stronger tissues. Lengthening forms a major part of rehabilitation methodologies and, on a local level, of trigger point deactivation.

2. *Compression loading* shortens and widens tissue, increasing pressure and influencing fluid movement significantly. Over time a degree of lengthening may also occur in the direction of pressure if the underlying structures allow this (i.e. limited by any bony surface beneath the compression). As well as affecting circulation, compression also influences neurological structures (mechanoreceptors, etc.) and encourages endorphin release.

3. *Rotation loading* produces a variety of tissue effects since it is effectively elongating (some fibers) and compressing simultaneously, with the circulatory and/or neurological influences outlined above. Techniques which produce a 'wringing' effect on soft tissues, or in which joints are rotated as they are articulated, will cause this form of loading on soft tissues. Manual methods such as 'S' bends (in which tissues are stretched in two directions at the same time by, for example, the action of opposing thumbs; see Chapter 12) can be seen to be simultaneously compressing, elongating and, in those fibers close to the transition, applying rotation loading.

4. *Bending loading* is in effect a combination of com-

pression (on the concave side) and tension (on the convex side). This has both a lengthening and a circulatory influence. On a local soft tissue level a 'C'-shaped bending of tissues which can be held to encourage elongation is commonly applied.

5. *Shearing loading* which translates or shifts tissue laterally in relation to other tissue. This is most used in joint articulation but insofar as it involves soft tissues, has the effect of compression and elongation in the region of transition.

6. *Combined loading* involves the application of combined variations of the modes of loading listed above, leading to complex patterns of adaptive demands on tissues. For example, Lederman (1997) points out that a stretch which is combined with a sidebend is more effective than either a sidebend or a stretch alone, something which most manual therapists will recognize.

7. Apart from the variations in loading that are chosen (push, pull, twist, bend, shift) additional permutations include the following.

- How hard? What is the degree of force being employed (from grams to kilos)?
- How large? What is the size of the area to which force is being applied (lentil-sized nodule or whole limb or even whole body)?
- How far? What is the intended amplitude of the induced movement? The degree of force largely determines the amplitude – how far the tissues are being taken (millimeters or centimeters).
- How fast? What is the speed with which force is applied (from extremely rapid to subtly slow)?
- How long? What is the length of time force is maintained (from milliseconds to minutes)?
- How rhythmic? What is the rhythmic quality of applied force (from rapid to deliberate to synchronous with, for example, breath or pulse rate)?
- How steady? Does the applied force involve movement or is it static (sustained pressure or gliding action)?
- Active, passive or mixed? Is the patient active in any of the processes (assisting in stretching, for example, or resisting applied force)?

The reader might usefully reflect on which of the variations of loading – and the permutations as to refining these as listed above – is involved in any particular method or technique currently employed. It will be rare indeed to find direct methods which do not incorporate these elements.

NUTRITION AND PAIN: A BIOCHEMICAL PERSPECTIVE

A variety of nutritional influences can be noted in relation to pain in general and myofascial trigger point evolution and behavior in particular. These include:

- nutritional deficiency
- allergy/intolerance
- antiinflammatory tactics.

Nutritional treatment strategies

Robert Gerwin (1993), Assistant Professor of Neurology at Johns Hopkins University, states that while manual methods (pressure, needling, etc.) can deactivate myofascial trigger points:

Management of recurrent myofascial pain syndrome (MPS) requires addressing the perpetuating factors of mechanical imbalances (structural, postural, compressive) and systemic biochemical abnormalities which interfere with the ability of the muscle to recover or which continuously stress muscle, reactivating the trigger point. (Travell & Simons 1983, 1992)

Among the 'systemic biochemical abnormalities' identified are 'hypothyroidism, folic acid insufficiency and iron insufficiency'. These deficiency states are seen to be important because of their influence on enzyme systems.

Vitamins act as cofactors in different enzyme systems that may be functioning at different rates at any one time. The optimum level of a vitamin is that which permits maximum function for each enzyme for which it is an essential cofactor. The vitamin requirements therefore change with time and circumstances. The daily vitamin intake should thus support optimum function ... [and is] affected by host factors such as smoking or by competitive inhibition by drugs.

Travell & Simons are absolutely clear in their insistence that nutritional balance has to be restored if myofascial pain is to be adequately dealt with:

Nearly half of the patients whom we see with chronic myofascial pain require resolution of vitamin inadequacies for lasting relief ... nutritional factors must be considered in most patients if lasting relief of pain is to be achieved.

Specific nutrients and myofascial pain

Folic acid (associated with the enzyme tetrahydrofolate)

It is suggested that levels should be measured in serum together with B12, as well as in red blood cells (Gerwin 1993). When in the low normal range, symptoms may include:

- feeling unnaturally cold (as in hypothyroidism but with low cholesterol levels rather than high)
- a tendency to diarrhea (rather than constipation which is associated with B12 deficiency)
- a tendency to restless legs, headache and disturbed sleep
- type II muscle fibers in the upper body are most likely to develop trigger points.

Iron (associated with various blood enzymes including cytochrome oxidase)

Serum ferritin levels should be measured to evaluate current levels. Deficiency may be noted more frequently in premenopausal women whose diet is inadequate to replace iron lost during menstruation. Blood loss may also be associated with taking of NSAIDs. Symptoms include:

- unnatural fatigue (iron is needed to convert thyroid hormone T4 into its active T3 form which may be an added fatigue factor if either is deficient)
- exercise-induced muscular cramping
- intolerance to cold.

Selenium and vitamin E

In a double-blind study 140 mg selenium and 100 mg alpha-tocopherol were supplemented daily and compared with placebo. Glutathione peroxidase levels increased in 75% of 81 patients with disabling muscular and osteoarthritic pain. Pain score reductions were more pronounced in the treated patients (Jameson 1985).

Additional nutritional deficiencies, including vitamins C and B complex, have been identified by Simons et al (1998) as being implicated in myofascial trigger point evolution and activity. It is self-evident that the ideal source of nutrients is well-selected and appropriately prepared food. Whether an omnivorous or a vegetarian (or other variant) dietary pattern is chosen, the key elements remain the need for adequate nutrient-rich protein, complex carbohydrate (fresh vegetables, pulses and grains), essential fatty acids, fruit and liquid. Food choices may be limited by economic factors, food intolerance issues (see below), ignorance or, more commonly, ignoring what is known to be appropriate, something most people are aware of as a personal issue at times. It is suggested that, at the very least, a well-formulated multivitamin mineral supplement should be incorporated into any self-care advice offered to patients with musculoskeletal dysfunction.

Allergy and intolerance: additional biochemical influences on pain

In the 1920s and 1930s, Dr A H Rowe demonstrated that widespread chronic muscular pains – often associated with fatigue, nausea, gastrointestinal symptoms, weakness, headaches, drowsiness, mental confusion and slowness of thought as well as irritability, despondency and widespread bodily aching – commonly had an allergic etiology. He called the condition 'allergic toxemia' (Rowe 1930, 1972).

Theron Randolph (1976) described 'systemic allergic reaction' as being characterized by a great deal of pain, either muscular and/or joint related, as well as numerous associated symptoms. He has studied the muscular pain phenomenon in allergy and his plea for this possibility to be considered by clinicians was based on his long experience of it being ignored.

The most important point in making a tentative working diagnosis of allergic myalgia is to think of it. The fact remains that this possibility is rarely ever considered and is even more rarely approached by means of diagnostico-therapeutic measures capable of identifying and avoiding the most common environmental incitants and perpetuants of this condition – namely, specific foods addictants, environmental chemical exposures and house dust.

Randolph points out that when a food allergen is withdrawn from the diet it may take days for the 'withdrawal' symptoms to manifest.

During the course of comprehensive environmental control [fasting or multiple avoidance] as applied in clinical ecology, myalgia and arthralgia are especially common withdrawal effects, their incidence being exceeded only by fatigue, weakness, hunger and headache.

The myalgic symptoms may not appear until the second or third day of avoidance and start to recede after the fourth day. Randolph warns that in testing for (stimulatory) reactions to food allergens (as opposed to the effects of withdrawal), the precipitation of myalgia and related symptoms may not take place for between 6 and 12 hours after ingestion (of a food which contains an allergen), which can confuse matters as other foods eaten closer to the time of the symptom exacerbation may then appear to be at fault. Other signs which can suggest that myalgia is allied to food intolerance include the presence of a common associated symptom, restless legs (Ekbom 1960).

When someone has an obvious allergic reaction to a food this may be seen as a causal event in the emergence of other symptoms. If, however, the reactions occur many times every day and responses become chronic, the cause-and-effect link may be more difficult to make. If a connection between particular foods and symptoms such as muscular pain can indeed be made, the major question remains – what is the cause of the allergy? One possibility is that the gut mucosa may have become excessively permeable, so allowing large molecules into the bloodstream where a defensive reaction is both predictable and appropriate.

Treatment for 'allergic myalgia'

Randolph states his position – 'Avoidance of incriminated foods, chemical exposures and sometimes lesser environmental excitants'. How this is achieved in a setting other than a clinic or hospital poses a series of major hurdles for the practitioner – and the person. If foods or other irritants can be identified, it makes perfect sense for these to be avoided, whether or not underlying causes

(such as possible gut permeability issues) can be, or are being, addressed.

According to the Fibromyalgia Network, the official publication of fibromyalgia patient support groups in the USA, the most commonly identified foods which cause muscular pain for many people are wheat and dairy products, sugar, caffeine, aspartame, alcohol and chocolate (Fibromyalgia Network Newsletter 1993).

Maintaining a wheat-free, dairy-free diet for any length of time is not an easy task, although many manage it. Issues involving concordance (a term currently suggested as being more appropriate than commonly used words such as 'compliance' or 'adherence', which denote passive obedience) deserve special attention, since the way information is presented and explained can make a major difference to the determination displayed by already distressed people as they embark on potentially stressful modifications to their lifestyles.

Anti-inflammatory nutritional (biochemical) strategies

Dietary strategies exist which have an anti-inflammatory influence because they reduce levels of arachidonic acid (a major leukotriene source which leads to superoxide release by neutrophils and which is a major contributing factor to the degree of inflammation being experienced). The first priority in an anti-inflammatory diet is to cut down or eliminate dairy fat.

- Fat-free or low-fat milk, yogurt and cheese should be eaten in preference to full-fat varieties, and butter avoided altogether (Moncada 1986).
- Meat fat should be completely avoided and since much fat in meat is invisible, meat itself can be left out of the diet for a time (or permanently). Poultry skin should be avoided.
- Hidden fats in products such as biscuits and other manufactured foods should be looked for on packages and avoided.
- Eating fish or taking fish oil is beneficial.

Some fish, mainly those from cold-water areas such as the North Atlantic or Alaska, contain high levels of eicosapentenoic acid (EPA), which helps cut levels of arachidonic acid, so helping to reduce inflammation, whether this is in a joint or the digestive tract or in a skin condition (such as eczema) or any other violent allergic reaction involving inflammation. Fish oil exerts these anti-inflammatory effects without interfering with the useful roles which some prostaglandins have, such as protection of delicate stomach lining and maintaining the correct level of blood clotting (unlike some anti-inflammatory drugs).

Research has shown that the use of EPA in rheumatic and arthritic conditions offers relief from swelling, stiffness and pain although benefits do not usually become evident until after 3 months of fish oil supplementation, reaching their most effective level after around 6 months. An experimental blinded study showed that after 6 months both pain and function of osteoarthritic patients (male and female, age range 52–85) improved with EPA (10 ml daily plus ibuprofen) compared with placebo, in patients who had not previously responded to ibuprofen alone (1200 mg daily) (Ford-Hutchinson 1985, Stammers 1989). To follow this strategy (but not if there is an allergy to fish) the individual should:

- eat fish such as herring, sardine, salmon and mackerel (but not fried) at least twice weekly
- take EPA capsules (10–15 daily) when inflammation is at its worst until relief appears and then a maintenance dose of six capsules daily
- consider a vegetarian option with supplementation with flax seed oil (same quantities as fish oil above).

PSYCHOSOCIAL FACTORS IN PAIN MANAGEMENT: THE COGNITIVE DIMENSION

Chiropractor Craig Liebenson (1996), an expert in spinal rehabilitation, states that:

Motivating patients to share responsibility for their recovery from pain or injury is challenging. Skeptics insist that patient compliance with self-treatment protocols is poor and therefore should not even be attempted. However, in chronic pain disorders where an exact cause of symptoms can only be identified 15% of the time the patient's participation in their treatment program is absolutely essential (Waddell 1998). Specific activity modification advice aimed at reducing exposure to repetitive strain is one aspect of patient education (Waddell et al 1996). Another includes training in specific exercises to perform to stabilize a frequently painful area (Liebenson 1996, Richardson & Jull 1995). Patients who feel they have no control over their symptoms are at greater risk of developing chronic pain (Kendall et al 1997). Teaching patients what they can do for themselves is an essential part of caring for the person who is suffering with pain. Converting a pain patient from a passive recipient of care to an active partner in their own rehabilitation involves a paradigm shift from seeing the doctor as healer to seeing him or her as helper (Waddell et al 1996). When health-care providers promise to fix or cure a pain problem they only perpetuate the idea that something is wrong that can be fixed (i.e. put back in place). In pain medicine the likelihood of recurrence is high (over 70%) and therefore it is important to show a person how to care for them self in addition to offering palliative care. Simple advice regarding activity is often better than more sophisticated forms of conservative care including mobilization or ergonomics (Malmivaara et al 1995). Promoting a positive state of mind and avoiding the disabling attitudes which accompany pain is crucial to recovery (Liebenson 1996). People who are at the greatest risk of developing chronic pain often have poorly developed coping skills (Kendall et al 1997). They may tend to catastrophize their illness and feel there is nothing that they can do themselves. It is easy for them to become dependent

on manipulation, massage, medication and various physical therapy modalities. A key to getting a person to become active in their own rehabilitation program is to shift them from being a pain avoider to a pain manager (Troup & Videman 1989, Waddell et al 1996). In a severely painful or unstable acute injury it may be appropriate to equate hurt and harm. But, in less severe cases, or certainly in the subacute or recovery phase, hurt should not be automatically associated with harm. In fact, the target of treatment may be the stiffness caused by the patient overprotecting themselves during the acute phase. Muscles and joints which lose their mobility while the patient restricts their activities during acute pain should be expected to cause discomfort and remobilizing them may hurt but certainly won't harm.

GUIDELINES FOR PAIN MANAGEMENT
(Bradley 1996)

- Assist the person in altering beliefs that the problem is unmanageable and beyond her control.
- Inform the person about the condition.
- Assist the person in moving from a passive to an active role.
- Enable the person to become an active problem solver and to develop effective ways of responding to pain, emotion and the environment.
- Help the person to monitor thoughts, emotions and behaviors and to identify how internal and external events influence these.
- Give the person a feeling of competence in the execution of positive strategies.
- Help the person to develop a positive attitude to exercise and personal health management.
- Help the person to develop a program of paced activity to reduce the effects of physical deconditioning.
- Assist the person in developing coping strategies that can be continued and expanded once contact with the pain management team or health-care provider has ended.

Group pain management

In pain clinics group work is often involved to achieve the objectives in the list immediately above. Possible reasons for excluding someone from group pain management include the following (all these are better dealt with individually rather than in group settings).

- Major psychiatric or psychological problems (psychotic patients, those with current major depressive illness, etc.).
- Major substance abuse including prescription drugs.
- Major cardiorespiratory disease.
- Severe structural deformity.

The litigation factor

Ongoing litigation or the receipt of large sums in wages

compensation is not necessarily a barrier to pain management, provided that the person is aware of the consequences of improved health on their financial position and can demonstrate that they are sufficiently motivated to change, despite these considerations and consequences (Watson 2000). Additionally, the litigation process itself, including depositions, medical improvement testing, court appearances and other procedures, may impose stresses – and distresses – which create emotional challenges that stimulate and provoke the pain response. This situation often results in setbacks in the recovery process.

Other barriers to progress in pain management (Gil et al 1988, Keefe et al 1996)

- Distorted perceptions of the person (and/or their partner or family) about the nature of their pain and disability.
- Beliefs based on previous (possibly incorrect) diagnosis and treatment failure ('But the specialist said…').
- Lack of hope created by practitioners (who often do not understand the myofascial pain responses) whose prognosis was limiting ('You will have to learn to live with it').
- Dysfunctional beliefs about pain and activity ('It's bound to get worse if I exercise').
- Negative expectation about the future ('It's bound to get worse whatever I do').
- Psychological disorders that may contribute to the experience of pain (e.g. depression and anxiety).
- The person's lack of awareness of the control they have over the pain.
- The possibility that disability offers secondary gains (what benefit does the person receive from maintaining their pain or limitations?).

Stages of change in behavior modification

DiClementi & Prochaska (1982) have developed a useful model which explains stages of change.

- Those who do not see their current behavior as a problem needing change or who are unwilling to change are described as *precontemplative*.
- A person who sees the need for change is in the stage of *contemplation*.
- Precontemplative individuals are unlikely to change their behavior.
- Those who are contemplating change need help to start to plan the necessary changes.
- Program attendance is part of this process of change and individuals are expected to also plan to make changes in their home and social environment.
- Putting these plans into action is the next stage, where behavioral change is enacted and agreed goals are set.
- People often relapse into old patterns if faced by additional or new stresses and challenges, such as a pain flare-up, and should be prepared for this.
- Health-care providers need to enable the person to acquire the knowledge, skills and strategies to avoid sliding back into old ways.

WELLNESS EDUCATION (Vlaeyen et al 1996)

Education regarding illness and wellness starts at the first consultation. Initial education in pain management should give the person information to help them make an informed decision about participating in a program. Such a program should offer the person a credible rationale for engaging in pain management, as well as information regarding:

- the condition itself (a major factor in rehabilitation)
- a simple guide to pain physiology (how pain is transmitted; where it is felt; what it means)
- separating the link between 'hurting' and 'harming' (a revelation for some people; 'I thought that if it hurt it was doing harm')
- ergonomic influences on pain, including education and advice about safe lifting and working postures, how to sit and lie safely without creating strain
- the effects of deconditioning and the benefits of exercise and healthy lifestyles.

GOAL SETTING AND PACING (Bucklew 1994, Gil et al 1988)

Pacing rehabilitation exercise is a strategy to enable people to control exacerbations in pain by learning to regulate activity and, once a regime of paced activity is established, to gradually increase the activity level. Part of the process of recovery necessarily involves empowerment, the sense of being in control, and this can be rapid or slow. The control learned by experiencing the effect of rehabilitation exercises on the condition is a powerful force in this empowerment process, since how often, how hard, how long, etc. an individual applies the program will be under *their* control and so to a large extent will the outcomes.

Rehabilitation goals should be set in three separate fields.

1. *Physical* – the person follows and sets the number of exercises to be performed, or the duration of the exercise, and the level of difficulty.
2. *Functional tasks* – this relates to the achievement of functional tasks of everyday living, such as housework or hobbies and tasks learned on the program.
3. *Social* – where the person is encouraged to set goals

relating to the performance of activities in the wider social environment. Goals should be personally relevant, interesting, measurable and, above all, achievable.

Physical exercise (Bennett 1996)

- Physical exercise should aim to redress the negative effects of deconditioning.
- The key to participation and acceptance of the beneficial effects of exercise is a reduction in the fear of activity ('It may hurt but it won't do harm').
- Activities should be incorporated that are meaningful to the person, such as those related to hobbies or interests (e.g. gardening), with some adaptation, which will increase activity levels and encourage more consistent participation.

Objectives of a physical activity

- Overcome the effects of deconditioning.
- Challenge and reduce the person's fear of engaging in physical activity.
- Reduce physical impairment and focus on recoverable function.
- Increase physical activity in a safe and graded manner.
- Help the person to accept responsibility for increasing functional capacity.
- Promote a positive view of physical activity in the self-management of health.
- Introduce challenging, functional activities to rehabilitation.

Exercise should be designed to:

- stretch, to increase soft tissue length
- mobilize joints
- increase fitness.

Low back pain rehabilitation

In regard to rehabilitation from painful musculoskeletal dysfunction (this text is related to low back problems but the principles are universal), Liebenson (1996) states:

The basic progressions to facilitate a 'weak link' and improve motor control include the following:

- train awareness of postural (neutral range joint) control during activities
- prescribe beginner ('no brainer') exercises
- facilitate automatic activity in 'intrinsic' muscles by reflex stimulation
- progress to more challenging exercises (i.e. labile surfaces, whole-body exercises)
- transition to activity-specific exercises
- transition to health club exercise options.

Concordance

It is of major concern that concordance (aka compliance, adherence, participation) is extremely poor regarding exercise programs (as well as other health enhancement self-help programs), even when the individuals felt that the effort was producing benefits. Research indicates that most rehabilitation programs report a reduction in participation in exercise (Lewthwaite 1990, Prochaska & Marcus 1994).

Wigers et al (1996) found that 73% of patients failed to continue an exercise program when followed up, although 83% felt they would have been better if they had done so. There is no record of whether patient-centered goal setting was part of this research. Participation in exercise is more likely if the individual finds it interesting and rewarding.

Research into patient participation in their recovery program in fibromyalgia settings has noted that a key element is that whatever is advised (exercise, self-treatment, dietary change, etc.) needs to make sense to the individual, in their own terms, and that this requires consideration of cultural, ethnic and educational factors (Burckhardt 1994, Martin 1996).

In general, most experts, including Lewit (1992), Liebenson (1996) and Lederman (1997) (see Further reading), highlight the need (in treatment and rehabilitation of dysfunction) to move as rapidly as possible from passive (operator-controlled) to active (patient-controlled) methods. The rate at which this happens depends largely on the degree of progress, pain reduction and functional improvement.

Patient advice and concordance (compliance) issues

Individuals should be encouraged to listen to their bodies and to never do more than they feel is appropriate in order to avoid what can be severe setbacks in progress when they exceed their current capabilities. It is vital that rehabilitation strategies are very carefully explained, as active participation is not high when novel routines or methods are suggested unless they are well understood.

Routines and methods (homework) should be explained in terms which make sense to the person and their carer(s). Written or printed notes, ideally illustrated, help greatly to support and encourage compliance with agreed strategies, especially if simply translated examples of successful trials can be included as examples of potential benefit. Information offered, spoken or written, needs to answer in advance questions such as:

- Why is this being suggested?
- How often, how much?
- How can it help?
- What evidence is there of benefit?

- What reactions might be expected?
- What should I do if there is a reaction?
- Can I call or contact you if I feel unwell after exercise (or other self-applied treatment)?

It is useful to explain that *all* treatment makes a demand for a response (or several responses) on the part of the body and that a 'reaction' (something 'feels different') is normal and expected and is not necessarily a cause for alarm but that it is OK to make contact for reassurance.

It may be useful to offer a reminder that symptoms are not always bad and that change in a condition towards normal may occur in a fluctuating manner, with minor setbacks along the way.

It can be helpful to explain, in simple terms, that there are many stressors being coped with and that progress is more likely to come when some of the 'load' is lightened, especially if particular functions (digestion, respiratory, circulation, etc.) are working better.

A basic understanding of homeostasis is also helpful ('broken bones mend, cuts heal, colds get better – all examples of how your body always tries to heal itself') with particular emphasis on explaining processes at work in their condition.

REFERENCES

Bennett R M 1996 Multidisciplinary group treatment programmes to treat fibromyalgia patients. Rheumatic Diseases Clinics of North America 22 (2):351–367

Bradley L A 1996 Cognitive therapy for chronic pain. In: Gatchel R J, Turk D C (eds) Psychological approaches to pain management. Guilford Press, New York, ch 6, pp 131–147

Bucklew S P 1994 Self efficacy and pain behaviour among subjects with fibromyalgia. Pain 59:377–384

Burckhardt C 1994 Randomized controlled clinical trial of education and physical training for women with fibromyalgia. Journal of Rheumatology 21(4):714–720

Carlstedt C, Nordin M 1989 Biomechanics of tendons and ligaments. In: Nordin M, Frankel V (eds) Basic biomechanics of the musculoskeletal system Lea and Febiger, London

DiClementi C, Prochaska J 1982 Self change and therapy change of smoking behaviour: a comparison of processes in cessation and maintenance. Addictive Behaviours 7:133–144

Ekbom K 1960 Restless legs syndrome. Neurology 10:868

Feldenkrais M 1972 Awareness through movement. Harper and Row, New York

Fibromyalgia Network Newsletter 1993 October, p12, Tucson

Ford-Hutchinson A 1985 Leukotrienes: their formation and role as inflammatory mediators. Fe. Proc. 44:25–29

Gerwin R 1993 The management of myofascial pain syndromes. Journal of Musculoskeletal Pain 1(3/4):83–94

Gil K M, Ross S L, Keefe F J 1988 Behavioural treatment of chronic pain: four pain management protocols. In: France R D, Krishnan K R R (eds) Chronic pain. American Psychiatric Press, Washington, pp 317–413

Hanna T 1988 Somatics, Addison-Wesley, New York

Jameson S 1985 Pain relief and selenium balance in patients with connective tissue disease and osteoarthrosis – a double blind study. Nutrition Research 1(Suppl):391–397

Janda V 1982 Introduction to functional pathology of the motor system. Proceedings of the VII Commonwealth and International Conference on Sport. Physiotherapy in Sport 3:39

Keefe F J, Beaupre P M, Gil K M 1996 Group therapy for patients with chronic pain. In: Gatchel R J, Turk D C (eds) Psychological approaches to pain management. Guilford Press, New York

Kendall N, Linton S J, Main C J 1997 Guide to assessing psychosocial yellow flags in acute low back pain: risk factors for long-term disability and work loss. Accident Rehabilitation & Compensation Insurance Corporation of New Zealand and the National Health Committee, Wellington, NZ. Available from http://www.nhc.govt.nz

Knaster M 1996 Discovering the body's wisdom. Bantam, New York

Lederman E 1997 Fundamentals of manual therapy. Churchill Livingstone, Edinburgh

Lewit K 1992 Manipulative therapy in rehabilitation of the locomotor system. Butterworths, London

Lewit K 1996 Role of manipulation in spinal rehabilitation. In: Liebenson C (ed) Rehabilitation of the spine. Williams and Wilkins, Baltimore

Lewthwaite R 1990 Motivational considerations in physical therapy involvement. Physical Therapy 70(12):808–819

Liebenson C (ed) 1996 Rehabilitation of the spine. Williams and Wilkins, Baltimore

Malmivaara A, Hakkinen U, Aro T 1995 The treatment of acute low back pain – bed rest, exercises, or ordinary activity? New England Journal of Medicine 332:351–355

Martin A 1996 An exercise program in treatment of fibromyalgia. Journal of Rheumatology 23(6):1050–1053

Moncada S 1986 Leucocytes and tissue injury: the use of eicosapentenoic acid in the control of white cell activation. Wien Klinische Wochenschrift 98(4):104–106

Myers T 1997 Anatomy trains. Journal of Bodywork and Movement Therapies 1(2):91–101 and 1(3):134–145

Prochaska J O, Marcus B H 1994 The transtheoretical model: applications to exercise. In: Dishman R K (ed) Advances in exercise adherence. Human Kinetics, New York, pp 161–180

Randolph T 1976 Stimulatory withdrawal and the alternations of allergic manifestations. In: Dickey L (ed) Clinical ecology. Charles C Thomas, Springfield, Illinois

Richardson C A, Jull G A 1995 Muscle control-pain control. What exercises would you prescribe? Manual Therapy 1(1):2–10

Rowe A 1930 Allergic toxemia and migraine due to food allergy. California West Medical Journal 33:78

Rowe A 1972 Food allergy – its manifestation and control. Charles C Thomas, Springfield, Illinois

Ruddy T J 1962 Osteopathic rapid rhythmic resistive technic. Academy of Applied Osteopathy Yearbook, Carmel, California, pp 23–31

Simons D, Travell J, Simons L 1998 Myofascial pain and dysfunction: the trigger point manual, vol 1: upper half of body, 2nd edn. Williams and Wilkins, Baltimore

Stammers T 1989 Fish oil in osteoarthritis. Lancet 2:503

Trager M 1987 Mentastics. Station Hill, Mill Valley, CA

Travell J, Simons D 1983 Myofascial pain and dysfunction: the trigger point manual vol 1: upper half of body. Williams and Wilkins, Baltimore

Travell J, Simons D 1992 Myofascial pain and dysfunction: the trigger point manual, vol 2: lower extremities. Williams and Wilkins, Baltimore

Troup J D G, Videman T 1989 Inactivity and the aetiopathogenesis of musculoskeletal disorders. Clinical Biomechanics 4:173–178

Van Wingerden J-P 1997 The role of the hamstrings in pelvic and spinal function. In: Vleeming A, Mooney V, Dorman T, Snijders C, Stoekart R (eds) Movement, stability and low back pain. Churchill Livingstone, Edinburgh

Vlaeyen J W, Teeken-Gruben N J, Goossens M E et al 1996 Cognitive-educational treatment of fibromyalgia: a randomized clinical trial. I. Clinical effects. Journal of Rheumatology 23(7):1237–1245

Vleeming A, Van Wingerden J, Snijders C 1989 Load application to the sacrotuberous ligament: influences on sacroiliac joint mechanics. Clinical Biomechanics 4:204–209

Waddell G 1998 The back pain revolution. Churchill Livingstone, Edinburgh

Waddell G, Feder G, McIntosh A, Lewis M, Hutchinson A 1996 Low back pain: evidence review. Royal College of General Practitioners, London

Ward R (ed) 1997 Foundations of osteopathic medicine. Williams and Wilkins, Baltimore

Watson P 2000 Interdisciplinary pain management in fibromyalgia. In: Chaitow L (ed) Fibromyalgia syndrome – a practitioner's guide. Churchill Livingstone, Edinburgh

Wigers S H, Stiles T C, Vogel P A 1996 Effects of aerobic exercise versus stress management treatment in fibromyalgia: a 4.5 year prospective study. Scandinavian Journal of Rheumatology 25:77–86

FURTHER READING

Pizzarno J 1996 Total wellness. Prima, Rocklin, California

For more detailed descriptions of the functional organization of the motor system and of therapeutic considerations (note that these texts do not always agree on which manual methods are most helpful!), the following are recommended for further reading.

Lederman E 1997 Fundamentals of manual therapy. Churchill Livingstone, Edinburgh

Lewit K 1992 Manipulative therapy in rehabilitation of the locomotor system. Butterworths, London

Liebenson C (Ed) 1996 Rehabilitation of the spine. Williams and Wilkins, Baltimore

9

Modern neuromuscular techniques

Box 9.1   The roots of modern neuromuscular techniques

Neuromuscular therapy techniques have emerged in both Europe and North America almost simultaneously over the last 50 years. First developed by Stanley Lief and Boris Chaitow, European-style NMT first emerged between the mid-1930s and early 1940. Trained in chiropractic and naturopathy, these cousins developed integrated concepts learned from teachers like Dewanchand Varma and Bernarr Macfadden.

Lief and Chaitow developed and refined what they called 'neuromuscular techniques' as a means of assessing and treating soft tissue dysfunction, in Lief's world-famous health resort, Champneys, at Tring in Hertfordshire, England. Many osteopaths and naturopaths have taken part in the evolution and development of European neuromuscular therapy, including Peter Lief, Brian Youngs, Terry Moule, Leon Chaitow and others. NMT is now taught widely in osteopathic and sports massage settings in Britain and forms an elective module on the Bachelor of Science (BSc(Hons)) degree courses in Complementary Health Sciences, University of Westminster, London.

A few years after neuromuscular techniques developed in Europe, across the ocean in America, Raymond Nimmo and James Vannerson began writing of their experiences with what they termed 'noxious nodules', in their newsletter, *Receptor-Tonus Techniques*. A step-by-step system began to emerge, supported by the writings of Janet Travell and David Simons. Travell and Simons' work impacted the medical, dental, massage and other therapeutic communities with documentation, research and references for a whole new field of study – myofascial trigger points.

Several of Nimmo's students began teaching their own NMT protocols, based on Nimmo's work. In the USA the acronym NMT signified neuromuscular *therapy* rather than *technique*. NMT St John Method and NMT American Version became two prominent systems which still today retain a strong focus on Nimmo's original techniques.

European and American versions of NMT have subtle differences in their hands-on applications while retaining similar foundations in their theoretical platform. North American-style neuromuscular therapy uses a medium-paced thumb or finger glide to uncover contracted bands or muscular nodules whereas European-style neuromuscular techniques use a slow-paced, thumb drag method of discovery. They also have slightly different emphasis on the method of application of ischemic compression in treating trigger points. Both versions emphasize a home care program and the patient's participation in the recovery process. In this text, the American version of NMT is offered as the foundation for developing palpatory skills and treatment techniques while the European version accompanies it to offer an alternative approach.

Box 9.2 Semantic confusion

A confusing element relating to the term NMT emerges from its use by some European authors when they describe what are in effect variations on the theme of isometric contractions (Dvorak et al 1988). These methods, all of which form part of what is known as muscle energy technique (MET) in osteopathic medicine, will be outlined in Box 9.11.

Dvorak et al (1988) have listed various MET methods as NMT, as follows.

- Methods which involve active self-mobilization, in order to encourage movement past a resistance barrier, are called 'NMT 1' by Dvorak et al.
- Isometric contraction, involving postisometric relaxation and subsequent passive stretching of agonist muscles is described as 'NMT 2'.
- Isometric contraction of antagonists involving reciprocal inhibition followed by stretching, is called 'NMT 3' by Dvorak et al.

Naming these methods NMT 1, 2 and 3 would seem to add to (rather than reduce) semantic confusion since they are adequately named already in general manual medicine and osteopathic texts. In reality, almost all manual methods which address either soft tissue or joint dysfunction involve a degree of both muscular and neural elements and could therefore receive a 'neuromuscular' designation. However, there would seem to be little to be gained via such an exercise.

In this text, when the letters NMT are used in relation to the American version, it should be understood to indicate *neuromuscular therapies* as described in this book in general and this chapter in particular (i.e. a broad approach to addressing musculoskeletal dysfunction, including myofascial trigger points). When NMT is used in relation to the European approach it should be understood to refer only to the *technique* of assessment and treatment of local musculoskeletal dysfunction, mainly involving myofascial trigger points utilizing finger and/or thumb techniques, and not the eclectic selection of complementary approaches incorporated under the American NMT label.

NEUROMUSCULAR THERAPY – AMERICAN VERSION

Neuromuscular therapy (NMT) American version, as presented in this volume, will attempt to address (or at least take account of) a number of features which are all commonly involved in causing or intensifying pain (Chaitow 1996a). These include, among others, the following factors which affect the whole body:

- nutritional imbalances and deficiencies
- toxicity (exogenous and endogenous)
- endocrine imbalances
- stress (physical or psychological)
- posture (including patterns of use)
- hyperventilation tendencies

as well as locally dysfunctional states such as:

- hypertonia
- ischemia
- inflammation
- trigger points
- neural compression or entrapment.

These 'components of pain and dysfunction' are particularly significant areas of influence on the perception of pain, its intensity and its spread throughout the body, as well as on the maintenance of dysfunctional states. These and other factors can be broadly clustered under the headings of:

- *biomechanical* (postural dysfunction, hyperventilation tendencies, hypertonicity, neural compression, trigger point activity)
- *biochemical* (nutrition, ischemia, inflammation, hyperventilation tendencies)
- *psychosocial* (stress, hyperventilation tendencies).

It is necessary to address whichever of these (or additional) influences on musculoskeletal pain can be identified in order to remove or modify as many etiological and perpetuating influences as possible (Simons et al 1998), without creating further distress or requirement for excessive adaptation. Unless this is comprehensively and effectively achieved, results of therapeutic intervention may be unsatisfactory (DeLany 1999).

Biomechanical factors

Trigger points (TrP) are located primarily in myofascial tissues. These points are hyperirritable spots found in taut bands which are usually painful on compression and (when active) give rise to referred pain (and other sensations), tenderness, motor disturbances and autonomic responses in other body tissues (see Chapter 6). Myofascial trigger points may form in muscle bellies (central trigger points) or tendons and periosteal attachments (attachment trigger points). Trigger points may also occur in skin, fascia, ligaments, periosteum, joint surfaces and, perhaps, in visceral organs. However, none of these would be considered myofascial TrPs since they are apparently different from the mechanisms associated with motor endplate dysfunction in myofascial tissues (Simons et al 1998).

It is not yet fully understood how trigger points develop but their locations are fairly predictable, as are their patterns of referral. NMT identifies and deactivates trigger points by means of ischemic compression methods (also known as trigger point pressure release). Lengthening the shortened fibers in which the points lie (stretching) is also part of the process of treating the trigger points as well as abolishing the underlying factors which helped create them (Simons et al 1998).

Nerve entrapments/compression can result from pressure on neural structures by soft tissue including muscle, tendon, disc, ligament, fascia or skin or via more direct osseous pressure (arthritic spur, for example). The structure(s) interfering with normal neural function are known as the 'mechanical interface'. The underlying cause of these entrapment/compression situations may lie in traumatic incidents or they may be the result of overuse or misuse patterns (work, sport, postural habits, etc.).

In order to evaluate the possibility of such entrapment/ compression, it is necessary to be aware of neural pathways as well as which hard tissues may crowd the nerve and/or which soft tissues may entrap them (see notes on Butler's work, in Chapter 13, p. 369, as it relates to shoulder and arm pain). For example, when considering pain in the arm, pressure may have been placed on nerve roots at the cord level by herniated discs, osteophytes or subluxations; by the scalene muscles, as the nerves travel between or through them; by the clavicle or first rib; by pectoralis minor; or by upper extremity tissues, such as the triceps or supinator muscles. Additionally, the position of the upper extremity itself may create tension and drag on the brachial plexus and its fascial ensheathment. NMT attempts to identify such entrapments and compressions and to use manual methods and rehabilitation exercises to modify or correct them when possible.

Postural (and use) influences. Debate continues as to the extent to which there is an anatomically 'correct' degree of alignment of the musculoskeletal system, a so-called 'correct' posture. Experts, including Feldenkrais (1972) and Hanna (1988), suggest that a degree of asymmetry is, in fact, the norm but that within that asymmetry there ought to be a relatively 'normal' functional balance, range of motion, etc., taking account of genetic characteristics (hyperflexibility, for example), body type and age.

Janda (1982) and Lewit (1992), among others, have identified patterns of dysfunction which modify regions in relation to each other (see crossed syndrome discussion in Chapter 5, p. 55). NMT seeks to correct dysfunctional postural patterns by releasing stressful tension in muscular and fascial tissues. An individualized home care program is usually developed, which includes awareness of undesirable as well as improved postural and use habits, appropriate stretching and strengthening procedures. Under the general heading of 'postural influences', habits of use need to be considered, whether these involve overuse, disuse or abuse (repetitive strain, hyperventilation breathing tendencies, improper sitting, standing or sleeping positions).

Biochemical factors

Ischemia is an insufficiency of blood flow (therefore of oxygen and nutrients) commonly caused by muscular spasm or contracture. If ischemia is prolonged, metabolic waste products accumulate and pool within the tissues, which increases neuroexcitability (Cailliet 1996). This may predispose toward a local energy crisis developing within the muscle tissue and a resultant decrease in ATP supplies while the tissue's energy needs increase (see Chapter 6) (Simons et al 1998).

NMT assesses and treats ischemia by using effleurage

(gliding techniques), pressure release methods and lengthening of the shortened myofascial fibers (stretching), which will encourage blood flow and a return to normal muscle length.

Nutrition is an area of consideration in musculoskeletal pain and dysfunction which includes all the processes involved in the intake of nutrients necessary for cellular metabolism, repair and normal reproduction of cells in the body as a whole. It includes ingestion, digestion, absorption and assimilation and the multitude of processes associated with these functions. Sound nutrition also considers avoidance of substances which are irritating and stimulating to the nervous system or toxic to the body (caffeine, smoke, chemical exposures, etc.).

Nutritional imbalances may perpetuate the existence of ischemia, trigger points, neuroexcitation and the resultant postural distortions (Simons et al 1998). Vitamin and mineral status should be considered, adequate fluid intake ensured and breathing habits evaluated (since both oxygen and carbon dioxide are critical factors in the nourishment of the body). Additionally, obvious or hidden ('masked') food intolerances and allergies should be identified in order to minimize the numerous negative effects such reactions can have, including increased nociception and lymphatic congestion (Randolph 1976).

Additional biochemical influences which require consideration include endocrine balance/imbalance (most particularly thyroid in the case of myofascial pain) (Ferraccioli 1990, Lowe & Honeyman-Lowe 1998) and inflammatory processes (discussed in detail in Chapter 7). A critical biochemical influence on pain involves the balance between oxygen and carbon dioxide in the body, which is intimately connected to breathing patterns – a biomechanical function with huge psychosocial overlays. This 'three-way' interaction is discussed in greater detail in Chapter 4.

Psychosocial factors

The influence of emotional stress on the musculoskeletal system is beyond doubt (see Chapter 4). It is sufficient at this stage to restate that there exists a fundamental requirement for stress factors, whether self-generated or externally derived, to be considered as a part of the 'load' to which the individual is adapting. The degree to which anyone can be helped in regard to emotional stress relates directly to how much of the load can be removed as well as to how efficiently adaptation is occurring. The same can, of course, be said for biochemical and biomechanical stresses.

The role of the practitioner may be seen to involve teaching and encouraging the individual (and their self-regulating, homeostatic functions) to handle the load more efficiently, as well as alleviating the stress burden as far as possible. This would involve improving functional efficiency and removing negative influences, manually and by means of rehabilitation, and nowhere is this seen more graphically than in the changes associated with breathing dysfunction (Chaitow 2000, Selye 1956).

Biomechanical, biochemical and psychosocial interaction

The influences of a biomechanical, biochemical and psychosocial nature do not produce single changes. Their interaction with each other is profound.

• Hyperventilation modifies blood acidity, alters neural reporting (initially hyper and then hypo), creates feelings of anxiety and apprehension and directly impacts on the structural components of the thoracic and cervical region, both muscles and joints (Gilbert 1998).
• Altered chemistry (hypoglycemia, acidosis, etc.) affects mood directly while altered mood (depression, anxiety) changes blood chemistry, as well as altered muscle tone and, by implication, trigger point evolution (Brostoff 1992).
• Altered structure (posture, for example) modifies function (breathing, for example) and therefore impacts on chemistry (e.g. O_2: CO_2 balance, circulatory efficiency and delivery of nutrients, etc.) which impacts on mood (Gilbert 1998).

Within these categories – biochemical, biomechanical and psychosocial – are to be found most major influences on health, with 'subdivisions' (such as ischemia, postural imbalance, trigger point evolution, neural entrapments and compressions, nutritional and emotional factors) being of particular interest in NMT.

NMT attempts to identify these altered states, insofar as they impact on the person's condition, and either offers therapeutic intervention which reduces the 'load' and/or assists the self-regulatory functions of the body (homeostasis) or, if this is inappropriate or outside the practitioner's scope of practice, offers referral to appropriate health-care professionals.

A *home care program* should be designed for both physical relief of the tissues (stretching, self-help therapies, hydrotherapies, postural awareness) and removal of perpetuating factors including nutritional choices, postural habits, work and recreational practices, stress and lifestyle factors (rest, exercise, etc.) (see notes on concordance in Chapter 8, p. 104). Lifestyle changes are encouraged to eliminate influences resulting from habits and potentially harmful choices made in the past.

NMT techniques contraindicated in initial stages of acute injury

If an injury has occurred within 72 hours of therapy, great care must be taken to protect the tissues and modulate blood flow and swelling. The body will, in most cases, naturally splint the area and often produces swelling as part of the recovery process (Cailliet 1996). The acronym RICE indicates appropriate care for the first 72 hours following a soft tissue injury – Rest, Ice, Compression and Elevation. NMT techniques should not be applied directly on the injured tissues within the first 72 hours following the injury, as this would tend to encourage increased blood flow to the already congested tissues and reduce the natural splinting which is needed in this phase of recovery.

The patient should be referred for qualified medical, osteopathic or chiropractic care, when indicated, and techniques such as lymphatic drainage and certain movement therapies may be used to encourage the natural healing process. Additionally, NMT techniques may be used in other parts of the body to reduce overall structural distress which often accompanies injuries. For instance, when an ankle is sprained, compensatory gait changes, crutch usage and redistribution of weight may stress the lower back, hip and even cervical or mandibular muscles. NMT applications to these muscles may help reduce structural adaptations which will not be needed beyond the acute phase and help to decrease the overall effects of the injury.

After 72 hours, NMT may be carefully applied to the injured tissues and applications to the supporting structures and muscles involved in compensating patterns should be continued. If range of motion work is questionable, such as when a moderate or severe whiplash has occurred, consultation with the attending physician is suggested to avoid further compromise to the structures (in this case, cervical discs, ligaments or vertebrae) which may have been damaged in the injury.

NMT for chronic pain

Chronic pain is considered to be that which remains at least 3 months after the injury or tissue insult (*Stedman's medical dictionary* 1998) Subacute stages lie between acute and chronic, at which time a degree of reorganization has started and the acute inflammatory stage is past. Active treatment appropriate to the person's current condition is constantly evaluated and adjusted as the tissue health changes. It is important to keep in mind that it is the degree of current pain and inflammation which defines which of these stages the tissue is in, not just the length of time since the injury.

Once acute inflammation subsides, a number of rehabilitation stages of soft tissue therapy are suggested in the order listed.

• Appropriate soft tissue techniques should be applied with the aim of decreasing spasm and ischemia, enhancing drainage of the soft tissues and deactivating trigger points.

- Appropriate active, passive and self-applied stretching methods should be introduced to restore normal flexibility.
- Appropriately selected forms of exercise should be encouraged to restore normal tone and strength.
- Conditioning exercises and weight-training approaches should be introduced, when appropriate, to restore overall endurance and cardiovascular efficiency.
- Normal proprioceptive function and coordination should be assisted by use of standard rehabilitation approaches.
- Methods for achieving improved posture and body use should be taught and/or encouraged as well as exercises for restoring normal breathing patterns. Posture, body usage and breath work may be addressed at any stage along with the other approaches listed above.

The sequence in which these recovery steps (see Box 9.3) are introduced is important (DeLany 1994). The last two may be started at any time, if appropriate; however, the first four should be sequenced in the order listed in most cases. Clinical experience suggests that recovery can be compromised and symptoms prolonged if all elements of this suggested rehabilitation sequence are not taken into account. For instance, if exercise or weight training is initiated before trigger points are deactivated and contractures eliminated, the condition could worsen and recovery be delayed. In cases of recently traumatized tissue, deep tissue work and stretching applied too early in the process could further damage and reinflame the recovering tissues.

Once traumatized tissues are no longer inflamed or particularly painful, the initial elements of reducing spasm and ischemia, encouraging drainage, commencing (cautious) stretching, as well as toning and strengthening exercises, can usually be safely introduced at the first treatment session. Pain should always be respected as a signal that whatever is being done is inappropriate in relation to the current physiological status of the area.

Tissues which respond painfully to active or passive movement need to be treated with particular care and caution, especially when that pain is elicited with little provocation. Gentle passive movement can usually safely accompany soft tissue manipulation but more compre-

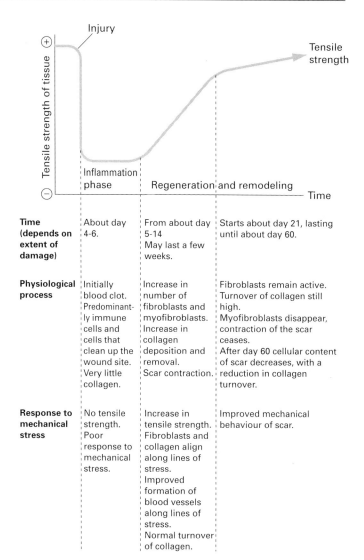

Figure 9.1 Stages of the repair process.

	Inflammation phase	Regeneration and remodeling	
Time (depends on extent of damage)	About day 4-6.	From about day 5-14. May last a few weeks.	Starts about day 21, lasting until about day 60.
Physiological process	Initially blood clot. Predominantly immune cells and cells that clean up the wound site. Very little collagen.	Increase in number of fibroblasts and myofibroblasts. Increase in collagen deposition and removal. Scar contraction.	Fibroblasts remain active. Turnover of collagen still high. Myofibroblasts disappear, contraction of the scar ceases. After day 60 cellular content of scar decreases, with a reduction in collagen turnover.
Response to mechanical stress	No tensile strength. Poor response to mechanical stress.	Increase in tensile strength. Fibroblasts and collagen align along lines of stress. Improved formation of blood vessels along lines of stress. Normal turnover of collagen.	Improved mechanical behaviour of scar.

hensive exercises, especially any involving weights, should be left until the tissues respond to active and passive movement without pain.

Palpation and treatment

The NMT techniques described in later chapters include step-by-step procedures for treatment of each muscle discussed. These are based on a generalized framework of assessment and treatment. The selection of alternative or additional treatment approaches will depend upon the practitioner's training so that, in a given situation, a number of manual approaches might each be effective in releasing excessive tone, easing pain and improving range of motion. Specific recommendations for soft tissue manipulations will therefore be accompanied by suggestions of alternative or supportive modalities and methods which will be described in detail nearby.

Box 9.3 Summary of rehabilitation sequencing

- Decrease spasm and ischemia, enhance drainage, deactivate trigger points
- Restore flexibility (lengthen)
- Restore tone (strengthen)
- Improve overall endurance and cardiovascular efficiency
- Restore proprioceptive function and coordination
- Improve postural positioning, body usage (active and stationary) and breathing

Based on the clinical experience of the authors (and of those experts cited in the text), it is suggested that the following be used as a general guideline when addressing most myofascial tissue problems.

• The most superficial tissue is usually treated before the deeper layers.
• The proximal portions of an extremity are treated ('softened') before the distal portions are addressed so that proximal restrictions of lymph flow are removed before distal lymph movement is increased.
• In a two-jointed muscle, both joints are assessed; in multijointed muscles, all involved joints are assessed. For instance, if triceps is examined, both glenohumeral and elbow joints are assessed; if extensor digitorum, then wrist and all phalangeal joints being served by that muscle would be checked.
• Most myofascial trigger points either lie in the endplate zone (mid-fiber) of a muscle or at the attachment sites (see Chapter 6) (Simons et al 1998).
• Other trigger points may occur in the skin, fascia, periosteum and joint surfaces.
• Knowledge of the anatomy of each muscle, including its innervation, fiber arrangement, nearby neurovascular structures and overlying and underlying muscles, will greatly assist the practitioner in quickly locating the appropriate muscles and their trigger points.
• Where multiple areas of pain are present, a general 'rule of thumb', based on clinical experience, is suggested.
1. Treat the most proximal,
2. most medial, and
3. most painful trigger points first.
4. Avoid overtreating the whole structure as well as the individual tissues.
5. Treatment of more than five active points at any one session might place an adaptive load on the individual which could prove extremely stressful. If the person is frail or demonstrating symptoms of fatigue and general susceptibility, common sense suggests that fewer than five active trigger points should be treated at any one session.

NMT examination and treatment, while being extremely effective, can be uncomfortable for the recipient as one objective is to locate and then to introduce an appropriate degree of pressure into tender localized areas of dysfunctional soft tissue. Applied compression has the effect of reducing inappropriate degrees of hypertonicity apparently by releasing the contracted sarcomeres in the TrP nodule (Simons et al 1998), therefore allowing more normal function of the involved tissues. Temporary discomfort may be produced, which needs to be monitored and adjusted to in order to avoid excessive treatment.

A 'discomfort scale' can usefully be established with the patient which allows them a degree of control over the process and which will help avoid the use of too much

---

Box 9.4 Effects of applied compression

When digital pressure is applied to tissues a variety of effects are simultaneously occurring.

1. A degree of ischemia results as a result of interference with circulatory efficiency, which will reverse when pressure is released (Simons et al 1998).
2. Neurological inhibition (osteopathic term) is achieved by means of the sustained barrage of efferent information resulting from the constant pressure (Ward 1997).
3. Mechanical stretching of tissues occurs as the elastic barrier is reached and the process of 'creep' commences (Cantu & Grodin 1992).
4. A possible piezoelectric influence occurs modifying relatively sol tissues toward a more gel-like state (Athenstaedt 1974, Barnes 1996) as colloids change state when shearing forces are applied (see Connective tissue, pp 3–4).
5. Mechanoreceptors are stimulated, initiating an interference with pain messages (gate theory) reaching the brain (Melzack & Wall 1988).
6. Local endorphin release is triggered along with enkephalin release in the brain and CNS (Baldry 1993).
7. Direct pressure often produces a rapid release of the taut band associated with trigger points (Simons et al 1998).
8. Acupuncture and acupressure concepts associate digital pressure with alteration of energy flow along hypothesized meridians (Chaitow 1990).

Box 9.5 Establishing a myofascial pain index

Note: This concept is discussed more fully in Chapter 6.

• The term 'pressure threshold' is used to describe the least amount of pressure required to produce a report of pain and/or referred symptoms.
• It is useful to know whether the degree of pressure utilized changes before and after treatment.
• In diagnosing fibromyalgia the criteria for a diagnosis depend upon 11 of 18 specific test sites testing as positive (hurting severely) on application of 4 kilograms of pressure (American College of Rheumatology 1990).
• An algometer (pressure meter) can be used as an objective measurement of the degree of pressure required to produce symptoms.
• An algometer is also a useful tool to assist a practitioner in training themselves to apply a standardized degree of pressure and to 'know' how hard they are pressing.
• Belgian researchers Jonkheere & Pattyn (1998) have used algometers to identify what they term the myofascial pain index (MPI).
• In order to achieve this, various standard locations are tested (for example, the 18 test sites used for fibromyalgia diagnosis, listed in Chapter 6). Based on the results of this (total poundage required to produce pain divided by the number of points tested), a myofascial pain index (MPI) is calculated.
• The calculation of the MPI determines the maximum degree of pressure which should be required to evoke pain in an active trigger point.
• If greater pressure than the MPI is needed to evoke symptoms the point is not regarded as 'active'.

The Belgian researchers based their approach on earlier work by Hong et al. (1996) who investigated pressure thresholds of trigger points and the surrounding soft tissues.

pressure. A scale is suggested in which 0 = no pain and 10 = unbearable pain. With regard to pressure techniques, it is best to avoid pressures which induce a pain level of between 8 and 10.

The person is instructed to report back, when requested or when they wish, if the level of their perceived discomfort varies from what they judge to be a score of between 5 and 7. Below 5 usually represents inadequate pressure to facilitate an adequate therapeutic response from the tissues, while prolonged pressure which elicits a report of pain above a score of 7 may provoke a defensive response from the tissues, such as reflexive shortening or exacerbation of inflammation (see reporting stations, Chapter 3).

Soft tissue treatment techniques often involve the use of a lubricant to prevent skin irritation and to facilitate smooth movement. Any dry-skin work to be done, such as would be used in myofascial release, skin assessments (seeking evidence of moisture, roughness, temperature) or skin rolling (*bindegewebsmassage*, connective tissue massage), is therefore best performed first. NMT often involves dry-skin techniques prior to lubricated ones, especially in the shoulder girdle region. If the skin or muscles need to be lifted following lubrication, this can be accomplished through a cover sheet or a piece of cloth, paper towel or tissue placed on the skin. The lubricant may also be removed using an appropriate alcohol-based medium.

Gliding techniques

Lightly lubricated gliding strokes (effluerage) are an important and powerful component of the manual applications of NMT. Such strokes are ideal for exploring the tissue for ischemic bands and/or trigger points and may also follow compression or manipulation techniques. While increasing blood flow, 'flushing' tissues and creating a mechanical counterpressure to the tension within the tissues, they also help the practitioner to become familiar with the individual quality, internal (muscle) tension and degree of tenderness in the tissues being assessed or treated.

- To glide most effectively on the tissues, the practitioner's fingers are spread slightly and 'lead' the thumbs.
- The fingers support the weight of the hands and arms which relieves the thumbs of that responsibility. As a result, the pressure exerted by the thumb is more easily controlled and can be changed as varying tensions are matched in the tissues.
- The fingers stabilize (steady) the hands while the thumbs are the actual treatment tool in most cases.
- The wrist needs to remain stable so that the hands

move as a unit, with little or no motion taking place in the wrist or the thumb joints. Excessive movement in the wrist or thumb may result in joint inflammation, irritation and dysfunction.

- When two-handed glides are employed, the lateral aspects of the thumbs are placed side by side or one slightly ahead of the other with both pointing in the same direction, that being the direction of the glide (Fig. 9.2A).
- Pressure is applied through the wrist and longitudinally through the thumb joints, not against the medial aspects of the thumbs, as would occur if the gliding stroke were performed with the thumb tips touching end to end (Fig. 9.2B).

During assessment strokes, the practitioner is constantly aware of information which is being received as variable

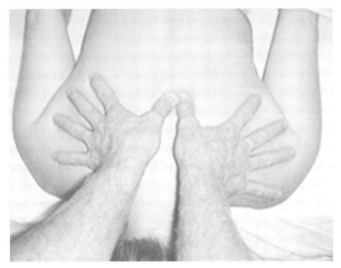

A

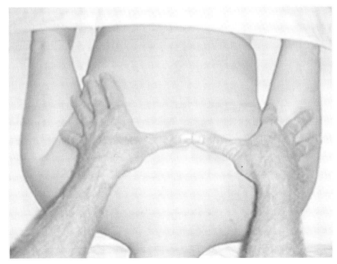

B

Figure 9.2 A: The fingers offer support and enhance control as the thumbs apply pressure or glide. B: Incorrect application of techniques which stresses the thumb joints.

pressure is being applied. As palpation skills develop, this awareness becomes second nature and does not require constant conscious thought, as it may during the early stages of manual development.

The variation in pressure is determined by a constantly fluctuating stream of information regarding the status of the tissues. As the thumb or fingers move from normal tissue to tense, edematous, fibrotic or flaccid tissue, the amount of pressure required to 'meet and match' it will vary. Some areas will feel 'hard' or tense and pressure should actually be lightened rather than increased, so that the quality and extent of the dense tissue can be evaluated. After assessment of the extent of tissue involvement (i.e. the size of area involved, a sense of depth of tissue involvement, degree of tenderness), pressure can be increased only if appropriate. Some areas will feel doughy, although they may be extremely tender (as in the tender points of fibromyalgia), while others may feel 'stringy' or 'ropy'.

Indurations may be felt as the thumb glides transversely across taut bands. Once the bands are located, assessment longitudinally along the band will help determine mid-fiber range where most central trigger points form. Palpation can then be altered to include compression and pincer palpation, depending upon the tissue's availability to be grasped.

Nodules are often embedded in (sometimes extensive) areas of dense (thick) tissue congestion and may not be felt clearly when the hands first encounter the tissue. As the tissue softens from repetitions of the gliding strokes, short applications of heat (when appropriate) or from tissue elongation (all of which encourage a change of state of the colloidal matrix), palpation of distinct bands and nodules becomes clearer.

The practitioner moves from assessment to treatment and back to assessment again as the palpating digits uncover dysfunctional tissues. If trigger points are found, modalities can be applied, including trigger point pressure release, various stretching techniques, heat or ice, vibration or movements, which will encourage the release of the taut fibers housing the trigger point.

Clinical experience indicates that the best result usually comes from gliding on the tissues repetitively (6–8 times) before working elsewhere. Gliding repeatedly on areas of hypertonicity:

- often changes the degree and intensity of the dysfunctional patterns
- reduces the time and effort needed to modify them in subsequent treatments
- tends to encourage the tissue to become more defined, which particularly assists in evaluation of deeper structures
- allows for a more precise localization of taut bands and trigger point nodules

- encourages hypertonic bands commonly found to become softer, smaller and less tender than before.

If the taut bands tend to become more tender after the gliding techniques, especially if this is to a significant degree, the tissue may be revealing an inflamed condition for which ice applications would be indicated. It is suggested that friction, excessive elongation methods, heat, deep gliding strokes or other modalities which might increase an inflammatory response be avoided in such circumstances, as they may aggravate matters. Positional release methods, gentle myofascial release, cryotherapy, lymph drainage or other antiinflammatory measures would be more appropriate.

Speed of gliding movements. Unless the tissue being treated is excessively tender or sensitive, the gliding stroke should cover 3–4 inches per second; if the tissue is sensitive, a slower pace and reduced pressure are suggested. It is important to develop a moderate gliding speed in order to feel what is present in the tissue. Movement that is too rapid may skim over congestion and other changes in the tissues or cause unnecessary discomfort while movement that is too slow may make identification of individual muscles difficult. A moderate speed will also allow for numerous repetitions which will significantly increase blood flow and soften fascia for further manipulation.

Unless contraindicated by excessive tenderness, redness, heat, swelling or other signs of inflammation, a moist hot pack placed on the tissues between gliding repetitions further enhances the effects. Ice may also be used and is especially effective on attachment trigger points where a constant concentration of muscle stress tends to provoke an inflammatory response (Simons et al 1998, *Stedman's medical dictionary* 1998).

The therapeutic benefits of water applications to the body, and particularly of thermal stimulations associated with them, should not be underrated in both clinical and home application. An extensive discussion of hydrotherapies occurs in Chapter 10 (beginning on p. 131) and a brief summary of the effects of hot and cold applications is given in Box 9.7.

Palpation and compression techniques

Flat palpation (Fig. 9.3) is applied by the whole hand, finger pads or finger tips through the skin and begins

---

Box 9.6 Two important rules of hydrotherapy

- There should almost always be a short cold application or *immersion* after a hot one and preferably also before it (unless otherwise stated).
- When heat is applied, it should never be hot enough to scald the skin and should always be bearable.

Box 9.7 The general principles of hot and cold applications

- Hot is defined as 98–104° Fahrenheit or 36.7–40° Centigrade. *Anything hotter than that is undesirable and dangerous.*
- Cold is defined as 55–65°F or 12.7–18.3°C.
- Anything colder is very cold and anything warmer is:
  cool (66–80°F or 18.5–26.5°C)
  tepid (81–92°F or 26.5–33.3°C)
  neutral/warm (93–97°F or 33.8–36.1°C).
- Short cold applications (less than a minute) stimulate circulation.
- Long cold applications (more than a minute) depress circulation and metabolism.
- Short hot applications (less than 5 minutes) stimulate circulation.
- Long hot applications (more than 5 minutes) depress both circulation and metabolism.
- Because long hot applications vasodilate and can leave the area congested and static, they require a cold application or massage to help restore normality.
- Short hot followed by short cold applications cause alternation of circulation followed by a return to normal.
- Neutral applications or baths at body heat are very soothing and relaxing.

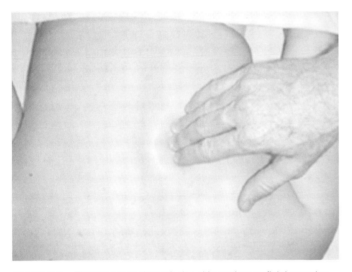

Figure 9.3 Fingers press through the skin and superficial muscles to evaluate deeper layers against underlying structures using deep flat palpation.

by sliding the skin over the underlying fascia to assess for restriction (see Skin palpation in Chapter 6, p. 81).

The skin overlying dysfunctional, reflexively active tissue (where trigger points often form) is almost always more adherent, 'stuck' to the underlying tissue. Whether this is revealed by sliding the skin (as described here and in Chapter 6) or by lifting and rolling it between the fingers and thumb (as in connective tissue massage, *bindegewebsmassage*), the lack of skin flexibility may indicate a suspicious zone which may either house a trigger point or be the target referral pattern for one (Simons et al 1998). Because of increased sympathetic activity in these tissues there will be a higher level of sweat activity

(increased hydrosis) and the superficial feel of the skin, on light unlubricated palpation, will reveal a sense of friction as the finger passes over the trigger point site. This identifies what Lewit (1992) calls a hyperalgesic skin zone, the precise superficial evidence of a trigger point.

Regarding these adherent tissues, Simons et al (1998) state:

In panniculosis, one finds a broad, flat thickening of the subcutaneous tissue with an increased consistency that feels coarsely granular. It is not associated with inflammation. Panniculosis is usually identified by hypersensitivity of the skin and the resistance of the subcutaneous tissue to 'skin rolling'. ... The particular, mottled, dimpled appearance of the skin in panniculosis indicates a loss of normal elasticity of the subcutaneous tissue, apparently due to turgor and congestion.

Panniculosis should be distinguished from panniculitis (which is an inflammation of subcutaneous adipose tissue), adiposa dolorosa and fat herniations. Skin-rolling techniques and myofascial release often dramatically soften and loosen the affected tissues; however, they should not be applied if inflammation is indicated.

Indurations in underlying muscles may be felt as the pressure is increased to compress the tissue against bony surfaces or muscles which lie deep to those being palpated. Pressure may be increased to evaluate deeper tissues and underlying structures, seeking soft tissues which feel congested, fibrotic, indurated or in any way altered. The finger or hand pressure meets and matches the tension found in the tissues. When tissue with excessive tension is found, two or three fingers can direct pressure into or against the tissue until the slack is taken out. The tissue may then be examined with these finger tips for tension levels, trigger point nodules, fibrosis or excessive tenderness. When pressure is being directed in search of deeply situated trigger points in well-muscled areas, it is often useful to apply this at an angle of around 45° to the surface and to offer slight 'support' to any tissues which might have a tendency to shift or roll away from the applied pressure. Flat palpation is used primarily when the muscles (such as the rhomboids) are difficult to lift or compress (see below) or to add information to that obtained by compression. For instance, the belly of biceps brachii can be easily lifted but its tendons cannot; they are best palpated against the underlying humerus.

Pincer compression techniques involve grasping and

Box 9.8 Compression definitions

- Compression techniques involve grasping and compressing the tissue between the thumb and fingers with either one hand or two.
- *Flat compression* (like a clothes pin) will provide a broad general assessment and release.
- *Pincer compression* (like a C-clamp) will compress smaller, more specific sections of the tissue.

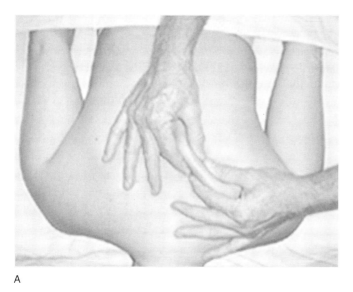

A

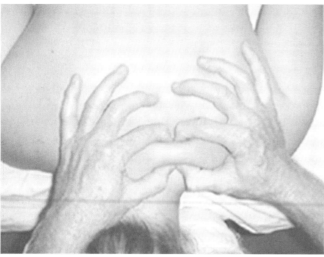

B

Figure 9.4 A&B: Pincer compression may be applied precisely with the finger tips or with finger pads for a more general release.

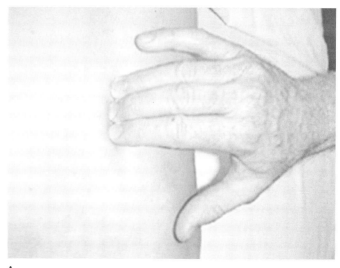

A

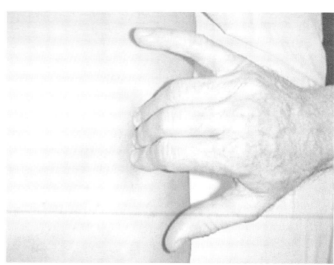

B

Figure 9.5 Snapping palpation may sometimes elicit a local twitch response (confirmatory of a trigger point location) and may be useful on more fibrotic tissue as a treatment technique when (if appropriate) it is applied repeatedly to the same fiber.

compressing the tissue between the thumb and fingers with either one hand or two. The finger pads (flattened like a clothes pin) (Fig. 9.4A) will provide a broad general assessment and release while the finger tips (curved like a C-clamp) (Fig. 9.4B) will compress smaller, more specific sections of the tissue. The muscle or skin may then be manipulated by sliding the thumb across the fingers with the tissue held between them or by rolling the tissues between the thumb and fingers.

Snapping palpation (Fig. 9.5) is a technique used to elicit a twitch response which confirms the presence of a trigger point. The fingers are placed approximately mid-fiber and quickly snap transversely across the taut fibers (similar to plucking a guitar string). While a twitch response confirms the presence of a trigger point meeting the minimal criteria, the lack of one does not rule out

a trigger point as this technique is extremely difficult to apply correctly and assess adequately. It may also be used repetitively as a treatment technique, which is often effective in reducing fibrotic adhesions.

Central trigger point (CTrP) palpation and treatment

Palpating trigger points

• When assessing the tissues for central trigger points or to treat a central trigger point which is not associated with an inflamed attachment site, the tissue is placed in a relaxed position by slightly (passively) approximating its ends (for example, the forearm would be passively supinated and elbow slightly flexed for biceps brachii).

The approximate center of the fibers should be located with a thumb or finger contact.

- Tendons should be ignored; only the length of the fibers is considered when locating the center of the fibers, which is also the endplate zone of most muscles and the usual location of central trigger points (CTrP).
- Digital pressure (flat or pincer compression) should be applied to the center of taut muscle fibers where trigger point nodules are found.
- The tissue may now be treated in this position or a slight stretch may be added as described below, which may increase the palpation level of the taut band and nodule.
- As the tension becomes palpable, pressure should be increased into the tissues to meet and match it.
- The fingers should then slide longitudinally along the taut band near mid-fiber to assess for a palpable (myofascial) nodule or thickening of the associated myofascial tissue.
- An exquisite degree of spot tenderness is usually reported near or at the trigger point sites.
- Sometimes stimulation from the examination may produce a local twitch response, especially when a transverse snapping palpation is used. When present, the local twitch response serves as a confirmation that a trigger point has been encountered.
- When pressure is increased (gradually) into the core of the nodule (CTrP), the tissue may refer sensations (usually pain) which the person either recognizes (active trigger point) or does not (latent trigger point). Sensations may also include tingling, numbness, itching or burning, although pain is the most common referral.
- The degree of pressure should be adjusted so that the person reports a mid-range number between 5 and 7 on their discomfort scale, as the pressure is maintained.
- *Note*: Alternative protocols for application of pressure to trigger points are described in the discussion of European NMT later in this chapter (see variable ischemic compression and INIT, pp. 119 and 123).
- Since the tenderness of the tissue will vary from person to person and even from tissue to tissue within the same person, the pressure needed may range from less than an ounce to several pounds but should always provoke between a 5 and 7 on the patient's discomfort scale when the correct pressure is used.
- The practitioner should feel the tissues 'melting and softening' under the sustained pressure. The person frequently reports that they believe the practitioner is reducing the pressure on the tissue.
- Pressure can usually be mildly increased as tissue relaxes and tension releases, provided the discomfort scale is respected.
- The length of time pressure is maintained will vary but tension should ease within 8–12 seconds and the discomfort level should drop.

- If it does not begin to respond within 8–12 seconds, the amount of pressure should be adjusted accordingly (usually lessened), the angle of pressure altered or a more precise location sought (move a little one way and then the other to find heightened tenderness or more distinct nodule).
- Since the tissues are being deprived of normal blood flow while pressure is ischemically compressing (blanching) them, it is suggested that 20 seconds is the maximum length of time to hold the pressure.

Adding stretch to the palpation. Slightly stretching the muscle tissue often makes the taut fibers much easier to palpate. However, caution should be exercised if movement produces pain or if palpation of the attachment sites reveals excessive tenderness which may represent an attachment trigger point and inflammation. Placing more tension on these already distressed tissues may provoke an inflammatory response. Additionally, care must be taken to avoid aggressive applications, such as strumming or friction, while the tissue is being stretched as injury is more likely in a stretched position.

- Manually commence a process of slowly elongating the muscle fibers (stretching the muscle slowly by separating the ends) while palpating for the first sign of tissue resistance (tension).
- As the muscle fibers are stretched, the first fibers to become taut may be shortened fibers and may house trigger points.
- As the taut fibers present themselves, the tissues are held in that position as the fibers are treated as noted above.
- As the tissue tension reduces, the tissue may be further stretched until more taut fibers are felt.
- The same procedure is used to release these until either full range of motion is restored or a barrier is met which does not respond to this procedure.

Other trigger point treatment considerations

- Trigger points frequently occur in 'nests' and 3–4 repetitions of the protocol as described above may need to be applied to the same area.
- Each time that digital pressure is released, blood flushes into the tissue and brings with it nutrients and oxygen while removing metabolic waste. If the colloidal state has changed sufficiently, the tissue will be more porous, a better medium for diffusion to take place (Oschman 1997).
- The treatment as described above is usually followed with several passive elongations (stretches) of the tissue to that tissue's range of motion barrier.
- The person is then asked to perform at least 3–4 active repetitions of the stretch, which they should be encouraged to continue to do as 'homework'.
- It is important to avoid excessive treatment at any

one session as a degree of microtrauma is undoubtedly inherent in the processes described.

• Residual discomfort, as well as the adaptive demands which this form of therapy imposes on repair functions, calls for treatment to be tailored to the individual's ability to respond, which is a judgment the practitioner needs to make.

• Treatment of the point directly, as described, should be followed by range of motion work, as well as by one or more forms of hydrotherapy, for example, heat (unless inflamed), ice, contrast hydrotherapy or mild a combination of heat to the belly and ice to the tendons (see hydrotherapy in Chapter 10 and Boxes 9.6 and 9.7 above).

Stretches should be performed before any prolonged applications of cold as fascia elongates best when warm and more liquid. The elastic components of muscle and fascia are less pliable when cold and less easily stretched (Lowe 1995). If the tissue is cold, it is helpful to rewarm the area with a hot pack or mild movement therapy before stretches are applied. These precautions do not apply for brief exposures to cold, such as spray and stretch or ice-stripping techniques (see hydrotherapy in Chapter 10).

Attachment trigger point (ATrP) location and palpation

As the taut band is being palpated (see above), it can be followed to the attachment sites on each end of the band. Palpation should be performed cautiously as these sites may be inflamed and/or extremely sensitive. Attachment trigger points form as the result of excessive, unrelieved tension on the attachment tissues, whether that site is musculotendinous or periosteal.

If found to be very tender, further tension should not be applied to the attachments, such as would be involved in stretching techniques. Undue stress to these tissues may provoke or increase an inflammatory response.

Attachment trigger points usually respond well once the associated central trigger point has been released. In the interim, cryotherapy (ice therapy) can be used on the attachment trigger points and manual traction applied locally to the taut fibers near the central trigger point to elongate the shortened sarcomeres.

Gliding strokes are usually effective in lengthening the shortened fibers. It is especially useful to apply 'stripping' strokes, using one or both thumbs. These gliding strokes may be started at the center of the fibers and stroked toward one attachment and then repeated toward the other attachment or by using both thumbs and gliding from the center to both ends simultaneously (Fig. 9.6).

At further sessions, the attachment trigger points should be reexamined. If they have responded to therapy and are non-tender or only mildly tender, passive and active range of motion can be added to the protocol.

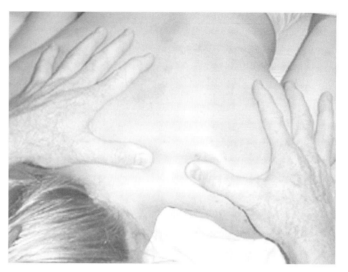

Figure 9.6 The thumbs, when gliding in opposite directions, provide precise traction of the fibers and a local myofascial release.

Box 9.9 Summary of American NMT assessment protocols

• Glide where appropriate.
• Assess for taut bands using pincer compression techniques.
• Assess attachment sites for tenderness, especially where taut bands attach.
• Return to taut band and find central nodules or spot tenderness.
• Elongate the tissue slightly if attachment sites indicate this is appropriate or tissue may be placed in neutral or approximated position.
• Compress CTrP for 8–12 seconds (using pincer compression techniques or flat palpation).
• The patient is instructed to exhale as the pressure is applied, which often augments the release of the contracture.
• Appropriate pressure should elicit a discomfort scale response of 5–7.
• If a response in the tissue begins within 8–12 seconds, it can be held for up to 20 seconds.
• Allow the tissue to rest for a brief time.
• Adjust pressure and repeat, including application to other taut fibers.
• Passively elongate the fibers.
• Actively stretch the fibers.
• Appropriate hydrotherapies may accompany the procedure.
• Advise the patient as to specific procedures which can be used at home to maintain the effects of therapy.

Treatment tools

Several treatment tools have been developed by practitioners in an attempt to preserve the practitioner's thumbs and hands and to more easily access attachments which lie under bony protrusions (such as infraspinatus attachment under the spine of the scapula) or between bony structures (such as the interossei between the metacarpal bones). While many of these tools offer unique qualities, the ones which remain the 'tools of the trade' of neuromuscular therapy are a set of pressure bars (Fig. 9.7), apparently introduced to the work by Dr Raymond Nimmo

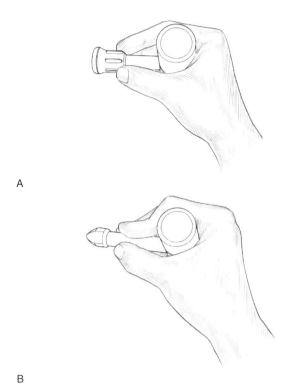

A

B

Figure 9.7 Stress on the practitioner's thumbs may be reduced with properly held treatment tools, such as the pressure bars shown here (reproduced, with permission, from Chaitow (1996a)).

(1957) associated with his receptor-tonus techniques. While tableside training is required to use the bars safely, they have been included in this text for those who have been adequately trained in their use. They may be used in addition to (or in place of) finger or thumb pressure, unless contraindicated (some contraindications are listed below).

Pressure bars are constructed of light wood and comprise a 1-inch dowel horizontal (top) crossbar and a 1/4-inch vertical shaft. They have either a flat or a beveled rubber tip at the end of the vertical shaft. (They somewhat resemble a 'T' with a stopper on the bottom.) The large flat tip is used to glide on flat muscle bellies, such as the anterior tibialis, or to press into large muscle bellies, such as the gluteals. The small bevelled tip is used under the spine of the scapula, in the lamina groove and to assess tendons and small muscles which are difficult to reach with the thumb (such as the intercostals). The beveled end of a flat 'typewriter' eraser can be used in a similar manner.

The pressure bars are never used at vulnerable nerve areas such as the lateral aspects of the neck, under the clavicle, on extremely tender tissues or to 'dig' into tissues. Ischemic tissues, fibrosis and bony surfaces along with their protuberances may be 'felt' through the bars just as a grain of sand or a crack in the table under writing paper may be felt through a pencil when writing. The tools (pressure bars, erasers or other tools which touch

the skin) should be scrubbed with an antibactericidal soap after each use or cleaned with cold sterilization or other procedures recommended by their manufacturers.

The descriptions above relate to American neuromuscular therapy. In order to avoid confusion a separate description is offered below of European (Lief's) neuromuscular technique. The reader may reflect on similarities and differences between them and experiment with aspects with which they are currently unfamiliar.

EUROPEAN (LIEF'S) NEUROMUSCULAR TECHNIQUE (NMT) (Chaitow 1996a)

Neuromuscular technique, as the term is used in this book, refers to the manual application of specialized (usually) digital pressure and strokes, most commonly applied by finger or thumb contact. These digital contacts can have either a diagnostic (assessment) or therapeutic objective and the degree of pressure employed varies considerably between these two modes of application.

Therapeutically, NMT aims to produce modifications in dysfunctional tissue, encouraging a restoration of functional normality, with a particular focus of deactivating focal points of reflexogenic activity, such as myofascial trigger points.

An alternative focus of NMT application is toward normalizing imbalances in hypertonic and/or fibrotic tissues, either as an end in itself or as a precursor to joint mobilization.

NMT aims to:

- offer reflex benefits
- deactivate myofascial trigger points
- prepare for other therapeutic methods such as exercise or manipulation
- relax and normalize tense fibrotic muscular tissue
- enhance lymphatic and general circulation and drainage
- simultaneously offer the practitioner diagnostic information.

There exist many variations of the basic technique as developed by Stanley Lief, the choice of which will depend upon particular presenting factors or personal preference.

NMT can be applied generally or locally and in a variety of positions (seated, supine, prone, etc.). The sequence in which body areas are dealt with is not regarded as critical in general treatment but is of some consequence in postural reintegration, much as it is in Rolfing™ and Hellerwork™.

The NMT methods described are in essence those of Stanley Lief DC and Boris Chaitow DC (1983). The latter has written:

To apply NMT successfully it is necessary to develop the art of palpation and sensitivity of fingers by constantly feeling the appropriate areas and assessing any abnormality in tissue structure for tensions, contractions, adhesions, spasms. It is important to acquire with practice an appreciation of the 'feel' of normal tissue so that one is better able to recognize abnormal tissue. Once some level of diagnostic sensitivity with fingers has been achieved, subsequent application of the technique will be much easier to develop. The whole secret is to be able to recognize the 'abnormalities' in the feel of tissue structures. Having become accustomed to understanding the texture and character of 'normal' tissue, the pressure applied by the thumb in general, especially in the spinal structures, should always be firm but never hurtful or bruising. To this end the pressure should be applied with a 'variable' pressure, i.e. with an appreciation of the texture and character of the tissue structures and according to the feel that sensitive fingers should have developed. The level of the pressure applied should not be consistent because the character and texture of tissue is always variable. The pressure should therefore be so applied that the thumb is moved along its path of direction in a way which corresponds to the feel of the tissues. This variable factor in finger pressure constitutes probably the most important quality a practitioner of NMT can learn, enabling him to maintain more effective control of pressure, develop a greater sense of diagnostic feel, and be far less likely to bruise the tissue.

NMT thumb technique

Thumb technique as employed in NMT, in either assessment or treatment modes, enables a wide variety of therapeutic effects to be produced.

The tip of the thumb can deliver varying degrees of pressure via any of four facets:

- the very tip may be employed for extremely focused contacts
- the medial or lateral aspect of the tip can be used to make contact with angled surfaces or for access to intercostal structures, for example
- for more general (less localized and less specific) contact, of a diagnostic or therapeutic type, the broad surface of the distal phalange of the thumb is often used.

It is usual for a light, non-oily lubricant to be used to facilitate easy, non-dragging passage of the palpating digit.

In thumb technique application, the hand should be spread for balance and control. The tips of the fingers provide a fulcrum or 'bridge', with the palm arched (Fig. 9.8). This allows free passage of the thumb toward one of the finger tips as it moves in a direction which takes it away from the practitioner's body.

During a single stroke, which covers between 2 and 3 inches (5–8 cm), the finger tips act as a point of balance while the chief force is imparted to the thumb tip, via controlled application of body weight through the long axis of the extended arm. The thumb and hand seldom impart their own muscular force except in dealing with small localized contractures or fibrotic 'nodules'.

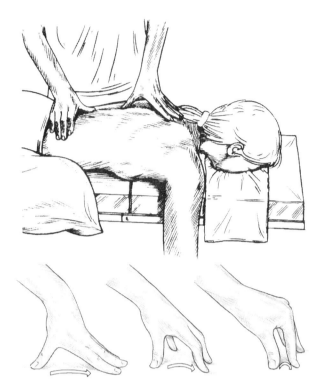

Figure 9.8 NMT thumb technique (reproduced, with permission, from Chaitow (2000)).

The thumb therefore never leads the hand but always trails behind the stable fingers, the tips of which rest just beyond the end of the stroke.

Unlike many bodywork/massage strokes, the hand and arm remain still as the thumb, applying variable pressure, moves through the tissues being assessed or treated.

The extreme versatility of the thumb enables it to modify the direction of imparted force in accordance with the indications of the tissue being tested/treated. As the thumb glides across and through those tissues it should become an extension of the practitioner's brain. For the clearest assessment of what is being palpated the practitioner should have the eyes closed so that every change in the tissue texture or tone can be noted.

In order that pressure/force be transmitted directly to its target, the weight being imparted should travel in as straight a line as possible, which is why the arm should not be flexed at the elbow or the wrist by more than a few degrees.

The positioning of the practitioner's body in relation to the area being treated is of importance in order to achieve economy of effort and comfort. The optimum height *vis-à-vis* the couch and the most effective angle of approach to the body areas being addressed should be considered (Fig. 9.9).

The degree of pressure imparted will depend upon the nature of the tissue being treated, with changes in pressure being possible, and indeed desirable, during strokes across and through the tissues. When being treated,

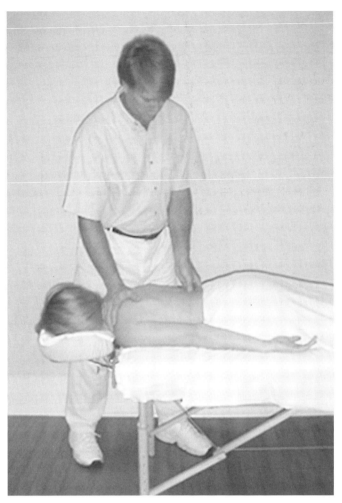

Figure 9.9 The practitioner's position for application of NMT. Note the straight arm for application of force via bodyweight and overall ease of posture.

the patient should not feel pain but a general degree of discomfort is usually acceptable, as the seldom stationary thumb varies its penetration of dysfunctional tissues.

A stroke or glide of 2–3 inches (5–8 cm) will usually take 4–5 seconds, seldom more unless a particularly obstructive indurated area is being dealt with. If myofascial trigger points are being treated, a longer stay will usually be required at a single site (or intermittent pressure may be applied) but in normal diagnostic and therapeutic use the thumb continues to move as it probes, decongests and generally treats the tissues.

It is impossible to state the exact pressures necessary in NMT application because of the very nature of the objective, which in assessment mode attempts to precisely meet and match the tissue resistance, to vary the pressure constantly in response to what is being palpated.

In subsequent or synchronous (with assessment) treatment of whatever is uncovered during evaluation, a greater degree of pressure is used and this will vary depending upon the objective, whether this is to inhibit neural

activity or circulation, to produce localized stretching, to decongest and so on (see Box 9.4).

Lief's NMT finger technique

In certain areas the thumb's width prevents the degree of tissue penetration suitable for successful assessment and/or treatment. Where this happens the middle, or index, finger can usually be suitably employed. This is most likely when access to the intercostal musculature is attempted or when trying to penetrate beneath the scapula borders, in tense or fibrotic conditions.

Working from the contralateral side, finger technique is also a useful approach to curved areas, such as the area above and below the pelvic crest or the lateral thigh. The middle or index finger should be slightly flexed and, depending upon the direction of the stroke and density of the tissues, should be supported by one of its adjacent members.

The angle of pressure to the skin surface should be between 40° and 50°. As the treating finger strokes, with a firm contact and a minimum of lubricant, a tensile strain is created between its tip and the tissue underlying it. The tissues are stretched and lifted by the passage of the finger which, like the thumb, should continue moving unless, or until, dense indurated tissue prevents its easy passage.

These strokes can be repeated once or twice as tissue changes dictate. The finger tip should never lead the stroke but should always follow the wrist, the palmar surface of which should lead as the hand is drawn toward the practitioner. It is possible to impart a great degree of traction on underlying tissues and the patient's reactions must be taken into account in deciding on the degree of force being used.

Transient pain or mild discomfort is to be expected, but no more than that. Most sensitive areas are indicative

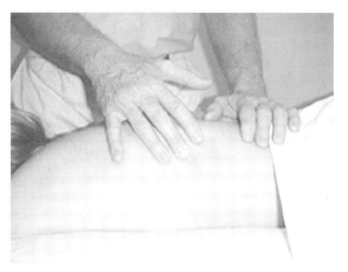

Figure 9.10 NMT finger technique.

of some degree of associated dysfunction, local or reflex. It is therefore important that their presence be recorded.

Unlike the thumb technique, in which force is largely directed away from the practitioner's body, in finger treatment the stroke is usually toward the practitioner. The arm position therefore alters, since elbow flexion is necessary to ensure that the stroke of the finger, across the lightly lubricated tissues, is balanced. Unlike the thumb, which makes a sweep toward the finger tips while the rest of the hand remains relatively stationary, the whole hand will move when a finger stroke is applied. Some variation in the degree of angle between finger tip and skin is in order during a stroke and some slight variation in the degree of 'hooking' of the finger may be necessary.

The treating finger should be supported by one of its neighbors if tissue resistance is marked.

Use of lubricant

The use of a lubricant during NMT application facilitates the smooth passage of the thumb or finger. A suitable balance between lubrication and adherence is found by mixing two parts of rapeseed (or almond) oil to one part lime water. It is important to avoid excessive oiliness or the essential aspect of slight traction, from the contact digit, will be lost.

If a frictional effect is required, for example in order to achieve a rapid vascular response, then no lubricant should be used.

Variations

Depending upon the presenting symptoms and the area involved, any of a number of procedures may be undertaken as the hand moves from one site to another. There may be:

- superficial stroking in the direction of lymphatic flow
- direct pressure along or across the line of axis of stress fibers
- deeper alternating 'make and break' stretching and pressure or traction on fascial tissue
- sustained or intermittent ischemic ('inhibitory') pressure, applied for specific effects.

As variable pressure is being applied, during assessment strokes, the practitioner needs to be almost constantly aware of information which is being received. It is this constantly fluctuating stream of information regarding the status of the tissues which determines the variations in pressure and the direction of force to be applied. As the thumb or finger moves from normal tissue to tense, edematous, fibrotic or flaccid tissue, so the amount of pressure required to 'meet and match' it will vary. As the thumb or finger passes through such tissues, varying its applied pressure as described, if a 'hard' or tense area is

sensed, pressure should actually lighten rather than increase, since to increase pressure would override the tension in the tissues, which is not the objective in assessment.

The metaphor of a boat's sail, filled with wind, can help to make this concept clearer. Standing on the full side of the sail, a hand or finger contacting it would require minimal pressure to sense the force of the wind on the other side. However, if the wind was light and the sail not fully extended, a hand contact could apply much more pressure before, having taken out the slack, a sense of the force of wind on the other side would be gained.

In just this way, NMT assessment is used to sense the 'tension' in tissue. A light contact achieves this whereas in slack tissue greater pressure is required to feel what lies beyond that slack.

In evaluating for myofascial trigger points, when a sense of something 'tight' is noted just ahead of the contact digit as it strokes through the tissues, pressure lightens and the thumb/finger slides over the 'tight' area and deeper penetration is made to sense for the characteristic taut band and the trigger point, at which time the patient is asked whether it hurts and whether there is any radiating or referred pain. As the assessment stroke is made, any alteration in direction or in the degree of applied pressure should take place gradually, without any sudden change, which could irritate the tissues or produce a defensive contraction.

Should trigger points be located, as indicated by the reproduction in a target area of an existing pain pattern, then a number of choices are possible.

- The point should be marked and noted (on a chart and if necessary on the body with a skin pencil).
- Sustained ischemic/inhibitory pressure, or 'make and break' pressure, can be used, discussed immediately below.
- Application of a positional release approach (strain/counterstrain) will reduce activity in the hyperreactive tissue, as outlined below.
- Initiation of an isometric contraction followed by stretch could be used – see MET details in Chapter 10.
- A combination of pressure, positional release and MET (integrated neuromuscular inhibition technique – INIT) can be introduced – see below and Fig. 9.11.
- Spray and stretch methods can be used (Vapocoolant or icing technique as discussed in Chapter 10).
- An acupuncture needle or a procaine injection can be used.

Variable ischemic compression

Pressure applied to a myofascial trigger point may be variable, i.e. deep pressure, sufficient to produce the referred pain symptoms, for approximately 5 seconds followed by an easing of pressure for 2–3 seconds and then repeating the stronger pressure and so on. This alternation is repeated until the local or the reference pain diminishes or until 2 minutes have elapsed.

Further easing of the hyperreactive patterns in a trigger point can be achieved by introduction of a positional release 'ease' position for 20–30 seconds or by means of ultrasound (pulsed) or application of a hot towel to the area, followed by effluerage. Whichever subsequent method is used, a final absolute requirement is to stretch the tissues to help them regain their normal resting length potential (Simons et al 1998).

Note: Whichever approach is used a trigger point will only be effectively deactivated if the muscle in which it lies is restored to its normal resting length and stretching methods such as MET can assist in achieving this.

A framework for assessment

Lief's basic spinal treatment followed a set pattern. The fact that the same order of tissue assessment is suggested at each session does not mean that the treatment is necessarily the same each time. The pattern suggests a framework and useful starting and ending points but the degree of therapeutic response offered to the various areas of dysfunction encountered varies, depending on individual considerations. This is what makes each treatment different.

Areas of dysfunction should be recorded on a case card, together with all relevant material and additional diagnostic findings, such as active or latent trigger points (and their reference zones), areas of sensitivity, hypertonicity, restricted motion and so on. Out of such a picture, super-

imposed on an assessment of whole-body features such as posture, as well as the patient's symptom picture and general health status, a therapeutic plan should emerge.

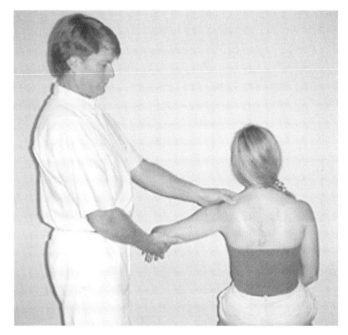

B

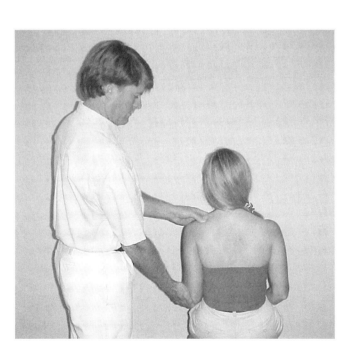

A

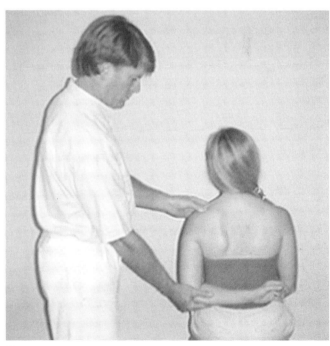

C

Figure 9.11 A: Ischemic compression is applied to trigger point in supraspinatus. B: Position of ease is located and held for 20–30 seconds. C: Following isometric contraction, the muscle housing the trigger point is stretched.

Integrated neuromuscular inhibition technique (Bailey & Dick 1992, Chaitow 1994, Jacobson 1989, Korr 1974, Rathbun & Macnab 1970)

In an attempt to develop a treatment protocol for the deactivation of myofascial trigger points a sequence has been suggested.

• The trigger point is identified by palpation methods

after which ischemic compression is applied, sufficient for the patient to be able to report that the referred pattern of pain is being activated.

• The preferred sequence after this is for that same degree of pressure to be maintained for 5–6 seconds, followed by 2–3 seconds of release of pressure.

• This pattern is repeated for up to 2 minutes until the patient reports that the local or referred symptoms (pain)

Box 9.10 Positional release techniques

Strain/counterstrain (Chaitow 1996b, Jones 1981, Walther 1988)

There are many different methods involving the positioning of an area, or the whole body, in such a way as to evoke a physiological response which helps to resolve musculoskeletal dysfunction. The means whereby the beneficial changes occur seem to involve a combination of neurological and circulatory changes which occur when a distressed area is placed in its most comfortable, its most 'easy', most pain-free position.

Walther (1988) describes how Laurence Jones DO first observed the phenomenon.

Jones' initial observation of the efficacy of counterstrain was with a patient who was unresponsive to treatment. The patient had been unable to sleep because of pain. Jones attempted to find a comfortable position for the patient to aid him in sleeping. After 20 minutes of trial and error, a position was finally achieved in which the patient's pain was relieved. Leaving the patient in this position for a short time, Jones was astonished when the patient came out of the position and was able to stand comfortably erect. The relief of pain was lasting and the patient made an uneventful recovery.

The position of 'ease' which Jones found for this patient was an exaggeration of the position in which spasm was holding him, which provided Jones with an insight into the mechanisms involved.

All areas which palpate as inappropriately painful are responding to or are associated with some degree of imbalance, dysfunction or reflexive activity which may well involve acute or chronic strain. Jones identified positions of tender points relating to particular strain positions but it makes just as much sense to work the other way round. Any painful point found during soft tissue evaluation could be treated by positional release, whether the strain pattern (acute or chronically adaptive) which produced or maintains it can be identified or not.

Common basis

All PRT methods move the patient or the affected tissues away from any resistance barriers and toward positions of comfort. The shorthand terms used for these two extremes are 'bind' and 'ease'.

One can imagine a situation in which the use of Jones' 'tender points as a monitor' method would be inappropriate (lost ability to communicate verbally or someone too young to verbalize). In such a case there is a need for a method which allows achievement of the same ends without verbal communication. This is possible using 'functional' approaches which involve finding a position of maximum ease by means of palpation alone, assessing for a state of 'ease' in the tissues.

Method

Strain/counterstrain (SCS) involves maintaining pressure on the

monitored tender point or periodically probing it, as a position is achieved in which:

• there is no additional pain in whatever area is symptomatic, and
• the monitor pain point has reduced by at least 75%.

This is then held for an appropriate length of time (90 seconds according to Jones).

SCS rules of treatment

The following 'rules' are based on clinical experience and should be borne in mind when using positional release (SCS, etc.) methods in treating pain and dysfunction, especially where the patient is fatigued, sensitive and/or distressed.

• Never treat more than five 'tender' points at any one session and treat fewer than this in sensitive individuals.
• Forewarn patients that, just as in any other form of bodywork which produces altered function, a period of physiological adaptation is inevitable and that there will therefore be a 'reaction' on the day(s) following even this extremely light form of treatment. Soreness and stiffness are therefore to be anticipated.
• If there are multiple tender points, as is inevitable in fibromyalgia, select those most proximal and most medial for primary attention; that is, those closest to the head and the center of the body rather than distal and lateral pain points.
• Of these tender points, select those that are most painful for initial attention/treatment.
• If self-treatment of painful and restricted areas is advised – and it should be if at all possible – apprise the patient of these rules (i.e. only a few pain points to be given attention on any one day, to expect a 'reaction', to select the most painful points and those closest to the head and the center of the body) (Jones 1981).

The general guidelines which Jones gives for relief of the dysfunction with which such tender points are related involve directing the movement of these tissues toward ease which commonly involves the following elements.

• For tender points on the anterior surface of the body, flexion, side bending and rotation should be toward the palpated point, followed by fine tuning to reduce sensitivity by at least 70%.
• For tender points on the posterior surface of the body, extension, side bending and rotation should be away from the palpated point, followed by fine tuning to reduce sensitivity by 70%.
• The closer the tender point is to the midline, the less side bending and rotation should be required and the further from the midline, the more side bending and rotation should be required, in order to effect ease and comfort in the tender point (without any additional pain or discomfort being produced anywhere else).
• The direction toward which side bending is introduced when trying to find a position of ease often needs to be away from the side of the palpated pain point, especially in relation to tender points found on the posterior aspect of the body.

Box 9.11 Muscle energy techniques (DiGiovanna 1991, Greenman 1989, Janda 1989, Lewit 1986, Liebenson 1989/1990, Mitchell 1967, Travell & Simons 1992)

Note: MET is described more fully in Chapter 10, with additional variations.

Assessments and use of MET

1. When the term 'restriction barrier' is used in relation to soft tissue structures, it indicates the first signs of resistance (as palpated by sense of 'bind' or sense of effort required to move the area or by visual or other palpable evidence), *not* the greatest possible range of movement available.
2. Assistance from the patient is valuable when movement is made to or through a barrier, providing the patient can be educated to gentle cooperation and not to use excessive effort.
3. When MET is applied to a joint restriction, *no stretching* is involved, merely a movement to a new barrier following the isometric contraction.
4. There should be no pain experienced during application of MET although mild discomfort (stretching) is acceptable.
5. The methods recommended provide a sound basis for the application of MET to specific muscles and areas. By developing the skills with which to apply MET, as described, a repertoire of techniques can be acquired offering a wide base of choices appropriate in numerous clinical settings.
6. Breathing cooperation can and should be used as part of the methodology of MET. Basically, if appropriate (the patient is cooperative and capable of following instructions), the patient should inhale as they slowly build up an isometric contraction,

hold the breath for the 7–10 second contraction and release the breath on slowly ceasing the contraction. They should be asked to inhale and exhale fully once more following cessation of all effort as they are instructed to 'let go completely'. During this last exhalation the new barrier is engaged or the barrier is passed as the muscle is stretched. A note to 'use appropriate breathing', or some variation on it, will be found in the text describing various MET applications.
7. Various eye movements are sometimes advocated during, or instead of, isometric contractions and during stretches (these will be described in treatment protocols for particular muscle treatments using MET, specifically in relation to the scalenes).

Isometric contraction using reciprocal inhibition

Indications

- Relaxing muscular spasm or contraction
- Stretching muscle housing trigger point

Contraction starting point – Commence contraction just short of first sign of resistance as tissues are taken through their range of movement.

Method – Antagonists to affected muscle(s) are used in isometric contraction so obliging shortened muscles to relax via reciprocal inhibition. Patient is attempting to push through the barrier of restriction against operator's precisely matched counterforce.

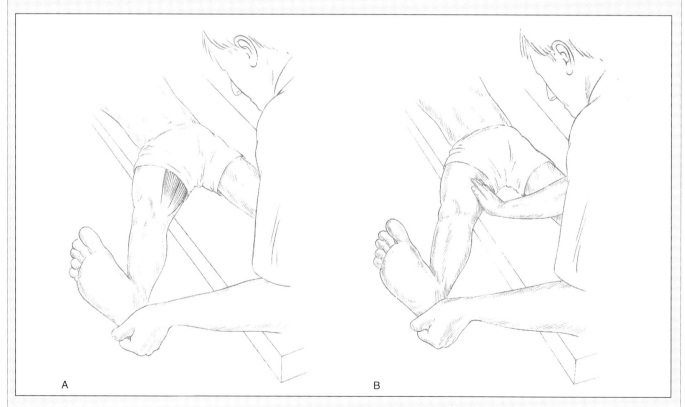

Figure 9.12 A: Assessment of 'bind'/restriction barrier assessed by practitioner's perception of transition from easy movement to 'effort' required. B: Same point ('first sign of resistance' barrier) is located by means of palpated sense of tension entering previously relaxed ('easy') tissues as leg is passively abducted (reproduced, with permission, from Chaitow L 1996 *Muscle Energy Techniques*. Churchill Livingstone, Edinburgh).

Box 9.11 *(cont'd)*

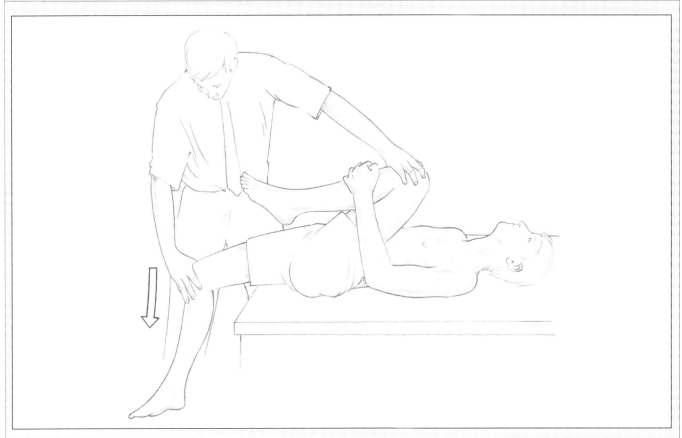

Figure 9.13 MET treatment of psoas following isometric contraction (reproduced, with permission, from Chaitow L 1996 *Muscle Energy Techniques*. Churchill Livingstone, Edinburgh).

Forces – Operator's and patient's forces are matched. Initial effort involves approximately 20% or less of patient's strength; increase to no more than 50% on subsequent contractions if appropriate. Increasing the duration of the contraction – up to 20 seconds – may be more effective than any increase in force.

Duration of contraction – 7–10 seconds initially, increasing up to 20 seconds in subsequent contractions if greater effect required.

Action following contraction – Area (muscle) is taken to light stretch after ensuring complete relaxation, with patient participation if possible. Perform movement to new barrier on an exhalation. Stretch is held for not less than 20 seconds.

Repetitions – Little gain is likely after third repetition.

Isometric contraction using postisometric relaxation (also known as postfacilitation stretching)

Indications

- Relaxing muscular spasm or contraction
- Stretching muscle housing trigger point

Contraction starting point – At or just short of resistance barrier.

Method – The affected muscles (agonists) are used in the isometric contraction. The shortened muscles subsequently relax via postisometric relaxation. Operator is attempting to push through barrier of restriction against the patient's precisely matched countereffort.

Forces – Operator's and patient's forces are matched. Initial effort involves approximately 20% of patient's strength; an increase to no more than 50% on subsequent contractions is appropriate. Increase of the duration of the contraction – up to 20 seconds – may be more effective than any increase in force.

Duration of contraction – 7–10 seconds initially, increasing to up to 20 seconds in subsequent contractions, if greater effect required.

Action following contraction – Area (muscle) is taken to light stretch after ensuring complete relaxation, with patient participation if possible. Perform movement to new barrier on an exhalation. Stretch is held for not less than 20 seconds.

Repetitions – Little gain is likely after third repetition.

Isotonic eccentric contraction (isolytic)

Indications

- Stretching tight fibrotic musculature housing trigger points

Contraction starting point – A little short of restriction barrier.

Method – The muscle to be stretched is contracted and is prevented from doing so by the operator, via superior operator effort, and the contraction is overcome and reversed, so that a contracting muscle is stretched. Origin and insertion do not approximate. Muscle is stretched to, or as close as possible to, full physiological resting length.

Box 9.11 (*cont'd*)

Forces – Operator's force is greater than patient's. Less than maximal patient's force is employed at first. Subsequent contractions build toward this, if discomfort is not excessive.

Duration of contraction – 2–4 seconds.

Repetitions – Once is adequate as microtrauma is being induced.

Caution – Avoid using isolytic contractions on head/neck muscles or at all if patient is frail, very pain sensitive or osteoporotic.

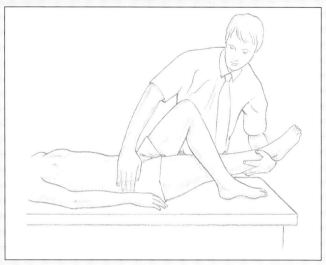

Figure 9.14 Isolytic MET treatment of TFL in which contraction and stretch of muscle are simultaneously applied (reproduced, with permission, from Chaitow L 1996 *Muscle Energy Techniques*. Churchill Livingstone, Edinburgh).

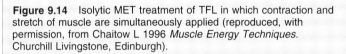

have reduced or that the pain has increased, a rare but significant event sufficient to warrant ceasing application of pressure.

• If, therefore, on reapplication of pressure during this make-and-break sequence, reported pain decreases or increases (or if 2 minutes elapse with neither of these changes being reported), the ischemic compression aspect of the INIT treatment ceases.

• At this time pressure is reintroduced and whatever degree of pain is noted is ascribed a value of 10 and the patient is asked to offer feedback information in the form of 'scores' as to the pain value, as the area is repositioned according to the guidelines of positional release methodology (Box 9.10). A position is sought which reduces reported pain to a score of 3 or less.

• This 'position of ease' is held for not less than 20 seconds, to allow neurological resetting, reduction in nociceptor activity and enhanced local circulatory interchange.

• At this stage an isometric contraction, focused into the musculature around the trigger point, is initiated (see muscle energy technique, Box 9.11) and following this, the tissues are stretched both locally and, where possible, in a manner which involves the whole muscle.

• In some instances it is also found useful to add a reeducational activation of antagonists to the muscle housing the trigger point using Ruddy's methods (see Box 9.12) to complete the treatment.

• This is the integrated neuromuscular inhibition technique (INIT) protocol.

INIT rationale

• When a trigger point is being palpated by direct

Box 9.12 Ruddy's pulsed muscle energy technique

A promising addition to this sequence takes account of the potential offered by the methods developed some years ago by osteopathic physician T J Ruddy (1962). In the 1940s and 1950s Ruddy developed a method of rapid pulsating contractions against resistance which he termed 'rapid rhythmic resistive duction'. For obvious reasons, the short-hand term 'pulsed muscle energy technique' is now applied to Ruddy's method.

Its simplest use involves the dysfunctional tissue or joint being held at its restriction barrier, at which time the patient ideally (or the practitioner if the patient cannot adequately cooperate with the instructions) introduces a series of rapid (two per second), *minute* efforts toward the barrier, against the resistance of the practitioner. The barest initiation of effort is called for, with (to use Ruddy's words) 'no wobble and no bounce'.

The application of this 'conditioning' approach involves, in Ruddy's words, contractions which are 'short, rapid and rhythmic, gradually increasing the amplitude and degree of resistance, thus conditioning the proprioceptive system by rapid movements'.

Ruddy suggests that the effects are likely to include improved oxygenation, venous and lymphatic circulation through the area being treated. Furthermore, he believed that the method influences both static and kinetic posture because of the effects on proprioceptive and interoceptive afferent pathways, so helping to maintain 'dynamic equilibrium', which involves 'a balance in chemical, physical, thermal, electrical and tissue fluid homeostasis'.

In a setting in which tense hypertonic, possibly shortened musculature has been treated by stretching, it is important to begin facilitating and strengthening the inhibited, weakened antagonists. This is true whether the hypertonic muscles have been treated for reasons of shortness/hypertonicity alone or because they accommodate active trigger points within their fibers.

The introduction of a pulsating muscle energy procedure, such as Ruddy's, involving these weak antagonists offers the opportunity for:

• proprioceptive reeducation
• strengthening facilitation of the weak antagonists
• further inhibition of tense agonists
• enhanced local circulation and drainage
• and, in Liebenson's (1996) words, 'reeducation of movement patterns on a reflex, subcortical basis'.

finger or thumb pressure and when the very tissues in which the trigger point lies are positioned in such a way as to take away (most of) the pain, during positional release application, the most stressed fibers in which the trigger point is housed will be in a position of relative ease.

- At this time the trigger point would have already received and would again be under direct inhibitory, ischemic pressure and would have been positioned so that the tissues housing it are relaxed (relatively or completely).

- Following a period of 30–60 seconds of this position of ease, the patient introduces an isometric contraction into the tissues and holds this for 7–10 seconds, involving the precise fibers which had been repositioned to obtain the positional release.

- The effect of this would be to produce (following the contraction) a reduction in tone in these tissues. These tissues could then be stretched locally or in a manner to involve the whole muscle, depending on their location, so that the specifically targeted fibers would be stretched.

REFERENCES

American College of Rheumatology 1990 Criteria for the classification of fibromyalgia. Arthritis and Rheumatism 33:160–172

Athenstaedt H 1974 Pyroelectric and piezoelectric properties of vertebrates. Annals of New York Academy of Sciences 238:68–110

Bailey M, Dick L 1992 Nociceptive considerations in treating with counterstrain. Journal of the American Osteopathic Association 92:334–341

Baldry P 1993 Acupuncture, trigger points and musculoskeletal pain. Churchill Livingstone, Edinburgh

Barnes M 1997 The basic science of myofascial release. Journal of Bodywork and Movement Therapies 1(4):231–238

Brostoff J 1992 Complete guide to food allergy. Bloomsbury, London

Cailliet R 1996 Soft tissue pain and disability, 3rd edn. F A Davis, Philadelphia

Cantu R, Grodin A 1992 Myofascial manipulation. Aspen Publications, Gaithersburg, Maryland

Chaitow B 1983 Personal communication

Chaitow L 1990 Acupuncture treatment of pain. Healing Arts Press, Rochester, Vermont

Chaitow L 1994 Integrated neuromuscular inhibition technique. British Journal of Osteopathy 13:17–20

Chaitow L 1996a Modern neuromuscular techniques. Churchill Livingstone, New York, ch 11, p 154

Chaitow L 1996b Positional release techniques. Churchill Livingstone, Edinburgh

Chaitow L 2000 Fibromyalgia syndrome: a practitioner's guide. Churchill Livingstone, Edinburgh

DeLany J 1994 NMT course manuals: applications pack. NMT Center, Saint Petersburg

DeLany J 1999 Clinical perspectives: breast cancer reconstructive rehabilitation: NMT. Journal of Bodywork and Movement Therapies 3(1):5–10

DiGiovanna E 1991 Osteopathic diagnosis and treatment. Lippincott, Philadelphia

Dvorak J, Dvorak V, Schneider W 1988 Manual medicine therapy. Georg Thieme Verlag, Stuttgart

Feldenkrais M 1972 Awareness through movement. Harper and Row, New York

Ferraccioli G 1990 Neuroendocrinologic findings in fibromyalgia and in other chronic rheumatic conditions. Journal of Rheumatology 17:869–873

Gilbert C 1998 Hyperventilation and the body. Journal of Bodywork and Movement Therapies 2(3):184–191

Greenman P 1989 Principles of manual medicine. Williams and Wilkins, Baltimore

Hanna T 1988 Somatics. Addison-Wesley, New York

Hong C-Z, Chen Y-N, Twehouse D, Hong D 1996 Pressure threshold for referred pain by compression on trigger point and adjacent area. Journal of Musculoskeletal Pain 4(3):61–79

Jacobson E 1989 Shoulder pain and repetition strain injury. Journal of the American Osteopathic Association 89:1037–1045

Janda V 1982 Introduction to functional pathology of the motor system. Proceedings of the VII Commonwealth and International Conference on Sport. Physiotherapy in Sport 3:39

Janda V 1989 Muscle function testing. Butterworths, London

Jones L 1981 Strain and counterstrain. Academy of Applied Osteopathy, Colorado Springs

Jonkheere P, Pattyn J 1998 Myofascial muscle chains. Trigger vzw, Brugge, Belgium

Korr I 1974 Proprioceptors and somatic dysfunction. Journal of the American Osteopathic Association 74:638–650

Lewit K 1986 Muscular patterns in thoraco-lumbar lesions. Manual Medicine 2:105

Lewit K 1992 Manipulative therapy in rehabilitation of the locomotor system. Butterworths, London

Liebenson C 1989 and 1990 Active muscular relaxation techniques (parts 1 and 2). Journal of Manipulative and Physiological Therapeutics 12(6):446–451 and 13(1):2–6

Liebenson C 1996 Rehabilitation of the spine. Williams and Wilkins, Baltimore

Lowe J, Honeyman-Lowe G 1998 Facilitating the decrease in fibromyalgic pain during metabolic rehabilitation Journal of Bodywork and Movement Therapies 2(4):208–217

Lowe W 1995 Looking in depth: heat and cold therapy. In: Orthopedic and sports massage reviews. Orthopedic Massage Education and Research Institute, Bend, Oregon

Melzack R, Wall P 1988 The challenge of pain, 2nd edn. Penguin, Harmondsworth, Middlesex

Mitchell F Snr 1967 Motion discordance. Academy of Applied Osteopathy Yearbook, Carmel, California, pp 1–5

Nimmo R 1957 Receptors, affectors and tonus. Journal of the American Chiropractic Association 27(11):21

Oschman J L 1997 What is healing energy? Pt 5: gravity, structure, and emotions. Journal of Bodywork and Movement Therapies 1(5):307–308

Randolph T 1976 Stimulatory withdrawal and the alternations of allergic manifestations. In: Dickey L (ed) Clinical ecology. Charles C Thomas, Springfield, Illinois

Rathbun J, Macnab I 1970 Microvascular pattern at the rotator cuff. Journal of Bone and Joint Surgery 52:540–553

Ruddy T J 1962 Osteopathic rapid rhythmic resistive technic. Academy of Applied Osteopathy Yearbook, Carmel, California, pp 23–31

Selye H 1956 The stress of life. McGraw Hill, New York

Simons D, Travell J, Simons L 1998 Myofascial pain and dysfunction: the trigger point manual, vol 1: the upper half of body, 2nd edn. Williams and Wilkins, Baltimore

Stedman's electronic medical dictionary, version 4.0 1998 Williams and Wilkins, Baltimore

Travell J, Simons D 1992 Myofascial pain and dysfunction: the trigger point manual, vol 2: The lower extremities. Williams and Wilkins, Baltimore

Walther D 1988 Applied kinesiology synopsis. Systems DC, Pueblo, Colorado

Ward R 1997 Foundations of osteopathic medicine. Williams and Wilkins, Baltimore

10

Associated therapeutic modalities and techniques

The techniques described in this chapter represent those methods which the authors see as most usefully combining with NMT (either Lief's or American version as described in Chapter 9). This is not meant to suggest that other methods which address soft tissue dysfunction are necessarily less effective or inappropriate. It does, however, mean that the methods described and incorporated throughout the clinical applications text, such as variations on the theme of muscle energy technique (MET), positional release technique (PRT) and myofascial release technique (MFR), are known to be helpful as a result of the clinical experience of the authors. Traditional massage methods are also frequently mentioned, as are applications of lymphatic drainage techniques. All these methods require appropriate training and the descriptions and explanations offered in this chapter are not meant to replace that requirement.

The material in this chapter describes both the methods employed in the different techniques as well as some of the underlying principles which may help to explain their mechanisms. Those methods which will be described are (in alphabetical order):

- acupuncture/acupressure (see Box 10.1)
- hydrotherapy/cryotherapy
- integrated neuromuscular inhibition technique (INIT) including Ruddy's reciprocal antagonist facilitation (RRAF)
- lymphatic drainage
- massage
- mobilization techniques
- muscle energy technique (MET)
- myofascial release techniques (MFR)
- positional release techniques (PRT, including strain/counterstrain (SCS))
- Ruddy's pulsed muscle energy technique
- stretching techniques (other than MET).

Box 10.1 Acupuncture and trigger points

Acupuncture points are sited at fairly precise anatomical locations, which can be corroborated by electrical detection, each point being evidenced by a small area of lowered electrical resistance (Mann 1963). When 'active', due presumably to reflex stimulation, these points become even more easily detectable, as the electrical resistance lowers further. The skin overlying them also alters and becomes hyperalgesic and easy to palpate as differing from surrounding skin. In this way they mimic the characteristics of trigger points (see Chapter 6 for discussion of skin characteristics in relation to trigger points).

Active acupuncture points also become sensitive to pressure and this is of value in assessment since the finding of sensitive areas during palpation or treatment is of diagnostic importance. Sensitive and painful areas may well be 'active' acupuncture points (or *tsubo*, in Japanese) (Serizawa 1980). Not only are these points detectable and sensitive but they are also amenable to treatment by direct pressure techniques (see below).

Serizawa (1980) discusses a 'nerve reflex' theory for the existence of these points.

The nerve reflex theory holds that, when an abnormal condition occurs in an internal organ, alterations take place in the skin and muscles related to that organ by means of the nervous system. These alterations occur as reflex actions. The nervous system, extending throughout the internal organs, like the skin, the subcutaneous tissues, and the muscles, constantly transmits information about the physical condition to the spinal cord and the brain. These information impulses, which are centripetal in nature, set up a reflex action that causes symptoms of the internal organic disorder to manifest themselves in the surface areas of the body. ... the intimate relation between internal organs and external ones has a reverse effect as well; that is, stimulation to the skin and muscles affects the condition of the internal organs and tissues.

A conceptual link between the forces underlying tsubo/acupuncture points and the explanations of facilitation (Chapter 6) is clearly evident.

Are acupuncture points and trigger points the same phenomenon?

Pain researchers Wall & Melzack (1989), as well as Travell & Simons (1992), maintain that there is little, if any, difference between acupuncture points and most trigger points. Since they spatially occupy the same positions in at least 70% of cases (Wall & Melzack 1989) there is often a coincidence of treatment in that a trigger point could be 'mistaken' for an active acupuncture point and vice versa. Wall & Melzack have concluded that 'trigger points and acupuncture points, when used for pain control, though discovered independently and labeled differently, represent the same phenomenon'.

Baldry (1993) claims differences in their structural make-up, however. He states:

It would seem likely that they are of two different types, and their close spatial correlation is because there are A-delta afferent-innervated [fast transmitting receptors with a high threshold and sensitive to sharply pointed stimuli or heat-produced stimulation] acupuncture points in the skin and subcutaneous tissues immediately above the intramuscularly placed predominantly C afferent-innervated [slow transmitting, low threshold, widely

distributed and sensitive to chemical – such as those released by damaged cells – mechanical or thermal stimulus] trigger points.

Clearly stimulation of an area which contains both an acupuncture and a trigger point will influence both types of neural transmission and both 'points'. Which route of reflex stimulation is producing a therapeutic effect or whether other mechanisms altogether are at work – endorphin release, for example – is therefore open to debate. This debate can be widened if we include the vast array of other reflex influences identified by other systems and workers including neurolymphatic and neurovascular reflexes (Chaitow 1996b).

Whereas traditional Oriental concepts focus on energy (*Qi*) imbalances in reaction to acupuncture points, there also exist a number of Western interpretations. Melzack (1977) assumed that acupuncture points represent areas of abnormal physiological activity, producing a continuous, low-level input into the CNS. He suggests that this might eventually lead to a combining with noxious stimuli deriving from other structures, innervated by the same segments, to produce an increased awareness of pain and distress. He found it reasonable to assume that trigger points and acupuncture points represented the same phenomenon, having found that the location of trigger points on Western maps and acupuncture points used commonly in painful conditions showed a remarkable 70% correlation in position.

Lewith & Kenyon (1984) point to a variety of suggestions as to the mechanisms via which acupuncture (or acupressure) achieves its pain-relieving results. These include neurological explanations such as the gate control theory. This in itself is seen to be an incomplete explanation and humoral (endorphin release, etc.) and psychological factors are also shown to be involved in modifying the patient's perception of pain. A combination of reflex and direct neurological elements, as well as the involvement of a variety of secretions such as enkephalins and endorphins, is thought to be the modus operandi of acupressure. Some of these influences are also considered to be operating during manual treatment of trigger points (see Chapter 6).

Ah Shi points

Acupuncture methodology also includes the treatment of points which are not listed on the meridian maps, known as Ah Shi points. These include all painful points which arise spontaneously, usually in relation to particular joint problems or disease. For the duration of their sensitivity they are regarded as being suitable for needle or pressure treatment. These points may therefore be thought of as identical to the 'tender' points described by Laurence Jones (1995) in his strain and counterstrain method, which also frequently coincide with established trigger point sites (see p. 150).

It is not the intention of this book to provide instruction in acupuncture methodology, nor to necessarily endorse the views expressed by traditional acupuncture in relation to meridians and their purported connection with organs and systems. However, it would be shortsighted to ignore the accumulated wisdom which has led many thousands of skilled practitioners to ascribe particular roles to these points. As far as a manual therapy is concerned, there seems to be value in having awareness of the reported roles of particular acupuncture points and of incorporating this into diagnostic and therapeutic settings. As we palpate and search through the soft tissues, in basic neuromuscular technique, we are bound to come across areas of sensitivity which relate to these points.

HYDROTHERAPY AND CRYOTHERAPY

(Boyle & Saine 1988, Chaitow 1999, Kirchfeld & Boyle 1994, Licht 1963)

How water works on the body

When anything *warm or hot is applied* to tissues, muscles relax and blood vessels dilate. This causes more blood to reach those tissues. Unless there is then activity (such as would occur with muscles contracting and relaxing during exercise or with gliding strokes of effleurage massage) or unless a cold application of some sort follows application of heat, the tissues will tend to become congested. For this reason a cold application almost always follows a hot one in hydrotherapy methodology.

When a *short cold* application is applied to tissues it causes vasoconstriction of the local blood vessels. This has the effect of decongesting tissues and is rapidly followed by a reaction in which blood vessels dilate and tissues are flushed with fresh, oxygen-rich blood.

Alternate hot and cold applications produce circulatory interchange and improved drainage and oxygen supply to the tissues, whether these be muscles, skin or organs.

Two important rules of hydrotherapy are that:

- there should almost always be a short cold application, or *immersion*, after a hot one and preferably also before it (unless otherwise stated), and
- when heat is applied, it should never be hot enough to scald the skin and should always be bearable.

The general principles of hot and cold applications are as follows.

- Short cold applications (less than a minute) stimulate circulation.
- Long cold applications (more than a minute) depress circulation and metabolism.
- Long hot applications (more than 5 minutes) vasodilate and can leave the area congested and static and require a cold application or massage to help restore normality.
- Short hot applications (less than 5 minutes) stimulate circulation but long hot applications (more than 5 minutes) depress both circulation and metabolism.
- Short hot followed by short cold applications cause alternation of circulation followed by a return to normal.
- Hot is defined as 98–104° Fahrenheit or 36.7–40° Centigrade. *Anything hotter than that is undesirable and dangerous.*
- Neutral applications or baths at body heat are very soothing and relaxing.
- Cold is defined as 55–65°F or 12.7–18.3°C.
- Anything colder is very cold and anything warmer is: cool (66–80°F or 18.5–26.5°C)

tepid (81–92°F or 26.5–33.3°C)
neutral/warm (93–97°F or 33.8–36.1°C).

Warming compress

This is called a 'cold compress' in Europe and is a simple but effective method. It involves use of a piece of cold, wet material (cotton is best), well wrung out in cold water and then applied to an area which is immediately covered in a way that insulates it and allows body heat to warm the cold material. Plastic is often used to prevent the damp from spreading and to further insulate the material.

A reflex stimulus takes place when the cold material first touches the skin, leading to a flushing of blood and a return of fresh, oxygenated blood. As the compress slowly warms there is a deeply relaxing effect and a reduction of pain. This is an ideal method for self-treatment or first aid for any of the following:

- painful joints
- mastitis
- sore throat (compress on the throat from ear to ear and supported over the top of the head)
- backache (see trunk pack below)
- sore tight chest from bronchitis.

Materials

- A single or double piece of cotton sheeting large enough to cover the area to be treated (double for people with good circulation and vitality, single for people with only moderate circulation and vitality)
- One thickness of woolen or flannel material (toweling will do but is not as effective) *larger* than the cotton material so that it can cover it completely with no edges protruding
- Plastic material of the same size as the woolen material
- Safety pins
- Cold water

Method

- The cotton material is well wrung out in cold water so that it is damp but not dripping wet.
- This is placed over the painful area and immediately covered with the woolen or flannel material, and also the plastic material if used, and pinned in place.
- The compress should be firm enough to ensure that there is no access for air to cool it but not so tight as to impede circulation.
- The cold material should rapidly warm and feel comfortable and after several hours, it should be virtually dry.
- The cotton material should be washed before reuse as it will absorb acid wastes from the body.

- A local (single joint) warming compress is used up to four times daily with at least an hour between applications. Ideally it is left on overnight.

Caution

If for any reason the compress is still cold after 20 minutes (the compress may be too wet or too loose or the vitality may not be adequate to the task of warming it), then remove it and give the area a brisk rub with a towel.

Trunk pack – an example of a warming compress

A trunk pack has no contraindications and is useful in either acute or chronic stages of back pain. Materials include:

- one or two thicknesses of cotton (tear up an old sheet) wide enough to measure from the underarm to the pelvis and long enough to pass just once around the body without overlapping
- one thickness of woolen or flannel material, almost the same dimension as the cotton but a little wider and a little longer so that none of the cotton material has access to air
- safety pins and cold water
- a warm room.

The cotton material is wrung out using cold water so that the material is just damp, not dripping, and is wrapped around the trunk so that it covers the area from the underarm to the pelvis. It is *immediately* covered with the dry wool/flannel material and pinned firmly so that it completely covers the damp cotton with no edges protruding. The patient is asked to lie down and is covered with a blanket. This method can be used for a few hours during the day or overnight.

- Within about 5 minutes any sense of cold should vanish and the material should feel comfortable. If it still feels cold after 5 minutes, the compress is removed.
- After about 20 minutes the compress should start to feel hot and this should be maintained for several hours until it 'bakes' itself dry.
- The initial cold has a decongesting effect, followed by a period of neutral temperature (at around body temperature) which relaxes the muscles, followed by the period of damp warmth which further enhances this relaxation.
- If the patient has a strong constitution and good vitality and is not adversely influenced by cold, two thicknesses of damp cotton are used, following all the same guidelines, to get a more powerful effect.
- This method is used three or four times weekly (alternate days) during either acute or chronic stages of back pain.
- The cotton material should be thoroughly washed

before reuse as it will absorb acid wastes from the body which can irritate the skin.

Alternate heat and cold: constitutional hydrotherapy (home application)

Effects

Constitutional hydrotherapy has a non-specific 'balancing' effect, reducing chronic pain, enhancing immune function and promoting healing. There are no contraindications since the degree of temperature contrast in its application can be modified to take account of any degree of sensitivity, frailty, etc.

Materials

- Somewhere for the patient to lie down
- A full-sized sheet folded in two or two single sheets
- Two blankets (wool if possible)
- Two bath towels (when folded in two, each should be able to reach from side to side and from shoulders to hips)
- Two small towels (each should as a single layer be the same size as the large towel folded in two)
- Hot and cold water (see temperature in notes below)

This method cannot be self-applied, assistance is needed.

Method

1. Patient undresses and lies supine between sheets and under blanket.
2. Two hot folded bath towels (four layers) are placed directly onto the skin of the patient's trunk – shoulders to hips, side to side.
3. The patient is covered with sheet and blanket and left for 5 minutes.
4. Helper returns with a small hot towel and a small cold towel.
5. The 'new' hot towel is placed on top of the four 'old' hot towels and the stack of towels is 'flipped' so that the hot towel is on the skin. The old towels are discarded.
6. Immediately the cold towel is placed onto the new hot towel and these are flipped so that the cold towel is on the skin. The small hot towel is discarded.
7. The patient is covered with a sheet and left for 10 minutes or until the cold towel is warmed.
8. The previously cold (now warm) towel is removed and the patient turns to lie prone.
9. Steps 2–7 are repeated to the back of the patient.

Notes

- If using a bed, precautions should be taken to avoid it getting wet.

• 'Hot' water in this context is a temperature high enough to prevent a hand remaining in it for more than 5 seconds.

• The coldest water from a running tap is adequate for the 'cold' towel. In hot summers adding ice to the water in which this towel is wrung out is acceptable if the temperature contrast is acceptable to the patient.

• If the patient feels cold after the cold towel is placed, back, foot or hand massage should be applied (through the blanket and towel) to warm her.

• By varying the differential between hot and cold, so that the contrast is small for someone whose immune function and overall degree of vulnerability is poor, for example, and using a large contrast, very hot and very cold, for someone whose constitution is robust, the application of the method can be tailored to meet individual cases.

• The method is used once or twice daily, if needed.

Neutral bath

A neutral bath, in which body temperature is the same as that of the water, has a profoundly relaxing influence on the nervous system. This was the main method of calming violent and disturbed patients in mental asylums in the 19th century. A neutral bath is useful in all cases of anxiety, for feelings of 'stress' and for relieving chronic pain and insomnia.

Contraindications

People with skin conditions which react badly to water or who have serious cardiac disease should avoid this method.

Materials

• A bathtub
• Water
• Bath thermometer

Method

• The bath as filled with water as close to 97°F (36.1°C) as possible.
• The bath has its effect by being as close to body temperature as can be achieved.
• Immersion in water at this neutral temperature has a profoundly relaxing, sedating effect on nervous system activity.
• The patient submerges in the bath so that the water covers the shoulders. The back of the head should rest on a towel or sponge.
• The thermometer should be in the bath to ensure

that the temperature does not drop below 92°F (33.3°C).

• The water can be 'topped up' periodically *but must not exceed the 97°F/36.1°C limit.*

• The duration of the bath should be anything from 30 minutes to 2 hours.

• After the bath the patient should rest in bed for at least an hour.

Alternate bathing

By alternating hot and cold water in different ways it is possible to have profound effects on circulation.

• Alternate bathing is useful for all conditions that involve congestion and inflammation, locally or generally, and for an overall tonic effect.

• Alternating sitz baths are ideal for varicose veins and hemorrhoids.

Contraindications

Alternate bathing should not be used if there is hemorrhage, colic and spasm, acute or serious chronic heart disease or acute bladder and kidney infections.

Materials

• Containers suitable for holding hot and cold water
• If the whole pelvic area is to be immersed, then a large plastic or other tub (an old-fashioned hip bath is best) is required, along with a smaller container for simultaneous immersion of the feet
• A bath thermometer
• Hot and cold water

Method

• If a local area such as the arm, wrist or ankle is receiving treatment, then that part should be alternately immersed in hot and then cold water following the timings given below for alternating sitz baths.

• For local immersion treatment ice cubes can be placed in the cold water for greater contrast.

• If the area is unsuitable for treatment by immersion (a shoulder or a knee could prove awkward), then application of hot and cold temperatures is possible by using towels, soaked in water of the appropriate temperature and lightly wrung out, again following the same timescales as for sitz baths, given below.

Alternating sitz baths

These baths involve the immersion of the pelvic area (buttocks and hips up to the navel) in water of one temperature, while the feet are in water of the same or a contrasting temperature. The sequence to follow in alternating pelvic sitz baths is:

- 1–3 minutes seated in hot water (106–110°F or 41–43°C)
- 15–30 seconds in cold (around 60°F/15°C)
- 1–3 minutes hot
- 15 seconds cold.

During the hip immersions the feet should, if possible, be in water of a contrasting temperature, so that when the hips are in hot water, the feet are in cold and vice versa. If this is difficult to organize, the alternating hip immersions alone should be used.

Ice pack

Ice causes vasoconstriction in tissues it is in contact with because of the large amount of heat it absorbs as it turns from solid into liquid.

Ice treatment is helpful for:

- all sprains and injuries
- bursitis and other joint swellings or inflammations (unless cold aggravates the pain)
- toothache
- headache
- hemorrhoids
- bites.

Contraindications

Applications of ice are contraindicated on the abdomen during acute bladder problems, over the chest during acute asthma or if any health condition is aggravated by cold.

Materials

- A piece of flannel or wool material large enough to cover the area to be treated
- Towels
- Ice
- Safety pins
- Plastic
- Bandage

Method

- Crushed ice is placed on a towel, to form a thickness of an inch.
- The towel is then folded and pinned to contain the ice.
- A layer of wool or flannel material is placed onto the site of the pain and the ice pack is placed onto this.

- The pack is then covered with plastic and the bandage is used to hold it all in place.
- Clothing and bedding should be protected with additional plastic and towels.
- The ice pack is left in place for up to half an hour and repeated after an hour, if helpful.

Ice coolants as a form of trigger point treatment

Chilling and stretching a muscle housing a trigger point rapidly assists in deactivation of the abnormal neurological behavior of the site. Travell (1952) and Mennell (1974) have described these effects in detail. Simons et al (1998) state that 'Spray and stretch is the single most effective non-invasive method to inactivate acute trigger points' and that the stretch component is the action and the spray is a distraction. They also point out that the spray is applied before or during the stretch and *not* after the muscle has already been elongated.

Travell & Simons (1992; Simons et al 1998) have discouraged the use of vapocoolants to chill the area due to environmental considerations relating to ozone depletion and have instead urged the use of stroking with ice in a similar manner to the spray stream to achieve the same ends. The objective is to chill the surface tissues while the underlying muscle housing the trigger is simultaneously stretched.

- A container of an environmentally friendly vapocoolant spray with a calibrated nozzle which delivers a moderately fine jet stream (or a source of ice) is needed.
- 'Gebauer Spray and Stretch' is an environmentally friendly spray that is undergoing testing at this time (Simons et al 1998). In the meantime, fluorimethane has a temporary medical acceptance for use in the US and is preferred over ethyl chloride, which is health hazardous and colder than desired for this treatment (Simons et al 1998).
- The jet stream should have sufficient force to carry in the air for at least 3 feet (a mist-like spray is less effective).
- A cylinder of ice may be used instead, formed by freezing water in a paper cup and then peeling the cup down to expose the ice edge. A wooden handle can be frozen into the ice to allow for ease of application, as the thin, cold edge of the ice is applied in unidirectional parallel strokes from the trigger toward the referred area in a series of sweeps.
- Travell & Simons (1992) have, however, pointed out that the skin should remain dry for this method to be successful as dampness retards the rate of cooling of the skin and may also delay rewarming. Wrapping the ice in thin plastic (bag or wrap) will prevent moisture from touching the skin (a factor which Dr Janet Travell insisted,

in a personal communication to JD, was of particular importance), but reduces the efficacy somewhat over that of vapocoolants.

• One author (LC) has found that a cold drink can which has been partially filled with water and then frozen is a good substitute. The ice-cold metal container can be rolled over the skin and will adequately retain its chilling potential without excessive moisture touching the skin.

• Cryostimulators (smooth-ended metal 'hot dog' shaped instruments which are frozen prior to use) are effective and do not produce much moisture.

• Another substitute for the vapocoolant spray is a neurologist's pin wheel run in a similar manner in parallel sweeps which creates a prickling sensation rather than the cold sensation (Simons et al 1998).

• Whichever method is chosen, the patient should be comfortably supported to promote muscular relaxation and should be warm. If the person is cold elsewhere on the body, a blanket or heating pads may be used to assist in her comfort and to discourage muscular tightening.

• If a spray is used, the container is held 1–2 feet away from the surface, in such a manner that the fine jet stream meets the body surface at an acute angle, not perpendicularly. This lessens the shock of the impact. For the same reason, the stream is sometimes started in air or on the practitioner's hand and is gradually brought into contact with the skin overlying the trigger point.

• The fine stream, or the ice-stroking/frozen canister, is applied only in unidirectional parallel sweeps, not back and forth, from the trigger point through the reference zone.

• Each sweep is started slightly proximal to the trigger point and is moved slowly and evenly through the reference zone to cover it and extend slightly beyond it.

• It is advantageous to spray or ice-chill both trigger and reference areas, since secondary trigger points are likely to have developed within reference zones when pain is very strong. This type of sweep also addresses both central and attachment trigger points (Simons et al 1998).

• The direction of movement is usually in line with the muscle fibers toward their insertion.

• The optimum speed of movement of the sweep/roll over the skin seems to be about 4 inches (10 cm) per second. The sweeps are repeated in a rhythm of a few seconds on and a few seconds off, until all the skin over trigger and reference areas has been covered once or twice.

• If aching or 'cold pain' develops or if the application of the spray or ice/canister activates a reference of pain, the interval between applications is lengthened. Care is taken not to frost or blanch the skin.

• During the application of cold or directly after it, the taut fibers should be passively stretched. The fibers should not be stretched in advance of the cold.

• Steady, gentle stretching is usually essential if a satisfactory result is to be achieved.

• As relaxation of the muscle occurs, continued stretch should be maintained for 20–30 seconds and after each series of cold applications, active motion is tested.

• The patient is asked to move in the directions which were restricted before spraying or which were painful to activate.

• An attempt should be made to restore the full range of motion, but always within the limits of pain, since sudden overstretching can increase existing muscle spasm.

• The treatment is continued in this manner until the trigger points (often several are present or a 'nest' of them) and their respective pain reference zones have been treated.

• The entire procedure may occupy 15–20 minutes and should not be rushed.

• Simple exercises which utilize the principle of passive or active stretch should be outlined to the patient, to be carried out several times daily, after the application of gentle heat (hot packs, etc.) at home. Usual precautions should be mentioned, such as avoiding use of heat if symptoms worsen or if there is evidence of inflammation.

These examples of the wide variety of hydrotherapy methods available for both clinical and home application should provide a basis for recommendations to patients. A key caution is that wherever heat is applied, cold should follow as the final application. The referenced texts are all recommended for further reading on the subject, particularly *Naturopathic hydrotherapy* by Wayne Boyle and Andre Saine (1988).

INTEGRATED NEUROMUSCULAR INHIBITION TECHNIQUE (Chaitow 1994)

INIT involves using the position of ease as part of a sequence which commences with the location of a tender/trigger point, followed by application of ischemic compression (optional – avoided if pain is too intense or the patient too sensitive) followed by the introduction of positional release. After an appropriate length of time during which the tissues are held in 'ease' (20–30 seconds), the patient is guided to introduce an isometric contraction into the tissues housing the trigger point and hold it for 7–10 seconds, after which these tissues are stretched (or they may be stretched at the same time as the contraction, if fibrotic tissue calls for such attention).

An additional sequence can often be usefully introduced, involving rhythmic contractions of the antagonist to the muscle housing the trigger point, which will introduce an inhibitory effect on excessive fiber tone as well as strengthening inhibited antagonists. This sequence is described below in detail.

Box 10.2 A summary of soft tissue approaches to FMS (Chaitow 2000)

When people are very ill (as in fibromyalgia syndrome – FMS and chronic fatigue syndrome – CFS), where adaptive functions have been stretched to their limits, any treatment (however gentle) represents an additional demand for adaptation (i.e. it is yet another stressor to which the person has to adapt).

It is therefore essential that treatments and therapeutic interventions are carefully selected and modulated to the patient's current ability to respond, as well as this can be judged.

When symptoms are at their worst only single changes, simple interventions, may be appropriate, with time allowed for the body/mind to process and handle these.

It may also be worth considering general, whole-body, constitutional, approaches (dietary changes, hydrotherapy, non-specific 'wellness' massage, relaxation methods, etc.), rather than specific interventions, in the initial stages and during periods when symptoms have flared. Recovery from FMS is slow at best and it is easy to make matters worse by overenthusiastic and inappropriate interventions. Patience is required by both the health-care provider and the patient, avoiding raising false hopes while realistic therapeutic and educational methods are used which do not make matters worse and which offer ease and the best chance of improvement.

Identification of local dysfunction

- Off-body scan for temperature variations (cold may suggest ischemia, hot may indicate irritation/inflammation).
- Evaluation of fascial adherence to underlying tissues, indicating deeper dysfunction.
- Assessment of variations in local skin elasticity, where loss of elastic quality indicates hyperalgesic zone and probable deeper dysfunction (e.g. trigger point) or pathology.
- Evaluation of reflexively active areas (triggers, etc.) by means of very light single-digit palpation seeking phenomenon of 'drag' (Lewit 1992).
- NMT palpation utilizing variable pressure, which 'meets and matches' tissue tonus.
- Functional evaluation to assess local tissue response to normal physiological demand, e.g. as in functional shoulder evaluation as described in Chapter 5.

Short postural muscles

- Sequential assessment and identification of specific shortened

postural muscles, by means of observed and palpated changes, functional evaluation methods, etc. (Greenman 1989).
- Subsequent treatment of short muscles by means of MET or self-stretching will allow for regaining of strength in antagonist muscles which have become inhibited. At the same time, gentle toning exercise may be appropriate.

Treatment of local (i.e. trigger points) and whole muscle problems

- Tissues held at elastic barrier to await physiological release (skin stretch, C bend, S bend, gentle NMT, etc.).
- Use of positional release methods – holding tissues in 'dynamic neutral' (strain/ counterstrain, functional technique, induration technique, fascial release methods, etc.) (Jones 1981).
- Myofascial release methods – gently applied.
- MET methods for local and whole muscle dysfunction (involving acute, chronic and pulsed [Ruddy's] MET variations as described in this chapter).
- Vibrational techniques (rhythmic/rocking/oscillating articulation methods; mechanical or hand vibration).
- Deactivation of myofascial trigger points (if sensitivity allows) utilizing INIT or other methods (acupuncture, ultrasound, etc.) (Baldry 1993).

Whole-body approaches

- Wellness massage and/or aromatherapy
- Hydrotherapy
- Cranial techniques
- Therapeutic touch
- Lymphatic drainage

Reeducation/rehabilitation/self-help approaches

- Postural (Alexander, etc.)
- Breathing retraining (Garland 1994)
- Cognitive behavioral modification
- Aerobic fitness training
- Yoga-type stretching, tai chi
- Deep relaxation methods (autogenics, etc.)
- Pain self-treatment (e.g. self-applied SCS)

Sound nutrition and endocrine balancing

INIT method 1

In an attempt to develop a treatment protocol for the deactivation of myofascial trigger points, a sequence has been suggested.

- The trigger point is identified by palpation methods.
- Ischemic compression is applied in either a sustained or intermittent manner.
- When referred or local pain begins to diminish, the tissues housing the trigger point are taken to a position of ease and held for approximately 20–30 seconds, to allow neurological resetting, reduction in nociceptor activity and enhanced local circulatory interchange.
- An isometric contraction focuses into the

musculature around the trigger point followed by the tissues being stretched both locally and (where possible) in a manner which involves the whole muscle.

- The patient assists in the stretching movements (whenever possible) by activating the antagonists and facilitating the stretch.

INIT rationale

When a trigger point is being palpated by direct finger or thumb pressure and when the very tissues in which the trigger point lies are positioned in such a way as to take away the pain (entirely or at least to a great extent), the most (dis)stressed fibers, in which trigger points are housed, are in a position of relative ease. The trigger point is under direct inhibitory pressure (mild or perhaps intermittent) while positioned so that the tissues housing it are relaxed (relatively or completely).

Following a period of 20–60 seconds of this position of ease and (constant or intermittent) inhibitory pressure, the patient is asked to introduce a mild (20% of strength) isometric contraction into the tissues (against the practitioner's resistance) and to hold this for 7–10 seconds while using the precise fibers involved in the positional release.

Following the contraction, a reduction in tone will have been induced in the tissues. The hypertonic or fibrotic tissues could then be stretched (as in any muscle energy procedure) so that the specifically targeted fibers would be lengthened. Wherever possible, the patient assists in this stretching movement in order to activate the antagonists and facilitate the stretch. Ruddy's RRAF method could then usefully be introduced (see below).

Ruddy's reciprocal antagonist facilitation (RRAF)

Liebenson (1996b) summarizes the way in which dysfunctional patterns in the musculoskeletal system can be corrected.

- Identify, relax and stretch overactive, tight muscles.
- Mobilize and/or adjust restricted joints.
- Facilitate and strengthen weak muscles.
- Reeducate movement patterns on a reflex, subcortical basis.

This sequence is based on sound biomechanical knowledge and research (Jull & Janda 1987, Lewit 1992) and serves as a useful basis for patient care and rehabilitation. Use of either postisometric relaxation (PIR) or reciprocal inhibition (RI) mechanisms, in order to induce a reduction in tone prior to stretching, is an integral part of muscle energy technique, as initially used in osteopathy and subsequently by most schools of manual medicine (DiGiovanna 1991, Greenman 1989, Mitchell 1967).

In the 1940s and 1950s Ruddy developed a method of rapid pulsating contractions against resistance which he termed 'rapid rhythmic resistive duction'. For obvious reasons the short-hand term 'pulsed muscle energy technique' is now applied to Ruddy's method.

Its simplest use involves the dysfunctional tissue or joint being held at its restriction barrier, at which time the patient (or the practitioner if the patient cannot adequately cooperate with the instructions) introduces a series of rapid (two per second) tiny efforts. These miniature contractions toward the barrier are ideally practitioner resisted. The barest initiation of effort is called for with (to use Ruddy's term) 'no wobble and no bounce'.

The application of this 'conditioning' approach involves contractions which are 'short, rapid and rhythmic, gradually increasing the amplitude and degree of resistance, thus conditioning the proprioceptive system by rapid movements' (Ruddy 1962).

Ruddy suggests the effects are likely to include improved oxygenation, venous and lymphatic circulation through the area being treated. Furthermore, he believed that the method influences both static and kinetic posture because of the effects on proprioceptive and interoceptive afferent pathways, so helping to maintain 'dynamic equilibrium' which involves, 'a balance in chemical, physical, thermal, electrical and tissue fluid homeostasis'.

In a setting in which tense hypertonic, possibly shortened musculature has been treated by stretching, it is important to begin facilitating and strengthening the inhibited, weakened antagonists. This is true whether the tight muscles have been treated for reasons of shortness/hypertonicity alone or because they accommodate active trigger points within their fibers.

The introduction of a pulsating muscle energy procedure, such as Ruddy's, involving these weak antagonists offers the opportunity for:

- proprioceptive reeducation
- strengthening facilitation of the weak antagonists
- reciprocal inhibition of tense agonists
- enhanced local circulation and drainage
- and, in Liebenson's words, 'reeducation of movement patterns on a reflex, subcortical basis'.

Consider the example of a shortened, hypertonic upper trapezius muscle. Whether this contains active trigger points or not (and most do according to Simons et al (1998) since this is the most commonly found trigger point site in the body), a form of stretching (MET or other) would almost certainly form part of a treatment approach to normalizing the dysfunctional pattern with which it is associated.

It is suggested that following the appropriate stretching of upper trapezius, a rehabilitation and proprioceptive reeducation element be introduced (as part of the INIT sequence). Ruddy's methods could be applied as follows:

1. The operator places a single digit contact very lightly against the lower medial scapula border, on the side of the treated upper trapezius of the seated or standing patient. The patient is asked to attempt to ease the scapula, at the point of digital contact toward the spine.
2. The request is made, 'press against my finger and toward your spine with your shoulder blade, just as hard as I am pressing against your shoulder blade, for less than a second'.
3. Once the patient has managed to establish control over the particular muscular action required to achieve this (which can take a significant number of

attempts) and can do so repetitively for a second at a time, it is time to begin the Ruddy sequence.

4. The patient is told something such as, 'Now that you know how to activate the muscles which push your shoulder blade lightly against my finger, I want you to do this 20 times in 10 seconds, starting and stopping, so that no actual movement takes place, just a contraction and a stopping, repetitively'.

5. These repetitive contractions will activate the rhomboids and the middle and lower trapezii while producing an automatic reciprocal inhibition of upper trapezius.

6. The patient can then be taught to place a light finger or thumb contact against her own medial scapula so that home application of this method can be performed.

A degree of creativity can be brought to bear when designing similar applications of RRAF for use elsewhere in the body. These methods complement stretching procedures and trigger point deactivation and can initiate an educational and rehabilitation phase of care, especially if the patient undertakes homework.

LYMPHATIC DRAINAGE TECHNIQUES

Lymphatic drainage expert Bruno Chikly (1999) suggests that practitioners who have had advanced lymph drainage training can learn to accurately follow (and augment) the specific rhythm of lymphatic flow. With sound anatomical knowledge, specific directions of drainage can be plotted, usually toward the node group responsible for evacuation of a particular area (lymphotome). Chikly emphasizes that hand pressure used in lymph drainage should be very light indeed, less than an ounce (28 g) per cm^2 (under 8 oz per inch^2), in order to encourage lymph flow without increasing blood filtration.

Stimulation of lymphangions leads to reflexively induced contraction of the lymphangions (internally stimulated), thereby producing peristaltic waves along the lymphatic vessel. There are also external stretch receptors which may be activated by manual methods of lymph drainage which create a similar peristalsis. However, shearing forces (as those created by deep-pressure gliding techniques) can lead to temporary inhibition of lymph flow by inducing spasms of lymphatic musculature. Lymph movement is also augmented by respiration as movements of the diaphragm 'pump' the lymphatic fluids through the thoracic duct.

Specific protocols have been devised for the most efficient treatment of lymphatic stasis. For example, movements are usually applied proximally first and gradually moved to distal (retrograde) in order to drain and prepare (empty) the lymphatic pathway before congested regions are 'evacuated' of lymph through that

same path. After the distal portion is treated, the practitioner proceeds back through the pathway proximally to encourage further (and more complete) drainage of the lymph.

A variety of extremely important cautions and contraindications are attached to lymphatic drainage usage (see p. 20). For this reason no attempt is made in this text to describe the methodology. The lymphatic pathways have been illustrated in each regional overview of this text.

- Practitioners who are trained in lymphatic drainage are reminded by these illustrations to apply lymphatic drainage techniques before NMT procedures to prepare the tissues for treatment and after NMT to remove excessive waste released by the procedures.

- Practitioners who are not trained in lymphatic techniques may (with consideration of the precautions and contraindications on p. 20) apply very light effleurage strokes along the lymphatic pathways before and after NMT techniques. Proximal portions of the extremity are always addressed before distal (i.e. thigh before lower leg).

Lymphatic drainage, which can usefully be assisted by coordination with the patient's breathing cycle, enhances fluid movement into the treated tissue, improving oxygenation and the supply of nutrients to the area.

The authors encourage practitioners to undertake lymphatic drainage training with qualified instructors, as this method of treatment is a useful adjunct to most manual therapies.

MASSAGE

Soft tissue techniques, apart from those specifically associated with NMT, might usefully include the following.

Petrissage

This involves wringing and stretching movements which attempt to 'milk' the tissues of waste products and assist in circulatory interchange. The manipulations press and roll the muscles under the hands. Petrissage may be performed with one hand, where the area requiring treatment is small or, more usually, with two hands. In extremely small areas (base of the thumb, for example) it can be performed by two fingers or finger and thumb. It is applicable to skin, fascia and muscle. In a relaxing mode, the rhythm should be around 10–15 cycles per minute and to induce stimulation, this can rise to around 35 cycles per minute. It is usually a crossfiber activity rather than following fiber direction.

Unhurried, deep pressure is the usual mode of application in large muscle masses, which require stretching and relaxing. The thenar eminence or the hypothenar eminence are the main strong contacts but fingers or the whole of the hand may be involved. An example of this movement, as applied to the low back, would be as follows.

- Both hands are placed on one side of the prone patient, one at the level of the upper gluteals, the other several inches higher.
- Each hand describes anticlockwise circles.
- As one hand starts to move away from the spine, the other hand begins to move toward it, from a point a little higher on the back.
- The contact is the flat hand or the thenar or hypothenar eminences.
- This series of overlapping, circular, anticlockwise hand movements rhythmically stretches and relaxes the soft tissues of the area.

One-handed petrissage may involve treatment of an arm, for example. In this, the treatment hand lifts and squeezes the tissues, making a small circular motion. Many other variations exist in this technique, which is mainly aimed at achieving general relaxation of the muscles and improved circulation and drainage.

Kneading

This is used to improve fluid exchange and to achieve relaxation of tissues. The hands shape themselves to the contours of the area being treated. The tissues between the hands, as they approximate each other, are lifted and pressed downwards and together. This squeezes and kneads the tissues. Each position receives three or four cycles of this sort before the adjacent tissues are given the same attention. Little lubricant is required, as the hands should cling to the part being manipulated, lifting it and pressing and sliding only when changing position. A few deep strokes are then used to encourage venous drainage.

Inhibition

Also known as ischemic compression or trigger point pressure release, this involves application of pressure directly to the belly or origins or insertions of contracted muscles or to local soft tissue dysfunction for a variable amount of time or in a 'make-and-break' (pressure applied and then released) manner, to reduce hypertonic contraction or for reflexive effects.

Effleurage (stroking)

Effleurage is used to induce relaxation and reduce fluid congestion and is applied superficially or at depth. This is a relaxing drainage technique which should be used, as appropriate, to initiate or terminate other manipulative methods. Pressure is usually even throughout the strokes,

which are applied with the whole hand in contact. Any combination of areas may be treated in this way. Superficial tissues are usually rhythmically treated by this method. Since drainage is one of its main aims, peripheral areas are often treated with effleurage to encourage venous or lymphatic fluid movement toward the center. Lubricants are usually used. Fluid may be directed along the lines of lymph channels (shown in the techniques portion of this book) with superficial effleurage to enhance general drainage (see lymphatic drainage precautions on p. 20). These strokes may also be applied with fingers or thumbs.

A variation for the lower back is to stroke horizontally across the tissues. The practitioner stands facing the side of the prone patient at waist level. The caudad hand rests on the upper gluteals and the cephalad hand on the area just above the iliac crest. One hand strokes from the side closest to the practitioner away to the other side as the other hand applies a pulling stroke from the far side toward the practitioner. The two hands pass and then, without changing position, reverse direction and pass each other again. The degree of pressure used is variable and the technique can be continued in one position for several strokes, before moving the hands cephalad on the back.

This is but one of many variations on the theme of stroking, a technique which is relaxing to the patient and useful in achieving fluid movement.

Vibration and friction

Used near origins and insertions and near bony attachments for relaxing effects on the muscle as a whole and to reach layers deep to the superficial tissues. It is performed by small circular or vibratory movements, with the tips of fingers or thumb. The heel of the hand may also be used. The aim is to move the tissues under the skin and not the skin itself. It is applied, for example, to joint spaces, around bony prominences and near well-healed scar tissue to reduce adhesions. Pressure is applied gradually, until the tolerance of the patient is reached. The minute circular or vibratory movement is introduced and maintained for several seconds, before gradual release and movement to another position. Stroking techniques are used subsequently, to drain tissues and to relax the patient. Vibration can also be achieved with mechanical devices which may have varying oscillation rates that may affect the tissue differently (see thixotropy, p. 4).

Transverse friction

This is performed along or across the belly of muscles using the heel of the hand, thumb or fingers applied slowly and rhythmically. Crossfiber friction is one such approach which involves pressure across the muscle fibers and in this form, the stroke moves across the skin, in a series of short deep strokes. One thumb following the other in a series of such strokes, laterally from the spinous processes, aids in reduction of local contraction and fibrous changes. Short strokes along the fibers of muscle may also be used, in which the skin contact is maintained and the tissues under the skin are moved. This requires deep short strokes and is useful in areas of fibrous change. Thumbs are the main contact in this variation.

Another variation on the treatment of fibrotic change is the use of deep friction, which may be applied to muscle, ligament or joint capsule, across the long axis of the fibers, using the thumb or any variation of the finger contacts. The index finger (supported by the middle finger) or the middle finger (with its two adjacent fingers supporting it) makes for a strong treatment unit. Precise localization of target tissues is possible with this sort of contact.

The methods listed above do not represent a comprehensive description of massage-based soft tissue techniques but are meant to indicate some of the basic movements available. Some or all of these can be usefully employed in treatment of most soft tissue problems. Other methods which we would associate with the above techniques of traditional massage might include the various applications of NMT, MET and MFR, as described in this text.

Effects explained

How are the various effects of massage and soft tissue manipulation explained? A combination of physical effects occur, apart from the undoubted anxiety-reducing influences (Sandler 1983) which involve a number of biochemical changes. For example, plasma cortisol and catecholamine concentrations alter markedly as anxiety levels drop and depression is also reduced (Field 1992). Serotonin levels rise as sleep is enhanced, even in severely ill patients – preterm infants, cancer patients and people with irritable bowel problems as well as HIV-positive individuals (Acolet 1993, Ferel-Torey 1993, Ironson 1993, Weinrich & Weinrich 1990).

On a physical level, pressure (as applied in deep kneading or stroking along the length of a muscle) tends to displace fluid content. Venous, lymphatic and tissue drainage is thereby encouraged. The replacement of this with fresh oxygenated blood aids in normalization via increased capillary filtration and venous capillary pressure. This reduces edema and the effects of pain-inducing substances which may be present (Hovind 1974, Xujian 1990). Massage also produces a decrease in the sensitivity of the gamma efferent control of the muscle spindles and thereby reduces any shortening tendency of the muscles (Puustjarvi 1990).

Fascial influences include provoking a transition from gel to sol as discussed in Chapter 1. Colloids respond to appropriately applied pressure and vibration by changing state from a gel-type consistency to a solute, which increases internal hydration and assists in the removal of toxins from the tissue (Oschman 1997).

Pressure techniques, such as are used in NMT and MET, have a direct effect on the Golgi tendon organs, which detect the load applied to the tendon or muscle. These effects have an inhibitory capability, which can cause the entire muscle to relax.

The Golgi tendon organs are set in series in the muscle and are affected by both active and passive contraction of the tissues. The effect of any system which applies longitudinal pressure or stretch to the muscle will be to evoke this reflex relaxation. The degree of slow stretch, however, has to be great as there is little response from a small degree of stretch. The effect of MET, articulation techniques and various functional balance techniques depends to a large extent on these tendon reflexes (Sandler 1983).

Lewit (1986) discusses aspects of what he describes as the 'no man's land' which lies between neurology, orthopedics and rheumatology which, he says, is the home of the vast majority of patients with pain derived from the locomotor system and in whom no definite pathomorphological changes are found. He makes the suggestion that these be termed cases of 'functional pathology of the locomotor system'. These include most of the patients receiving therapy from osteopathic, chiropractic and physiotherapy practitioners.

The most frequent symptom of individuals whose condition is of unknown etiology is pain, which may be reflected clinically by reflex changes such as muscle spasm, myofascial trigger points, hyperalgesic skin zones, periosteal pain points or a wide variety of other sensitive areas which have no obvious pathological origin. Since the musculoskeletal system is the largest energy user in the body, it is not surprising that fatigue is a feature of chronic changes in the musculature.

A major role of NMT is to help in both identifying such areas and offering some help in differential diagnosis. NMT and other soft tissue methods are then capable of normalizing many of the causative aspects of these myriad sources of pain and disability.

MOBILIZATION AND ARTICULATION

The simplest description of articulation (or mobilization) is that it involves taking a joint through its full range of motion, using low velocity (slow moving) and high amplitude (largest magnitude of normal movement). This is an exact opposite approach to a high-velocity thrust (HVT) manipulation approach, in which amplitude is very small and speed is very fast.

The therapeutic goal of articulation is to restore freedom of range of movement where it has been reduced.

The rhythmic application of articulatory mobilization effectively releases much of the soft tissue hypertonicity surrounding a restricted joint. However, it will not reduce fibrotic changes which may require more direct manual methods.

Brian Mulligan (1992), New Zealand physiotherapist, has developed a number of extremely useful mobilization procedures for painful and/or restricted joints. He describes some simple guidelines based on his vast experience of the methods rather than on clinical trials which, as with most manual medicine techniques, remain to be carried out.

The basic concept of Mulligan's mobilization with movement (MWM) is that a painless, gliding, translation pressure is applied by the practitioner, almost always at right angles to the plane of movement in which restriction is noted, while the patient actively (or sometimes the practitioner passively) moves the joint in the direction of restriction or pain (see 'Finger (or wrist) joint MWM' in the section on clinical applications for the forearm and hand – p. 408).

Mulligan (1992) has also described effective MWM techniques for the spinal joints. In this summary only those relating to the cervical spine are detailed, although precisely the same principles apply wherever they are used. Mulligan highly recommends that the work of Kaltenborn (1985) relating to joint articulation be studied, especially that relating to end-feel. These mobilization methods carry the acronym SNAGs, which stands for 'sustained natural apophyseal glides'. They are used to improve function if any restriction or pain is experienced

on flexion, extension, side flexion or rotation of the cervical spine, usually from C3 and lower (there are other more specialized variations of these techniques for the upper cervicals, not described in this text). In order to apply these methods to the spine, it is essential for the practitioner to be aware of the facet angles of those segments being treated. These are discussed in Chapter 12. It should be recalled that the facet angles of C3 to C7 lie on a plane which *angles toward the eyes*. Rotation of the lower five cervical vertebrae therefore follows the facet planes, rather than being horizontal (Kappler 1997, Lewit 1986, Mulligan 1992).

Notes on sustained natural apophyseal glides (SNAGs)

- Most applications of sustained natural apophyseal glides commence with the patient weight bearing, usually seated.
- They are movements which are *actively* performed by the patient, in the direction of restriction, while the practitioner *passively* holds an area (in the cervical spine, it is the segment immediately cephalad to the restriction) in an anteriorly translated direction.
- In the cervical spine the direction of translation is almost always anteriorly directed, along the plane of the facet articulation, i.e. toward the eyes.
- In none of the SNAGs applications should any pain be experienced, although some residual stiffness/soreness is to be anticipated on the following day, as with most mobilization approaches.
- In some instances, as well as actively moving the head and neck toward the direction of restriction while the practitioner maintains the translation, the patient may usefully apply 'overpressure' in which a hand is used to reinforce the movement toward the restriction barrier.
- The patient is told that at no time should pain be experienced and that if it is, all active efforts should cease.
- The reason for pain being experienced could be because:
  1. the facet plane may not have been correctly followed
  2. the incorrect segment may have been selected for translation
  3. the patient may be attempting movement toward the barrier with excessive strength.
- If a painless movement through a previously restricted barrier is achieved while the translation is held, the same procedure is performed several times more.
- There should be an instant, and lasting, functional improvement.
- The use of these mobilization methods is enhanced by normalization of soft tissue restrictions and shortened musculature, using NMT, MFR, MET, etc.
- See Chapter 11, Fig. 11.38, pp. 202–203, for descriptions of application of SNAGs.

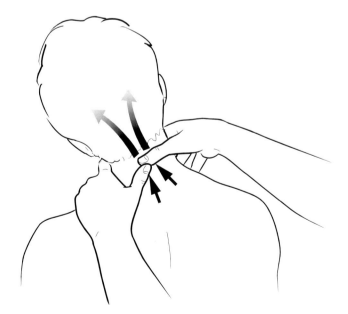

Figure 10.1 SNAG (sustained natural apophyseal glide) hand position for mobilization of mid-cervical dysfunction.

MUSCLE ENERGY TECHNIQUES (MET) AND VARIATIONS (DiGiovanna 1991, Greenman 1989, Janda 1989, Lewit 1986, Liebenson 1989/1990, Mitchell 1967, Travell & Simons 1992)

Muscle energy techniques (MET) are soft tissue manipulative methods in which the patient, on request, actively uses her muscles from a controlled position, in a specific direction, with mild effort against a precise counterforce. The counterforce can match the patient's effort (isometrically) or fail to match it (isotonically) or overcome it (isolytically), depending upon the therapeutic effect required. Depending upon the relative acuteness of the situation, the contraction will be commenced from or short of a previously ascertained barrier of resistance.

In order to apply the MET methods effectively there are several basic 'rules' which need to be well understood and applied.

- The 'barrier' described refers to the very first sign of palpated or sensed resistance to free movement, as soft tissues are taken toward the direction of their restriction (as palpated by sense of 'bind' or sense of effort required to move the area or by visual or other palpable evidence). This will be well short of the physiological or pathophysiological barrier and literally means that the very first sign of perceived restriction needs to be identified and respected.

- It is from this barrier that MET is applied in *acute* conditions, acute being defined as anything that is acutely painful or which relates to trauma which occurred within the last 3 weeks or so.

- Following an isometric contraction (see below) of the agonist or antagonist, in *acute* conditions the tissue is passively moved to the new barrier (first sign of resistance) without any attempt to stretch. Additional contraction followed by movement to a new barrier is repeated until no further gain is achieved.

- When MET is applied to joints the acute model is always used, i.e. no stretching, simply movement to the new barrier and repetition of isometric contraction of agonist or antagonist.

- In *chronic* conditions (non-acute) the same barrier is identified but the isometric contraction (see below) is commenced from short of it (for patient comfort and safety, avoidance of cramp, etc.).

- Following the contraction, in *chronic* conditions, the tissues are moved beyond (a short way only) the new barrier and are held in that stretched state for 10–20 seconds (or longer), before being returned to a position short of the new barrier for a further isometric contraction.

- Wherever possible, the patient assists in the stretching movement in order to activate the antagonists and facilitate the stretch.

- There are times when 'co-contraction' is useful, involving contraction of both the agonist and the antagonist. Studies have shown that this approach is particularly useful in treatment of the hamstrings, when both these and the quadriceps are isometrically contracted prior to stretch (Moore 1980).

Neurological explanation for MET effects

1. When a muscle is contracted isometrically, a load is placed on the Golgi tendon organs which, on cessation of effort, results in a phenomenon known as postisometric relaxation (PIR). This is a period of relative hypotonicity, lasting in excess of 15 seconds, during which a stretch of the tissues involved will be more easily achieved than before the contraction (Lewit 1986, Mitchell et al 1979).

2. During and following an isometric contraction of a muscle, its antagonist(s) will be reciprocally inhibited (RI), allowing tissues involved to be more easily stretched (Levine 1954, Liebenson 1996a).

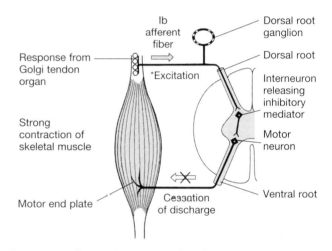

Figure 10.2 Schematic representation of mechanisms involved in postisometric relaxation response to a MET isometric contraction involving the agonist (reproduced, with permission, from Chaitow (1996c)).

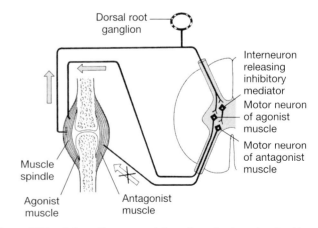

Figure 10.3 Schematic representation of mechanisms involved in reciprocal inhibition relaxation response to a MET isometric contraction involving the antagonist (reproduced, with permission, from Chaitow (1996c)).

3. Contractions are kept light in MET methodology (15–20% of available strength) as clinical experience indicates this is as effective as a strong contraction in achieving the desired effects (PIR or RI). Light contractions are also easier to control and far less likely to provoke pain or cramping. There is evidence that greater strength use recruits phasic muscle fibers (type II) rather than postural (type 1) fibers, with the latter being the ones which will have shortened and require stretching (see Chapter 4) (Lewit 1992).

Use of breathing cooperation (Gaymans & Lewit 1975)

Breathing cooperation can and should be used as part of the methodology of MET if appropriate (i.e. if the patient is cooperative and capable of following instructions).

- The patient should inhale as she slowly builds up an isometric contraction.
- Hold the breath for the 7–10 second contraction.
- Release the breath on slowly ceasing the contraction.
- The patient is asked to inhale and exhale fully once more following cessation of all effort as she is instructed to 'let go completely'.
- During this last exhalation the new barrier is engaged or the barrier is passed as the muscle is stretched.

Use of eye movement (Lewit 1986)

Various eye movements are sometimes advocated during contractions and stretches and these will usually be described in the text. The use of eye movement relates to the increase in muscle tone in preparation for movement when the eyes move in a given direction. Thus, if the eyes look down there will be a general increase in tone (slight but measurable) in the flexors of the neck and trunk. The reader might experiment by fixing their gaze to the left as they attempt to turn their head to the right. Follow this by gazing right and simultaneously turning to the right, in order to appreciate the influence of eye movement on muscle tone.

Muscle energy technique variations

Isometric contraction using reciprocal inhibition (acute setting, without stretching)

Indications

- Relaxing acute muscular spasm or contraction
- Mobilizing restricted joints
- Preparing joint for manipulation

Contraction starting point – For acute muscle or any joint problem, commence at 'easy' restriction barrier, (first sign of resistance).

Method – Antagonist to affected muscle(s) is used in isometric contraction so obliging shortened muscles to relax via reciprocal inhibition. Patient is attempting to push toward the barrier of restriction against practitioner's precisely matched counterforce.

Forces – Practitioner's and patient's forces are matched. Initial effort involves approximately 20% of patient's strength (or less); increase to no more than 50% on subsequent contractions, if appropriate. Increasing the duration of the contraction – up to 20 seconds – may be more effective than any increase in force.

Duration of contraction – 7–10 seconds initially, increasing to up to 20 seconds in subsequent contractions, if greater effect required and if no pain is induced by the effort.

Action following contraction – Area (muscle/joint) is passively taken to its new restriction barrier *without stretch* after ensuring complete relaxation. Perform movement to new barrier on an exhalation.

Repetitions – 3–5 times or until no further gain in range of motion is possible.

Isometric contraction using postisometric relaxation (acute setting, without stretching)

Indications

- Relaxing acute muscular spasm or contraction
- Mobilizing restricted joints
- Preparing joint for manipulation

Contraction starting point – At resistance barrier.

Method – The affected muscles (agonists) are used in the isometric contraction, therefore the shortened muscles subsequently relax via postisometric relaxation. If there is pain on contraction this method is contraindicated and the previous method (use of antagonist) is used. Practitioner is attempting to push toward the barrier of restriction against the patient's precisely matched countereffort.

Forces – Practitioner's and patient's forces are matched. Initial effort involves approximately 20% of patient's strength; an increase to no more than 50% on subsequent contractions is appropriate. Increase of the duration of the contraction – up to 20 seconds – may be more effective than any increase in force.

Duration of contraction – 7–10 seconds initially, increasing to up to 20 seconds in subsequent contractions, if greater effect required.

Action following contraction – Area (muscle/joint) is passively taken to its new restriction barrier *without stretch* after ensuring patient has completely relaxed. Perform movement to new barrier on an exhalation.

Repetitions – 3–5 times or until no further gain in range of motion is possible.

Isometric contraction using postisometric relaxation (chronic setting, with stretching, also known as postfacilitation stretching)

Indications

- Stretching chronic or subacute restricted, fibrotic, contracted, soft tissues (fascia, muscle) or tissues housing active myofascial trigger points

Contraction starting point – Short of resistance barrier, in mid-range.

Method – Affected muscles (agonists) are used in the isometric contraction, therefore the shortened muscles subsequently relax via postisometric relaxation, allowing an easier stretch to be performed. Practitioner is attempting to push through barrier of restriction against the patient's precisely matched countereffort.

Forces – Practitioner's and patient's forces are matched. Initial effort involves approximately 30% of patient's strength; an increase to no more than 50% on subsequent contractions is appropriate. Increase of the duration of the contraction – up to 20 seconds – may be more effective than any increase in force.

Duration of contraction – 7–10 seconds initially, increasing to up to 20 seconds in subsequent contractions, if greater effect required.

Action following contraction – Rest period of 5 seconds or so, to ensure complete relaxation before commencing the stretch. On an exhalation the area (muscle) is taken to its new restriction barrier and a small degree beyond, painlessly, and held in this position for at least 10 seconds. The patient should, if possible, participate in helping move the area to and through the barrier, effectively further inhibiting the structure being stretched and retarding the likelihood of a myotatic stretch reflex.

Repetitions – 3–5 times or until no further gain in range of motion is possible with each isometric contraction commencing from a position short of the barrier.

Isometric contraction using reciprocal inhibition (chronic setting, with stretching)

Indications

- Stretching chronic or subacute restricted, fibrotic, contracted, soft tissues (fascia, muscle) or tissues housing active myofascial trigger points
- This approach is chosen if contraction of the agonist is contraindicated because of pain

Contraction starting point – Short of resistance barrier, in mid-range.

Method – Antagonist(s) to affected muscles are used in the isometric contraction, therefore the shortened muscles subsequently relax via reciprocal inhibition, allowing an easier stretch to be performed. Patient is attempting to push through barrier of restriction against the practitioner's precisely matched countereffort.

Forces – Practitioner's and patient's forces are matched. Initial effort involves approximately 30% of patient's strength; an increase to no more than 50% on subsequent contractions is appropriate. Increase of the duration of the contraction – up to 20 seconds – may be more effective than any increase in force.

Duration of contraction – 7–10 seconds initially, increasing to up to 20 seconds in subsequent contractions, if greater effect required.

Action following contraction – Rest period of 5 seconds or so, to ensure complete relaxation before commencing the stretch. On an exhalation the area (muscle) is taken to its new restriction barrier and a small degree beyond, painlessly, and held in this position for at least 10 seconds. The patient should if possible participate in helping move the area to, and through, the barrier, effectively further inhibiting the structure being stretched and retarding the likelihood of a myotatic stretch reflex.

Repetitions – 3–5 times or until no further gain in range of motion is possible with each isometric contraction commencing from a position short of the barrier.

Isotonic concentric contraction (for toning or rehabilitation)

Indications

- Toning weakened musculature.

Contraction starting point – In a mid-range, easy position.

Method – The contracting muscle is allowed to do so, with some (constant) resistance from the practitioner.

Forces – The patient's effort overcomes that of the practitioner since patient's force is greater than practitioner resistance. Patient uses maximal effort available but force is built slowly, not via sudden effort. Practitioner maintains constant degree of resistance.

Duration – 3–4 seconds.

Repetitions – 5–7 times or more if appropriate.

Isotonic eccentric contraction (isolytic, for reduction of fibrotic change, to introduce controlled microtrauma)

Indications

- Stretching tight fibrotic musculature.

Contraction starting point – A little short of restriction barrier.

Method – The muscle to be stretched is contracted and is prevented from doing so by the practitioner, via superior practitioner effort, and the contraction is overcome and reversed, so that a contracting muscle is stretched. Origin and insertion do not approximate. Muscle is stretched to, or as close as possible to, full physiological resting length.

Forces – Practitioner's force is greater than patient's. Less than maximal patient's force is employed at first. Subsequent contractions build toward this, if discomfort is not excessive.

Duration of contraction – 2–4 seconds.

Repetitions – 3–5 times if discomfort is not excessive.

Caution – Avoid using isolytic contractions on head/neck muscles or at all if patient is frail, very pain sensitive or osteoporotic.

Isokinetic (combined isotonic and isometric contractions)

Indications

- Toning weakened musculature
- Building strength in all muscles involved in particular joint function
- Training and balancing effect on muscle fibers

Contraction starting point – Easy mid-range position.

Method – Patient resists with moderate and variable effort at first, progressing to maximal effort subsequently, as practitioner puts joint rapidly through as full a range of movements as possible. This approach differs from a simple isotonic exercise by virtue of whole ranges of motion, rather than single motions being involved, and because resistance varies, progressively increasing as the procedure progresses.

Forces – Practitioner's force overcomes patient's effort to prevent movement. First movements (for instance, taking an ankle into all its directions of motion) involve moderate force, progressing to full force subsequently.

An alternative is to have the practitioner (or machine) resist the patient's effort to make all the movements.

Duration of contraction – Up to 4 seconds.

Repetitions – 2–4 times.

MYOFASCIAL RELEASE TECHNIQUES (MFR) (Barnes 1996, 1997, Shea 1993)

John Barnes PT (1997) writes: 'Studies suggest that fascia, an embryological tissue, reorganizes along the lines of tension imposed on the body, adding support to misalignment and contracting to protect tissues from further trauma'. Having evaluated where a restriction area exists, MFR technique calls for a sustained pressure (gentle usually) which engages the elastic component of the elasticocollagenous complex, stretching this until it ceases releasing (this can take some minutes).

This barrier is held until release recommences as a result of what is known as the viscous flow phenomenon, in which a slowly applied load (pressure) causes the viscous medium to become more liquid ('sol') than would be allowed by rapidly applied pressure. As fascial tissues distort in response to pressure, the process is known

by the short-hand term 'creep' (Twomey & Taylor 1982). Hysteresis is the process of heat and energy exchange by the tissues as they deform (see Chapter 1 on fascia, pp. 4–5) (*Dorlands medical dictionary* 1985).

Mark Barnes MPT (1997) describes the simplest MFR treatment process as follows.

Myofascial release is a hands-on soft tissue technique that facilitates a stretch into the restricted fascia. A sustained pressure is applied into the tissue barrier; after 90 to 120 seconds the tissue will undergo histological length changes allowing the first release to be felt. The therapist follows the release into a new tissue barrier and holds. After a few releases the tissues will become softer and more pliable.

Shea (1993) explains this phenomenon as follows.

The components of connective tissue (fascia) are long thin flexible filaments of collagen surrounded by ground substance. The ground substance is composed of 30–40% glycosaminoglycans (GAG) and 60–70% water. Together GAG and water form a gel … which functions as a lubricant as well as to maintain space (critical fiber distance) between collagen fibers. Any dehydration of the ground substance will decrease the free gliding of the collagen fibers. Applying pressure to any crystalline lattice increases its electrical potential, attracting water molecules, thus hydrating the area. This is the piezoelectric effect of manual connective tissue therapy.

By applying direct pressure (of the appropriate degree) at the correct angle (angle and force need to be suitable for the particular release required), a slow lengthening of restricted tissue occurs.

A number of different approaches are used in achieving this (note that some have a strong resemblance to the methodology of Lief's NMT as described in Chapter 9).

- A pressure is applied to restricted myofascia using a 'curved' contact and direction of pressure in an attempt to glide or slide against the restriction barrier.

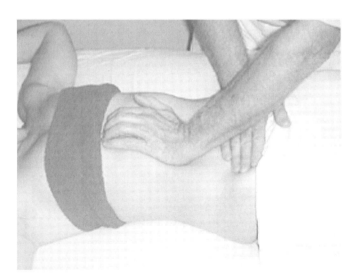

Figure 10.4 Hand positions for myofascial release of psoas.

- The patient may be asked to assist by means of breathing tactics or by moving the area in a way which enhances the release, based on practitioner instructions.
- As softening occurs, the direction of pressure is reassessed and gradually applied to move toward a new restriction barrier.

Mock (1997) describes a hierarchy of MFR stages or 'levels'.

1. Level 1 involves treatment of tissues without introducing tension. The practitioner's contact (which could involve thumb, finger, knuckle or elbow) moves longitudinally along muscle fibers, distal to proximal, with the patient passive.
2. Level 2 is precisely the same as the previous description but in this instance, the glide is applied to muscle which is in tension (at stretch).
3. Level 3 involves the introduction to the process of passively induced motion, as an area of restriction is compressed while the tissues being compressed are taken passively through their fullest possible range of motion.
4. Level 4 is the same as the previous description but the patient actively moves the tissues through the fullest possible range of motion, from shortest to longest, while the operator offers resistance.

It can be seen from the descriptions offered that there are different models of myofascial release, some taking tissue to the elastic barrier and waiting for a release mechanism to operate and others in which force is applied to induce change. Whichever approach is adopted, MFR technique is used to improve movement potentials, reduce restrictions, release spasm, ease pain and to restore normal function to previously dysfunctional tissues. This text offers samples of many of these variations within the treatment sections.

Exercise 1 Longitudinal paraspinal myofascial release

- The practitioner stands to the side of the prone patient at chest level.
- The cephalad hand is placed on the paraspinal region in the contralateral side, fingers facing caudad.
- The caudad hand is placed, fingers facing cephalad, so that the heels of the hands are a few centimeters apart and on the same side of torso.
- The arms will be crossed. Light compression is applied into the tissues to remove the slack by separation of the hands until each individually reaches the elastic barrier of the tissues being contacted. Pressure is *not* applied into the torso. Instead, traction occurs on the superficial tissues, which lie between the two hands.
- These barriers are held for not less than 90 seconds,

and commonly between 2 and 3 minutes, until a sense of separation of the tissues is noted.
- The tissues are followed to their new barriers and the light, sustained separation force is maintained until a further release is noted.
- The superficial fascia will have been released and the status of associated myofascial tissues will have altered.

Exercise 2 Freeing subscapularis from serratus anterior fascia

- The patient is sidelying with the affected side uppermost.
- The arm is lying along the side so that the back of the wrist is on the hip, which internally rotates the arm or as illustrated in Fig. 10.5.
- The practitioner stands behind the person and slides a hand (palm up) under the arm toward the axilla.
- The finger tips engage the apex of the axilla while the finger pads gently touch the anterior surface of the scapula.
- This contact should be in touch with subscapularis (or possibly teres major and/or latissimus more laterally).
- The fingers and side of hand should slowly be eased as far as possible into the division between subscapularis and serratus anterior, without causing pain.
- When all slack has been removed the patient is asked to slowly lift the arm toward the ceiling and to externally rotate the arm at the shoulder.

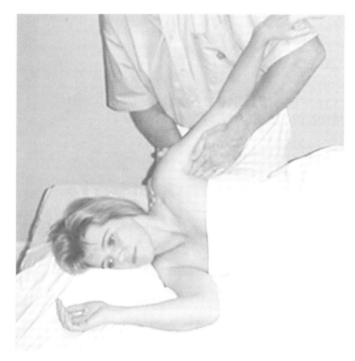

Figure 10.5 Subscapularis myofascial release from serratus.

- This movement should be slowly and deliberately performed, several times.
- This form of myofascial release involves the practitioner locating and stabilizing restricted tissues, with the patient performing the movements which stretch and free them.

POSITIONAL RELEASE TECHNIQUES (PRT) (Chaitow 1996a)

There are many different methods involving the positioning of an area, or the whole body, in such a way as to evoke a physiological response which helps to resolve musculoskeletal dysfunction. The beneficial results seem to be due to a combination of neurological and circulatory changes which occur when a distressed area is placed in its most comfortable, its most 'easy', most pain free position.

The proprioceptive hypothesis (Korr 1947, 1974, Mathews 1981)

Laurence Jones DO (1964) first observed the phenomenon of spontaneous release when he 'accidentally' placed a patient who was in considerable pain and some degree of compensatory distortion into a position of comfort (ease) on a treatment table. Despite no other treatment being given, after just 20 minutes resting in a position of relative ease, the patient was able to stand upright and was free of pain.

The pain-free position of ease into which Jones had helped the patient was one which exaggerated the degree of distortion in which his body was being held. He had taken the patient into the direction of ease (as opposed to 'bind') since any attempt to correct or straighten the body would have been met by both resistance and pain. In contrast, moving the body further into distortion was acceptable and easy and seemed to allow the physiological processes involved in the resolution of spasm to operate. This 'position of ease' is the key element in what later came to be known as Strain and counterstrain.

Example

The events which occur at the moment of strain provide the key to understanding the mechanisms of neurologically induced positional release.

- Someone bending forward from the waist has positioned the flexor muscles short of their resting length.
- The muscle spindles in these muscles would be reporting little or no activity, with no change of length taking place.
- Simultaneously the antagonists, the spinal erector group, would be stretched or stretching and firing rapidly.

- Any sudden stretch increases the rate of reporting from the affected muscle spindles which would trigger further contraction via the myotatic stretch reflex.
- This further increases the tone in that muscle together with an instant inhibition of its antagonists.
- This feedback link with the central nervous system is known as the primary muscle spindle afferent response and it is modulated by an additional muscle spindle function, the gamma efferent system which is controlled from higher centers (Mathews 1981).
- If under these circumstances an emergency situation arose (the person loses her footing while stooping or the load she is lifting shifts) there would be demands for stabilization from both sets of muscles (the short, relatively 'quiet' flexors and the stretched, relatively actively firing extensors).
- The two muscle groups would be in quite different states of preparedness for action, with the flexors 'unloaded', inhibited, relaxed and providing minimal feedback to the cord, while the spinal extensors would be at stretch, providing a rapid outflow of spindle-derived information, some of which would ensure that the relaxed flexor muscles remained relaxed due to inhibitory activity.
- The central nervous system would at this time have minimal information as to the status of the relaxed flexors and at the moment that the crisis demand for stabilization occurred, these shortened/relaxed flexors would be obliged to stretch quickly to a length in order to balance the already stretched extensors, which would be contracting rapidly.
- As this happened the annulospiral receptors in the short (flexor) muscles would respond to the sudden stretch demand by contracting even more – the stretch reflex again.
- The neural reporting stations in these shortened muscles would be firing impulses as if the muscles were being stretched even when the muscle remained well short of its normal resting length.
- At the same time the extensor muscles which had been at stretch, and which in the alarm situation were obliged to rapidly shorten, would remain longer than their normal resting length as they attempted to stabilize the situation (Korr 1978).
- Korr has described what happens in the abdominal muscles (flexors) in such a situation. He says that because of their relaxed status short of their resting length, there occurs a silencing of the spindles. However, due to the demand for information from the higher centers, gamma gain is increased reflexively so that, as the muscle contracts rapidly to stabilize, the central nervous system receives information saying that the muscle, which is actually short of its neutral resting length, is being stretched.
- In effect, the muscles would have adopted a re-

stricted position as a result of inappropriate propriocep-tive reporting. As DiGiovanna (1991) explains: 'Since this inappropriate proprioceptor response can be maintained indefinitely, a somatic dysfunction has been created'.

• The joint(s) involved would not have been taken beyond their normal physiological range and yet the normal range would be unavailable due to the shortened status of the flexor group (in this particular example). Going further into flexion, however, would present no problems or pain.

• Walther (1988) summarizes the situation as follows: 'When proprioceptors send conflicting information there may be simultaneous contraction of the antagonists ... without antagonist muscle inhibition, joint and other strain results ... a reflex pattern develops which causes muscle or other tissue to maintain this continuing strain. It [strain dysfunction] often relates to the inappropriate signaling from muscle proprioceptors that have been strained from rapid change that does not allow proper adaptation'.

• This situation would be unlikely to resolve itself spontaneously and is the 'strain' position in Jones' Strain/counterstrain method.

• This is a time of intense neurological and proprio-ceptive confusion. This is the moment of 'strain'.

• Using positional release methodology, the affected tissues are placed into an 'ease' position and maintained there for a minute or more, offering an opportunity for neurological resetting to occur, with partial or total resolution of the dysfunctional state.

The nociceptive hypothesis (Bailey & Dick 1992, Van Buskirk 1990)

If someone were involved in a simple whiplash-like neck stress as their car came to an unexpected halt, the neck would be thrown backwards into hyperextension, provoking all the factors described above involving the flexor group of muscles in the bending forward strain.

The extensor group would be rapidly shortened and the various proprioceptive changes leading to strain and reflexive shortening would operate. At the time of the sudden braking of the car, hyperextension would occur and the flexors of the neck, scalenes, etc. would be violently stretched, inducing actual tissue damage.

Nociceptive responses would occur (which are more powerful than proprioceptive influences) and these multi-segmental reflexes would produce a flexor withdrawal, increasing tone in the flexor muscles.

The neck would now have hypertonicity of both the extensors and the flexors, pain, guarding and stiffness would be apparent and the role of clinician would be to remove these restricting influences layer by layer.

Where pain is a factor in strain, this has to be consid-ered as producing an overriding influence over whatever

other more 'normal' reflexes are operating. In reality, matters are likely to be even more complicated, since a true whiplash would introduce both rapid hyper-extension and hyperflexion and a multitude of layers of dysfunction.

As Bailey & Dick (1992) explain:

Probably few dysfunctional states result from a purely proprioceptive or nociceptive response. Additional factors such as autonomic responses, other reflexive activities, joint receptor responses or emotional states must also be accounted for.

Fortunately the methodology of positional release does not demand a complete understanding of what is going on neurologically, since what Jones and his followers, and those clinicians who have evolved the art of Strain and counterstrain to newer levels of simplicity, have shown is that by a slow, painless return to the position of strain, aberrant neurological activity can often resolve itself.

Resolving restrictions using PRT (DiGiovanna 1991, Jones 1964, 1966)

• If someone has been in a flexed position and they find it painful to straighten, as in the example discussed above under the heading 'Proprioceptive hypothesis', they would be locked in flexion with an acute low back pain.

• The resulting spasm in tissues 'fixed' by this or other similar neurologically induced 'strains' causes the fixation of associated joint(s) and prevents any attempt to return to neutral.

• Any attempt to force this toward its anatomically correct position would be strongly resisted by the shortened fibers.

• It is, however, usually not difficult or painful to take the joint(s) further toward the position in which the strain occurred (flexion in this case), thus shortening the fibers, now in spasm, even further.

• Joints affected in this way behave in an apparently irrational manner, in that they do the converse of what a relaxed, normal joint would do. When a strained joint is placed in a position which exaggerates its deformity, it feels more comfortable.

Toward 'ease'

• Jones (1964, 1981) found that by taking the distressed joint (area) close to the position in which the original strain took place, proprioceptive functions were given an opportunity to reset themselves, to become coherent again, during which time pain in the area lessened.

• This is the 'counterstrain' element of Jones' ap-proach. If the position of ease is held for a period (Jones suggests 90 seconds), the spasm in hypertonic, shortened tissues commonly resolves, following which it is usually possible to return the joint/area to a more normal resting position, if this action is performed extremely slowly.

• The muscles which had been overstretched might remain sensitive for some days, but for all practical considerations the joint would be normal again.

• Since the position achieved during Jones' therapeutic methods is the same as that of the original strain, the shortened muscles are repositioned so as to allow the dysfunctioning proprioceptors to cease their inappropriate activity.

Korr's (1975) explanation for the physiological normalization of tissues brought about through positional release is that:

The shortened spindle nevertheless continues to fire, despite the slackening of the main muscle, and the CNS is gradually able to turn down the gamma discharge and, in turn, enables the muscles to return to 'easy neutral', at its resting length. In effect, the physician has led the patient through a repetition of the lesioning process with, however, two essential differences. First it is done in slow motion, with gentle muscular forces, and second there have been no surprises for the CNS; the spindle has continued to report throughout.

Jones' approach to positioning requires verbal feedback from the patient as to tenderness in a 'tender' point the practitioner is palpating (which is being used as a monitor) while attempting to find a position of ease. There is also a need for a method which allows achievement of the same ends without verbal communication. It is also possible to use 'functional' approaches which involve finding a position of maximum ease by means of palpation alone.

Circulatory hypothesis

We know from the research of Travell & Simons (1992) that in stressed soft tissues there are likely to be localized areas of relative ischemia, lack of oxygen, and that this can be a key factor in production of pain and altered tissue status, which leads to the evolution of myofascial trigger points.

Studies on cadavers have shown that a radioopaque dye injected into a muscle is more likely to spread into the vessels of the muscle when a 'counterstrain' position of ease is adopted as opposed to when it is in a neutral position. Rathbun & Macnab (1970) demonstrated this by injecting a suspension into the arm of a cadaver while the arm was maintained at the side. No filling of blood vessels occurred. When, following injection of a radioopaque suspension, the other arm was placed in a position of flexion, abduction and external rotation (position of ease for the supraspinatus muscle), there was almost complete filling of the blood vessels as a result.

Jacobson (1989) suggests that, 'Unopposed arterial filling may be the same mechanism that occurs in living

tissue during the 90 second counterstrain treatment'. It is likely, therefore, that in taking a distressed, strained (chronic or acute) muscle or joint into a position which is not painful for it and which allows for a reduction in tone in the tissues involved, some modification of neural reporting takes place as well as local circulation being improved.

The end result of such positioning, if slowly performed and held for an appropriate length of time, is a reduction in hyperreactivity of the neural structures which resets these to painlessly allow a more normal resting length of muscle to be achieved and circulation to be enhanced.

Variations of PRT

Exaggeration of distortion (an element of SCS methodology)

Consider the example of an individual bent forward in psoas spasm/'lumbago'.

• The patient is in considerable discomfort or pain, posturally distorted into flexion together with rotation and side bending.

• Any attempt to straighten toward a more physiologically normal posture would be met by increased pain.

• Engaging the barrier of resistance would therefore not be an ideal first option, in an acute setting such as this. Moving the area away from the restriction barrier is, however, not usually a problem.

• The position required to find ease for someone in this state normally involves painlessly increasing the degree of distortion displayed, placing them (in the case of the example given) into some variation based on forward bending, until pain is found to reduce or resolve.

• After 60–90 seconds in this position of ease, a slow return to neutral would be carried out and commonly in practice the patient will be partially or completely relieved of pain and spasm.

Replication of position of strain (an element of SCS methodology)

Take as an example someone who is bending to lift a load when an emergency stabilization is required and strain results (the person slips or the load shifts). The patient could be locked into the same position of 'lumbago-like' distortion as in the above.

• If, as SCS suggests, the position of ease equals the position of strain then the patient needs to go back into flexion in slow motion until tenderness vanishes from the monitor/tender point and/or a sense of ease is perceived in the previously hypertonic shortened tissues.

• Adding small, fine-tuning positioning to the initial position of ease achieved by flexion usually produces a maximum reduction in pain.

- This position is held for 60–90 seconds before slowly returning the patient to neutral, at which time a partial or total resolution of hypertonicity, spasm and pain should be noted.
- The position of strain, as described, is probably going to be similar to the position of exaggeration of the apparent distortion.

Patients can rarely describe precisely in which way their symptoms developed. Nor is obvious spasm such as torticollis or acute anteflexion spasm ('lumbago') the norm and so ways other than 'exaggerated distortion' and 'replication of position of strain' are needed in order to easily be able to identify probable positions of ease.

Strain/counterstrain: using tender points as monitors

Over many years of clinical experience, Jones (1981) and his colleagues compiled lists of specific tender point areas relating to every imaginable strain of most of the joints and muscles of the body. These are his 'proven' (by clinical experience) points.

The tender points are usually found in tissues which were in a shortened state at the time of strain, rather than those which were stretched.

New points are periodically reported in the osteopathic literature; for example, the identification of sacral foramen points relating to sacroiliac strains (Ramirez 1989).

Jones and his followers have also provided strict guidelines for achieving ease in any tender points which are being palpated (the position of ease usually involving a 'folding' or crowding of the tissues in which the tender point lies). This method involves maintaining pressure on the monitor tender point, or periodically probing it, as a position is achieved in which:

- there is no additional pain in whatever area is symptomatic, and
- the monitor point pain has reduced by at least 75%.

This is then held for an appropriate length of time (90 seconds according to Jones; however, variations are suggested for the length of time required in the position of ease, as will be explained).

In the example of a person with acute low back pain who is locked in flexion, tender points will be located on the anterior surface of the abdomen, in the muscle structures which were short at the time of strain (when the patient was in flexion). The position which removes tenderness from this point will usually require flexion and probably some fine tuning involving rotation and/or side bending.

If there is a problem with Jones' formulaic approach, it is that while he is frequently correct as to the position of ease recommended for particular points, the mechanics of the particular strain with which the practitioner

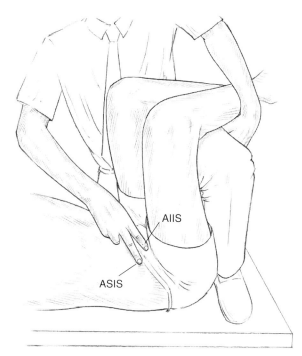

Figure 10.6 Position of ease for tender point associated with flexion strain of lower thoracic region (reproduced, with permission, from Chaitow (1996a)).

is confronted may not coincide with Jones' guidelines. A practitioner who relies solely on these 'menus' or formulae could find difficulty in handling a situation in which Jones' prescription failed to produce the desired results. Reliance on Jones' menu of points and positions can therefore lead the practitioner to become dependent on them and it is suggested that a reliance on palpation skills and other variations on Jones' original observations offers a more rounded approach to dealing with strain and pain.

Fortunately Goodheart (and others) have offered less rigid frameworks for using positional release.

Goodheart's approach (Goodheart 1984, Walther 1988)

George Goodheart DC (the developer of applied kinesiology) has described an almost universally applicable guide which relies more on the individual features displayed by the patient and less on rigid formulae as used in Jones' SCS approach.

- Goodheart suggests that a suitable tender point be sought (palpated for) in the tissues opposite those 'working' when pain or restriction is noted.
- If pain/restriction is reported/apparent on any given movement, muscles antagonistic to those operating at the time pain is noted will be those housing the tender point(s).
- Thus, for example, pain (wherever it is felt) which occurs when the neck is being turned to the left will

suggest that a tender point be located in the muscles which turn the head to the right.

• In the case of a person locked in forward bending with acute pain and spasm, using Goodheart's approach, pain and restriction would be experienced as the person moved toward extension, from their position of enforced flexion.

• This action (straightening up) would usually cause pain in the back but, irrespective of where the pain is noted, a tender point would be sought (and subsequently treated by being taken to a state of ease) in the muscles opposite those working when pain was experienced, i.e. it would lie in the flexor muscles (probably psoas) in this example.

It is important to emphasize this factor, that tender points which are going to be used as 'monitors' during the positioning phase of this approach are not sought in the muscles opposite those where pain is noted but in the muscles opposite those which are actively moving the patient, or area, when pain or restriction is noted.

Functional technique (Bowles 1981, Hoover 1969)

Osteopathic functional technique relies on a reduction in palpated tone in stressed (hypertonic/spasm) tissues as the body (or part) is being positioned or fine-tuned in relation to all available directions of movement in a given region.

• One hand palpates the affected tissues (molded to them, without invasive pressure).

• This is described as the 'listening' hand since it assesses changes in tone as the practitioner's other hand guides the patient or part through a sequence of positions which are aimed at enhancing 'ease' and reducing 'bind'.

• A sequence is carried out involving different directions of movement (e.g. flexion/extension, rotation right and left, side bending right and left, etc.) with each movement starting at the point of maximum ease revealed by the previous evaluation or combined point of ease of a number of previous evaluations. In this way one position of ease is 'stacked' on another until all movements have been assessed for ease.

• Were the same previous fictional patient with the low back problem being treated using functional technique, the tense tissues in the low back would be palpated.

• All possible planes of movement are introduced, one by one, in each case seeking the position during the movement (say, during flexion and extension) which caused the palpated tissues to feel most relaxed ('ease') to the palpating, 'listening' hand

• Once a position of ease is identified, this is maintained (i.e. no further flexion or extension), with the subsequent assessment for the next ease position being sought (say, involving side flexion to each side), with that

ease position then being stacked onto the first one and so on through all variables (rotation, translation, etc.).

• A full sequence would involve flexion/extension, side bending and rotating in each direction, translation right and left, translation anterior and posterior, as well as compression/distraction, so involving all available directions of movement of the area.

• Finally a position of maximum ease would be arrived at and the position held for 90 seconds.

• A release of hypertonicity and reduction in pain should result.

The precise sequence in which the various directions of motion are evaluated is irrelevant, as long as all possibilities are included.

Theoretically (and often in practice) the position of palpated maximum ease (reduced tone) in the distressed tissues should correspond with the position which would have been found were pain being used as a guide, as in either Jones' or Goodheart's approach, or using the more basic 'exaggeration of distortion' or 'replication of position of strain'.

Any painful point as a starting place for SCS

• All areas which palpate as painful are responding to, or are associated with, some degree of imbalance, dysfunction or reflexive activity which may well involve acute or chronic strain.

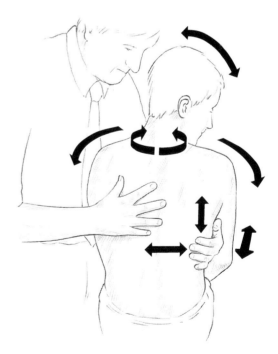

Figure 10.7 Functional palpation in which one hand assesses tissue changes, seeking 'ease', as body or part is sequentially taken in all possible directions of motion. A compound, 'stacked' position of maximum ease is found and held to allow physiological changes to commence (reproduced, with permission, from Chaitow (1996a)).

- Jones identified positions of tender points relating to particular strain positions.
- It makes just as much sense to work the other way around and to identify where the 'strain' is likely to have occurred in relation to any pain point which has been identified.
- It could therefore be considered that any painful point found during soft tissue evaluation could be treated by positional release, whether it is known what strain produced it or not and whether the problem is acute or chronic.

Experience and simple logic tell us that the response to positional release of a chronically fibrosed area will be less dramatic than from tissues held in simple spasm or hypertonicity. Nevertheless, even in chronic settings, a degree of release can be produced, allowing for easier access to the deeper fibrosis.

This approach, of being able to treat any painful tissue using positional release, is valid whether the pain is being monitored via feedback from the patient (using reducing levels of pain in the palpated point as a guide) or whether the concept of assessing a reduction in tone in the tissues is being used (as in functional technique).

A 60–90 second hold is recommended as the time for maintaining the position of maximum ease.

Facilitated positional release (FPR) (Schiowitz 1990)

This variation on the theme of functional and SCS methods involves the positioning of the distressed area into the direction of its greatest freedom of movement starting from a position of 'neutral' in terms of the overall body position.

- The seated patient's sagittal posture might be modified to take the body or the part (neck, for example) into a more neutral position – a balance between flexion and extension – following which an application of a facilitating force (usually a crowding, compression of the tissues) is introduced.
- No pain monitor is used but rather a palpating/listening hand is applied (as in functional technique) which senses for changes in 'ease' and 'bind' in distressed tissues as the body/part is carefully positioned and repositioned.
- The final crowding of the tissues, to encourage a slackening of local tension, is the facilitating aspect of the process (according to its theorists).
- This crowding might involve compression applied through the long axis of a limb, perhaps, or directly downwards through the spine via cranially applied pressure or some such variation.
- The length of time the position of ease is held is usually suggested at just 5 seconds. It is claimed that altered tissue texture, either surface or deep, can be successfully treated in this way.

SCS rules of treatment

The following 'rules' are based on clinical experience and should be borne in mind when using positional release (SCS, etc.) methods in treating pain and dysfunction, especially where the patient is fatigued, sensitive and/or distressed.

- Never treat more than five 'tender' points at any one session and treat fewer than this in sensitive individuals.
- Forewarn patients that, just as in any other form of bodywork which produces altered function, a period of physiological adaptation is inevitable and that there may be a 'reaction' on the day(s) following even this extremely light form of treatment. Soreness and stiffness are therefore to be anticipated.
- If there are multiple tender points, as is inevitable in fibromyalgia, select those most proximal and most medial for primary attention; that is, those closest to the head and the center of the body rather than distal and lateral pain points.
- Of these tender points, select those that are most painful for initial attention/treatment.
- If self-treatment of painful and restricted areas is advised – and it should be if at all possible – apprise the patient of these rules (i.e. only a few pain points to be given attention on any one day, to expect a 'reaction', to select the most painful points and those closest to the head and the center of the body).

The guidelines which should therefore be remembered and applied are:

- locate and palpate the appropriate tender point or area of hypertonicity
- use minimal force
- use minimal monitoring pressure
- achieve maximum ease/comfort/relaxation of tissues
- produce no additional pain anywhere else.

These elements need to be kept in mind as positional release/SCS methods are learned and are major points of emphasis in programs which teach it (Jones 1981).

The general guidelines which Jones gives for relief of the dysfunction with which such tender points are related involves directing the movement of these tissues toward ease, which commonly involves the following elements.

- For tender points on the anterior surface of the body, flexion, side bending and rotation should be toward the palpated point, followed by fine tuning to reduce sensitivity by at least 70%.
- For tender points on the posterior surface of the body, extension, side bending and rotation should be away from the palpated point, followed by fine tuning to reduce sensitivity by 70%.
- The closer the tender point is to the midline, the less side bending and rotation should be required and the

further from the midline, the more side bending and rotation should be required, in order to effect ease and comfort in the tender point (without any additional pain or discomfort being produced anywhere else).

- The direction toward which side bending is introduced when trying to find a position of ease often needs to be away from the side of the palpated pain point, especially in relation to tender points found on the posterior aspect of the body.

REHABILITATION

Rehabilitation implies returning the individual toward a state of normality which has been lost through trauma or ill health. Issues of patient compliance and home care are key features in recovery and these have been discussed elsewhere in this text (see Chapter 8).

Among the many interlocking rehabilitation features involved in any particular case are the following.

- Normalization of soft tissue dysfunction, including abnormal tension and fibrosis. Treatment methods might include massage, NMT, MET, MFR, PRT and/or articulation/mobilization and/or other stretching procedures, including yoga.
- Deactivation of myofascial trigger points, possibly involving massage, NMT, MET, MFR, PRT, spray and stretch and/or articulation/mobilization. Appropriately trained and licenced practitioners might also use injection or acupuncture in order to deactivate trigger points.
- Strengthening weakened structures, involving exercise and rehabilitation methods, such as Pilates.
- Proprioceptive reeducation utilizing physical therapy methods (e.g. wobble board) and spinal stabilization exercises, as well as methods such as those devised by Trager (1987), Feldenkrais (1972), Pilates (Knaster 1996), Hanna (1988) and others.
- Postural and breathing reeducation, using physical therapy approaches as well as Alexander, yoga, tai chi and other similar systems.
- Ergonomic, nutritional and stress management strategies, as appropriate.
- Psychotherapy, counseling or pain management techniques such as cognitive behavior therapy.
- Occupational therapy which specializes in activating healthy coping mechanisms, determining functional capacity, increasing activity that will produce greater concordance than rote exercise and developing adaptive strategies to return the individual to a greater level of self-reliance and quality of life (Lewthwaite 1990).
- Appropriate exercise strategies to overcome deconditioning (Liebenson 1996b).

A team approach to rehabilitation is called for where referral and cooperation allow the best outcome to be achieved.

ADDITIONAL STRETCHING TECHNIQUES

The methods of stretching described in this text are largely based on osteopathic MET methodology which is itself, in part, a refinement of proprioceptive neuro-muscular facilitation (PNF) methodology. Aspects of PNF are described in some of the stretching exercises, notably spiral upper limb movements, modified into an MET format (see pp. 370–371).

Why are we, as authors, not embracing and describing other forms of stretching? There are excellent alternative methods available (see below) and we do utilize other forms of stretching in practice. However, in the clinical applications sections of the book where particular areas and muscles are being addressed, with NMT protocols being described, sometimes with both a European and an American version being offered, as well as MET, MFR and PRT additions and alternatives, it was impractical to include the many variations available.

The stretching method chosen for this text (MET) is one which carries the endorsement of David Simons (Simons et al 1998) as well as some of the leading world experts in rehabilitation medicine (Lewit 1992, Liebenson 1996b).

The authors use, and recommend, other stretching approaches (if appropriately studied and applied), including facilitated stretching, active isolated stretching and yoga. These and several other approaches are summarized below.

Facilitated stretching

This active stretching approach represents a refinement of PNF and is largely the work of Robert McAtee LMT (McAtee & Charland 1999). This approach uses strong isometric contractions of the muscle to be treated, followed by active stretching by the patient. The main difference between this and MET lies in the strength of the contraction and the use of spiral, diagonal patterns (see MET notes on pp. 142, 370). The debate as to how much strength should be used is unresolved. MET prefers lighter contractions than facilitated stretching and PNF because:

- it is considered that once a greater degree of strength than 25% of available force is used, recruitment is occurring of phasic muscle fibers, rather than the postural fibers which will have shortened and require stretching (Liebenson 1996a)
- it is far easier for the practitioner to control light contractions than strong ones
- there is far less likelihood of provoking cramp, tissue damage or pain when light contractions rather than strong ones are used
- researchers, such as Karel Lewit (1992), have demonstrated that very light isometric contractions, utilizing breathing and eye movements alone, are

often sufficient to produce postisometric relaxation and in this way to facilitate subsequent stretching.

For these reasons, the modified facilitated stretches which have been described in this text are far lighter than the recommendations in McAtee's excellent text.

Proprioceptive neuromuscular facilitation (PNF) variations

These include hold-relax and contract-relax (Surburg 1981, Voss et al 1985).

Most PNF variations involve stretching which is either passive or passive assisted, following a strong contraction. The same reservations listed above in the facilitated stretching discussion apply to these methods. There are excellent aspects to their use but the authors consider MET, as detailed in this text, to have distinct advantages and no drawbacks.

Active isolated stretching (AIS) (Mattes 1995)

Flexibility is encouraged in AIS by using active stretching (by the patient) to incorporate RI mechanisms. The stretch, which is performed with the muscle to be stretched in a non-loadbearing state, can be assisted by the practitioner or performed independently. It incorporates an active full range of fluid movement of the joint at a medium speed which eludes the stretch reflex mechanism by being held just past its barrier for only 2 seconds or slightly less.

MET (as detailed in this text) offers the use of either RI or PIR as well as active patient participation. While AIS does not utilize the benefits of PIR as MET does, its inhibitory effect is rapidly achieved by its use of active full range of movement. The deliberately induced irritation in the stretched tissues is mild and soreness commensurate with the degree of irritation produced. However, when the tissue is overstretched (beyond light irritation) or held for too long (beyond 2 seconds), some degree of microtrauma can result, which Mattes (1995) suggests is not an acceptable exchange and should be avoided. Additionally, the stretch (myotatic) reflex can be inappropriately stimulated which will result in reflexive spasming due to stimulation of muscle proprioceptors. This is particularly the case in hard, bouncy, high-velocity movements, which are to be avoided.

AIS employs the following factors to (at least in part) achieve its results.

• Repetitive isotonic contractions (as utilized in AIS) increase blood flow, oxygenation and nutritional supply to tissues.
• When tissues are loaded and unloaded heat will be produced as energy is lost due to friction. Heat is one of the factors which can induce a colloid (the matrix of the myofascial tissue) to change state from a gel to a sol (see hysteresis discussion in relation to connective tissue, p. 5).
• Movement encourages the collagen fibers to align themselves along the lines of structural stress as well as improving the balance of glycosaminoglycans and water and therefore lubricating and hydrating the connective tissue.

Yoga stretching (and static stretching)

Adopting specific postures, based on traditional yoga, and maintaining these for some minutes at a time (combined with deep relaxation breathing as a rule) allows a slow release of contracted and tense tissues to take place. A form of self-induced, viscoelastic, myofascial release (see discussion of 'creep' in Chapter 1, p. 4) seems to be taking place as tissues are held, unforced, at their resistance barrier. Yoga stretching, applied carefully after appropriate instruction, represents an excellent means of home care. There are superficial similarities between yoga stretching and static stretching as described by Anderson (1984). Anderson, however, maintains stretching at the barrier for short periods (usually no more than 30 seconds) before moving to a new barrier. In some settings the stretching aspect of this method is assisted by the practitioner.

Ballistic stretching (Beaulieu 1981)

A series of rapid, 'bouncing', stretching movements are the key feature of ballistic stretching. Despite claims that it is an effective means of lengthening short musculature rapidly, the risk of irritation or frank injury makes this method undesirable in our view.

REFERENCES

Acolet D 1993 Changes in plasma cortisol and catecholamine concentrations on response to massage in preterm infants. Archives of Diseases in Childhood 68:29–31

Anderson B 1984 Stretching. Shelter, Bolinas, California

Bailey M, Dick L 1992 Nociceptive considerations in treating with counterstrain. Journal of the American Osteopathic Association 92:334–341

Baldry P 1993 Acupuncture, trigger points and musculoskeletal pain. Churchill Livingstone, Edinburgh

Barnes J 1996 Myofascial release in treatment of thoracic outlet syndrome. Journal of Bodywork and Movement Therapies 1(1):53–57

Barnes M 1997 The basic science of myofascial release. Journal of Bodywork and Movement Therapies 1(4):231–238

Beaulieu J 1981 Developing a stretching program. Physician and Sports Medicine 9(11):59–69

Bowles C 1981 Functional technique – a modern perspective. Journal of the American Osteopathic Association 80(3):326–331

Boyle W, Saine A 1988 Naturopathic hydrotherapy. Buckeye Naturopathic Press, East Palestine, Ohio

Chaitow L 1994 Integrated neuromuscular inhibition technique. British Journal of Osteopathy 13:17–20

Chaitow L 1996a Positional release techniques. Churchill Livingstone, Edinburgh

Chaitow L 1996b Modern neuromuscular techniques. Churchill Livingstone, Edinburgh

Chaitow L 1996c Muscle energy techniques. Churchill Livingstone, Edinburgh

Chaitow L 1999 Hydrotherapy. Element, Shaftesbury, Dorset

Chaitow L 2000 Fibromyalgia syndrome: a practitioner's guide. Churchill Livingstone, Edinburgh

Chikly B 1999 Clinical perspectives: breast cancer reconstructive rehabilitation: LDT. Journal of Bodywork and Movement Therapies 3(1):11–16

DiGiovanna E 1991 Osteopathic diagnosis and treatment. Lippincott, Philadelphia

Dorlands medical dictionary 1985 26th edn. W B Saunders, Philadelphia

Feldenkrais M 1972 Awareness through movement. Harper and Row, New York

Ferel-Torey A 1993 Use of therapeutic massage as a nursing intervention to modify anxiety and perceptions of cancer pain. Cancer Nursing 16(2):93–101

Field T 1992 Massage reduces depression and anxiety in child and adolescent psychiatry patients. Journal of the American Academy of Adolescent Psychiatry 31:125–131

Garland W 1994 Somatic changes in hyperventilating subject. Presentation at Respiratory Function Congress, Paris

Gaymans F, Lewit K 1975 Mobilization techniques. In: Lewis K, Gutman G (eds) Functional pathology of the motor system. Rehabilitacia Supplementum 10–11, Bratislava

Goodheart G 1984 Applied kinesiology. Workshop procedure manual, 21st edn. Privately published, Detroit

Greenman P 1989 Principles of manual medicine. Williams and Wilkins, Baltimore

Hanna T 1988 Somatics. Addison-Wesley, New York

Hoover H 1969 Collected papers. Academy of Applied Osteopathy Yearbook, Carmel, California

Hovind H 1974 Effects of massage on blood flow in skeletal muscle. Scandinavian Journal of Rehabilitation Medicine 6:74–77

Ironson G 1993 Relaxation through massage associated with decreased distress and increased serotonin levels. Touch Research Institute, University of Miami School of Medicine, unpublished ms

Jacobson E 1989 Shoulder pain and repetition strain injury. Journal of the American Osteopathic Association 89:1037–1045

Janda V 1989 Muscle function testing. Butterworths, London

Jones L 1964 Spontaneous release by positioning. The DO 4:109–116

Jones L 1966 Missed anterior spinal lesions: a preliminary report. The DO 6:75–79

Jones L 1981 Strain and counterstrain. Academy of Applied Osteopathy, Colorado Springs

Jones L 1995 Jones strain-counterstrain. Jones SCS Inc, Boise, Indiana

Jull G, Janda V 1987 Muscles and motor control in low back pain. In: Twomey L, Taylor J (eds) Physical therapy for the low back. Clinics in physical therapy. Churchill Livingstone, New York

Kaltenborn F 1985 Mobilization of the extremity joints. Olaf Norlis Bokhandel, Oslo

Kappler R 1997 Cervical spine. In: Ward R (ed) Foundations of osteopathic medicine. Williams and Wilkins, Baltimore

Kirchfeld F, Boyle W 1994 Nature doctors. Medicina Biologica, Portland, Oregon

Knaster M 1996 Discovering the body's wisdom. Bantam, New York

Korr I 1947 The neural basis of the osteopathic lesion. Journal of the American Osteopathic Association 48:191–198

Korr I 1974 Proprioceptors and somatic dysfunction. Journal of the American Osteopathic Association 74:638–650

Korr I 1975 Proprioceptors and somatic dysfunction. Journal of the American Osteopathic Association 74:638–650

Levine M 1954 Relaxation of spasticity by physiological techniques. Archives of Physical Medicine and Rehabilitation 35:214

Lewit K 1986 Postisometric relaxation in combination with other methods. Manuelle Medezin 2:101

Lewit K 1992 Manipulative therapy in rehabilitation of the locomotor system. Butterworths, London

Lewith G, Kenyon J 1984 Comparison between needling and manual pressure on acupuncture points. Social Science in Medicine 19 (12):1367–1376

Licht S 1963 Medical hydrology. Elizabeth Licht, New Haven, Connecticut

Liebenson C 1989/1990 Active muscular relaxation techniques (parts 1 and 2). Journal of Manipulative and Physiological Therapeutics 12(6):446–451 and 13(1):2–6

Liebenson C 1996a Manual resistance. In: Liebenson C (ed) Rehabilitation of the spine. Williams and Wilkins, Baltimore

Liebenson C 1996b Active rehabilitation protocols. In: Liebenson C (ed) Rehabilitation of the spine. Williams and Wilkins, Baltimore

Mann F 1963 The treatment of disease by acupuncture. Heinemann Medical, London

Mathews P 1981 Muscle spindles. In: Brooks V (ed) Handbook of physiology. Section 1 the nervous system, vol 2. American Physiological Society, Bethesda, Maryland, pp 189–228

Mattes A 1995 Active isolated stretching. Privately published, Sarasota, Florida

McAtee R, Charland J 1999 Facilitate Stretching, Human Kinetics, Champaigne, IL

Melzack R 1977 Trigger points and acupuncture points of pain. Pain 3: 3–23

Mennell J 1974 Therapeutic use of cold. Journal of the American Osteopathic Association 74(12)

Mitchell F Sr 1967 Motion discordance. Academy of Applied Osteopathy Yearbook, Carmel, California, pp 1–5

Mitchell F Jr, Moran P, Pruzzo N 1979 An evaluation of osteopathic muscle energy procedures. Pruzzo, Valley Park

Mock L 1997 Myofascial release treatment of specific muscles of the upper extremity (levels 3 and 4). Clinical Bulletin of Myofascial Therapy 2(1):5–23

Moore M 1980 Electromyographic investigation manual of muscle stretching techniques. Medical Science in Sports and Exercise 12:322–329

Mulligan B 1992 Manual therapy. Plane View Services, Wellington, New Zealand

Oschman J L 1997 What is healing energy? Pt 5: gravity, structure, and emotions. Journal of Bodywork and Movement Therapies 1(5):307–308

Puustjarvi K 1990 Effects of massage in patients with chronic tension headaches. Acupuncture and Electrotherapeutics Research 15:159–162

Ramirez M 1989 Low back pain – diagnosis by six newly discovered sacral tender points and treatment with counterstrain technique. Journal of the American Osteopathic Association 89(7):905–913

Rathbun J, Macnab I 1970 Microvascular pattern at the rotator cuff. Journal of Bone and Joint Surgery 52:540–553

Ruddy T J 1962 Osteopathic rapid rhythmic resistive technic. Academy of Applied Osteopathy Yearbook, Carmel, California, pp 23–31

Sandler S 1983 The physiology of soft tissue massage. British Osteopathic Journal 15:1–6

Schiowitz S 1990 Facilitated positional release. Journal of the American Osteopathic Association 90(2):145–156

Serizawa K 1980 Tsubo: vital points for Oriental therapy. Japan Publications, Tokyo

Shea M 1993 Myofascial release – a manual for the spine and extremities. Shea Educational Group, Juno Beach, Florida

Simons D, Travell J, Simons L 1998 Myofascial pain and dysfunction: the trigger point manual, vol 1: upper half of body, 2nd edn. Williams and Wilkins, Baltimore

Surburg P 1981 Neuromuscular facilitation techniques in sports medicine. Physician and Sports Medicine 9(9):115–127

Trager M 1987 Mentastics. Station Hill, Mill Valley, California

Travell J 1952 Ethyl chloride spray for painful muscle spasm. Archives of Physical Medicine 33:291–298

Travell J, Simons D 1992 Myofascial pain and dysfunction: the trigger point manual, vol 2: the lower extremities. Williams and Wilkins, Baltimore

Twomey L, Taylor J 1982 Flexion, creep, dysfunction and hysteresis in the lumbar vertebral column. Spine 7(2):116–122

Van Buskirk R 1990 Nociceptive reflexes and the somatic dysfunction. Journal of the American Osteopathic Association 90:792–809

Voss D, Ionta M, Myers B 1985 Proprioceptive neuromuscular facilitation, 3rd edn. Harper and Row, Philadelphia

Wall P, Melzack R 1989 Textbook of pain. Churchill Livingstone, London

Walther D 1988 Applied kinesiology. SDC Systems, Pueblo, Colorado

Weinrich S, Weinrich M 1990 Effect of massage on pain in cancer patients. Applied Nursing Research 3:140–145

Xujian S 1990 Effects of massage and temperature on permeability of initial lymphatics. Lymphology 23:48–50

FURTHER READING

Chaitow L 1996 Muscle energy techniques. Churchill Livingstone, Edinburgh

Chaitow L 1996 Modern neuromuscular techniques. Churchill Livingstone, Edinburgh

Chaitow L 1996 Positional release techniques. Churchill Livingstone, Edinburgh

Greenman P 1989 Principles of manual medicine. Williams and Wilkins, Baltimore

Jones L 1981 Strain and counterstrain. Academy of Applied Osteopathy, Colorado Springs

Lewit K 1999 Manipulative therapy in rehabilitation of the locomotor system, 3rd edn. Butterworths, London

Liebenson C (ed) 1996 Rehabilitation of the spine. Williams and Wilkins, Baltimore

Mattes A 1995 Active isolated stretching. Privately published, Sarasota, Florida

McAtee R, Charland J 1999 Facilitated stretching. Human Kinetics, Champaign, Illinois

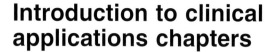

Introduction to clinical applications chapters

In each region, descriptions are presented of the region's structure and function, as well as detailed assessment and treatment protocols. It is assumed that all previous 'overview' chapters have been read since what is detailed in the clinical applications chapters builds organically from the information and ideas previously outlined. Numerous specific citations are included in the following chapters but the authors wish to acknowledge, in particular, the following primary sources: *Gray's anatomy* (35th and 38th editions), *Clinical biomechanics* by Schafer, Ward's *Foundations of osteopathic medicine*, Lewit's *Manipulative therapy in rehabilitation of the motor system*, Liebenson's *Rehabilitation of the spine*, Simons et al's *Myofascial pain and dysfunction: the trigger point manual, Vol. 1*, 2nd edn, *The physiology of the joints, vols I & III* by Kapandji, *Color atlas/text of human anatomy: locomotor system, Vol 1*, 4th edn by Platzer and Cailliet's 'Pain Series' textbooks.

11

The cervical region

THE VERTEBRAL COLUMN: A STRUCTURAL WONDER

The vertebral column represents an impressive structure, fulfilling two diverse roles simultaneously. It must provide *rigidity* so that the structure is able to maintain an upright posture and at the same time provide *plasticity* for an extremely wide range of movements. To accomplish this seemingly contradictory task, its design is made so that smaller structures are superimposed upon one another, held together by an array of ligaments and muscles. Since the tensile forces of the musculature must both erect the structure and provide its movement, dysfunctions within the musculature can cause structural repositioning as well as loss of range of movement, both locally and at a distance.

Intervertebral disc structure (discussed in greater detail below) (Fig. 11.2)

- There is an outer annulus fibrosus, comprising concentric fibrocartilaginous lamellae which are oriented at angles to adjacent layers (forming a crisscross pattern).
- There is an inner nucleus pulposus, a semifluid mucopolysaccharide gel which becomes less hydrated under sustained compressive force.
- Endplates are sheets of thin cortical bone and hyaline cartilage separating the disc from the vertebral bodies above and below.
- The discs are bound to the bodies of the vertebrae above and below, strongly at the periphery and weakly at the core.

The intervertebral discs:

- offer shock-absorbing potential
- provide enhanced flexibility, but not uniformly, varying from region to region of the spine, with least motion in the thoracic spine
- operate according to the laws governing viscoelastic structures (see discussion of creep and hysteresis in

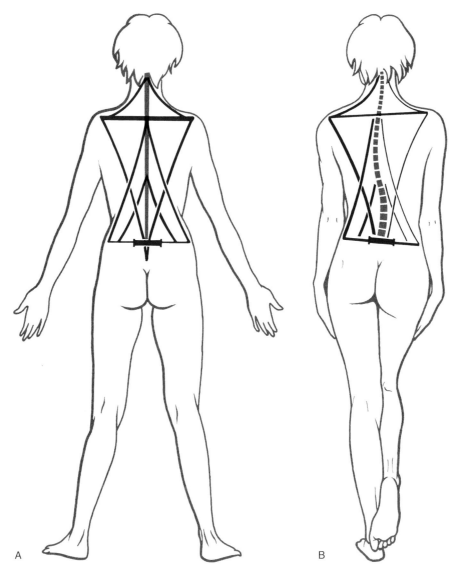

Figure 11.1 A&B: The framework and form of the body have both a solid rigidity and fluid plasticity due to the interaction of skeletal struts and myofascial tensional forces (reproduced, with permission, from Kapandji (1998)).

Chapter 1) so that the greater the degree of load applied, the greater the deformation process in a healthy disc

• are avascular, making repair and regeneration slow, should tears occur in the annulus.

When degeneration occurs these features are lost; shock-absorbing and flexibility features diminish.

There is a popular appreciation of the spine as representing nothing more than a tower created by stacking blocks one upon the other. This is a model which is commonly clinically applied: the tower is misaligned, 'blocks' are out of place and, working in a biomechanical manner, an attempt can be made to 'put back in place what is out'. The authors believe that this simplistic purview may not offer the most useful way of understanding the spine.

A different perspective is offered by Buckminster

Fuller and his tensegrity principle. When applied to the human body, this architectural model is characterized by:

a continuous tensional network (tendons), connected by a discontinuous set of compressive elements (struts, i.e. bones), forming a stable yet dynamic system that interacts efficiently and resiliently with the forces acting upon it. (Oschman 1997)

In relation to the spine, the tensegrity principle suggests that when the soft tissues around the spine are under appropriate tension, they can 'lift' each vertebra off the one below it. This viewpoint sees the spine as a tensegrity mast, rather than a stack of blocks (Robbie 1977). The suggestion which emerges from this theoretical model is that, if the strength and tone of ligaments and the soft tissues generally can be enhanced, the spine can become more 'tensegrous' and functional.

When viewed from an anterior or posterior position,

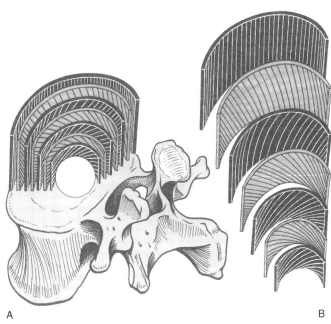

A   B

Figure 11.2   A&B: Multiple layers of annular fibers overlap each other diagonally to enclose a gelatinous nucleus which is held under pressure within its casing (reproduced, with permission, from Kapandji (1998)).

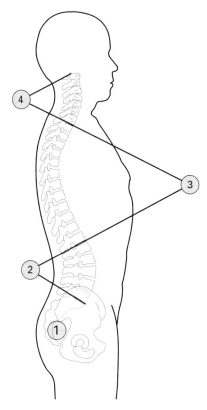

Figure 11.3   Points where relatively rigid structures meet flexible ones are the most unstable while points of deepest concavity are sites of greatest osteophyte formation (reproduced, with permission, from Kapandji (1998)).

the normal spine is seen to be straight. But when viewed from the side (coronal), four superincumbent curves are immediately obvious (Fig. 11.3).

Two lordotic curves (concave posteriorly) are found, one each in the cervical and lumbar regions, while the thorax and sacrum display kyphotic curvature (convex posteriorly). The first three are flexible curves while the fourth, the sacral curve, is inflexible, being composed of fused joints. Each curve is not only interdependent on the position of the others, they are also each subservient to the center of gravity (Cailliet 1991). Centered atop this flexible (indeed, bendable) mast is 8–12 pounds of additional compressional force – the cranium.

Kapandji (1974), who often presents the body from an 'architectural' point of view, tells us:

the curvatures of the vertebral column increase its resistance to axial compressional forces. Engineers have shown that the resistance of a curved column is directly proportional to the square of the number of curvatures plus one. If we take as reference a straight column (number of curvatures = 0), with resistance equal to 1, it follows that a column with one curvature has a resistance equal to 2, a column with 2 curvatures has a resistance equal to 5 and a column with 3 flexible curvatures – like the vertebral column with its lumbar, thoracic and cervical [flexible] curvatures – has a resistance of 10, i.e. *ten times that of a straight column*.

While curvatures do provide tremendous resistance to compressional forces, such as gravity or the weight of the cranium, at the same time, curves also present their own collection of structural challenges. For instance, the site of greatest concavity will also be the region of greatest

osteophyte formation (Cailliet 1991). Additionally, while some curvature is good, excessive curvature requires excessive muscular support and therefore additional energy expenditure.

The entire spinal column does not rest directly in the center of the body; however, the weight-bearing structures, such as the cervical region which bears the weight of the head and the lumbar region which bears the weight of the entire upper body, do ideally lie centrally, with the center of gravity running through their bodies. When optimal postural positioning is achieved, standing should be effortless and require little energy.

Cailliet (1991) tells us that:

Normal posture implies:

1. there is essentially minimal or no muscular activity needed to support the head
2. the intervertebral discs maintained in proper alignment experience no excessive anterior or posterior vertebral disc annular compression
3. the nucleus remains in its proper physiologic center
4. the zygapophyseal joints are properly aligned and do not bear excessive weight upon the body assuming the erect posture
5. the intervertebral foramina remain appropriately open and the nerve roots emerge with adequate space.

There are four regions of relative instability in the spine, which require particular attention. These are areas where relatively rigid structures are in direct opposition to more flexible structures, allowing for greater mobility as well as a greater potential for dysfunction. These are:

1. the occipitoatlantal joint – where the rigid skull meets the highly mobile atlas
2. the cervicothoracic junction – where the relatively mobile cervical spine meets the more rigid thoracic spine
3. the lumbodorsal junction – where the relatively rigid thoracic spine meets the more flexible lumbar spine
4. the lumbosacral junction – where the relatively mobile lumbar spine meets the more rigid sacrum.

It is important to consider whole-body posture rather than local factors alone, when assessing biomechanical dysfunction, and also the need for awareness of previous adaptations. While some compensatory patterns can be seen as common, almost 'normal' (see notes on Zink in Chapter 2 and later in this chapter), how the body adjusts itself when traumas (even minor ones) and new postural strains are imposed will be determined by the stresses which already exist. In other words, there is a degree of unpredictability where compensations are concerned, especially when recent demands are overlaid onto existing adaptation patterns.

Structural compensations can involve a variety of influences, for example as the body attempts to maintain the eyes and ears in an ideally level position. Such adaptations will almost always involve the cervical region and will be superimposed on whatever additional adaptive changes have occurred in that region. The practitioner therefore has to keep in mind that what is presented and observed may represent acute problems evolving out of chronic adaptive patterns. 'Unpeeling' the layers of the problem to reveal core, treatable obstacles to normal function involves patience and skill.

The second volume of this text examines posture and postural compensations in more depth when the pelvis and feet, the very foundations of the body's structural support, are discussed. However, for the purpose of understanding the cervical region, a look at its structural make-up and common postural dysfunctions – especially forward head posture – is imperative.

Cervical vertebral structure

The cervical spine is composed of two functional units – the upper unit (atlas and axis) and the lower unit (C3–7). Of these seven cervical vertebrae, C1 (atlas), C2 (axis) and C7 (vertebra prominens) are each unique in design, while the remaining vertebrae (C3–6) are considered to be typical cervical vertebrae, with only small differences between them.

Each typical vertebra (Fig. 11.4) has two major components: the vertebral body anteriorly and the vertebral arch posteriorly. Weight is borne on these components throughout the entire vertebral column onto three supporting 'pillars'. The major pillar is located anteriorly and is composed of the vertebral bodies and the intervertebral discs. Two minor pillars are located more posteriorly and are composed of the articular processes and their interposed arthrodial joints. In between these pillars lies the fluid-filled spinal canal where the spinal cord is housed.

Between all vertebral bodies (none between C1 and C2 since C1 has no body) are intervertebral discs, each disc having a fluid-filled nucleus which is surrounded by 12 layers of lamellae called the *annulus fibrosus* (Cailliet 1991). These annular fibers offer containment for the fluid as well as providing a highly mobile construction.

Regarding the discs, in normal, healthy conditions:

- the annulus is composed of sheets of collagen, each fiber being a trihelix chain of numerous amino acids, which gives it an element of elasticity
- the fibers may be stretched to their physiological length and will recoil when the force is released
- if stretched beyond physiological length, the amino acid chains may be damaged and will no longer recoil
- the annular fibers course on a diagonal to connect adjacent vertebral endplates
- each layer of fibers lies in the opposite direction to the previous layer so that when one layer is stretched by rotation or shearing forces, the adjacent layer is relaxed
- the cartilaginous endplates of adjacent vertebrae serve as the top and bottom of the disc with the annular fibers firmly attached to both endplates
- though the discs have a vascular supply in early stages of life, by the third decade, the disc is avascular
- nutrition to the disc is thereafter in part supplied through imbibition, where alternating compression and relaxation creates a spongelike induction of fluids
- the nucleus, a proteoglycan gel, is approximately 80% water
- the nucleus is completely contained within the compressed center of the annulus
- as long as the container remains elastic, the gel cannot be compressed but can merely reform in response to any external pressure applied to it
- the nucleus conforms to the laws of fluids under pressure
- when the disc is at rest, *external pressure applied to the disc will be transmitted in all directions*, according to Pascal's law
- when the disc is compressed by external forces, the nucleus deforms and the annular fibers, while remaining taut, bulge.

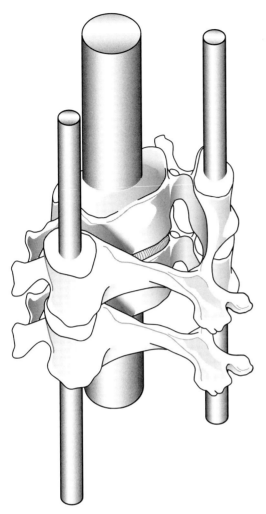

Figure 11.4 Three supporting pillars include one through the vertebral bodies with interposed discs and two minor pillars through the articular processes and their joints (reproduced, with permission, from Kapandji (1998)).

While the design offers optimal conditions of hydraulic support as well as numerous combinations of movements, postural distortions brought on by overuse, strain and trauma can lead to degenerative changes in the disc, usually accompanied by muscular dysfunction and often resulting in chronic pain. Postural dysfunction, once initiated, tends to lead to further postural compensation and a self-perpetuating pattern in which dysfunction begets ever greater dysfunction.

The pathology of the forward head posture is well explained by Cailliet (1991).

- In this pose the zygapophyseal (facet) joints become maximally weight bearing and their cartilage is exposed to persistent recurrent trauma.
- In this increased cervical lordotic posture the intervertebral foramina are closed and the nerve roots are potentially compressed.
- With prolonged unremitting compression from the posture, the zygapophyseal joint capsules can become constricted

and even adherent, thus leading to gradual structural limitation.
- With cartilaginous structural changes, a degenerative arthritic condition of the facet joints occurs.
- If there is also superimposed muscular tension, the compression is increased and structural tissue changes are precipitated.'

Juhan (1987) offers further insights.

Because of this posture, the normal supporting structures (the internal disc pressure, the intervertebral ligaments, the ligamentum nuchae, and so forth) now must be supplemented by sustained isometric muscular contraction of the extensor musculature. This muscular action is a compensatory muscular activity that is initiated by the neurologic mechanisms discussed earlier. The extrafusal muscular fiber contraction is gravity initiated and sustained and the normal physiologic neuromuscular reaction gradually becomes pathologic.

While maintaining 'perfect postural alignment' at all times is not possible, not even desirable due to its static nature, functioning posture itself is an expression of the attitude of the person, of their feelings about their experiences and who they are or see themselves to be. It is often modified by their occupation, recreational habits, illnesses and traumas which may, in turn, cause or influence structural integrity and lead to orthopedic or neurological syndromes or disease. Feldenkrais has coined the name *acture* to describe 'active posture' (Myers 1999).

In order to fully appreciate the compensatory nature of the postures of the cervical region, an understanding of the two functional units of the cervical spine (and cranium) is essential. Movement of the cervical spine and its adaptations to structural stress are based on these concepts.

The upper and lower cervical functional units

The cervical vertebral column is actually two segments, one set upon the other (Fig. 11.6): the superior segment, comprising C1 and C2, and the inferior segment, beginning with the inferior surface of C2 and ending at the superior surface of T1. These units have uniquely different designs but they functionally complement each other to provide pure movements of rotation, lateral flexion, flexion and extension of the cranium.

While the anatomy of these vertebrae is well covered in numerous books, the following points are important in understanding this region. The reader is referred to Kapandji (1974) for a detailed and well-illustrated discussion of the individual and complex movements of the cervical spine.

C1 (the atlas) (Fig. 11.7)

- This vertebra has no body and is simply a ring with two lateral masses.

Kapandji (1974) reports:

The nucleus rests on the centre of the vertebral plateau, an area lined by cartilage which is transversed by numerous microscopic pores linking the casing of the nucleus and the spongy bone underlying the vertebral plateau. When a significant axial force is applied to the column, as during standing, the water contained within the gelatinous matrix of the nucleus escapes into the vertebral body through these pores. As this static pressure is maintained throughout the day, by night the nucleus contains less water than in the morning so that the disc is perceptibly thinner. In a healthy individual this cumulative thinning of the discs can amount to 2 cm.

Conversely, during the night, when one lies flat, the vertebral bodies are subject, not to the axial force of gravity, but only to that generated by muscular tone, which is much reduced during sleep. At this time the water-absorbing capacity of the nucleus draws water back into the nucleus from the vertebral bodies and the disc regains its original thickness. Therefore, one is taller in the morning than at night. As the preloaded state is more marked in the morning the flexibility of the vertebral column is greater at this time. The imbibition pressure of the nucleus is considerable since it can reach 250 mmHg. With age the water-absorbing ability of the disc decreases, reducing its state of preloading. This explains the loss of height and flexibility in the aged.

Hirsch has shown that when a constant load is applied to a disc the loss of thickness is not linear, but exponential (first part of the curve), suggesting a dehydration process proportional to the volume of the nucleus. When the load is removed, the disc regains its initial thickness, once more exponentially, and the restoration to normal requires a finite time. If forces are applied and removed at too short intervals, the disc does not have the time to regain its initial thickness. Similarly, if these forces are applied or moved over periods that are too prolonged (even if one gives time for restoration), the disc does not recover its initial thickness. This results in a state analogous to ageing.

Rene Cailliet (1991) explains:

Disk nutrition has been well-studied (Maroudas & Stockwell 1975), and it is accepted that the vascular supply to the intervertebral disk is obliterated by calcification of the vertebral endplates at puberty. Disk nutrition is the response considered to occur by diffusion from variable solute concentrations which are transported into the disk via (1) blood vessels surrounding the disk and (2) blood vessels in the subchondral layers of the endplates.

By variations of alternating compressive forces, imbibition has been postulated to be as important in nutrition of the disk as it is in cartilage, but some questions regarding this mechanism in disk nutrition are arising. Studies (Maroudas & Stockwell 1975) have indicated that hydraulic permeability of the disk matrix is very low, whereas solute diffusivity is very high. This would indicate greater infusion of nutritive solutes via diffusion than by imbibition. The method by which the disk receives its nutrition is not yet confirmed.

• On the posterior surface of the anterior aspect of the ring is an oval-shaped cartilaginous facet which articulates with the odontoid process of C2.

• While the atlas has no spinous process, only a thickened tubercle at its posterior mid-line, its transverse processes are wider than the other cervical vertebrae.

• On these lateral masses are biconcave superior articular surfaces which receive the occipital condyles of the cranium superiorly and a second set which articulate with the axis inferiorly.

• The superior articular facets are shaped so that they allow flexion and extension of the head (as in nodding 'yes') while allowing only minimal rotation between these two bones.

C2 (the axis) (Fig. 11.8)

• This vertebra carries centrally on its body a projecting odontoid process (the *dens*) around which the atlas pivots.

• On the odontoid's anterior surface is an articular facet corresponding to the one on the internal aspect of the atlas' ring.

• A transverse ligament wraps the odontoid and, along with several other uniquely designed ligaments, secures it to the atlas.

• While these ligaments are intended to prevent the odontoid's posterior encroachment into the spinal cord, normal movement does allow a minute amount of flexion of the atlantoodontoid joint.

• C2 therefore has six articulating surfaces – two superior facets, two inferior facets and two odontoidal facets, though one of these articulates with a ligament, much as the superior radioulnar joint does at the elbow.

• On the superior and inferior aspects of the transverse process of C2 lie articular facets which receive the inferior articular facets of the atlas above and a second set which articulate with C3 below.

• The superior articular facets between C1 and C2 are designed to allow considerable rotation with very limited flexion and extension of the head or lateral flexion. Excessive movements in these directions might cause odontoidal encroachment upon the spinal cord.

• Minimal sidebending occurs above the C2–3 articulation.

The typical cervical vertebrae (Fig. 11.9)

• These vertebrae each have a body anteriorly and spinous processes posteriorly which usually are bifid, having two tubercles.

• The transverse processes are located somewhat posterolateral and have superior and inferior articular facets which correspond to the contacting vertebrae.

• A foramen transversarium is present in the transverse process of all cervical vertebrae, through which runs the vertebral artery and tributaries of the vertebral vein.

• On the anterior surface of the transverse process lies the foraminal gutter through which the nerve roots course en route to the upper extremity.

• At the proximal end of the gutter lies the intervertebral foramen.

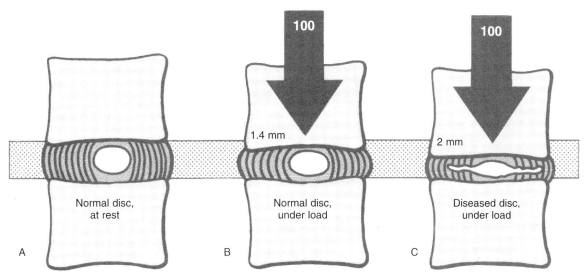

Figure 11.5 A diseased disc may fail to recover its full thickness after loading (reproduced, with permission, from Kapandji (1998)).

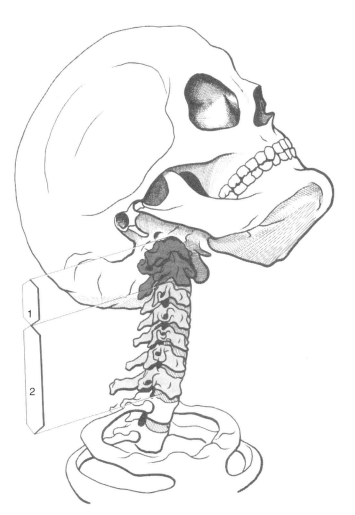

Figure 11.6 The upper and lower functional units are both anatomically and functionally distinct (reproduced, with permission, from Kapandji (1998)).

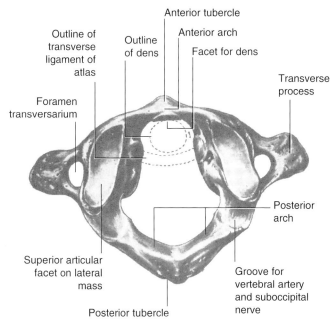

Figure 11.7 The atlas (C1) appears as a simple ring with the odontoid process of C2 filling the space where the vertebral body is missing. Flexion and extension of the head occurs between the occipital condyles and the superior articular facets of C1 (reproduced, with permission, from *Gray's anatomy* (1995)).

- The distal end of the gutter is composed of the anterior and posterior tubercles, to which the scalene muscles attach.

- Located just anterior to the foramen and on the body of the vertebra are the unique uncinate processes (also called uncovertebral bodies or Luschka's joints) which (to some degree) protect the vertebral artery and nerve roots from disc encroachment.

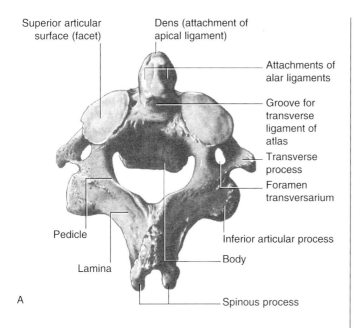

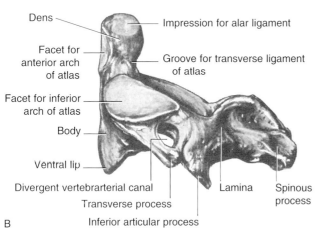

Figure 11.8 Rotation of the head primarily occurs between C1 and C2 as the atlas encircles the unique odontoid process of the axis. Flexion and extension occur between the atlas (C1) and the occiput (reproduced, with permission, from *Gray's anatomy* (1995)).

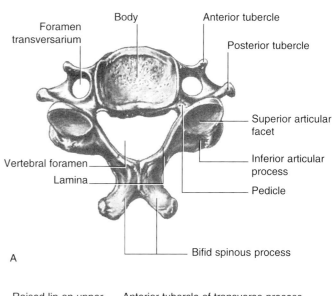

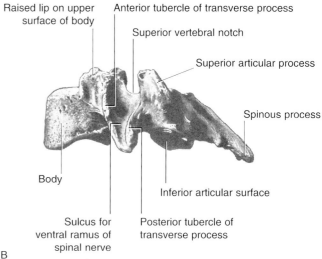

Figure 11.9 The lower functional unit is composed of typical cervical vertebrae and C7, where the cervical spine transitions to the thoracic spine (reproduced, with permission, from *Gray's anatomy* (1995)).

C7 (vertebra prominens)

• This vertebra has a long spinous process which is usually visible at the lower end of the cervical column.

• It has thick prominent transverse processes through which the vertebral artery *does not* pass, but vertebral veins do.

Except the atlas, all vertebrae have a spinous process which is palpable most of the time. The portion of the vertebra which lies between the spinous process and the transverse process is the lamina. When the vertebrae are addressed as a column, the lamina are contiguous with the next, forming a trough-like structure next to the spinous processes. This 'trench' is the attachment site of numerous muscles and is referred to in this text as the *lamina groove*.

MOVEMENTS OF THE CERVICAL SPINE

The movements of the cervical spinal column are complex, its function being to place the head in space in a variety of positions anteriorly, posteriorly, laterally and in rotation while functioning posturally to maintain the ears and eyes level with the horizon. While it is beyond the scope of this text to discuss these movements in detail, the following are important concepts to remember when considering cervical function.

• Extension is limited by the anterior longitudinal ligament, which is being stretched, and by the impaction of the articular process of the inferior vertebra against the transverse process of the one above and by the occlusion of the spinous processes posteriorly (see Fig. 11.10).

• During extension, the intervertebral disc is com-

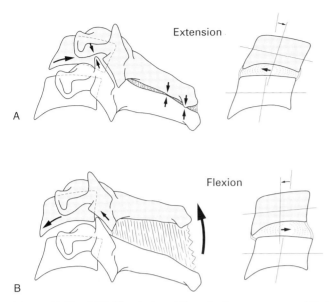

Extension

A

Flexion

B

Figure 11.10 A&B: The design of the articular processes and their associated ligaments allow movement while discouraging excessive translation of their joints (reproduced, with permission, from Kapandji (1998)).

pressed posteriorly as the overlying vertebra slides and tilts posteriorly, which drives the nucleus anteriorly.

- Flexion is limited by stretching of the posterior longitudinal ligament, by the impaction of the articular process of the inferior vertebra against the articular process of the superior one and by the posterior cervical ligaments (ligamenta flava, ligamentum nuchae, the posterior cervical ligaments and the capsular ligaments).

- During flexion, the intervertebral disc is compressed anteriorly as the overlying vertebra slides and tilts anteriorly. The nucleus is driven posteriorly, where it may endanger the spinal cord.

- While precise movements of nodding and rotating the head can occur in the upper functional unit, most movements of the head are combinations of both upper and lower cervical units.

- As the cervical column laterally flexes, there is a certain amount of automatic rotation of the vertebrae ('coupling') due to the angles of the facets between the segments, as well as the compression of the intervertebral discs and the stretching of the ligaments.

- The upper cervical unit compensates for the automatic rotation of the lower cervical unit by the contraction of the suboccipital (and other) muscles, which compensate with counterrotation.

- When the column becomes posturally distorted for lengths of time, for instance due to an uneven cushion on a favorite chair, the muscles must compensate more constantly. The resulting chronic contraction may eventually lead to the formation of trigger points and fibrosis.

- Chronic contractions may also lead to osseous changes and cervical pathologies as discussed in this chapter.

Upper cervical (occipitocervical) ligaments
(Schafer 1987)

- The *cruciate ligament* attaches to the odontoid process and comprises a triangular bilateral *transverse ligament* which passes posterior to the dens connecting the lateral masses of the atlas just anterior to the cord. It prevents the atlas from translating anteriorly.

- Additionally there exist two vertical ligamentous bands, one attaching the dens to the basiocciput superiorly and the other attaching the dens to the axis inferiorly. The strength of these ligaments is such that it is more likely, under stress, for the dens to fracture than for these to fail.

- The *accessory atlantoaxial ligaments* run superiorly and laterally, linking the inferior vertical cruciate, and thereby the dens, with C1.

- The *apical* and *alar ligaments* are situated anterior to the upper arm of the cruciate ligament. The slim apical ligament joins the tip of the dens to the anterior margin of the foramen magnum, while the more robust alar ligaments run from medial aspects of the condyles of the occiput to the dens. These three (two alar and one apical) ligaments, which restrict rotation and lateral flexion, are jointly known as the *dentate ligaments*.

- Connecting the anterior body of the axis with the inferior aspect of the anterior ring of the atlas is the *atlantoepistrophic ligament* while the *atlantooccipital ligament* links the superior aspect of the anterior ring of the atlas with the occipital tubercle.

- A structural link between the dens and the dura exists in the form of the fan-shaped *tectorial membrane* which is the termination of the *posterior longitudinal ligament* (see below). This structure runs from the base of the dens, up its posterior aspect, before changing direction to angle anteriorly and superiorly to merge with the dura at the basiocciput on the anterior surface of the foramen magnum. The tectorial membrane is said to have the function of checking excessive anteroposterior motion (Moore 1980). This structure would seem to be part of a number of structural 'check' ligaments which have a dural connection (see discussion of ligamentum nuchae below and the link between rectus capitis posterior minor in Chapter 3).

- The powerful *anterior longitudinal ligament* (see below) has as its superior aspect the *posterior atlantoaxial membrane* (12) which connects the posterior arch of the axis to the posterior ring of the atlas, before passing over the vertebral artery to terminate at the foramen magnum as the *atlantooccipital membrane*.

- Support is given to the atlantooccipital articulation by thin *capsular ligaments*, as well as to the C1–2 articulation where the capsular ligaments are thicker.

- A large triangular band, the *nuchal ligament*, runs on the cervical mid-line from the occiput to attach to the posterior atlas and all the spinous processes down to C7. Recent research in the UK has shown a bridge between the ligamentum nuchae and the cervical posterior dura and lateral occipital bone (Mitchell 1998). The role of this dural bridge would seem to be prevention of dural folding during extension and translation movements of the head. A strong link has been made between bodywide musculoskeletal pain (fibromyalgia, for example) and damage to associated 'bridges' to the dura formed by rectus capitis posterior minor, which lies immediately adjacent to the ligamentum nuchae, bilaterally (Hallgren et al 1994) (see Chapter 3).

Lower cervical ligaments

- There are four anterior and four posterior *intervertebral ligaments* associated with the lower five cervical vertebrae.
  - Anteriorly:
  1. The relatively thin *anterior longitudinal ligament* connects the anterior vertebral bodies, merging with the *annulus fibrosus* anterior to the discs. Its role is to limit extension.
  2. The *annulus fibrosus* is the peripheral aspect of the intervertebral disc, made up of laminated, concentric fibers, running in oblique directions near the core but tending toward a vertical orientation at the periphery where they bind the vertebral bodies together. The attachment to the bodies is very powerful at the periphery of the disc (*Sharpey's fibers*) where they merge with the posterior and anterior longitudinal ligaments.
  3. The *posterior longitudinal ligament* forms an anterior wall for the spinal cord, attaching strongly to the intervertebral discs (*annulus fibrosus*) but not to the vertebral bodies (apart from the lips). It is possible for ossification or thickening of this ligament to trespass on the vertebral canal. The role of the ligament is to restrict flexion.
  4. Running between adjacent vertebrae, connecting the inferior aspect of the transverse process above to the superior aspect of the transverse process below and just anterior to the vertebral artery, is the *intertransverse ligament*. Its role is to check lateral bending and rotational movement.
  - Posteriorly:
  1. Connecting the lamina of adjacent vertebrae is the powerful *ligamentum flavum*. The stabilizing potential of this ligament prevents any tendency to folding or buckling of the structures it supports.
  2. Connecting the spinous processes are the *interspinous* and the *supraspinous ligaments*. The latter is continuous with ligamentum nuchae posteriorly. The role of these ligaments is to

prevent undue displacement of the vertebrae during flexion and rotation.
  3. The *ligamentum nuchae* represents an inelastic supporting structure preventing undue cervical flexion, and by means of its bridge-like attachment to the dura, protects it from folding on translation of the head (see above).

ASSESSMENT OF THE CERVICAL REGION

It can be cogently argued that the success of any treatment method depends on how *appropriate* that treatment is (McPartland & Goodridge 1997). Understandably, where placebo is a major feature (and it is *always* a partial feature of all treatment), therapeutic appropriateness becomes less important, as long as it does no harm! (Melzack & Wall 1989). Just how accurate any given assessment method can be is therefore keenly linked to eventual therapeutic benefits (Johnston 1985). Since single assessments seldom offer sufficient information for selection of a therapeutic strategy, a number of pieces of information, gleaned from different observation, palpation and assessment procedures (which confirm each other), offer the most reassuring basis for clinical intervention.

The range of possible dysfunctional conditions relating to the spine (in general) and the cervical region (in particular) is vast and full discussion is beyond the scope of this text. This text offers multidisciplinary, practical assessment approaches relating to cervical function and dysfunction and the reader is responsible for determining which of these techniques lies within the scope of his or her license and skills. In later sections, clinical application of appropriate soft tissue manipulation methods, including NMT, will be described.

Osteopathic medicine has produced a useful sequence for assessing a distressed area by means of palpation, covered by the acronym TART (McPartland & Goodridge 1997, Ward 1997):

- **T**issue texture abnormality
- **A**symmetry, ascertained by static observation, as well as during motion, and by altered temperature, tone, etc.
- **R**estriction of normal motion
- **T**enderness or pain (in the area of abnormality).

If an area 'feels' different from usual and/or looks different symmetrically (one side from the other) and/or displays a restriction in normal range of motion and/or is tender to the touch, dysfunction and distress are present. These elements, together with the history and presenting symptoms, can then usefully be related to the degree of acuteness or chronicity, so that tentative conclusions can be reached as to the nature of the problem and what therapeutic interventions are most appropriate.

A cautionary note needs to be introduced regarding

standard methods of testing, for instance, of the effect of a particular movement on the patient's symptoms. McKenzie (1990), in particular, has highlighted the need in assessment for repetitive movement ('loading'), which simulates normal daily activities. Jacob & McKenzie (1996) summarize this viewpoint.

Standard range of motion examinations and orthopedic tests do not adequately explore how the particular patient's spinal mechanics and symptoms are affected by specific movements and/or positioning. Perhaps the greatest limitation of these examinations and tests is the supposition that each test movement need be performed only once [in order] to fathom how the patient's complaint responds. The effect of repetitive movements, or positions maintained for prolonged periods of time, are not explored, even though such loading strategies might better approximate what occurs in the 'real world'.

Patterns and coupling

Other 'real-world' factors also need to be kept in mind when assessing function and one of the most important of these is that movements should reproduce those actually performed in daily life. It is, of course, appropriate to evaluate single directions of motion – abduction of the arm, for example – in order to gain information about specific muscles. In daily life, however, abduction of the arm is a movement seldom performed on its own; it is usually accompanied by flexion or extension and some degree of internal or external rotation, depending on the reason for the movement.

This highlights the fact that many (most) body movements are compound and a great many have a spiral nature (to bring a cup to the mouth requires adduction, flexion and internal rotation of the arm).

McAtee & Charland (1999) quote from Hendrickson (1995) who discusses the way in which tissues, such as actin and myosin, are organized in spirals microscopically and that 'the gross structure of the tendon and ligament is also spiral. Tendons, ligaments and bones

are composed mostly of type 1 collagen, which is a triple helix. On the macroscopic level the long bones, such as the humerus, spiral along their axes'. Note also Myers' discussion in Chapter 1 of the spiral nature of fascial interaction throughout the body.

These observations reinforce the need, when performing assessments, to take account of movement patterns which approximate real-life activities, most of which are multidirectional. In the spine, for example, many movements are 'coupled'. It is virtually impossible for a spinal segment to move on its own without its neighbors being, to a degree, involved and it is quite impossible for a sideflexion movement to occur spinally without rotation also occurring (coupling) due to spinal biomechanics. This is discussed further in the section on cervical motion palpation (pp. 177–178) (and in the section covering thoracic motion, p. 425) (Ward 1997).

Landmarks

In order to palpate the cervical spine, its basic landmarks need to be identified (Mitchell et al 1979, Schafer 1987).

- The cervical vertebrae (as in the lumbar spine) lie in the same horizontal plane as their spinous processes (not true in thoracic spine).
- C1 is not palpable apart from between the mastoid process and lobe of the ear, where its transverse process can usually be located.

• C2 spinous process is easily palpated on the mid-line below the occiput, having the most bifid (double-headed) tip of all vertebrae.

• C3–5 spinous processes are not as easily palpated as C2 but careful introduction of slight flexion and extension allows palpation access, unless the cervical musculature is extremely heavy.

• C4 has the shortest spinous process and is usually level with the angle of the jaw. However, its transverse processes are readily palpable.

• C4 (Schafer 1987) or C3 (Hoppenfeld 1976) is at the same level as the hyoid bone anteriorly.

• C4–5 are at the same level as the thyroid cartilage.

• C6 transverse and spinous processes are both easily palpated, with a likelihood of a markedly bifid spinous process in half the population. C6 is at the same level as the cricoid cartilage anteriorly and presents the carotid tubercle on the anterior surface of its transverse process.

• C7 is often mistaken for T1, especially if the spinous process is being used for assessment, as neither C7 nor T1 is bifid. To ensure that contact is on C7, the practitioner contacts the transverse processes of what is thought to be C7 and asks the patient to extend the neck. If the contact is on C7, the contacts will move anteriorly. If on T1, only a minimal movement will be noted.

Functional features of the cervical spine
(Calais-Germain 1993, Jacob & McKenzie 1996, Kappler 1997, Lewit 1992, Schafer 1987)

• Anteroposterior movement of vertebrae occurs mainly at the fibrocartilaginous intervertebral discs and at the zygapophyseal joints, between the inferior facets of the superior vertebra and the superior facet of the one positioned below it.

• The flexibility of the disc and the angle of the facet, to a great extent, structurally govern the degree of movement possible.

• The superior aspect of the atlas is shaped to articulate with the occipital condyles.

• The body of C2 (axis) is modified superiorly to form a peg (odontoid or dens) onto which the atlas slots.

• The remaining five cervical vertebrae have a more typical structure with facets lying on a plane which angles toward the eyes. Rotation of the lower five cervical vertebrae therefore follows the facet planes rather than being horizontal.

• Full flexion of the cervical spine prevents any rotation below C2, allowing rotation to take place only at C1 and C2.

• Full extension of the cervical spine locks C1 and C2 and allows rotation to occur only below these.

Cervical biomechanics are unusual. Whereas in the spine below the cervical region, it is common for sidebending of a vertebral segment to be accompanied by rotation to the opposite side (type 1), this is not the case throughout the cervical spine (Van Mameren 1992).

• The atlantooccipital joint is type 1 so that as side-bending occurs, rotation will take place toward the opposite side (Hosono 1991).

• The axis–atlas joint is neutral, neither type 1 nor 2. It is largely devoted to rotation and, as stated previously, this occurs around the odontoid peg, the dens. Kappler (1997) reports that, 'Cineradiographic studies have shown that during rotation, anteriorly or posteriorly, the atlas moves inferiorly *on both sides*, maintaining a horizontal orientation'. Fully half of the entire rotation potential of the cervical spine takes place at this joint but it possesses minimal sidebending potential. Flexion and extension are seldom restricted here as true flexion and extension of this joint are limited due to the presence of the dens which, if flexion occurred, would compress the spinal cord.

• The spine from C2 to C7 displays type 2 mechanics in which sidebending and rotation take place to the same sides. As sidebending occurs between C2 and C7 a degree of translation ('side-slip' or shunt) takes place, toward the convexity. This offers a useful assessment tool in which translation is introduced as a means of safely assessing the relative freedom of sidebending and rotation at a particular segment (this will be described later in this section as an assessment protocol, see pp. 181–182).

Muscular and fascial features

• Important proprioceptive and protective functions are associated with some of the suboccipital muscles such as rectus capitis posterior major and minor, which are discussed in greater detail in Chapter 3.

• The prevertebral cervical muscles (longus colli and capitis, rectus capitis anterior and lateralis and, according to some experts, the scalenes) (Kapandji 1974), which lie anterior to the cervical spine, run from T3 and upwards, to the occiput.

• Scalenes attach at the lateral anterior cervical spine (anticus attaches from transverse processes of C3–6, medius attaches to C2–7 and posterior to C4–6) and the 1st and 2nd ribs and clavicles. Scalenes are both stabilizers and lateral flexors as well as accessory breathing muscles.

• Levator scapula attaches to the posterior tubercles of C1–4 and the upper angle of the scapula.

• Kappler (1997) states, 'The general investing fascia splits to cover the sternocleidomastoid muscle anteriorly (mastoid process and clavicle) and the trapezius muscle posteriorly. Since the trapezius muscle attaches to the scapula, it is the primary connection between the head and neck and the shoulder girdle. The process of lifting the upper extremity distributes force to the cervical spine'.

Box 11.4 Post-trauma fibromyalgia

Trauma to the cervical region is seen to be one of the major triggers for the onset of fibromyalgia syndrome (FMS). A diagnosis of 'secondary FMS' or 'posttraumatic FMS' distinguishes such patients from those who develop FMS spontaneously, without an obvious triggering event.

Whiplash as a trigger for fibromyalgia

A study involving over 100 patients with traumatic neck injury as well as approximately 60 patients with leg trauma evaluated the presence of severe pain (fibromyalgia syndrome) an average of 12 months posttrauma (Buskila & Neumann 1997). The findings were that 'Almost all symptoms were significantly more prevalent or severe in the patients with neck injury ... The fibromyalgia prevalence rate in the neck injury group was 13 times greater than the leg fracture group'.

Pain threshold levels were significantly lower, tender point counts were higher and quality of life was worse in the neck injury patients as compared with leg injury subjects. Over 21% of the patients with neck injury (none of whom had chronic pain problems prior to the injury) developed fibromyalgia within 3.2 months of trauma as against only 1.7% of the leg fracture patients (not significantly different from the general population). The researchers make a particular point of noting that, 'In spite of the injury or the presence of FMS, all patients were employed at the time of examination and that insurance claims were not associated with increased FMS symptoms or impaired functioning'.

Why should whiplash-type injury provoke FMS more effectively than other forms of trauma? One answer may lie in a particular muscle, part of the suboccipital group, rectus capitis posterior minor. For a fuller discussion of this topic, see p. 207.

Neurological features

• The spinal cord runs from the brain to the lumbar spine (L2) and therefore passes through the cervical spine. The cord is vulnerable to being injured traumatically in numerous ways and may also become ischemic due to cervical spinal stenosis, a narrowing of the neural canal, which may be exacerbated by osteophyte formation.

• Other factors which might cause impingement or irritation of the cord include cervical disc protrusion, as well as excessive laxity allowing undue degrees of vertebral translation anteroposteriorly and from side to side.

• The brachial plexus, which supplies the upper extremity, derives from the cord at the cervical level, which means that any nerve root impingement (disc protrusion, osteophyte pressure, etc.) of the cervical intervertebral foramina could produce both local symptoms and neurological effects on the entire upper extremity.

• Kappler (1997) reports that, 'Nociceptive input from the cervical spine produces palpable musculoskeletal changes in the upper thoracic spine and ribs as well as increased sympathetic activity from this area. Upper thoracic and upper extremity problems may have their origin in the cervical spine'.

Circulatory features and thoracic outlet syndrome

• The blood supply to the head derives from subclavian, carotid (anterior to cervical vertebrae) and vertebral arteries. **Extreme caution should be exercised in palpating the regions where these arteries lie**.

• A foramen exists in the lateral aspects of the first six cervical vertebrae through which the vertebral artery and three veins pass. The hard encasement of the transverse process offers some protection to the vessels but also exposes them to danger from ill-advised cervical movements or from chronically dysfunctional vertebral segments. Cailliet (1991) notes: 'The space difference between body and foramen (3–6 mm) and facet foramen (2–3 mm) indicates that vascular impingement is most commonly due to encroachment by the superior articular process and rarely due to changes of the uncovertebral joints'.

• Kappler (1997) reports that in normal individuals, extension and rotation of the occiput produce a functional occlusion of the opposite vertebral artery. Therefore, excessive or prolonged rotation of the cervical spine is to be avoided, particularly in the elderly, where even temporary occlusion of this vessel might significantly reduce cranial arterial flow or venous drainage.

• Circulatory return from the head and neck area can be compromised by various compression possibilities relating to thoracic outlet syndrome. These include crowding of neural and vascular structures by:
  1. anterior and middle scalenes
  2. clavicular and 1st rib dysfunction
  3. pectoralis minor and upper ribs.

• Lymphatic drainage from the cervical region which has to pass through the thoracic inlet/outlet is easily restricted by these same biomechanical features.

Cervical spinal dysfunction

While Janda (1988) acknowledges that it is not known whether dysfunction of muscles causes joint dysfunction or vice versa, he points to the undoubted fact that they greatly influence each other and that it is possible that a major element in the benefits noted following joint manipulation derives from the effects such methods have on associated soft tissues.

Steiner (1994) has discussed the influence of muscles in disc and facet syndromes. He describes a possible sequence as follows.

• A strain involving body torsion, rapid stretch or loss of balance produces a myotatic stretch reflex response (for example, in a part of the erector spinae).

• The muscles contract to protect excessive joint movement and spasm may result if there is an exaggerated response and they fail to assume normal tone following the strain. The reason for an 'exaggerated response' might be due to factors such as segmental facilitation (see notes on facilitation in Chapter 6).

- This limits free movement of the attached vertebrae, approximates them and causes compression and bulging of the intervertebral discs and/or a forcing together of the articular facets.
- Bulging discs might encroach on nerve roots producing disc syndrome symptoms.
- Articular facets, when forced together, produce pressure on the intraarticular fluid, pushing it against the confining facet capsule which becomes stretched and irritated.

- The sinuvertebral capsular nerves may therefore become irritated, provoking muscular guarding and initiating a self-perpetuating process of pain–spasm–pain.

Steiner continues, 'From a physiological standpoint, correction or cure of the disc or facet syndromes should be the reversal of the process that produced them, eliminating muscle spasm and restoring normal motion'. He argues that before discectomy or facet rhizotomy is attempted,

---

Box 11.5 Tests for circulatory dysfunction

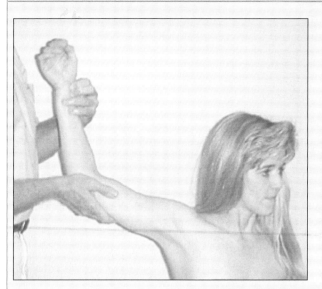

Figure 11.11 Adson's test for subclavian artery compression.

Adson's test for subclavian artery compression (Fig. 11.11)

- The patient is seated and the practitioner supports the arm at the elbow and with the other hand records the radial pulse rate.
- While continuing to monitor the pulse, the arm is abducted, extended and externally rotated.
- When these movements have been fully realized the patient is asked to inhale and hold the breath, while turning the head away from the side being assessed.
- If the radial pulse drops or vanishes or if paresthesia is reported within a few seconds, compression of the subclavian artery is implicated, probably as a result of shortening of anterior and/or middle scalene or possibly 1st rib restriction.
- A variation is to move the arm into full elevation and extension of the shoulder (arm above head and back of trunk) after initially taking the pulse. If the pulse rate drops or symptoms appear, pectoralis minor is implicated.
- Both variations should be performed since pectoralis minor and the scalenes might both be implicated.

Maigne's test for vertebral artery-related vertigo (Fig. 11.12)

- The patient is seated and the head is placed in extension and rotation.

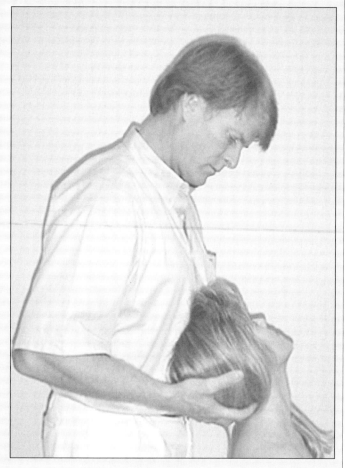

Figure 11.12 Maigne's test for vertebral artery function.

- Some practitioners prefer the patient to be supine with the head free of the end of the table, so that it can be held in extension and rotation.
- This position is held for approximately 30 seconds to evaluate the onset of dizziness, nausea or syncope resulting from ischemia.
- The indication of vertebrobasilar ischemia implicates the vertebral arteries on the *side opposite* that to which the head was turned.

Box 11.6   Tests for cervical spinal dysfunction

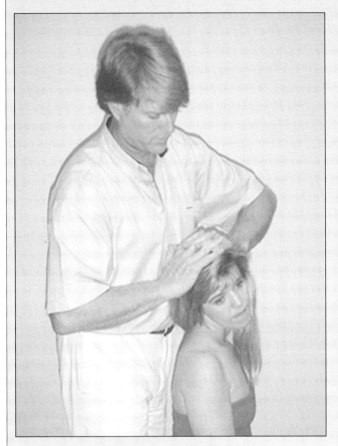

Figure 11.13   Cervical compression test.

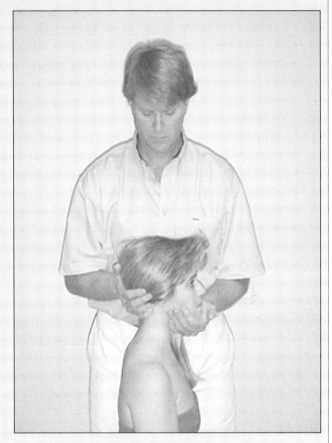

Figure 11.14   Decompression test.

Compression test (Fig. 11.13)

• The patient is seated and the practitioner stands behind her. One side is tested at a time.
• Initially, the patient will laterally flex and rotate the head slightly toward the first side to be tested.
• The practitioner interlocks his fingers and places his hands at the vertex of the patient's head and applies firm caudal pressure (2–3 kilos, 5 pounds).
• If there is a narrowing of an intervertebral foramen this compression test will aggravate the situation, producing pain which may mirror the patient's symptoms.
• An alternative procedure has all the same elements described above but in this instance the patient extends the head slightly before compression is applied.
• In this variation bilateral foraminal crowding will be induced with possible symptom reproduction, or exacerbation, confirming the etiological features of the problem (disc degeneration, etc.).

Decompression test (Fig. 11.14)

• The patient is seated, with the practitioner to one side.
• The practitioner cups the chin with one hand and the occiput with the other and introduces a slow, deliberate degree of traction, easing the head toward the ceiling, while sensing for any protective, defensive barrier which may be produced if tissues are being irritated by the maneuver.
• Extreme care is needed to avoid irritating tissues which may

have been traumatized, therefore the emphasis is on the key words 'slow and deliberate'.
• If pain and/or other radicular symptoms are relieved by this test the indication is that narrowing at one or more intervertebral foramen, bulging of the disc(s) into the spinal canal or cervical facet syndrome exists.

Hautant's test for disturbed equilibrium (Fig. 11.15)

• The patient is seated with her back supported and both arms outstretched in front (sleep-walking position).
• The practitioner stands in front with his thumbs extended, to act as 'markers' of the patient's starting hand positions.
• *Note*: The practitioner's hands do not touch those of the patient. They are used only as indicators as to the patient's original hand position.
• The patient closes her eyes and the practitioner observes for several (say 5) seconds, to note whether the patient's hands deviate relative to his own thumbs.
• The same procedure is carried out with the patient's head in different positions: flexed, extended, rotated, sideflexed, etc.
• The practitioner should hold the patient's hands in the neutral position whenever the patient is asked to change head position.
• This test has advantages over similar assessments made with the patient standing, in that the seated, supported posture reduces the chance of body sway being interpreted as arm deviation.
• Any deviation which does take place implicates the cervical spine.

Box 11.6 *(cont'd)*

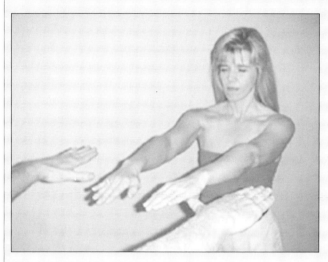

• 'Relief' positions can also be demonstrated in which deviations occur in the starting position (say, neutral) and are normalized in one or other of the head positions.
• Lewit (1985, p. 327) reports, 'The reaction to changed head position in cases of imbalance is so characteristic that we can speak of a "cervical pattern"'. He continues, 'A cervical factor [confirmed by Hautant's test] may be present in all forms of vertigo and dizziness ... In 72 examinations of 69 patients I found the most constant phenomenon was increased deviation of the forward-stretched arms, at rotation of the head, in the opposite direction to that of deviation [of the arm during Hautant's test], and at retroflexion [extension] of the head'. He found that deviation seldom occurred in the direction toward which the head was turning or on flexion. In a significant number of cases, Lewit reports, 'Deviation [of the arms] disappears after treatment of [associated cervical] movement restriction, or at least becomes much less marked, the effect being visible a few minutes after treatment'.

Figure 11.15 Hautant's test.

---

with the all-too-frequent 'failed disc syndrome surgery' outcome, attention to the soft tissues and articular separation to reduce the spasm should be tried, to allow the bulging disc to recede and/or the facets to resume normal motion. Clearly, osseous manipulation often has a place in achieving this objective but the evidence of clinical experience indicates that soft tissue approaches also produce excellent results in many instances.

Assessments

Strength tests (Daniels & Worthingham 1980)

A standard scale of, say, 5 (normal) to 0 (no contraction occurs) should be used to record findings of strength (see discussion below). These strength tests involve, by their nature, isometric contractions as the patient attempts to move against the resistance offered by the practitioner.

Lewit (1985) points out that such tests may induce pain which is likely to be of muscular origin. Although these tests are designed to evaluate muscular strength, if pain is induced, implicating particular muscles, this too should have diagnostic value. If muscles test as weak, the reason for this is often excessive tone in their antagonists which reciprocally inhibit them (Janda 1988). See upper and lower crossed syndromes in Chapter 5 for a full discussion of the implications of the chain reaction of influences as some muscles become excessively hypertonic and their antagonists are almost constantly inhibited.

In the absence of atrophy, weakness of a muscle may be due to:

• compensatory hypotonicity relative to increased tone in antagonistic muscles

• palpable trigger points in affected (weak) muscles, notably those close to the attachments
• trigger points in remote muscles for which the tested muscle lies in the target referral zone.

Muscle strength is most usually graded as follows.

• Grade 5 is normal, demonstrating a complete (100%) range of movement against gravity, with firm resistance offered by the practitioner.
• Grade 4 is 75% efficiency in achieving range of motion against gravity with slight resistance.
• Grade 3 is 50% efficiency in achieving range of motion against gravity without resistance.
• Grade 2 is 25% efficiency in achieving range of motion with gravity eliminated.
• Grade 1 shows slight contractility without joint motion.
• Grade 0 shows no evidence of contractility.

For efficient muscle strength testing, it is necessary to ensure that:

• the patient builds force slowly after engaging the barrier of resistance offered by the practitioner
• the patient uses maximum controlled effort to move in the prescribed direction
• the practitioner ensures that the point of muscle origin is efficiently stabilized
• care is taken to avoid use of 'tricks' by the patient, in which synergists are recruited.

Strength tests for the cervical region

• Assessment of *flexion* strength (Fig. 11.16A) evaluates sternocleidomastoid, longus colli and capitis, rectus capitis anterior and lateralis (and to a secondary degree

Box 11.7 Whiplash

True whiplash injuries are normally thought of as relating to 'non-impact' trauma. However, Taylor & Taylor (1996) state that:

A large proportion of cervical spinal injuries are secondary to head impact. A comparison of the nature and distribution of cervical spine injuries in those subjects with primary head impact, and those without head injury but with primary acceleration of the torso [i.e. whiplash], fails to reveal significant differences in the nature and distribution of injuries.

Whiplash-associated disorders (WAD) account for upwards of 20% of compensated traffic injury claims in some regions (Cassidy 1996). Cassidy states that when over 3000 whiplash claims were analyzed by the Quebec Task Force they found that 'The vast majority of WAD victims recovered quickly, but that 12.5% of claimants still [being] compensated 6 months after the collision accounted for 46% of the total cost to the insurance system'.

The Quebec Task Force has classified whiplash-related disorders as follows (Spitzer et al 1995).

- Category I: neck complaint *without* musculoskeletal signs such as loss of mobility
- Category II: neck complaint *with* musculoskeletal signs such as loss of mobility
- Category III: neck complaint with neurological signs
- Category IV: cervical fracture or dislocation

Research suggests that 75% of persons with significant whiplash injury recover in approximately 6 months and over 90% by the end of the first year following the accident, irrespective of age or gender, as demonstrated in Canadian, Swiss and Japanese studies (Cassidy 1996, Radanov 1994).

Variations in response to WAD

Why do some of these traumatic soft tissue sprains not heal when most do? The answer for some researchers suggests damage such as tearing of the endplates of discs and to facet joints (Taylor 1994).

A study involving over 100 patients with traumatic neck injury as well as approximately 60 patients with leg trauma evaluated the presence of severe pain (fibromyalgia syndrome) an average of 12 months posttrauma. (Buskila & Neumann 1997). The findings were that 'Almost all symptoms were significantly more prevalent or severe in the patients with neck injury ... The fibromyalgia prevalence rate in the neck injury group was 13 times greater than the leg fracture group'. Pain threshold levels were significantly lower, tender point counts were higher and quality of life was worse in the neck injury patients as compared with leg injury subjects. Over 21% of the patients with neck injury (none of whom had chronic pain problems prior to the injury) developed fibromyalgia within 3.2 months of trauma as against only 1.7% of the leg fracture patients (not significantly different from the general population). The researchers make a particular point of noting that, 'In spite of the injury or the presence of fibromyalgia, all patients were employed at the time of examination and that insurance claims were not associated with increased fibromyalgia symptoms or impaired functioning'.

Why should whiplash-type injury provoke fibromyalgia more effectively than other forms of trauma? One answer may lie in the role of rectus capitis posterior minor, part of the suboccipital group, details of which are found on pp. 34 and 207 (Hallgren et al 1993, 1994).

Treatment choices for whiplash?

With common whiplash symptoms ranging from radiating neck and arm pain to chronic headache and virtually incapacitating dizziness and imbalance, WAD has attracted a wide range of (apparently mostly useless) treatment strategies.

Collars are probably contraindicated for whiplash ... they irritate jaws, foster joint adhesions, and lead to tissue atrophy. Physicians can be blamed for prescribing too many drugs ... most of which are probably an ugly approach to whiplash. Physiotherapists are chided for excessive passive modalities which not only do no good, but by their repeated failure can help convince the poor suffering patients that all is lost. Among the chiropractors repeated manipulations can also foster illness behavior, but short-term manipulation and mobilization may be helpful. (Allen 1996)

Dr Allen, whose opinion is quoted above, is a world authority on whiplash and his views are based on both experience and research and are therefore deserving of respect. Contrary viewpoints (Schafer 1987) and clinical experience suggest that short-term use of cervical collars and NSAID medication during the acute phase, post-whiplash, *may* be helpful. However, it is our opinion that illness behavior and retardation of healing can certainly be promoted by anything other than a brief use of such approaches.

What happens in a collision?

Early studies suggested that in rear-end automobile accidents the trauma occurring in the cervical spine related to hyperextension and/or hyperflexion of the neck. Current seat and head support design tend to prevent hyperextension and yet whiplash injuries do not appear to have lessened and research has tried to assess the reasons for this apparent anomaly.

Cervical damage resulting from rear-end accidents seems to relate directly to the position initially adopted by the injured individual during the incident, with those leaning forward experiencing compressive stresses as well as hyperflexion injuries and those seated upright or reclining experiencing initial extension, with no compressive cervical damage. The speed of impact, as well as different directions of impact and car design features, all add obvious variations to these basic findings (Gough 1996).

All in the mind?

Lewit (1999) places whiplash in context when he says:

The high incidence of traumatic neurosis [following whiplash-type injuries] must be put down to mismanagement; in the vast majority of cases without gross neurological findings doctors not trained in the manual diagnosis of movement restriction and segmental reflex change come to the disastrous conclusion that there are no 'organic findings', and hence dismiss the trouble as 'functional', i.e. a psychological disturbance.

In treating patients with whiplash and concussion (the symptoms of which differ only in minor ways, according to Lewit), he found that out of a series of 65 patients, he achieved results which could be classified as 'excellent' in 37, 'fair' in 18, with 10 failures. 'Failure was most frequently due to ligament pain and anteflexion [i.e. flexion] headache; the most frequent site of blockage was between atlas and axis.' Lewit's methods in these cases involved 'manipulation', which incorporates, in his definition, soft tissue approaches such as MET and trigger point deactivation.

We believe that the methods outlined in this text, in which a comprehensive soft tissue approach is recommended, involving NMT, MET, PRT, MFR and massage, as well as rehabilitation methods, offer the best opportunity for successfully treating the majority of patients suffering the sequels of whiplash, as long as full and accurate assessments are undertaken before and during treatment. In some cases active manipulation (mobilization or high-velocity thrust) may also be required but it is strongly suggested that soft tissue approaches be attempted initially.

the scalenes and hyoid muscles). If a group of muscles tests as weak this could involve inhibitory influences from their antagonists.

• The practitioner places a hand on the forehead of the supine patient and the other hand on the sternum (to prevent thoracic flexion) as the patient slowly attempts to flex the neck against this resistance.

• Assessment of *extension* strength (Fig. 11.16B) evaluates upper trapezius, splenius capitis and cervicis, semispinalis capitis and cervicis, erector spinae (longissi-

mus capitis and cervicis) and, to a secondary degree, levator scapulae and the transversospinalis group. The practitioner places a stabilizing hand on the upper posterior thoracic region and the palm of the other hand on the occiput as the *prone* patient slowly extends the neck against this resistance. The suboccipital muscles are tested if this extension movement concludes with a 'tipping' backwards and caudad of the occiput.

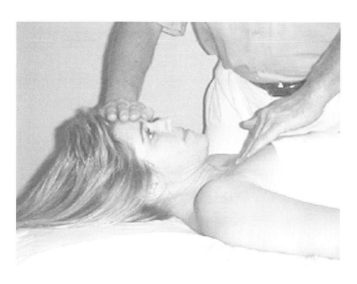

A

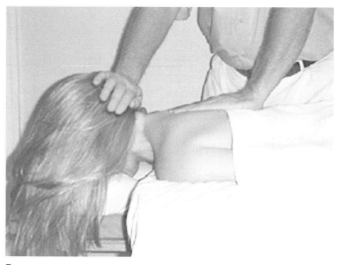

B

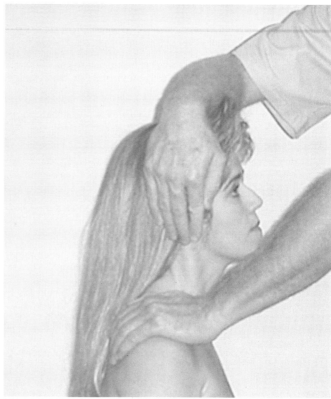

C

D

Figure 11.16 Various strength tests for the cervical region. A: Flexion. B: Extension. C: Rotation. D: Sidebending (lateral flexion).

• Assessment of *rotational* strength (Fig. 11.16C) evaluates sternocleidomastoid, upper trapezius, obliquus capitis inferior, levator scapula, splenius capitis and cervicis (and to a secondary degree the scalenes and transversospinalis group). The practitioner stands in front of the seated patient and places his stabilizing hand on the posterior aspect of the shoulder with the other hand on the patient's cheek on the same side, as the patient slowly turns the head ipsilaterally to meet the resistance offered by the hand.

• Assessment of *sidebending (lateral flexion)* strength (Fig. 11.16D) involves the scalenes and levator scapula (and to a secondary degree rectus capitis lateralis and the transversospinalis group). The practitioner places a stabilizing hand on the top of the shoulder to prevent movement and the other on the head above the ear as the seated patient attempts to flex the head laterally against this resistance.

Palpation of symmetry of movement – general (Fig. 11.17)

As so often is the case when comparing anatomy texts, there exists disagreement as to the normal ranges of motion of the structures of the cervical region. The authors have offered approximate ranges below which are intended to guide the practitioner in assessing joint motion.

Lewit (1985) suggests the patient be seated with the shoulder girdle stabilized with one hand as the other hand guides the head into flexion.

• The chin (mouth closed) should easily touch the sternum and any shortness in the posterior cervical musculature will prevent this.

• The normal range of *flexion* is approximately 50° (Mayer et al 1994). If pain is noted when full, unforced flexion has been achieved (and if meningitis and radicular pain have been ruled out), Lewit maintains that this probably indicates restriction of the occiput on the atlas. If, however, there is pain after the head has been in flexion for 15–20 seconds (see McKenzie notes, p. 169), it is probably ligamentous pain. This is especially common in individuals who display hypermobility tendencies. Headaches will be a likely presenting symptom with extreme sensitivity noted on palpation of the lateral tip of the transverse process of the axis.

• Normal range of *extension* is approximately 70° (Mayer et al 1994). Extension should be assessed but with caution relating to possible interference with cranial blood supply. During extension, an increased degree of 'bulging' of distressed intervertebral discs may occur, along with a folding of the dura and anteriorly directed pressure on the ligamentum flavum, any of which could produce a degree of increased symptomatology, including pain.

• The normal range of *lateral flexion* is 45° (Mayer et al 1994). When testing sidebending (lateral flexion) of the cervical spine, the side *toward* which lateral flexion is taking place is stabilized. If the shoulder on the side *from* which lateral flexion is taking place is stabilized, upper trapezius is being evaluated.

• The normal range of *rotation* is approximately 85° (Mayer et al 1994).

1. With the patient seated, gentle rotation around a vertical axis is carefully performed as symmetry and quality of movement are evaluated.
2. Full flexion rotation is then performed to assess

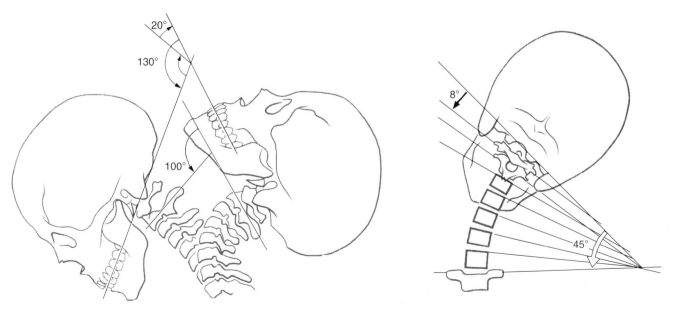

Figure 11.17 Though there is disagreement as to exact 'normal' degrees of cervical movement, these offer approximate ranges (reproduced, with permission, from Kapandji (1998)).

symmetry of rotational movement of the occiput and C2.

3. The practitioner is standing behind the seated patient. With the neck upright, the patient's chin is actively drawn toward the neck (without flexion of the remainder of the cervical spine) while the practitioner's other hand cradles the occiput in order to direct subsequent rotational movement of the head. Rotational restriction with the head in this position indicates dysfunction localized to C2 and C3.

4. With the head and neck in extension, rotation increasingly focuses on the lower cervicals (the greater the extension, the lower the segment involved). It is important in this assessment to avoid chin poking (which would induce anterior translation of the mid-cervicals), but to maintain the chin relatively fixed.

Functional evaluation of fascial postural patterns

Zink & Lawson (1979) have described methods for testing tissue preference.

• There are four crossover sites where fascial tensions can most easily be noted: occipitoatlantal (OA), cervicothoracic (CT), thoracolumbar (TL) and lumbosacral (LS).

• These sites are tested for rotation and sideflexion preference.

• Zink's research showed that most people display (assessing the occipitoatlantal pattern first) alternating patterns of rotatory preference, with about 80% of people showing a common pattern of left-right-left-right (L-R-L-R, termed the 'common compensatory pattern' or CCP).

• Zink observed that the 20% of people whose compensatory pattern did *not* alternate had poor health histories and low levels of 'wellness' and coped poorly with stress.

• Treatment of either CCP or uncompensated fascial patterns has the objective of trying as far as possible to create a symmetrical degree of rotatory motion at the key crossover sites.

• The methods used to achieve this range from direct muscle energy approaches to indirect positional release techniques and high-velocity thrusts.

Assessment of tissue preference

• Tissue preference is the sense of preferred direction(s) of movement the palpating hands derive from the tissues as they are moved.

• Evaluations of this sort are discussed under the heading Functional Technique in Chapter 10.

• The process of evaluation can be conceived as a series of 'questions' which are being asked as tissues are moved.

'Are you more comfortable moving in this direction, or that?'

• The terms 'comfort position', 'ease' and 'tissue preference' are synonymous.

• Positions of ease, comfort, preference are directly opposite to directions which engage barriers or move toward 'bind'.

1. Occipitoatlantal area

• The patient is supine.

• The practitioner is at the head of the table, facing the patient's head.

• One hand (caudal hand) cradles the occiput so that it is supported by the hypothenar eminence and the middle, ring and small fingers.

• The index finger and thumb are free to control either side of the atlas.

• The other hand is placed on the patient's forehead or crown of head to assist in moving this during the procedure.

• The neck is flexed to its fullest easy degree, locking the rotational potential of the cervical segments below C2.

• The contact hand on the occipitoatlantal joint evaluates the tissue preference as the area is slowly rotated left and right.

• By holding tissues in their 'loose' or ease positions or by holding tissues in their 'tight' or bind positions and introducing isometric contractions or by just waiting for a release, changes can be encouraged.

2. Cervicothoracic area (Fig. 11.18)

• The patient is seated in a relaxed posture; the practitioner stands behind with hands placed to cover the medial aspects of upper trapezius so that fingers rest over the clavicles.

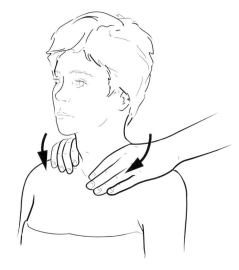

Figure 11.18 Assessment of tissue rotation preference in cervicothoracic region.

- Each hand independently assesses the area being palpated for its 'tightness/looseness' (see above) preferences, in rotation.
- By holding tissues in their 'loose' or ease positions or by holding tissues in their 'tight' or bind positions and introducing isometric contractions or by just waiting for a release, changes can be encouraged.

Variation

- With the patient supine, the cervicothoracic junction is assessed by the practitioner sliding the fingers under the transverse processes.
- An anterior compressive force is applied, first to one side then the other, assessing the response of the transverse process to an anterior, compressive, springing force.
- A sense should easily be achieved of one side having a tendency to move further anteriorly (and therefore more easily into rotation) compared with the other.

3. Thoracolumbar area (Fig. 11.19)

- The patient is supine; the practitioner stands facing caudally and places his hands over the lower thoracic structures, fingers along the lower rib shafts laterally.
- Treating the structure being palpated as a cylinder, the hands test its preference for rotating around its central axis, one way and then the other.
- Once this has been established, the preference to sidebend one way or the other is evaluated, so that combined ('stacked') positions of ease or bind can be established.

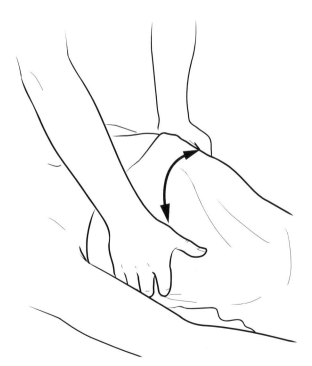

Figure 11.19 Assessment of tissue rotation preference in thoracolumbar (diaphragm) region.

- By holding tissues in their 'loose' or ease positions or by holding tissues in their 'tight' or bind positions and introducing isometric contractions or by holding at the barrier (bind position) without a contraction and just waiting for a release, changes can be encouraged.

4. Lumbosacral area

- The patient is supine; the practitioner stands below waist level facing cephalad and places his hands on the anterior pelvic structures, using the contact as a 'steering wheel' to evaluate tissue preference as the pelvis is rotated around its central axis, seeking information as to its 'tightness/looseness' (see above) preferences. Once this has been established, the preference to sidebend one way or the other is evaluated, so that combined ('stacked') positions of ease or bind can be established.
- By holding tissues in their 'loose' or ease positions or by holding tissues in their 'tight' or bind positions and introducing isometric contractions or by holding at the barrier (bind position) without a contraction and just waiting for a release, changes can be encouraged.

Assessment becomes treatment

The series of range of motion (and tissue preference) assessments outlined above offers a general impression. *Specific* localized evaluations should then also be performed which offer information directly linking the assessment procedure to a range of treatment options.

- If a movement in one direction is more restricted than the same movement in the opposite direction, a barrier will have been identified.
- This might be by means of a sense of bind, locking or restriction as compared with a sense of ease, comfort or freedom in the opposite direction.
- The palpated information might take the form of a difference in end-feel, or a contrast in the feel of tissue texture ('bind').

Once a barrier of resistance is identified, several treatment options are open to the practitioner.

1. If a shortened soft tissue structure is identified during assessment, holding tissues at their barrier of resistance and then waiting allows a slow passive myofascial release to occur (as in holding a yoga posture for several minutes and then being able to move further in that direction).

2. If a shortened soft tissue structure is identified during assessment, holding tissues at their barrier of resistance and having the patient attempt to push further in that direction, using no more than 20% of strength for 7 seconds, against the practitioner's resistance, produces an isometric contraction of the *antagonists* to the tissues restricting movement (the agonists) which would produce

a *reciprocal inhibition* effect (MET) and allow movement to a new barrier – or through it if stretching was being used.

3. If a shortened soft tissue structure is identified during assessment, holding the tissues at their barrier of resistance and having the patient attempt to push away from that barrier, using no more than 20% of strength for 7 seconds, against the practitioner's resistance, produces an isometric contraction of the *agonists* which would produce a *postisometric relaxation* effect (MET) and allow movement to a new barrier – or through it if stretching was being used.

4. In examples 2 and 3, an alternative is to introduce a series of very small rhythmic contractions (20 contractions in 10 seconds, rather than a 7-second sustained one) toward or away from the resistance barrier – *pulsed MET* (Ruddy's approach) – in order to achieve an increase in range of movement. If the pulsating contractions are toward the restriction barrier, this will effectively be activating the antagonists to the shortened soft tissues which are restricting movement. This action would therefore induce a series of minute reciprocal inhibition influences into the shortened tissues. *Note*: Ruddy's method should not be confused with ballistic stretching. Ruddy specifically warns against 'bounce' occurring during the pulsations, which because they involve the merest initiation and cessation of an action are *extremely* small in their amplitude, designed to both produce a series of small isometric contractions as well as reeducate proprioceptive function.

5. If a barrier of resistance was noted when (as an example) flexion of the neck was being tested, the cause might lie in a restriction (shortening of the muscles) which would move the area in the opposite direction, in this example the extensors. If the principles of *strain-counterstrain* (SCS) are being used as part of positional release methodology (PRT), an area of localized tenderness or pain should be sought in the shortened musculature (extensors) and this point should be used as a monitor (press and score '10') as the area is positioned to take the pain down to a score of '3' or less. This position of ease is then held for 90 seconds (see guidelines for SCS, including Goodheart's approach, in Chapter 10).

6. An alternative positional release method (PRT) might involve '*functional*' technique, in which the practitioner uses a series of movements involving all the variables available (flexion, extension, sideflexion both ways, rotation both ways, translation, compression, traction), seeking in each the most easy, relaxed, comfortable response from the tense, distressed tissues under palpation. Each tested direction of movement commences from the combined positions of ease previously identified, so that the final position represents a 'stack' of positions of ease. This is held for 90 seconds before a slow release and retesting occurs.

7. Changes of a dysfunctional nature (fibrotic, contracted, etc.) might be palpated in the shortened soft tissues and after the tissues had been placed in a shortened state, the area of restriction could be localized by a flat compression (thumb, finger, heel of hand). The patient then initiates a slow stretching movement which would take the muscle to its full length while compression is maintained, before returning it to a shortened state and then repeating the exercise. This is a form of *active myofascial release* (MFR).

8. The soft tissues of the area could be mobilized by means of *massage* techniques, including neuromuscular normalization of areas of dysfunction and reflexogenic activity discovered during palpation (NMT).

9. The joints and soft tissues of the area can be mobilized by careful *articulation* movements, which take the tissues through their normal ranges of motion in a rhythmic painless sequence, so encouraging greater range of motion. This approach actively releases and stretches the soft tissues associated with the joint, often effectively mobilizing the joint without recourse to manipulation.

10. A suitably trained and licensed individual could engage the restriction barrier identified during motion palpation and utilize a *high-velocity thrust* (HVT) to overcome the barrier.

All these examples indicate different ways in which assessment *becomes* treatment, as a seamless process of discovery leads to therapeutic action.

Caution

When MET is used in relation to joint restriction, no stretching should be introduced after an isometric contraction, only a movement to the new barrier. This is also true of MET treatment of acute soft tissue dysfunction. Therefore, for acute muscular problems and all joint restrictions:

- identify the barrier
- introduce MET
- move to the new barrier after release of the contraction.

Any sense that force is needed to move a joint, or that tissues are 'binding' as movement is performed, should inform the hands of the practitioner that the barrier has been passed or reached.

Only in chronic soft tissue conditions is stretching beyond the restriction barrier introduced, never in joint restrictions.

The following examples offer a means of exploring the therapeutic possibilities which emerge from assessment methods which uncover restrictions. The clinical language used derives from osteopathic medicine.

Upper cervical dysfunction assessment (Fig. 11.20)

- To test for dysfunction in the upper cervical region, the patient lies supine.
- The practitioner passively flexes the head on the neck fully, with one hand, while the other cradles the neck.
- Since flexion locks the cervical area below C2, evaluation is isolated to atlantoaxial rotation where half the gross rotation of the neck occurs.
- With the neck flexed (effectively 'locking' everything below C2), the head is then passively rotated to both left and right.
- If the range is greater on one side, then this is indicative of a probable restriction, which may be amenable to soft tissue manipulation treatment or HVT.
- If rotation toward the right is restricted compared with rotation toward the left, the indication is of a 'left rotated atlas' or, in osteopathic terminology, an atlas which is 'posterior left' (as the transverse process on the left has moved posteriorly).
- Treatment options discussed above can then be utilized by means of engaging the barrier and introducing MET variations (reciprocal inhibition, postisometric relaxation, pulsed MET) or considering PRT methods (in more acute settings, ideally).

Assessment and treatment of occipitoatlantal restriction (C0–C1) (Fig. 11.21)

- The patient is supine while the practitioner sits or stands at the head of the table.

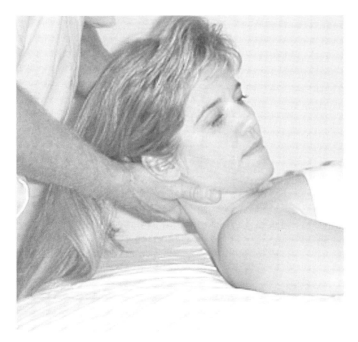

Figure 11.20 To assess dysfunction of the upper cervical unit, the head is first placed in flexion, which locks the area below C2 and isolates rotational movement to the upper unit. This step is omitted when posterior disc damage is present in the cervical region.

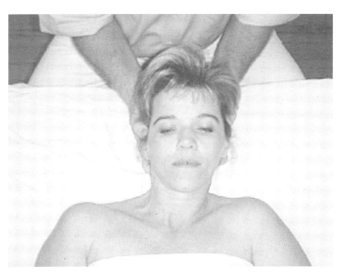

Figure 11.21 Ease of movement as well as changes in tissue texture and tone may be assessed using translation side to side (without imposing sidebending or rotation).

- The patient's head is supported in both the practitioner's hands with middle and/or index fingers immediately inferior to the occiput, bilaterally.
- The fingers assess tissue change as the hands take the head into lateral translation one way and then the other (a 'shunt' movement along an axis; simple translation side to side, without rotation or deliberate sideflexion).
- Translation assessment is performed with the head in a neutral position, as well as in flexion and also in extension.
- As translation occurs in a given direction (say, toward the right), a sideflexion is taking place to the left and therefore, in the case of the occiput/atlas, rotation is occurring to the right (refer to notes on spinal coupling earlier in this section, p. 167).
- It is far safer (and much simpler) to use translation in order to evaluate sideflexion and rotation than it would be to perform these movements at each articulation.
- Two sets of information are being received from the hands as the translation movement takes place.
  1. The relative ease of movement left and right as translation is performed.
  2. The changes in the tissue tone and texture as translation takes place. There may also be reported discomfort, either in response to the movement or to the palpation of suboccipital tissues.

Because spinal biomechanics decree that sidebending and rotation take place in opposite directions at the occipitoatlantal junction, the following findings would relate to any sense of restriction ('bind') noted (using the same example) during flexion and translation toward the right.

  1. The occiput is extended and rotated left and side-

flexed right (this describes the *positional* situation of the structure involved – the occiput in relation to the atlas).

2. This same restriction pattern can be described differently, by saying that there is a flexion, right rotation, left sideflexion restriction (this describes the *dysfunctional pattern*, i.e. the directions toward which movement is restricted).

Treatment choices might include the following.

• *NMT*. Application of soft tissue manipulation methods, deep massage and neuromuscular techniques to the soft tissues of the area which display altered tone or tissue texture, followed by reassessment of range of motion.

• *MET*. Takes the occiput/atlas to its restriction barrier, either using simple translation (as in the assessment) or into full flexion, right rotation, left sideflexion, in order to engage the restriction barrier before introducing a light isometric contraction toward or away from the barrier for 7 seconds, and then reassesses the range of motion.

• *PRT*. Takes the occiput/atlas away from its restriction barrier, either into translation to the left, in the direction opposite that in which restriction was noted, or into extension, left rotation, right sideflexion to disengage from the restriction barrier, and waits for 30–90 seconds for a positional release change to occur. Range of motion is then reassessed.

• *HVT*. A high-velocity thrust could be performed (by a suitably licensed individual) by taking the structures to their restriction barrier and then rapidly forcing them through the restriction barrier.

All these methods would be successful in certain circumstances. The MET and PRT choices, as well as the application of NMT, would be the least invasive. HVT may be the only choice if the less invasive measures fail.

Functional release of atlantooccipital joint

• The patient is supine.
• The practitioner sits at the corner of the head of the table, facing the patient's head from that corner.
• The caudal hand cradles the occiput with opposed index finger and thumb controlling the atlas.
• The other hand is placed on the patient's forehead.
• The caudal hand ('listening hand') searches for feelings of 'ease', 'comfort' or 'release' in the tissues surrounding the atlas as the hand on the forehead directs the head into a compound series of motions.
• As each motion is 'tested', a point is found where the tissues being palpated feel at their *most relaxed or easy*. This is used as the start point for the next sequence of assessment. In no particular order, the following ranges and directions of motion are tested, seeking always the easiest position to 'stack' onto the previously

identified positions of ease as evaluated by the 'listening hand'.

1. Flexion/extension
2. Sidebending left and right
3. Rotation left and right
4. Anteroposterior translation
5. Side-to-side translation
6. Compression/traction

• Once 'three-dimensional equilibrium' has been ascertained (known as *dynamic neutral*), the patient is asked to inhale and exhale fully, to identify which stage of the cycle increases 'ease', and then asked to hold the breath in that phase for 10 seconds or so.

• The combined position of ease is held for 90 seconds before slowly returning to neutral.

Note that the sequence of movements is not relevant, as long as as many variables as possible are employed in seeking a combined position of ease. The effect of this held position of ease is to allow neural resetting to occur, reducing muscular tension, and also to encourage dramatically better circulation through previously tense and possibly ischemic tissues. Following this sequence, a direct inhibitory method (such as cranial base release – see p. 209) is used to further release the suboccipital musculature.

Translation assessment for cervical spine (C2–7)

The following assessment sequence is based on the work of Philip Greenman DO (1989). In performing this exercise, it is important to recall that normal physiology dictates that sidebending and rotation in the cervical area below the axis are type 2, i.e. segments which are sidebending will automatically rotate toward the same side. Most cervical restrictions are compensations and will involve several segments, all of which will adopt this type 2 pattern. Exceptions occur if a restriction is traumatically induced by a direct blow to the joint, in which case there might be sidebending to one side and rotation to the other – type 1 – which is the physiological pattern for the rest of the spine.

• To easily palpate for sidebending and rotation, a side-to-side translation movement is used, with the neck in slight flexion or slight extension.

• When the neck is absolutely neutral (no flexion or extension, an unusual state in the neck) true translation side to side is possible.

• As a segment is translated to one side, it is automatically sidebending to the opposite side and because of the biomechanical rules which govern it, it will be rotating to the same side.

• The practitioner is seated or standing at the head of the supine patient.

- The index finger pads rest on the articular pillars of C6, medial and superior to the transverse processes of C7 (which can be palpated just anterior to the upper trapezius).
- The middle finger pads will be on C6 and the ring finger on C5 with the little finger pads on C3.
- With these contacts, it is possible to examine for sensitivity, fibrosis and hypertonicity as well as being able to apply lateral translation to cervical segments with the head in flexion or extension.
- In order to do this effectively, it is necessary to stabilize the superior segment to the one about to be examined with the finger pads.
- The heel of the hand controls movement of the head.
- With the head/neck in relative neutral (no flexion and no extension), translation to one side and then the

other is introduced by a combination of contact forces involving the finger pads on the articular pillars of the segment being assessed, as well as the supporting hands supporting the head, to assess freedom of translation movement (and, by implication, sidebending and rotation) in each direction.

- For example, C5 is being stabilized with the finger pads, as translation to the left is introduced. The ability of C5 to freely sidebend and rotate to the right on C6 is being evaluated with the neck in neutral.
- If the joint is normal this translation will cause a gapping of the left facet and a closing of the right facet as left translation is performed and vice versa. There will be a soft end-feel to the movement, without harsh or sudden breaking.
- If, say, translation of the segment toward the left from the right produces a sense of resistance or bind, then the segment is restricted in its ability to sidebend right and (by implication) also to rotate right.
- If such a restriction is noted, the translation should be repeated but this time with the head in extension instead of neutral. This is achieved by lifting the contact fingers on C5 (in this example) slightly toward the ceiling, before reassessing the side-to-side translation.
- The head and neck are then taken into flexion and right-to-left translation is again assessed.
- The objective is to ascertain which position creates the greatest degree of bind as the barrier is engaged. Is translation more restricted in neutral, extension or flexion?
- If this restriction is greater with the head extended, the diagnosis is of a joint locked in flexion, sidebent left and rotated left (meaning that there is difficulty in the joint extending, sidebending and rotating to the right).
- If this (C5 on C6 translation right to left) restriction is greater with the head flexed, then the joint is locked in extension and sidebent left and rotated left (meaning there is difficulty in the joint flexing, sidebending and rotating to the right).

Treatment choices

- Using MET and using the same example (C5 on C6 as above, with greatest restriction in extension).
- The hands palpate the articular pillars of the inferior segment of the pair which is dysfunctional.
- One hand stabilizes the C6 articular pillars, holding the inferior vertebra so that the superior segment can be moved on it.
- The other hand controls the head and neck above the restricted vertebra.
- The articular pillars of C6 should be eased toward the ceiling, introducing extension, while the other hand introduces rotation and sidebending until the restriction barrier is reached.

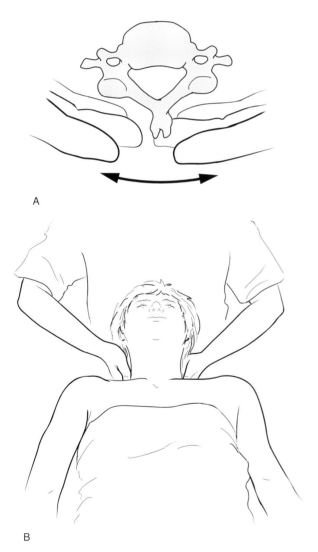

A

B

Figure 11.22 A: Finger positions in relation to articular pillars and spinous process. B: Individual segments of cervical spine (below C3) are taken into left and right translation, in order to evaluate ease of movement, in neutral, slight flexion and slight extension.

- A slight isometric contraction is introduced by the patient using sidebending, rotation or flexion (or all of these) either towards or away from the barrier.
- After 5–7 seconds the patient relaxes and extension, sidebending and rotation left are increased to the new resistance barrier.
- Repeat 2–3 times.

Alternative positional release approach

- As an alternative, the directions of *ease* of translation of the dysfunctional segment can be assessed in neutral, slight flexion and slight extension.
- Whichever position produces the greatest sense of palpated 'ease' is held for 90 seconds
- Following this reassessment, the area should show a degree of 'release' and increased range of motion.

SCS cervical flexion restriction method
(Fig. 11.23)

Note that Strain and counterstrain is an ideal approach for self-treatment of 'tender' points and can safely be taught to patients for home use.

- An area of local dysfunction is sought, using an appropriate form of palpation on the skin areas overlying the tips of the transverse processes of the cervical spine (Lewit 1992).
- Light compression is introduced to identify and establish a point of sensitivity (a 'tender point') which in this area represents (based on Jones' findings) an anterior (forward-bending) strain site.
- The patient is instructed in the method for reporting a reduction in pain during the positioning sequence which follows.
  1. Say to the patient, 'I want you to score the pain caused by my pressure, before we start moving your head into different positions, as a '10'. Please don't say anything apart from giving me the present score (out of 10) whenever I ask for it'.
  2. The aim is to achieve a reported score of '3' or less before ceasing the positioning process and to avoid conversation which would distract from the practitioner's focus on palpating tissue change and repositioning the tissues.
- The head/neck should then be passively taken lightly into flexion until some degree of 'ease' is reported in the tender point (based on the score reported by the patient) which is being constantly compressed at this stage (Chaitow 1991).
- When a reduction of pain of around 50% is achieved, a degree of fine tuning is commenced in which very small degrees of additional positioning are introduced in order

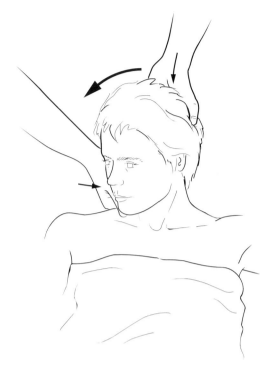

Figure 11.23 For cervical flexion strain using SCS, a tender point is monitored (right thumb) as the head is flexed and fine tuned (usually turning towards side of pain) to remove pain from the point.

to find the position of maximum ease, at which time the reported 'score' should be reduced by at least 70%.

- At this time the patient may be asked to inhale fully and exhale fully while observing for herself changes in the palpated pain point, in order to evaluate which phase of the cycle reduces the pain score still more. That phase of the breathing cycle in which she senses the greatest reduction in sensitivity is maintained for a period which is tolerable to the patient (holding the breath in or out or at some point between the two extremes, for as long as is comfortable) while the overall position of ease continues to be maintained and the tender/tense area monitored.
- This position of ease is held for 90 seconds in Jones' methodology.
- During the holding of the position of ease the direct compression can be reduced to a mere touching of the point along with a periodic probing to establish that the position of ease has been maintained.
- After 90 seconds the neck/head is very slowly returned to the neutral starting position. This slow return to neutral is a vital component of SCS since the neural receptors (muscle spindles) may be provoked into a return to their previously dysfunctional state if a rapid movement is made at the end of the procedure.
- The tender point/area, and any functional restriction, may be retested at this time and should be found to be improved.

SCS cervical extension restriction method
(Fig. 11.24)

- With the patient in a supine position and the head clear of the end of the table and fully supported by the practitioner, areas of localized tenderness are sought by light palpation alongside the tips of the spinous processes of the cervical spine.
- Having located a tender point, compression is applied to elicit a degree of sensitivity or pain which the patient notes as representing a score of '10'.
- The head/neck is then taken into light extension along with sidebending and rotation (usually away from the side of the pain if it is not on the mid-line) until a reduction of at least 50% is achieved in the reported sensitivity.
- The pressure on the tender point is constant at this stage.
- With fine tuning of position, a reduction in sensitivity should be achieved of at least 70%, at which time inhalation and exhalation are monitored by the patient to see which reduces sensitivity even more and this phase of the cycle is held for as long as is comfortable, during which the overall position of ease is maintained.
- Intermittent pressure on the point is applied periodically during the holding period in order to ensure that the position of ease has been maintained.
- After 90 seconds a very slow and deliberate return to neutral is performed and the patient is allowed to rest for several minutes.

- The tender point should be repalpated for sensitivity, or functional restriction retested, to assess for improvements.

Mobilization of the cervical spine

General, non-specific cervical mobilization as well as precise segmental releases, as appropriate, considerably enhance cranial function by reducing undue myofascial and mechanical stress in the region. The following methods, based on the work of Drs Greenman, Harakal and Stiles, incorporate safe non-invasive approaches which can be easily learned. Practitioners are again strongly advised to practice within the scope of their license.

Stiles' (1984) general procedure using MET for cervical restriction

- Stiles suggests a general maneuver, in which the patient is sitting upright.
- The practitioner stands behind and holds the head in the mid-line, with both hands stabilizing it and possibly employing his chest to prevent neck extension.
- The patient is told to try (gently) to flex, extend, rotate and sidebend the neck alternately in all directions.
- No particular sequence is necessary, as long as all directions are engaged, a number of times.
- Each muscle group should undergo slight contraction for 5–7 seconds, against unyielding force offered by the practitioner's hands (either toward or away from the

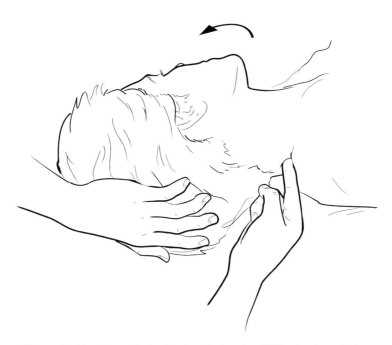

Figure 11.24 For cervical extension strain using SCS, a tender point is monitored (right finger) as the head is extended and fine tuned (usually turning away from the side of pain) to remove pain from the point.

direction of the barrier) once the barrier in any particular direction is engaged.

• This relaxes the tissues in a general manner. Traumatized muscles will relax without much pain via this method. After each contraction the patient eases the area to its new position (barrier) without stretching or force.

Harakal's (1975) cooperative isometric technique (MET) (Fig. 11.25)

The following technique is used when there is a specific or general restriction in a spinal articulation.

• The area should be placed in neutral (patient seated).
• The permitted range of motion should be determined by noting the patient's resistance to further motion.
• The patient should be rested for some seconds at a point just short of the resistance barrier, termed the 'point of balanced tension', in order to 'permit anatomic and physiologic response' to occur.
• The patient is asked to reverse the movement toward the barrier by 'turning back toward where we started' (thus contracting any agonists which may be influencing the restriction) and this movement is resisted by the practitioner.
• The degree of patient participation at this stage can be at various levels, ranging from 'just think about turning' to 'turn as hard as you would like' or by giving specific instructions ('use only about 20% of your strength').
• Following a holding of this isometric effort for a few seconds (5–7) and then relaxing completely, the patient is assisted to move further in the direction of the previous barrier to a new point of restriction determined by their resistance to further motion as well as tissue response (feel for 'bind').
• The procedure is repeated until no further gain is being achieved.
• It would also be appropriate to use the opposite direction of rotation; for example, asking the patient to 'turn further toward the direction you are moving', so utilizing the antagonists to the muscles which may be restricting free movement.

What if it hurts? Evjenth & Hamburg (1984) have a practical solution to the problem of pain being produced when an isometric contraction is employed.

• They suggest that the degree of effort be markedly reduced and the duration of the contraction increased, from 10 to up to 30 seconds.
• If this fails to allow a painless contraction then use of the antagonist muscle(s) for the isometric contraction is another alternative.
• Following the contraction, if a joint is being moved to a new resistance barrier and this produces pain, what variations are possible?

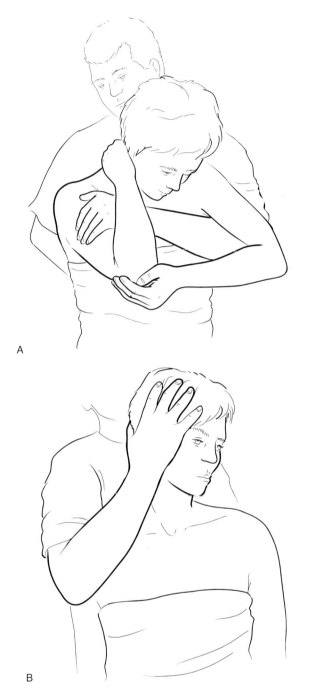

A

B

Figure 11.25 A: Harakal's approach requires the restricted segment to be taken to a position just short of the assessed restriction barrier before isometric contraction is introduced as the patient attempts to return to neutral, after which slack is removed and the new barrier engaged. B: Sidebending and rotation restriction of the cervical region is treated by holding the neck just short of the restriction barrier and having the patient attempt to return to neutral, after which slack is removed and the new barrier engaged.

• If following an isometric contraction and movement toward the direction of restriction there is pain, or if the patient fears pain, Evjenth & Hamburg suggest, 'Then the therapist may be more passive and let the patient actively move the joint'.

• Pain experienced may often be lessened considerably if the practitioner applies gentle traction while the patient actively moves the joint.

• Sometimes pain may be further reduced if, in addition to applying gentle traction, the practitioner simultaneously either aids the patient's movement at the joint or provides gentle resistance while the patient moves the joint.

CERVICAL TREATMENT: SEQUENCING

In the assessment section of this chapter, we have seen how it is possible to move from the gathering of information into treatment almost seamlessly. This is a characteristic of NMT. As the practitioner searches for information, the appropriate degree of pressure modification from the contact digit or hand can turn 'finding' into 'fixing'. This will become clearer as the methods and objectives of NMT and its associated modalities become more familiar. The authors feel it useful to suggest that where the tissues being assessed and treated are particularly tense, restricted and indurated, the prior use of basic muscle energy or positional release methods can reduce superficial hypertonicity sufficiently to allow better access for exploring, assessing and ultimately treating the dysfunctional tissues.

Sequencing is an important element in bodywork, as the discussion immediately below reinforces. What should be treated first? Where should treatment begin? To some extent this is a matter of experience but in many instances protocols and prescriptions based on clinical experience – and sometimes research – can be offered. Several concepts relating to sequencing may usefully be kept in mind when addressing upper body (and other) dysfunctions from an NMT perspective. Most of these thoughts are based on the clinical experience of the authors and those with whom they have worked and studied.

• Superficial muscles are addressed before deeper layers (see cervical planes below).

• The proximal portions of the body are released before the distal portions; therefore, the cervical region is treated before craniomandibular or other cranial myofascial techniques are used.

• The portion of the spinal column from which innervation to an extremity emerges is addressed with the extremity (i.e. cervical spine is treated when the upper extremity is addressed).

• Beginning in a supine position (especially the first session or two) allows the patient to communicate more easily when tenderness is found since the face is not obscured by the table. (European (Lief's) NMT applied to the posterior aspect of the body is almost always performed with the patient prone, from the outset.)

• A reclining position for the patient reduces the muscle's weight-bearing responsibilities and is usually preferred over upright postures (sitting or standing), although upright postures can be used in some areas.

• Alternative body positions such as sidelying postures may be substituted where appropriate, although they are not always described in this text.

• *Note*: The instructions in this text are given for the right side of the neck but both sides of the spine should always be treated to avoid instability and reflexive splinting, which may occur if only one side is addressed.

Cervical planes and layers

When addressing multiple muscles simultaneously, as occurs during the cervical lamina groove treatment, it is very useful to envision them in layers. If the direction of fibers is known for each muscle and the muscles residing in each layer are considered, it is much easier to ascertain which tissues are being palpated and which are involved when tenderness, contracture or fibrosis are revealed. These palpation skills are enhanced by a solid anatomy knowledge, particularly in regard to fiber arrangement and the muscle layers.

However, when considering movement (or movement dysfunctions) of the cervical region, it is also helpful to think in terms of muscular planes. In the posterior neck (Kapandji 1974), these would be:

• *superficial plane* – trapezius and sternocleidomastoid (posterosuperior part) (SCM anatomy with anterior cervical muscles, p. 213)
• *second plane* – splenius capitis, splenius cervicis, levator scapula (levator scapula anatomy given with prone position, p. 329)
• *third plane* – semispinalis capitis, semispinalis cervicis, transversus thoracis, longissimus thoracis, most superior portion of iliocostalis (thoracic muscles with thorax, p. 436)
• *fourth (deep) plane* – the suboccipital muscles, rotatores, multifidus, interspinalis muscles.

The muscles listed in the various planes, when contracting unilaterally, usually provide movements similar to others on the same plane (superficial plane – contralateral head rotation, second plane – ipsilateral head rotation, third plane – lateral flexion, fourth (deep) plane – fine contralateral rotation or sideflexion). All of these muscles, when contracting bilaterally, extend the spine or head, with the exception of rectus capitis posterior minor, which attaches to the dura via an anteriorly oriented bridge and pulls posteriorly on the dura mater to prevent it from folding on itself or on to the spinal cord during anterior translation of the head (Hallgren et al 1994).

Confusion may occur when considering the information offered above if the reader is thinking in terms of *layers of muscles*, rather than *muscular planes*. For example, when layers are considered, we see that the second layer at the superior aspect of the cervical lamina is semispinalis capitis (deep to trapezius), whereas in the lower cervical region the splenii comprise the second layer (also deep to trapezius) and semispinalis capitis there forms the third layer.

Developing palpation skills to provide quick reference to involved musculature is very useful in NMT. Understanding movement and relationships of synergists and antagonists is also helpful. Orientation to muscular planes (for movement dysfunctions) as well as muscular layers (for palpation) are both discussed and illustrated by Kapandji (1974). Knowing the direction and approximate length of fibers and tendons will assist in quickly locating trigger point sites.

Upper portions of the trapezius are included here with the posterior cervical muscles since it is the most superficial tissue layer of the posterior neck, where it plays a role as an extensor and rotator of the head and neck. However, since a primary function of the trapezius is to move the shoulder girdle, it is more fully discussed with the shoulder region. When trapezius is addressed in a prone position, treatment of the middle and lower portions of the muscle may be included (see p. 320). Later in this chapter treatment of upper trapezius in the prone position, using Lief's European NMT, is described as an alternative to American NMT. A sidelying position (see repose, p. 229) is also effective (in some cases advantageous) for examining the trapezius and many other cervical muscles and may be used as an alternative position for many of the techniques taught in this text.

Posterior cervical region

Upper trapezius (Fig. 11.26)

Attachments: Mid-third of nuchal line and ligamentum nuchae to the lateral third of the clavicle; in some people there is a merging of upper trapezius fibers with sternocleidomastoid (*Gray's anatomy* 1995)

Innervation: Accessory nerve (cranial nerve XI) supplies primarily motor while C2–4 supply mostly sensory

Muscle type: Postural (type 1), shortens when stressed

Function: Unilaterally, laterally flexes (sidebends) the head and neck to the same side when the shoulder is fixed, aids in contralateral extreme head rotation, elevation of the scapula via rotation of the clavicle, assists in carrying the weighted upper limb, assists to rotate the glenoid fossa upward; when contracting bilaterally, assists extension of the cervical spine

Synergists: SCM (head motions); supraspinatus, serratus anterior and deltoid (rotation of scapula during abduction); the trapezius pair are synergistic with each other for head or neck extension

Antagonists: *To scapular rotation*: levator scapula, rhomboids

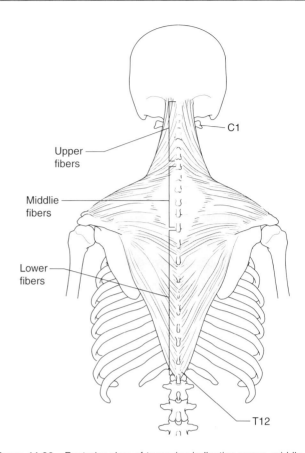

Figure 11.26 Posterior view of trapezius indicating upper, middle and lower portions as described in the text.

Indications for treatment

Upper fibers

- Headache over or into the eye or into the temporal area
- Pain in the angle of the jaw
- Neck pain and/or stiff neck
- Pain with pressure of clothing, purse or luggage strapped across upper shoulder area

Special notes

It is useful to divide the trapezius into three portions for both nomenclature and function (see Fig. 11.26). The upper portion of trapezius attaches the occiput and ligamentum nuchae to the lateral third of the clavicle. The middle fibers of trapezius attach the spinous processes and interspinous ligaments of C6–T3 to the acromion and spine of the scapula while the lower trapezius attaches the spinous processes and interspinous ligaments of T3–12 to the medial end of the spine of the scapula. Although most anatomy books name three divisions, there is inconsistency with the actual names as well as which fibers are included with each portion. For the purpose of describing these techniques, the middle trapezius may be outlined by drawing parallel lines from each end of the spine of the scapula toward the vertebral column. The fibers lying between these two lines are addressed as the middle trapezius. The fibers lying cephalad to the middle fibers are the upper trapezius while those lying caudad to the middle fibers are the lower trapezius. The upper, middle and lower portions of the muscle often function independently (*Gray's anatomy* 1995).

In describing treatment of the upper portion of trapezius, using MET for example (see later in this chapter), upper trapezius itself can usefully be functionally subdivided into anterior, middle and posterior fibers (see Fig. 11.27) with different head positions assisting to focus contractions into these aspects of the muscle. This is an approach, based on clinical experience, the effects of which the practitioner can easily palpate (Chaitow 1996b).

Upper trapezius is designated as a postural muscle. This means that, when dysfunctional, it will almost always be shorter than normal (Janda 1996) (see postural muscle discussion, Chapter 5). It assists in maintaining the head's position and serves as a 'postural corrector' for deviations originating further down the body (in the spine, pelvis or feet). Therefore, fibers of the upper trapezius may be active when the patient is sitting or standing, in order to make adaptive compensations for structural distortions or strained postures.

If the muscle is in a shortened state the occiput will be pulled inferolaterally via very powerful fibers. Due to its attachments, trapezius has the potential to directly influence occipital, parietal and temporal function, which should be noted in cranial therapy.

The motor innervation of trapezius is from the spinal portion of the XI cranial (spinal accessory) nerve. Originating within the spinal canal from ventral roots of the first five cervical segments (usually), it rises through the foramen magnum, exiting via the jugular foramen, where it supplies and sometimes penetrates sternocleidomastoid before reaching a plexus below trapezius (*Gray's anatomy* 1995). Upledger points out that hypertonus of trapezius can produce dysfunction at the jugular foramen with implications for accessory nerve function, so increasing and perpetuating trapezius hypertonicity (Upledger & Vredevoogd 1983).

Fibers of upper trapezius initiate rotation of the clavicle to prepare for elevation of the shoulder girdle. Any position which strains or places the trapezius in a shortened state for periods of time without rest may shorten the fibers and lead to dysfunction. Long telephone conversations, particularly those which elevate the shoulder to hold the phone itself, working from a chair set too low for the desk or computer terminal and elevation of the arm for painting, drawing, playing a musical instrument and computer processing, particularly for extended periods of time, can all shorten trapezius fibers. Overloading of fibers may activate or perpetuate trigger point activity or may make tissue more vulnerable to activation

when a minor trauma occurs, such as a simple fall, minor motor vehicle accident or when reaching (especially quickly) to catch something out of reach.

Trigger points in the upper trapezius (see Fig. 11.27) are some of the most prevalent and potent trigger points found in the body and are relatively easy to locate (Simons et al 1998). They are easily activated by day-to-day habits and abuses (such as repetitive use, sudden trauma, falls) and also by acceleration/deceleration injuries ('whiplash'). They are often predisposed to activation by postural asymmetries, including pelvic tilt and torsion which require postural compensations by these and other muscles (Simons et al 1998).

Assessment of upper trapezius for shortness

1. See scapulohumeral rhythm test (p. 62) which helps identify excessive activity or inappropriate tone in levator scapula and upper trapezius which, because they are postural muscles, indicates shortness.

2. The patient is seated and the practitioner stands behind with one hand resting on the shoulder of the side to be tested and stabilizing it. The other hand is placed on the ipsilateral side of the head and the head/neck is taken into contralateral sidebending without force while the shoulder is stabilized. The same procedure is performed on the other side with the opposite shoulder stabilized. A comparison is made as to which sidebending maneuver produced the greater range and whether the neck can easily reach 45° of sideflexion in each direction, which it should. If neither side can achieve this degree of sidebend then both upper trapezius muscles may be short. The relative shortness of one, compared with the other, is evaluated.

3. The patient is seated and the practitioner stands behind with a hand resting over the muscle on the side to be assessed. The patient is asked to extend the arm at the shoulder joint, bringing the flexed arm/elbow backwards. If the upper trapezius is stressed on that side it will inappropriately activate during this movement. Since it is a postural muscle, shortness in it can then be assumed (see discussion of postural muscle characteristics, Chapter 2).

4. The patient is supine with the neck fully (but not forcefully) sidebent contralaterally (away from the side being assessed). The practitioner is standing at the head of the table and uses a cupped hand contact on the ipsilateral shoulder (i.e. on the side being tested) to assess the ease with which it can be depressed (moved caudally). There should be an easy 'springing' sensation as the practitioner pushes the shoulder toward the feet, with a soft end-feel to the movement. If depression of the shoulder is difficult or if there is a harsh, sudden end-feel, upper trapezius shortness is confirmed.

5. This same assessment (always with full lateral

flexion) should be performed with the head fully rotated contralaterally, half turned contralaterally and slightly turned ipsilaterally, in order to assess the relative shortness and functional efficiency of posterior, middle and anterior subdivisions of the upper portion of the trapezius (see also p. 191).

NMT for upper trapezius in supine position

Cervical portion of upper trapezius. The most superficial layer of the posterior cervical muscles is the upper trapezius. Its fibers lie directly beside the spinous processes, while orienting vertically at the higher levels and turning laterally near the base of the neck. With the patient supine, these fibers may be grasped between the thumb and fingers and compressed, one side at a time or both sides simultaneously, at thumb-width intervals throughout the length of the cervical region. The head may be placed in slight extension to soften the tissue, which may enhance the grasp.

The occipital attachment may be examined with light friction and should be differentiated from the thicker semispinalis capitis which lies deep to it. This attachment will be addressed again with the suboccipital region (p. 205).

Upper trapezius. The patient is supine with the arm placed on the table with the elbow bent and upper arm abducted to reduce tension in the upper fibers of trapezius. This arm position will allow some slack in the muscle which will make it easier to grasp the fibers in the cervical and upper (horizontal) portions. If appropriate and needed, the fibers may be slightly stretched by placing the patient's arm closer to her on the massage table. This additional elongation may make the taut fibers more palpable and precise compression possible; however, it may also stretch taut fibers so much that they are difficult to palpate or are painful.

The center of the upper portion of the upper trapezius is grasped with the fibers held between thumb and two or three fingers (Fig. 11.27). This hand position will provide a general release and can be applied in thumb-width segments along the full length of the upper fibers to examine them in both broad and precise compression.

The fibers of the outermost portion of the trapezius may be 'uncoiled' by dragging 2–3 fingers on the anterior surface of the fibers while the fingers simultaneously press through the fibers and against anteriorly directed thumb pressure. As the fingers 'uncoil' directly across the hidden deep fibers, palpable bands, trigger point nodules and twitch responses may be felt. The practitioner's elbow should be maintained in a high position to avoid placing flexion stresses onto the wrist and to avoid accidentally, and probably painfully, flipping over the most anterior fibers. While controlled and specific snapping techniques can be developed and used as a treatment

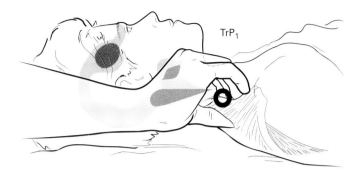

Figure 11.27 The outermost fibers of upper trapezius may be rolled between the thumb and fingers to identify taut bands. Elevation of the elbow of the treating hand may reduce strain on the wrist which may be indicated in this illustration.

modality or to elicit twitch responses for trigger point verification, they should not be accidentally applied to these vulnerable fibers.

A static pincer-like compression may be applied to taut bands, trigger points or nodules found in the upper fibers of trapezius. Toothpick-sized strands of the outermost portion of upper trapezius often produce noxious referrals into the face and eyes. Local twitch responses are readily felt in these easily palpable, often taut fibers.

The patient's arm is allowed to rest on the treatment table beside the patient or the hand may be secured under the patient's buttock. The practitioner is seated cephalad to the shoulder to be treated with the treating thumb placed at approximately the mid fiber level of the upper trapezius and used to glide laterally to the acromioclavicular joint (Fig. 11.28). This gliding motion is repeated several times. The practitioner returns to the middle of the muscle belly and glides medially toward C7 or T1, a process which is also repeated several times.

These alternating, gliding techniques may be repeated several times from the muscle's center toward its attachment sites, to spread the shortened sarcomeres and to elongate taut bands. A double-thumb glide applied by spreading the fibers from the center simultaneously toward the two ends (see Fig. 9.6) will traction the shortened central sarcomeres and may produce a profound release. Full-length glides may reveal remaining thickness within the tissue which needs to be readdressed with compression. Using the thumbs, fingers or palms to spread the tissues from the center, the glide may be applied as precisely as desired as a general or specific myofascial release to soften and elongate the upper fibers.

Central trigger points in these upper fibers refer strongly into the cranium and particularly into the eye. Attachment trigger points and tenderness may be associated with tension from central trigger points and may not respond well until central trigger points have been abolished.

Upper trapezius attachments. Static pressure or friction applied with the finger or thumb can be used directly

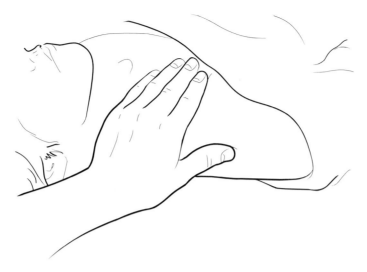

Figure 11.28 The upper trapezius fibers may be pressed against the underlying supraspinatus with gliding strokes in lateral or medial directions.

medial to and against the acromioclavicular joint for the upper fiber attachment of trapezius. Friction is avoided when moderate to extreme tenderness is present or when other symptoms indicate inflammation. Release of central trigger points usually relieves tension on attachment sites.

The pressure may be angled anteriorly against the trapezius attachment on the clavicle (Fig. 11.29) and static pressure or light transverse friction may be applied, increasing pressure only if appropriate. Pressure is applied only at the first finger width medial to the acromioclavicular joint as the brachial plexus lies deep to the clavicle and intrusion into the supraclavicular fossa might damage the nerves and accompanying blood vessels in this area.

Lubricated, gliding strokes may be used to soothe the tissues. Gliding strokes may be used along the superior aspect of the spine of the scapula to assess and treat trapezius attachments and to reveal areas of enthesitis and periosteal tension which, if present, may respond more favorably to applications of ice rather than heat.

 MET treatment of upper trapezius

• In order to treat all the fibers of upper trapezius, MET needs to be applied sequentially. The upper trapezius is subdivided here as anterior, middle and posterior fibers.

• The neck should be placed into different positions of rotation, coupled with the sidebending as described in the assessment above (p. 189), for precise treatment of the various fibers.

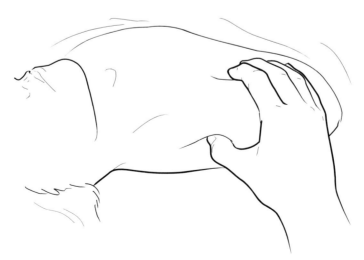

Figure 11.29 Pressure or friction to the clavicular attachment of trapezius is carefully applied to assess tenderness due to inflammation which is often associated with attachment trigger points.

Box 11.8 Lief's NMT for upper trapezius area

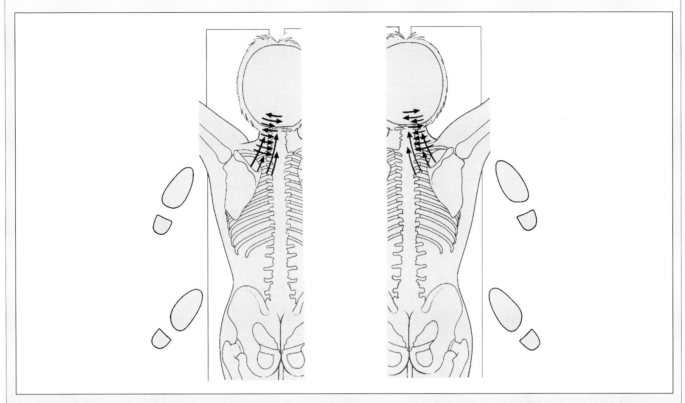

Figure 11.30 Lief's NMT 'maps' for the upper thoracic area (reproduced, with permission, from Chaitow (1996a)).

- In Lief's NMT the practitioner begins by standing half-facing the head of the table on the left of the prone patient with his hips level with the mid-thoracic area.
- The first contact to the left side of the patient's head is a gliding, light-pressured movement of the medial tip of the right thumb, from the mastoid process along the nuchal line to the external occipital protuberance. This same stroke, or glide, is then repeated with deeper pressure. The practitioner's left hand rests on the upper thoracic or shoulder area as a stabilizing contact.
- The treating/assessing hand should be relaxed, molding itself to the contours of tissues. The finger tips offer balance to the hand.
- After the first two strokes of the right thumb – one shallow and diagnostic, the second, deeper, imparting therapeutic effort – the next stroke is half a thumb width caudal to the first. A degree of overlap occurs as these strokes, starting on the belly of the sternocleidomastoid, glide across and through the trapezius, splenius capitis and posterior cervical muscles.
- A progressive series of strokes is applied in this way until the level of the cervicodorsal junction is reached. Unless serious underlying dysfunction is found it is seldom necessary to repeat the two superimposed strokes at each level of the cervical region. If underlying fibrotic tissue appears unyielding a third or fourth slow, deeper glide may be necessary.

- The practitioner now moves to the head of the table. The left thumb is placed on the right lateral aspect of the first dorsal vertebra and a series of strokes are performed caudad and laterally as well as diagonally toward the scapula (Fig. 11.46).
- A series of thumb strokes, shallow and then deep, is applied caudad from T1 to about T4 or 5 and laterally toward the scapula and along and across all the upper trapezius fibers and the rhomboids. The left hand treats the right side and vice versa, with the non-operative hand stabilizing the neck or head.
- By repositioning himself to one side, it is possible for the practitioner to more easily apply a series of sensitively searching contacts into the area of the thoracic outlet. Thumb strokes which start in this triangular depression move toward the trapezius fibers and through them toward the upper margins of the scapula.
- Several light palpating strokes should also be applied directly over the spinous processes, caudally toward the mid-dorsal area. Triggers sometimes lie on the attachments to the spinous processes or between them.
- Any trigger points located should be treated according to the protocol of integrated neuromuscular inhibition technique (INIT); see p. 123.

- The patient lies supine, head/neck sidebent contralaterally to just short of the restriction barrier, while the practitioner stabilizes the shoulder with one hand and cups the ear/mastoid area of the same side of the head with the other.

- With the neck fully sidebent and fully rotated contralaterally, the *posterior* fibers of upper trapezius are involved in the contraction which will be performed, as described below. This will facilitate subsequent stretching of this aspect of the muscle.

- With the neck fully sidebent and half rotated, the *middle* fibers are involved in the contraction.
- With the neck fully sidebent and slightly rotated toward the side being treated, the *anterior* fibers of upper trapezius are being treated.
- These various contractions and subsequent stretches can be performed with the practitioner's arms crossed, hands stabilizing the mastoid area and shoulder.
- The patient introduces a light resisted effort (20% of available strength) to take the stabilized shoulder toward the ear (a shrug movement) and the ear toward the shoulder. The double movement (or effort toward movement) is important in order to introduce a contraction of the muscle, from both ends simultaneously. The degree of effort should be mild and no pain should be felt.
- The contraction is sustained for 10 seconds (or so) and, upon complete relaxation of effort, the practitioner gently eases the head/neck into an increased degree of sidebending where it is stabilized, as the shoulder is stretched caudally. The tissues being treated are taken to, and then slightly through, the barrier of perceived resistance, if appropriate (i.e. not in an acute condition where stretching might be inappropriate).
- If stretching is introduced the patient can usefully assist in this phase of the treatment by initiating, on instruction, the stretch of the muscle ('As you breathe out please slide your hand toward your feet'). This reduces the chances of a stretch reflex being initiated.
- CAUTION: No stretch should be introduced from the cranial end of the muscle as this could stress the neck.

Myofascial release of upper trapezius

- The patient is seated erect. Feet are separated to shoulder width and placed flat on the floor below the knees; arms hang freely.
- The practitioner stands to the side and behind the patient with the proximal aspect of the forearm closest to the patient resting on the lateral aspect of the muscle to be treated (Fig. 11.31a). The forearm is allowed to glide slowly medially toward the scapula/base of the neck, all the while maintaining a firm but acceptable pressure toward the floor.
- By the time the contact arm is close to the medial aspect of the superior border of the scapula, the practitioner's treatment contact will be with the elbow itself.
- As this slow glide is taking place, the patient should equally deliberately be sidebending and turning the head away from the side being treated, having been made aware of the need to maintain an erect sitting posture all the while (Fig. 11.31b).
- The pressure being applied by the practitioner's

forearm/elbow contact should be transferred through the upright spine, toward the ischial tuberosities and ultimately the feet. No slump should be allowed to occur in the patient's posture.
- If areas of extreme tension are encountered by the practitioner's moving arm, it is useful to maintain firm pressure into the restricted area while the patient can be asked to slowly return the head to the neutral position and to make several slow rotations and lateral flexions of the neck away from the treated side, altering the degree of neck flexion as appropriate to ensure maximal tolerable stretching of the compressed tissues.
- Separately or concurrently, the patient can be asked to stretch the fingers of the open hand on the side being treated toward the floor, so adding to the fascial 'drag'

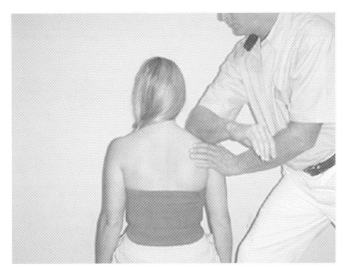

A

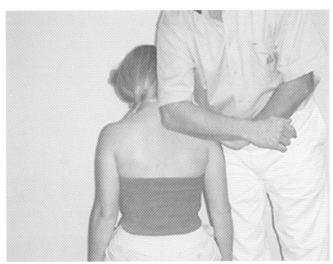

B

Figure 11.31 A: Myofascial release using forearm compression to upper trapezius. B: Myofascial release using elbow compression and patient-induced stretch to upper trapezius.

which ultimately achieves a degree of lengthening and release.

 ## Variation of myofascial release

- The patient lies supine, neck sidebent contralaterally to just short of the restriction barrier and head rotated contralaterally to the restriction barrier.
- The practitioner stabilizes the shoulder with his most medial hand and, crossing the forearms, places the most lateral hand on the lateral surface of the neck just below the mastoid area of the same side of the head.
- The practitioner applies light pressure with the palm through the skin and slides the skin on the neck toward the cranium until skin restriction is felt. This pressure will simultaneously stabilize the neck in its sidebent, rotated position.
- The practitioner laterally tractions the skin under the palm placed on the shoulder to its restriction barrier and simultaneously presses the shoulder caudally and laterally until a firm barrier of the skin and muscles lying between the hands is felt.
- The practitioner maintains the traction of the skin and myofascia of the region for 90–120 seconds. As the pressure is maintained, a softening of the tissues between the hands may be felt. As this occurs, the hands may traction the tissue further until the next barrier is encountered.
- Caution should be exercised with the cervical hand so as not to strain the neck. The shoulder-side hand is used to apply the most traction while the cervically placed hand stabilizes the neck and skin with only enough pressure to engage the skin to avoid undue stress on the cervical region.
- Varying the placement of the shoulder-side hand as well as the angle of lateral flexion will vary the fibers being addressed.
- The finger pads may be used and more precisely placed to address specific portions or bands found in the upper trapezius. The center of the muscle fibers may be stretched more precisely with this method.

As we look at the posterior cervical region, the trapezius, which lies superficial and extensively covers the upper back, is immediately obvious. With its removal, a complex, often confusing array of short and long extensors and rotators are revealed. While the names of these muscles are similar, their distinctions become apparent when the systems by which they are associated and differentiated are understood.

There are many useful ways to interpret these muscles and to group them by performance.

- One could group those muscles which erect and laterally flex the spinal column (erector spinae group) and which lie for the most part on a vertical line.

- Those muscles which traverse the spine on a diagonal line (transversospinal group) rotate the column.
- All of these muscles bilaterally extend the spine.

Platzer (1992) further breaks these two groups into lateral (superficial) and medial (deep) tracts, each having a vertical (intertransverse) and diagonal (transversospinal) component. It is useful to have this subdivision, especially when assessing rotational dysfunctions as the superficial rotators are synergistic with the contralateral deep rotators.

- The lateral tract consists of the iliocostalis and longissimus groups and the splenii muscles, with the vertical components extending the spine and the diagonal splenii rotating the spine ipsilaterally.
- The medial tract includes the spinalis group, the interspinalis and intertransversarii as the vertical components, and the semispinalis group, rotatores and multifidus comprising the deep diagonal group which rotate the spine contralaterally.

The erector spinae system is discussed more fully in the second volume of this text due to its substantial role in postural positioning and its origin in the lumbar and sacral region. However, its cervical components are included here and its thoracic portions are included later in this text, as they are treated when these regions are addressed.

Box 11.9 Summary of American NMT assessment protocols

- Glide where appropriate.
- Assess for taut bands using pincer compression techniques or flat palpation.
- Assess attachment sites for tenderness, especially where taut bands attach.
- Return to taut band and find central nodules or spot tenderness.
- Elongate the tissue slightly if attachment sites indicate this is appropriate or tissue may be placed in neutral or approximated position.
- Compress CTrP for 8–12 seconds (using pincer compression techniques or flat palpation).
- The patient is instructed to exhale as the pressure is applied, which often augments the release of the contracture.
- Appropriate pressure should elicit a discomfort scale response of 5, 6 or 7.
- If a response in the tissue begins within 8–12 seconds, it can be held for up to 20 seconds.
- Allow the tissue to rest for a brief time.
- Adjust pressure and repeat, including application to other taut fibers.
- Passively elongate the fibers.
- Actively stretch the fibers.
- Appropriate hydrotherapies may accompany the procedure.
- Advise the patient as to specific procedures which can be used at home to maintain the effects of therapy.

NMT: cervical lamina gliding techniques – supine

In the following steps the thumb is used to glide repeatedly (starting at the occiput and ending in the C7 region) in three or four rows with the first row placed beside the spinous processes and the last one placed on the posterior aspect of the transverse process. These gliding strokes should be repeated several times with progressively deeper pressure used to assess several layers of posterior cervical muscles (the number of layers varying depending upon the thumb's position – see cervical planes and layers, p. 187). Fibers of particularly the deeper muscles are not always distinguishable when the tissues are normal. However, when contractures exist within the deeper muscles, the taut bands are usually tender and vary from distinctly palpable to thick and undefined.

These descriptions are given for treating the right side with the patient supine and the practitioner seated cephalad to the head. All steps should be repeated for the other side as it is recommended by the authors that all spinal muscles are assessed and treated bilaterally.

- The lamina groove is lightly lubricated from the occiput to T1 and from the spinous processes to the transverse processes.
- The practitioner's left hand lifts and supports the head sufficiently for the right hand to fit underneath the neck and for the forearm to lie under the cranium. This position assists in aligning the thumb to avoid undue stress on its joints.
- The right hand fingers lie across the back of the neck at the occipital ridge with the forearm fully supinated.
- The pad of the thumb faces toward the ceiling and is placed just lateral to the spinous processes of C2.
- The hand position should be comfortable.
- The practitioner glides the thumb from C1 to T1 while simultaneously pressing into the tissues (toward the ceiling).
- The thumb is returned to C1 and the gliding movements are repeated 5–6 times.
- The practitioner's elbow is bent to approximately 90° and the arm should remain in the same plane as the spine.
- There should be no stress on the thumb joints as pressure is being applied through the length of the thumb without incurring lateral stress into the thumb joints (see p. 113).
- The practitioner may observe the head moving into extension as the thumb progresses down the neck.
- Then, the patient's head is rotated contralaterally (away from the side being treated) to approximately 60° from the mid-line and allowed to rest on the table while being stabilized by the opposite hand.

- Extreme head rotation is not recommended (particularly for the elderly) as it may cause occlusion of the vertebral artery within the transverse processes.
- The practitioner's thumb is moved laterally one thumb width (about 1") and the gliding movements are repeated 5–6 times.
- The head should not move in to flexion or extension as the thumb glides on the more lateral rows.
- The practitioner continues the gliding steps until the entire lamina groove has been treated.
- The thumb remains posterior to the transverse processes since the foraminal gutters (anterior and posterior tubercles) on the anterior surface of these processes are sharp and may damage the soft tissues and neural structures.
- When the head is rotated, the transverse processes lie on a diagonal from the ear lobe to the middle of the top of the shoulder at the base of the neck.
- Therefore, the final row of gliding strokes on the posterior aspect of the transverse processes will follow this diagonal line.

This entire procedure is repeated to the other side. Alternating between the two sides will allow brief pauses for enhanced drainage of the tissues. Deeper pressure may be applied progressively as the entire procedure is repeated several times to each side to assess layers of posterior cervical muscles. Applications of heat or ice

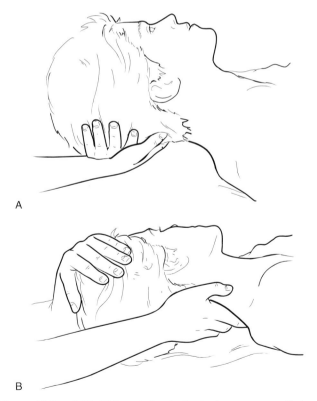

A

B

Figure 11.32 A&B: Gliding strokes to the lamina groove are first applied just lateral to the spinous processes while the most lateral glides are against the posterior aspect of the transverse processes.

(as appropriate – see guidelines on p. 131) may be used to augment the effects of the gliding strokes or to replace them if any layer is too tender to treat in this way. In some cases, treatment of the deeper layers may need to be delayed until future sessions.

Many of the following muscles are addressed with the gliding procedures described above. Some of these muscles have additional procedures given or supporting modalities suggested. Even though the gliding techniques described above are very simple to apply, they are extremely effective for addressing much of what is found in the posterior cervical musculature. Additionally, trigger point pressure release, stretching and other techniques may be used to address contractures and other dysfunctions discovered during the gliding steps.

Semispinalis capitis (Figs 11.33, 11.34)

Attachments: Articular processes of C3(4)–7 and the transverse processes of T1–6(7) to between the superior and inferior nuchal lines of the occiput
Innervation: Dorsal rami of the cervical nerves
Muscle type: Postural (type 1), shortens when stressed
Function: Head extension; controversy exists as to its role in rotation and flexion (Simons et al 1998)
Synergists: Longissimus capitis, suboccipital muscles, upper trapezius, splenius capitis
Antagonists: Head flexors, especially rectus capitis anterior and anterior fibers of sternocleidomastoid

Indications for treatment

- Headache like a band around the head and into the eye region
- Loss of flexion of head and neck
- Restriction of rotation (possibly)

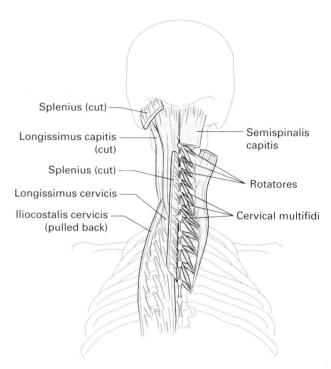

Figure 11.33 Direction of fiber and depth of pressure needed to palpate taut bands in posterior cervical region offer clues to identify taut bands.

Semispinalis cervicis

Attachments: Transverse processes of T1–5(6) to the spinous processes of C2–5
Innervation: Dorsal rami of the cervical nerves
Muscle type: Postural (type 1), shortens when stressed
Function: Unilaterally, flexes the neck to the same side and contralaterally rotates the cervical spine; bilaterally extends the spine
Synergists: *For rotation of the neck*: contralateral splenius cervicis and levator scapula, and ipsilateral multifidi and rotatores

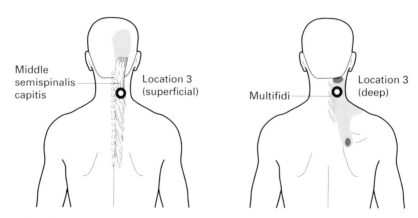

Figure 11.34 The location of trigger points for semispinalis capitis and multifidi overlie each other but their patterns of referral are notably different.

For extension of the neck: splenius cervicis, longissimus cervicis, semispinalis capitis, levator scapula, multifidi
Antagonists: *For extension of the neck*: anterior neck muscles, including infrahyoids and prevertebral muscles

Indications for treatment

- Headache (especially cervicogenic)
- Reduced flexion of head and neck
- Possibly other painfully restricted motion

Special notes

The semispinalis muscles are powerful extensors of the head and neck. They comprise the second and third muscular layer in the upper medial half of the posterior neck and the third and fourth layers in the lower medial half where the splenii overlie them.

The large, thick occipital attachment of semispinalis capitis is often mistaken as the trapezius tendon, which is thinner and overlies it. Trapezius and semispinalis capitis both have the ability to entrap the greater occipital nerve, which usually passes through them on its way to supply the scalp with sensory branches (Simons et al 1998, p. 455). This nerve also supplies motor branches to the semispinalis capitis itself.

The semispinalis capitis may be divided by one or more tendinous inscriptions which allow the fibers split by them to have separate endplate zones. Because of the varying lengths of fibers, trigger point occurrences will be widely distributed throughout the posterior cervical region. The gliding techniques described above will assess the upper half of both semispinalis capitis and cervicis, although in some areas they lie in the third and fourth layers, which makes them more difficult to distinguish.

In addition to the gliding techniques, unidirectional transverse friction (snapping across the fibers in one direction – see spinalis muscles, p. 199) may be used as long as care is taken not to impact the spinous processes. Elongation of the tissues after the gliding techniques as well as home care stretching is suggested for this region.

Splenii (Figs 11.35, 11.36)

Attachments: *Splenius capitis*: lower half of ligamentum nuchae, spinous processes and supraspinous ligaments of lower four cervical and upper 3–4 thoracic vertebrae, coursing diagonally to the mastoid process and occipital bone (just deep to the SCM)
Splenius cervicis: spinous processes of T3–6 coursing diagonally to the transverse processes of the upper two or three cervical vertebrae
Innervation: Dorsal rami of the middle and lower cervical nerves (varying from C1 to C6)
Muscle type: Postural (type 1), shortens when stressed

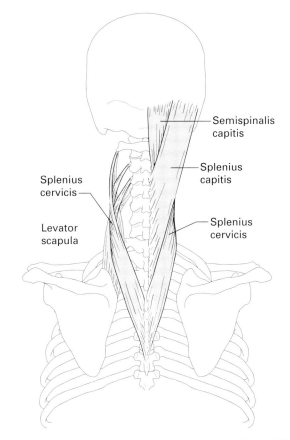

Figure 11.35 The diagonal bands of splenii are readily identified when gliding in the lamina groove, as no other muscles have a similar direction of fiber.

Function: Extension of the head and neck and ipsilateral rotation and flexion (questionable on capitis) of the head and neck
Synergists: *For extension*: posterior cervical group, especially semispinalis muscles
For rotation: contralateral SCM, trapezius, semispinalis cervicis, rotatores, multifidus and ipsilateral levator scapula
Antagonists: *To extension*: SCM, prevertebral muscles and hyoid muscles
To rotation: ipsilateral SCM, trapezius, semispinalis cervicis, rotatores, multifidus and contralateral levator scapula

Indications for treatment

- 'Stiff neck'
- Pain produced by rotation
- Pain in head, especially the eyes
- Blurred vision

Special notes

The splenii are often distinguished in the second layer

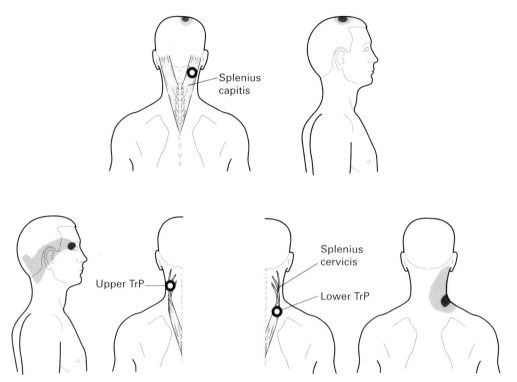

Figure 11.36 The combined patterns of splenii trigger point target zones of referral.

of the posterior cervical muscles as a diagonal band lying in the lamina groove which runs from the lower mid-line of the cervical region to the upper cervical transverse processes and to the mastoid process just under the posterior aspect of the sternocleidomastoid attachment. They (capitis more easily than cervicis) can often be palpated during the gliding techniques described above, as the thumb glides caudally on the second (sometimes third) row of the lamina since the two muscles lie directly under the skin in this area and are not obscured by other muscle fibers.

The cranial attachment of splenius capitis crosses the suture between the temporal and the occipital bones just posterior to the mastoid. As Upledger & Vredevoogd (1983) point out, contraction of splenius capitis causes the squamous portion of the temporal bone to rotate posteriorly while producing internal rotation of the petrous portion. Crowding of the occipitomastoid suture, they state, can contribute to a wide range of symptoms including head pain, dyslexia, gastrointestinal symptoms and personality problems. The cranial attachments are addressed with the suboccipital region on page 205.

Headache (to vertex of head) and neck pain as well as blurred vision can result from trigger point activity in splenius capitis (Simons et al 1998). Headache with explosive pressure 'in the eye' is a frequent complaint, therefore glaucoma and other eye pathologies should be ruled out in addition to addressing trigger points within these and other cervical and cranial muscles.

Cold wind or drafts across the neck tend to activate trigger points in these two muscles. Cervical articulation dysfunctions are often associated with splenii, particularly C1 and C2.

 NMT techniques for splenii tendons

The mid-bellies of the splenii are addressed in the gliding techniques previously discussed. Their cranial attachments are treated with the suboccipital assessment. However, the spinal attachments may be assessed here with a special procedure which allows the thumb to be placed deep to the trapezius and directly onto a portion of the spinal attachments. Dr Raymond Nimmo referred to this procedure as the 'corkscrew technique' (Chaitow 1996a).

- No pressure should be applied until the hand is correctly positioned and the head is rotated.
- The right-hand fingers cup across the back of the base of the neck, like a shirt collar (C6–7 area).
- The right thumb is placed anterior to the trapezius and posterior to the lower cervical transverse processes, pointing caudally.
- The left hand is used to rotate the head ipsilaterally, that is, toward the side being treated (Fig. 11.37A).
- As the left hand rotates the head, the right hand should rotate with the neck as if glued to the back of the neck.
- This rotating movement will 'open the pocket' by

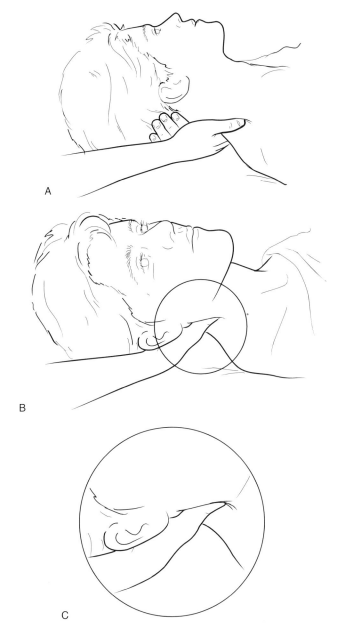

A

B

C

Figure 11.37 The thumb slides into a 'pocket' formed anterior to the trapezius while remaining posterior to the transverse process to directly palpate a portion of lower splenii.

passively shortening the upper trapezius fibers while angling the thumb toward the nipple of the contralateral breast and against the lateral surface of the spinous processes.

• The thumb pad should press toward the ceiling as the right thumb slides into the 'pocket' formed anterior to the trapezius.

• If the area does not allow penetration or if pressure of the thumb produces more than moderate discomfort, light sustained pressure is applied to the 'mouth' of the pocket until the tissues relax enough to slide in further (Fig. 11.37B,C).

• Pressure is directed toward the ceiling as the thumb is positioned just lateral to the spinous processes.

• Appropriate pressure is applied continuously for 8–12 seconds, which will often provoke a referral pattern if active trigger points are encountered.

• The thumb will be pressing into the tendons of the splenius capitis and splenius cervicis superficially.

• The thumb should then sink more deeply into the pocket (caudally) as the pressure release technique is repeated.

• When taut fibers stop the thumb's caudal movements, mild to moderate static pressure may produce more relaxation of the surrounding tissue and may allow the thumb to slide further down the spinal column. This step may also address a small portion of the rhomboid minor, serratus posterior superior, semispinalis capitis, cervicis and thoracis, spinalis cervicis, multifidi and rotatores, since these muscles attach within the lamina of this area.

• If tender, repeat the entire process 3–4 times during a single session.

• This step will help restore cervical rotation as well as reduce tilting pull on the transverse processes of C1–3.

• Surrounding tissue may also be treated by adjusting the thumb position and its direction of pressure.

Spinalis capitis and cervicis

Attachments: Spinous processes of C7–T2 and lower portion of ligamentum nuchae to the (cervicis) spinous process of C2–4 or (capitis) blending with the semispinalis capitis

Innervation: Dorsal rami of spinal nerves (C2–T10)

Muscle type: Postural (type 1), shortens when stressed

Function: Flexes the spine laterally to the same side and (bilaterally) extends the spine

Synergists: *For lateral flexion*: longissimus, semispinalis cervicis, splenius cervicis, iliocostalis cervicis
For extension: posterior cervical group

Antagonists: *For lateral flexion*: contralateral fibers of the same muscle and contralateral fibers of its synergists
For extension: prevertebral group

Indications for treatment

• Inability to fully flex the neck
• Loss of sidebending range of motion

Special notes

The spinalis muscles represent the most centrally located fibers of the three muscular columns commonly referred to as the erector spinae group. Longissimus components lie intermediately while iliocostalis has the most lateral influence on the positioning of the torso and spinal column.

The spinalis cervicis muscle is often absent and the spinalis capitis is only occasionally present and if so, usually blends to some extent with semispinalis capitis (*Gray's anatomy* 1995). When these muscles are present, they add bulk to the mass of lamina muscle fibers just lateral to the spinous processes, which is addressed with the first row of gliding strokes applied to the cervical lamina groove.

NMT for spinalis muscles

- Repeat the gliding steps for the lamina groove while increasing the pressure (if appropriate) to penetrate to the spinalis muscles which lie deep to the semispinalis muscles.
- When trigger point tenderness or contractures are revealed, individual examination and appropriate releases may be applied, such as static compression, muscle energy techniques and positional release.
- Transverse, snapping friction may be applied to tissues which have a more fibrotic quality as long as evidence of inflammation is not present.
- The finger tips of the contralateral hand (nails cut short) are used to apply the techniques.
- The hand lies across the back of the neck with the finger tips curled so that they lie in the lamina of the opposite side.
- While avoiding contact with the spinous processes, the finger tips are transversely snapped across the fibers as if plucking a guitar string.
- The snapping transverse friction is applied repeatedly to the most fibrotic fibers, which are then lengthened through stretching.
- Microtrauma of the tissues is an almost certain outcome of such attention, requiring appropriate attention to avoid excessive posttreatment discomfort.
- Ice applications can be used both immediately following treatment and also as home care, coupled with carefully employed active elongation of the involved muscles.
- Active movement methods may follow immediately in the treatment session and should also be added to the home care program.

Longissimus capitis

Attachments: Transverse processes of T1–5 and the articular processes of C4–7 and to the posterior mastoid process
Innervation: Dorsal rami of spinal nerves
Muscle type: Postural (type 1), shortens when stressed
Function: Rotates the head ipsilaterally, laterally flexes the head to the same side and extends the head when bilaterally active
Synergists: Semispinalis capitis, spinalis capitis, longissimus cervicis
Antagonists: Fibers of its contralateral synergists

Longissimus cervicis

Attachments: Transverse processes of T1–5 ascending to the transverse processes of C2–6
Innervation: Dorsal rami of spinal nerves
Muscle type: Postural (type 1), shortens when stressed
Function: Laterally flexes and ipsilaterally rotates the neck; bilaterally extends the neck
Synergists: Semispinalis capitis and cervicis, iliocostalis cervicis, longissimus capitis and cervicis, spinalis cervicis
Antagonists: Fibers of its contralateral synergists

Indications for treatment of longissimus muscles

- Loss of range of motion in flexion and rotation
- Pain behind, below or into the ear region, into the eye region and down the neck (trigger point referral pattern)

Special notes

The longissimus muscles represent the intermediate vertical column of muscular tension which erects the torso and head. The cranial attachment of longissimus capitis lies deep to both splenius capitis and sternocleidomastoid. It usually has a tendinous inscription transversing it so that its upper and lower fibers would have separate endplate zones and, therefore two locations for potential central trigger point formation.

The fibers of the longissimus muscles are addressed with the gliding strokes and transverse friction techniques previously mentioned within this section. The occipital attachment is addressed with the suboccipital techniques on p. 205. Hydrotherapy applications appropriate to the condition of the tissues as well as stretching techniques may be used both in the treatment session and at home.

Iliocostalis cervicis

Attachments: The superior aspect of the angles of the 3rd–6th ribs to the posterior tubercles of the transverse processes of C4–6
Innervation: Dorsal rami of lower cervical nerves (C6–8)
Muscle type: Postural (type 1), shortens when stressed
Function: Laterally flexes the spine and extends the spine when bilaterally active
Synergists: *For extension*: splenius cervicis, semispinalis cervicis, longissimus cervicis
For lateral flexion: scalenii, longus capitis, longus colli
Antagonists: Contralateral fibers of scalenii, longus capitis,

longus colli and fibers of contralateral iliocostalis cervicis

Special notes

The iliocostalis muscles represent the most lateral vertical column of muscles of the back. They extend segmentally from the most caudal attachments of the erector spinae group at the sacrum, iliac crest and thoracolumbar fascia to the cervical vertebrae. While no individual fibers span the entire length, these segments work dynamically to erect the spine. While iliocostalis does not attach to the cranium, it influences cranial positioning through its attachment to the cervical spine.

Fibers of iliocostalis cervicis are influenced in the most lateral gliding strokes of the posterior cervical lamina as the thumb glides along the posterior aspect of the transverse processes. Further applications of gliding as well as transverse friction are used in a prone position which is discussed later in this section (p. 232).

Multifidi

Attachments: From the articular processes of C4–7 these muscles cross 2–4 vertebrae and attach to the spinous processes of higher vertebrae
Innervation: Dorsal rami of spinal nerves
Muscle type: Postural (type 1), shortens when stressed
Function: When these contract unilaterally they produce ipsilateral flexion and contralateral rotation; bilaterally, they extend the spine
Synergists: *For rotation*: rotatores, semispinalis cervicis, scalenii, longus capitis, longus colli
Antagonists: Matching contralateral fibers of multifidi as well as contralateral rotatores, semispinalis cervicis, scalenii, longus capitis, longus colli

Indications for treatment

- Chronic instability of associated vertebral segments
- Reduced flexion of neck
- Restricted rotation (sometimes painfully)
- Suboccipital pain (referral zone)
- Vertebral scapular border pain (referral zone)

Rotatores longus and brevis

Attachments: From the transverse processes of each vertebra to the spinous processes of the second (longus) and first (brevis) vertebra above (ending at C2)
Innervation: Dorsal rami of spinal nerves
Muscle type: Postural (type 1), shortens when stressed
Function: When these contract unilaterally they produce contralateral rotation; bilaterally, they extend the spine
Synergists: Multifidi, semispinalis cervicis

Antagonists: Matching contralateral fibers of rotatores as well as contralateral multifidi and semispinalis cervicis

Indications for treatment

- Pain and tenderness at associated vertebral segments
- Tenderness to pressure or tapping applied to the spinous processes of associated vertebrae

Special notes

Multifidi and rotatores muscles comprise the deepest layer of posterior cervical muscles and are responsible for fine control of the rotation of vertebrae. They exist through the entire length of the spinal column and the multifidi also broadly attach to the sacrum after becoming appreciably thicker in the lumbar region.

These muscles are often associated with vertebral segments which are difficult to stabilize and should be addressed throughout the spine when scoliosis is presented. Discomfort or pain provoked by pressure or tapping applied to the spinous processes of associated vertebrae, a test used to identify dysfunctional spinal articulations, also often indicates multifidi and rotatores involvement.

Trigger points in rotatores tend to produce rather localized referrals whereas the multifidi trigger points refer locally and to the suboccipital region, medial scapular border and top of shoulder. These local (for both) and distant (for multifidi) patterns of referral continue to be expressed through the length of the spinal column. In fact, the lower spinal levels of multifidi may also refer to the anterior thorax or abdomen.

In addition to the deepest level of gliding techniques suggested above for the cervical lamina groove (when appropriate), the fibers may be treated with sustained digital pressure, such as that used in trigger point pressure release. Unless contraindicated, contrast hydrotherapy (alternating heat and cold applications) may be applied several times for short intervals (10–15 seconds), which often profoundly releases the overlying muscles so that these deeper tissues may be more easily palpated.

Interspinales

Attachments: Connects the spinous processes of contiguous vertebrae, one on each side of the interspinous ligament, in the cervical and lumbar regions
Innervation: Dorsal rami of spinal nerves
Muscle type: Postural (type 1), shortens when stressed
Function: Extends the spine
Synergists: All posterior muscles and especially multifidi, rotatores and intertransversarii
Antagonists: Flexors of the spine

Indications for treatment

- Tenderness between the spinous processes
- Loss of cervical flexion

Special notes

The interspinalis muscles are present in the cervical and lumbar regions and sometimes the extreme ends of the thoracic segment. In the cervical region, they sometimes span two vertebrae (*Gray's anatomy* 1995).

 NMT for interspinales

The tip of an index finger is placed between the spinous processes of C2 and C3. Mild pressure is applied or gentle transverse friction used to examine the tissues which connect the spinous processes of contiguous vertebrae. This process is gently applied to each interspinous muscle in the cervical region. The neck may be placed in passive flexion in order to slightly separate the spinous processes and allow a little more room for palpation.

The tissues being examined include the supraspinous ligament, interspinous ligament and interspinalis muscles. In the cervical region, the supraspinous ligament is altered to form the ligamentum nuchae.

We suggest that the small beveled pressure bar is *not* appropriate as a treatment tool in the cervical region due to the vulnerability of the vertebral artery in the sub-occipital region and the highly mobile nature of cervical vertebrae in general. While the tool can readily be used in the thoracic and lumbar region, the finger tips are safer and sufficient for addressing the cervical region.

Intertransversarii

Attachments: Anterior and posterior pairs of bilateral muscles which join the transverse processes of contiguous vertebrae
Innervation: Dorsal and ventral rami of spinal nerves
Muscle type: Not established
Function: Lateral flexion of the spine
Synergists: Interspinales, rotatores, multifidi
Antagonists: Spinal flexors of the contralateral side

Indications for treatment

- Cervical segments restricted in lateral flexion

Special notes

These short, laterally placed muscles most likely act as postural muscles which stabilize the adjoining vertebrae during movement of the spinal column as a whole. The pattern of movement of intertransversarii is unknown, but thought to be lateral flexion. Fibers may also extend the spine.

These muscles are difficult to reach and attempts to

Box 11.10 Spinal mobilization using mobilization with movement (MWM)

New Zealand physiotherapist Brian Mulligan (1992) has described a series of extremely effective mobilization with movement techniques for the spinal joints. In this summary only those relating to the cervical spine are detailed, although precisely the same principles apply wherever they are used. Mulligan highly recommends that the work of Kaltenborn (1985) relating to joint articulation be studied, especially that relating to end-feel (see Chapter 13).

These mobilization methods carry the acronym SNAGs, which stands for 'sustained natural apophyseal glides'. They are used to improve function if any restriction or pain is experienced on flexion, extension, sideflexion or rotation of the cervical spine, usually from C3 and lower. (There are other more specialized variations of these techniques for the upper cervicals, not described in this text.)

In order to apply these methods to the spine, it is essential for the practitioner to be aware of the facet angles of those segments being treated. These are discussed in the structure portion of this chapter. It should be recalled that the facet angles of C3–7 lie on a plane which *angles toward the eyes*. Rotation of the lower five cervical vertebrae therefore follows the facet planes, rather than being horizontal (Kappler 1997, Lewit 1985).

Notes on SNAGS

- Most applications of SNAGs commence with the patient weight bearing, usually seated.
- They are movements which are *actively* performed by the patient, in the direction of restriction, while the practitioner *passively*

holds an area (in the cervical spine it is the segment immediately cephalad to the restriction) in a translated direction.
- In the cervical spine the direction of translation is almost always anterior, along the plane of the facet articulation, i.e. toward the eyes.
- In none of the SNAGS applications should any pain be experienced, although some residual stiffness/soreness is to be anticipated on the following day, as with most mobilization approaches.
- In some instances, as well as actively moving the head and neck toward the direction of restriction while the practitioner maintains the translation, the patient may usefully apply 'overpressure' in which a hand is used to reinforce the movement toward the restriction barrier.
- The patient is told that at no time should pain be experienced and that if it is, all active efforts should cease.
- Reasons for pain being experienced could be:
1. the facet plane may not have been correctly followed
2. the incorrect segment may have been selected for translation
3. the patient may be attempting movement toward the barrier excessively strongly.
- If a painless movement through a previously restricted barrier is achieved while the translation is held, the same procedure is performed several times more.
- There should be an instant, and lasting, functional improvement.
- The use of these mobilization methods is enhanced by normalization of soft tissue restrictions and shortened musculature, using NMT, MFR, MET, etc.

Box 11.10 (cont'd)

Treatment of limited cervical rotation or pain on rotation

- The patient is seated with the practitioner standing behind.
- The restricted segments will have been identified using normal palpation methods.
- The practitioner places the medial aspect of the distal phalanx of one thumb against the spinous process of the vertebra, *cephalad* to the dysfunctional vertebra.
- This contact, against the tip of the spinous process, acts as a 'cushion', as the other thumb is placed against the lateral aspect of the 'cushion' thumb, reinforcing the contact.
- The practitioner's hands rest over the lateral aspect of the neck.
- The practitioner glides the spinous process along its articulation plane (toward the eyes) until slack has been removed (a very small amount of translation, glide, will be noted). The 'force' used is applied by the superimposed thumb, not the one in contact with the spinous process, which acts as a cushion to avoid discomfort on the spinous process tip.

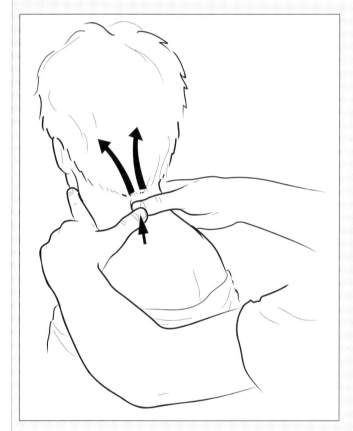

Figure 11.38 Mobilization for cervical rotation restriction using the SNAG method.

- The sustained glide/translation is maintained as the patient turns the head and neck in the direction of restriction or pain. This should be pain free and have a greater range, if the correct spinous process is receiving the appropriate translation. Mulligan says, 'Remember to try more than one [segmental] level if your first choice is painful. There is a tendency to locate on the spinous process below the appropriate one, or rather, this has often been so in my case'.
- If pain is still noted or the range is not painlessly increased, the practitioner should recheck and identify the correct segment and repeat the process.
- As rotation is carried out by the patient, the practitioner's hands follow the movement so that the angle of translation is constant.
- If a new range is achieved this should be held for several seconds before returning to the start position and repeating the process several times.

Identical mechanisms are used for treatment of sideflexion, flexion and extension restrictions. The anterior glide/translation is maintained as the restricted movement is actively introduced by the patient, with all the cautions and recommendations as above.

It is important to remember that as full flexion is achieved, the direction of glide will be more or less horizontal (always toward the eyes) and during extension it will be more vertical.

Mulligan reminds the reader to ensure that the end of range is maintained for several seconds before a return to neutral and that the glide/translation should be maintained until neutral is resumed.

An additional caution relating to extension dysfunction arises because as extension is introduced, the approximation of the spinous processes makes localization of contact more difficult. Mulligan states, 'This is especially true if the neck being treated is small and your thumbs are of a generous size. This is where "self SNAGs" are marvelous'.

Self-treatment using SNAGs

Mulligan suggests using a small hand-towel to engage the spinous process, with the patient holding the ends of the towel to introduce an anterior pull and therefore a glide/translation of the engaged segment. At the same time, the restricted movement is slowly performed.

We have found that this is even more effectively achieved if the patient places her hands behind her neck, with one middle (or index) finger on the appropriate spinous process (previously identified by the practitioner and shown to the patient). The other middle (or index) finger is superimposed on the initial contact and the patient glides the segment anteriorly, toward her eyes. This process will have been explained by, and practiced with, the practitioner.

The restricted movement is then carried out (sideflexion, rotation, etc.), while the translation is maintained. After the end of range has been achieved, the translation is sustained until a neutral neck position is resumed.

palpate them may endanger cervical nerves which exit the spine near the muscles. Additionally, the vertebral artery courses between each unilateral pair and pressure on this is to be avoided. The cervical portion of the intertransversarii may be elongated by active contralateral flexion, especially when combined with rotation, as when one attempts to touch the chin to the ipsilateral shoulder.

Levator scapula (Fig. 11.39)

Attachments: From the transverse processes of C1 and C2 and the dorsal tubercles of C3 and C4 to the medial scapular border between the superior angle and the medial end (root) of the spine of the scapula

Innervation: C3–4 spinal nerves and the dorsal scapular nerve (C5)

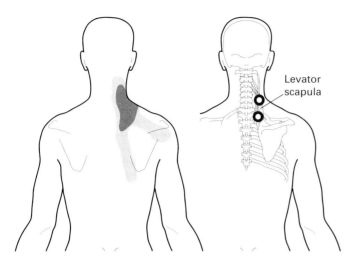

Figure 11.39 The referral pattern of levator scapula is a common complaint which is often mistaken as trapezius pain.

Muscle type: Postural (type 1), shortens when stressed

Function: Elevation of the scapula, resists downward movement of the scapula when the arm or shoulder is weighted, rotates the scapula medially to face the glenoid fossa downward, assists in rotation of the neck to the same side, bilaterally acts to assist extension of the neck and perhaps lateral flexion to the same side (Warfel 1985)

Synergists: *Elevation/medial rotation of the scapula*: rhomboids
Neck stabilization: splenius cervicis, scalenus medius

Antagonists: *To elevation*: serratus anterior, lower trapezius, latissimus dorsi.
To rotation of scapula: serratus anterior, upper and lower trapezius
To neck extension: longus colli, longus capitis, rectus capitis anterior, rectus capitis lateralis (Norkin & Levangie 1992)

Indications for treatment

- Neck stiffness or loss of range of cervical rotation
- Torticollis
- Postural distortions including high shoulder and tilted head
- Patient indicates upper angle area when complaining of discomfort

Special notes

The levator scapula usually spirals as it descends the neck to attach to the superior medial angle of the scapula. It is known to split into two layers, one attaching to the posterior aspect of the superior angle while the other merges its fibers anteriorly onto the scapula and the fascial sheath of serratus anterior (*Gray's anatomy* 1995,

p. 838, Simons et al 1998). Between the two layers of the proximal attachment, a bursa is often found which may be the site of considerable tenderness.

The transverse process attachments include scalene medius, splenius cervicis and intertransversarii, which may be addressed at the same time as levator scapula with laterally directed (unidirectional) transverse friction or static pressure. Medial frictional strokes are contraindicated since they could bruise the tissue against the underlying transverse processes. Caution must be exercised to stabilize the treating fingers to avoid pressing the nerve roots against sharp foraminal gutters.

The anterior surface of the superior angle, while often the source of deep ache, is usually neglected during treatment unless special accessing positions are used. These 'buried' fibers may be touched directly in the supine position as described below as well as the prone position as shown on p. 329 where levator scapula is discussed in detail with the shoulder.

Assessment for shortness of levator scapula

- The patient lies supine with the arm of the side to be tested stretched out with the supinated hand and lower arm tucked under the buttocks, to help restrain movement of the shoulder/scapula.
- The practitioner's contralateral arm is passed across and under the neck to cup the shoulder of the side to be tested with the forearm supporting the neck.
- The practitioner's other hand supports the head.
- The forearm is used to lift the neck into *full pain-free flexion* (aided by the other hand). The head is placed fully toward contralateral flexion and contralateral rotation.
- With the shoulder held caudally and the head/neck

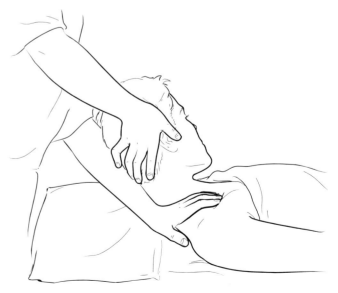

Figure 11.40 MET assessment and treatment of right levator scapula.

in the position described (each at its resistance barrier), stretch is placed on levator from both ends. If dysfunction exists and/or levator scapula is short, there will be discomfort reported at the attachment on the upper medial border of the scapula and/or pain reported near the spinous process of C2.

- The hand on the shoulder can gently 'spring' it caudally.
- If levator is short there will be a harsh, wooden feel to this action. If it is normal there will be a soft feel to the springing pressure.

 ## NMT for levator scapula

The patient is supine with the arm lying on the table. The practitioner sits or stands cephalad to the shoulder with one hand placed on the posterior aspect of the scapula, grasping its inferior angle lightly and displacing it cranially. Proper displacement is imperative.

The shoulder is passively shrugged and the scapula moved toward the head until its upper angle is available for palpation by the fingers of the practitioner's treating hand. The finger pads are placed onto the anterior aspect of the superior medial angle while the stabilizing hand continues to gently traction the scapula cranially (Fig. 11.41).

The trapezius usually displaces naturally toward the table but if its attachment on the clavicle is wide, it may overlie the upper angle of the scapula. The fingers should wrap all the way around the most anterior fibers of the trapezius to touch the upper anterior aspect of the scapula. Pressing through the trapezius will not achieve the same results and might irritate trigger points located in these fibers. Palpation of the anterior surface of the upper angle will assess fiber attachments of the levator scapula, serratus anterior and possibly a small portion of the subscapularis muscles. In some cases, angling the

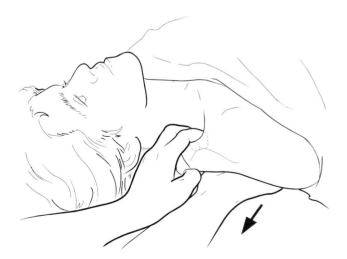

Figure 11.41 Direct contact of the anterior aspect of the upper angle of the scapula where levator scapula attaches.

fingers laterally may (rarely) contact the omohyoid attachment but it is doubtful that the rhomboid minor will be contacted medially. If tenderness is encountered, static pressure or gentle massage may be used to address these vulnerable tissues.

Static pressure or laterally applied unidirectional friction can be used on the transverse process attachments of levator scapula as well as other tissues attaching there. The most lateral glide of the previously discussed lamina groove treatment will also address fibers of levator scapula (p. 194).

 ## MET treatment of levator scapula
(see Fig. 11.40)

Treatment using MET for levator scapulae enhances the lengthening of the extensor muscles attaching to the occiput and upper cervical spine. The position described below is used for treatment, either at the limit of easily reached range of motion or well short of this, depending upon the degree of chronicity, which will also determine the degree of effort called for (20–30%) and the duration of each contraction (7–10 seconds or up to 30 seconds). The more acute the condition, the less resistance is offered.

- The patient lies supine with the arm of the side to be tested stretched out alongside the trunk with the hand supinated.
- The practitioner, standing at the head of the table, passes his contralateral arm under the patient's neck to rest on her ipsilateral shoulder, so that the practitioner's forearm supports the neck.
- The practitioner's other hand supports and directs the head into subsequent movement (below).
- The practitioner's forearm lifts the neck into full flexion (aided by the other hand). The head is turned fully toward contralateral sidebending and rotation.
- With the shoulder held caudally by the practitioner's hand and the head/neck in full flexion, sidebending and rotation (each at its resistance barrier), stretch is placed on levator from both ends. If dysfunction exists and/or it is short, there will be marked discomfort reported at the insertion on the upper medial border of the scapula and/or as pain near the spinous process of C2.
- The patient is asked to take the head back toward the table and slightly to the side from which it was turned, against the practitioner's unmoving resistance, while at the same time a slight (20% of available strength) shoulder shrug is also resisted.
- Following the 7–10-second isometric contraction and complete relaxation, slack is taken out as the shoulder is depressed further caudally with the patient's assistance ('As you breathe out, stretch your hand toward your feet'), while the neck is taken to (acute) or through (chronic) further flexion, sidebending and rotation.
- The stretch is held for at least 20 seconds.

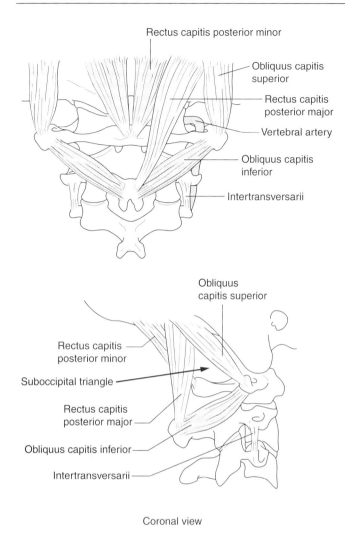

Coronal view

Figure 11.42 A&B: The suboccipitals, which are often discussed as a group, each have their own unique function in movements of the head.

• Caution is required to avoid overstretching this sensitive area.

Suboccipital region (Fig. 11.42)

Rectus capitis posterior minor (RCPMi) and major (RCPMa), obliquus capitis superior (OCS) and obliquus capitis inferior (OCI) (collectively called the suboccipital group) perform fine-tuning movements which are vital to the positioning of the head and counteractive to the composite triple movements of the lower functional unit of the cervical region. The suboccipital group, because of their attachments, are often directly involved in cranial suture crowding and/or temporal bone dysfunction, with the potential to negatively influence cranial function.

Unilateral contraction of the four muscles produces slight lateral flexion of the head with associated ipsilateral head rotation accompanied with extension – the three composite movements of the upper cervical unit (type II).

Bilateral contraction of all four muscles produces extension of the cranium and translation of the cranium anteriorly on the atlas. However, when acting alone, each of these muscles individually produces a fine control of stabilization or movement of the cranium on the atlas, the atlas on the axis or retraction of the dural tube within the spinal canal (see discussion of rectus capitis posterior minor on pp. 34, 207). Their functions can be more fully appreciated when they are viewed from above as well as from the side since the normal posterior view does not fully expose their oblique angles and, therefore, their full influence as head positioners. Their roles are discussed individually below.

Three of the four suboccipital muscles (all except RCPMi) form the suboccipital triangle. The vertebral artery lies relatively exposed in the lower aspect of this triangle and is to be avoided when pressure or friction is applied to this area, especially when the tissues are placed on stretch. The greater occipital nerve courses through the top of the triangle before penetrating the semispinalis capitis and trapezius muscles on its way to supply the posterior external cranium. The nerve may also penetrate obliquus capitis inferior.

Ideally, flexion (10°) and extension (25°) of the head occur between the occiput and atlas, as well as translation of the head upon the atlas. The degree of rotation or lateral flexion is only slight since more would be undesirable at this particular joint due to the risk of unwanted spinal encroachment of the odontoid process (the dens) on the spinal cord. The vertebral artery, which lies on the superior aspect of the lateral masses of the atlas, might also be crowded by excessive movements of the atlas. The transverse ligament retains the dens in position while allowing the atlas to rotate around it. The ligament articulates with the posterior aspect of the dens while the atlas articulates with its anterior surface.

Faulty head/neck mechanics, such as forward head posture, place high demand on the suboccipital muscles to maintain the head's position, while simultaneously crowding the space in which they operate, often physiologically shortening them in the process.

When suboccipital muscles house trigger points, these are usually accompanied by articular dysfunctions of the upper three cervical levels (Simons et al 1998). All the suboccipital muscles apart from obliquus capitis inferior connect the atlas or axis to the cranium, while the inferior attaches the atlas to the axis.

While the motor function of these four muscles is primarily to extend the head and to translate and rotate the head, their dysfunctions include involvement in the all-too-common forward head position. A number of researchers have shown that dysfunction of these small muscles in general, and RCPMi in particular (often resulting from whiplash), leads to marked increase in pain perception as well as reflex irritation of other cervical as well as jaw muscles (Hack et al 1995, Hallgren et al 1994, Hu et al 1995). An ultimate aim of postural compensation is to maintain the eyes and ears in an approximately level position. When the cranium is posteriorly rotated, the suboccipital group's role in sustaining this position is substantial. A forward head position involves a posteriorly rotated cranium which has then been brought to a position where the eyes and ears are level with the horizon. The suboccipital space is crowded and the muscles significantly shortened, which often leads to trigger point formation. The contractures associated with trigger points may then assist in maintaining the shortened position without excessive energy consumption.

Pain patterns and dysfunctional biomechanical patterns associated with trigger points may lead to compensatory changes in the lower functional unit and more distant structures. Until these muscles are considered and treated, attempts to restore the head to a balanced posture are unlikely to fully succeed. Similarly, addressing only these suboccipital muscles for forward head posture, while ignoring the role of other cervical tissues, pectoralis minor, the diaphragm, upper rectus abdominis and pelvic positioning, as well as more wide-ranging causes of postural imbalance, will produce short-term results at best.

The proprioceptive role of the muscles of the suboccipital region is directly related to the number of spindles per gram of muscle. There are an average of 36 spindles per gram in RCPMi, 30.5 spindles/gram in RCPMa, as compared, for example, with 7.6 spindles/gram in splenius capitis and just 0.8 in gluteus maximus (Peck et al 1984). McPartland & Brodeur (1999) suggest that 'The high density of muscle spindles found in the RCPM muscles suggests a value … [which] … lies not in their motor function, but in their role as "proprioceptive monitors" of the cervical spine and head'.

Hallgren et al (1994) suggest that damage to RCPMi, such as occurs in whiplash, would reduce its proprioceptive input, while facilitating transmission of impulses from a wide range of nociceptors which could develop into a chronic pain syndrome (such as fibromyalgia).

Forward head posture is discussed further in volume 2 of this text, where the influences of the lower half of the body on total body mechanics is more fully explored.

Rectus capitis posterior minor (Fig. 11.43)

Attachments: Medial part of the inferior nuchal line on the occipital bone and between the nuchal line and the foramen magnum to the tubercle on the posterior arch of the atlas

Innervation: Suboccipital nerve (C1)

Muscle type: Postural (type 1), shortens when stressed

Function: While most texts note that this muscle extends the head, recent research (Greenman 1997) has shown it to contract during translation of the head and to tense

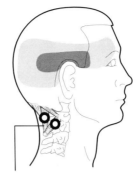 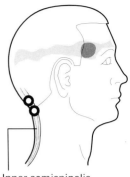

Suboccipitals   Upper semispinalis capitis

Figure 11.43 The referral patterns of the suboccipital muscles and the upper semispinalis capitis are similar.

a connective tissue attachment (fascial bridge) to the dura mater which retracts the dural tube and prevents it from folding onto the spinal cord. RCPMi may play a small part in head extension and translation but, as noted above, its main role would seem to be proprioceptive rather than motor.

Synergists: *In head extension*: rectus capitis posterior major, obliquus capitis superior, semispinalis capitis, longissimus capitis

Antagonists: Rectus capitis anterior, longus capitis

Indications for treatment

- Loss of suboccipital space
- Deep-seated posterior neck pain
- Headache wrapping around the side of the head to the eyes
- Trigger points in overlying muscles

Special notes

Recent research (Hack et al 1995) has demonstrated that a connective tissue extension links this muscle to the dura mater which provides it with potential for influencing the reciprocal tension membranes directly, with particular implications to cerebrospinal fluid fluctuation because of its site close to the posterior cranial fossa and the cisterna magna. It could also influence normal functioning of the vertebral artery and the suboccipital nerve which could further aggravate any hypertonus of the region. A fuller discussion of rectus capitis posterior minor is found on p. 34.

The researchers at the University of Maryland in Baltimore state:

In reviewing the literature, the subject of functional relations between voluntary muscles and dural membranes has been addressed by Becker (Upledger & Vredevoogd 1983) who suggests that the voluntary muscles might act upon the dural membranes via fascial continuity, changing the tension placed upon them, thus possibly influencing CSF pressure. Our observation that simulated contraction of the RCPM [rectus capitis posterior minor] muscle flexed the PAO membrane–spinal dural complex and produced CSF movement supports Becker's hypothesis ... During head extension the spinal dura is subject to folding, with the greatest amount occurring in the area of the atlantooccipital joint (Cailliet 1991). One possible [motor] function of the RCPM muscle may be to modulate dural folding, thus assisting in the maintenance of the normal circulation of the CSF. Trauma resulting in atrophic changes to the RCPM muscle may interfere with this suggested mechanism (Hallgren et al 1994). The observed transmission of tension created in the spinal dura to the cranial dura of the posterior cranial fossa is consistent with the described discontinuity between the spinal and intracranial parts of the dura mater (Penfield & McNaughton 1940). Not only has the dura lining the posterior cranial fossa been described as being innervated by nerves that subserve pain (Kimmel 1961) but also it has been demonstrated that pressure applied to the dura of the posterior cranial fossa in neurosurgical patients induces pain in the region of the posterior base of the skull (Northfield 1938). Therefore, one may postulate that the dura of the posterior cranial fossa can be perturbed and become symptomatic if stressed to an unaccustomed extent by the RCPM muscle acting on the dura mater.

McPartland & Brodeur (1999) hypothesize:

A disease cycle involving RCPMinor, initiated by injury or chronic somatic dysfunction ... leads to RCPMinor atrophy ... [which] ... may directly irritate the meninges via the posterior atlantooccipital membrane, and result in reduced proprioceptive output to higher centers. The lack of proprioceptive output causes a loss of standing balance and cervical vertigo ... chronic pain ... reflexive cervical and jaw muscle activity, directly affecting the biomechanics of the region.

Rectus capitis posterior major

Attachments: Lateral part of the inferior nuchal line on the occipital bone and the occipital bone immediately inferior to the nuchal line to attach to the spinous process of C2 (axis)
Innervation: Suboccipital nerve (C1)
Muscle type: Postural (type 1), shortens when stressed
Function: Ipsilateral head rotation, extension of the head
Synergists: *For rotation*: splenius capitis, contralateral SCM
For extension: rectus capitis posterior minor (questionable), obliquus capitis superior, semispinalis capitis, longissimus capitis
Antagonists: *For rotation*: contralateral mates of obliquus capitis inferior and rectus capitis posterior major
For extension: rectus capitis anterior, longus capitis

Indications for treatment

- Loss of suboccipital space
- Deep-seated posterior neck pain
- Headache wrapping around the side of the head to the eyes
- Trigger points in overlying muscles

Special notes

People who chronically place the neck in flexion or extension stress these 'check' muscles while encouraging the evolution of hypertonicity and trigger point activity. Referred pain from triggers has poor definition, radiating into the lateral head from the occiput to the eye. Upledger & Vredevoogd (1983) indicate that bilateral hypertonicity of rectus capitis posterior major and minor can retard occipital flexion while unilateral hypertonicity is said to be capable of producing torsion at the cranial base.

The possibility of such a torsion occurring, at the cranial base, in an adult skull is unlikely in the extreme once ossification of the sphenobasilar synchondrosis had taken place. It could, however, occur in the more malleable infant or young adult skull (Chaitow 1999).

Obliquus capitis superior

Attachments: Superior surface of the transverse process of C1 to the occipital bone between the superior and inferior nuchal lines
Innervation: Suboccipital nerve (C1)
Muscle type: Not established
Function: Extension of the head, minimal lateral flexion of the head
Synergists: *For extension*: rectus capitis posterior minor (questionable) and major, semispinalis capitis, longissimus capitis
For minimal lateral flexion: rectus capitis lateralis
Antagonists: *For extension*: rectus capitis anterior, longus capitis
For sidebending: contralateral obliquus capitis superior and contralateral rectus capitis lateralis

Indications for treatment

- Loss of suboccipital space
- Deep-seated posterior neck pain
- Headache wrapping around the side of the head to the eyes
- Unstable atlas, especially sidebend cranially

Obliquus capitis inferior

Attachments: Spinous process of C2 to the inferior aspect and dorsum of the transverse process of C1
Innervation: Suboccipital nerve (C1)
Muscle type: Not established
Function: Ipsilateral rotation of the atlas (and therefore cranium)
Synergists: *For rotation*: splenius capitis, contralateral SCM
Antagonists: *For rotation*: contralateral mates of obliquus capitis inferior, RCPMa and splenius capitis and the ipsilateral SCM

Indications for treatment

- Loss of rotation, such as looking over shoulder
- Deep-seated posterior neck pain
- Headache wrapping around the side of the head to the eyes
- Unstable atlas, especially sidebend inferiorly with rotation

Special notes

Gray's anatomy (1995) suggests that the superior oblique and the two recti muscles are probably postural rather than phasic muscles, which has implications regarding their response to 'stress' in that they are likely to shorten over time (Lewit 1992).

These two oblique muscles transmit tilting pull on the atlas, creating an unstable base for the head to rest upon. They will often be dysfunctional together contralaterally. That is, the superior oblique on one side and the inferior on the opposite side will be shortened by a tilted, rotated atlas. Since compensation by the upper functional cervical unit can be associated with any distortions occurring in the remainder of the spinal column, we recommend examination of the suboccipital region (and the cervical spine) when any spinal distortions are found further down the column. Likewise, when the upper unit is found to be dysfunctional, a full spinal examination may reveal associated distortions.

When tissues of the suboccipital region are too tender to be frictioned or when cranial techniques are to be applied, the static release techniques offered in Box 11.11 may be preferred over those appearing here. The cranial base release may also be used prior to the following steps or following them and is recommended to accompany craniomandibular therapy, especially when forward head posture is noted.

NMT for suboccipital group – supine
(Fig. 11.45)

The practitioner is seated at the head of the table with the patient lying supine. The palms of the practitioner's hands cradle the posterior cranium and the fingers cup the occipital bone with the finger pads resting on the inferior surface of the bone. The first two fingers of the treating hand address one side at a time as the person may be intolerant of two sides being treated at once. A ½–1″ space is usually palpable between the occipital ridge and the first vertebra (atlas). This area influences rocking and tilting of the head and, therefore, posterior rotation of the cranium.

The treating fingers are placed just lateral to the mid-line at the inferior aspect of the occipital bone and press into the trapezius muscle and its tendon. Static pressure for 8–12 seconds may be followed by medial to lateral friction

Box 11.11 Cranial base release

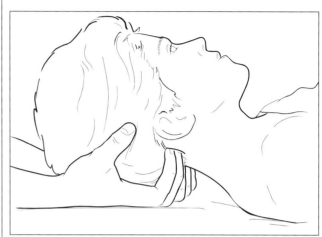

Figure 11.44 Hand positions for cranial base release.

This technique releases the soft tissues where they attach to the cranial base and may be used either before or following suboccipital NMT assessment.

- The patient is supine and the practitioner is seated at the head of the table with his arms resting on and supported by the table.
- The dorsum of the practitioner's hand rests on the table with finger tips pointing toward the ceiling, acting as a fulcrum on which the patient rests the occiput so that the back of the skull is resting on the practitioner's palm. The distal finger tips touch the suboccipital muscles while the palmar surfaces of the tips (finger pads) touch the occiput itself.
- The patient allows the head to lie heavily so that the pressure induces tissue release against the finger tips.
- As relaxation proceeds and the finger tips sink deeper into the tissues, the arch of the atlas may be palpated and it may be encouraged to disengage from the occiput by application of mild traction applied to the occiput, 'separating' it from the atlas (ounces of effort at most, applied cranially by the middle fingers). This would probably not be for some minutes after commencement of the exercise.
- The effect is to relax the attachments in the area being treated with benefit to the whole muscle. This 'release' of deep structures of the upper neck enhances drainage from the head and circulation to it, while reducing intercranial congestion.

directly on the trapezius attachment. Deeper pressure, if appropriate, will treat semispinalis capitis and RCPMi. Since the minor's attachment to the dura may be fragile, static pressure is preferred over the more aggressive frictional techniques when the pressure intrudes this deeply.

The fingers are moved laterally 1″ and static pressure and frictional movements repeated to influence the remainder of the trapezius, semispinalis capitis and RCPMa. The head may be rotated slightly away from the side being treated to make these muscles more palpable.

CAUTION: Extreme head rotation is not recommended for prolonged periods of time as the vertebral artery may be occluded within the transverse process, thereby reducing blood flow to the cranium.

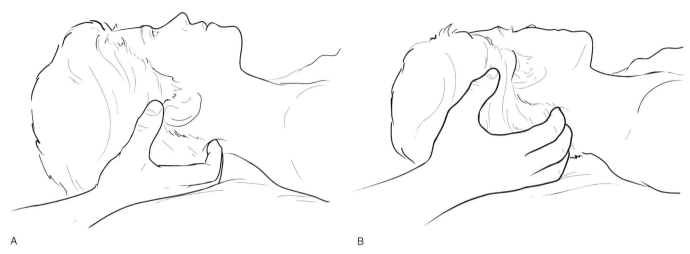

A   B

Figure 11.45   A&B: Friction may be applied to the suboccipitals and overlying muscles from the mid-line to the mastoid process. However, **CAUTION must be exercised to avoid deep friction to the rectus capitis posterior minor and to the vertebral artery, which is located in the suboccipital triangle**.

Box 11.12   Lief's NMT for the suboccipital region

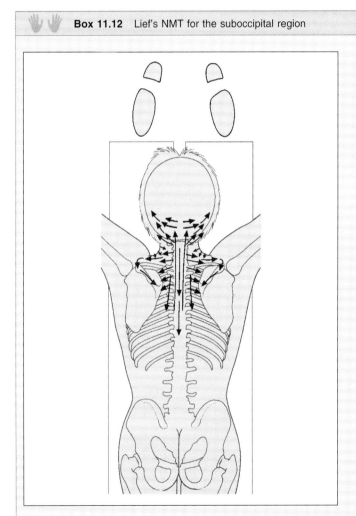

Figure 11.46   Lief's NMT 'map' for cervical and upper thoracic areas (reproduced, with permission, from Chaitow (1996a)).

• The patient is prone with her face in a cradle or face hole.
• The practitioner stands at the head of the table, resting the tips of his fingers on the lower, lateral aspect of the neck, the thumb tips placed just lateral to the first dorsal-spinal process.
• A degree of downward (toward the floor) pressure is applied via the thumbs which are then bilaterally drawn slowly cephalad alongside the lateral margins of the cervical spinous processes.
• This bilateral stroke culminates at the occiput where a lateral searching stretch is introduced across the bunched fibers of the muscles inserting into the base of the skull.
• The cephalad stroke should contain an element of pressure medially toward the spinous process so that the pad of the thumb is pressing downward (toward the floor) while the lateral thumb tip is directed medially/centrally, attempting to contact the bony contours of the spine, evaluating for tissue abnormalities, all the time being drawn slowly cephalad so that the stroke terminates at the occiput.
• This combination stroke is repeated two or three times. The finger tips which have been resting on the sternocleidomastoid may also be employed at this stage to lift and stretch the muscle posteriorly and laterally.
• The series of lateral strokes (bilaterally, performed singly, or simultaneously) across the occiput from its inferior margin to above the occipital protuberance attempt to evaluate the relative induration and contraction of the fibers attaching to the occiput.
• The thumb tips apply pressure to remove all slack into the medial fibers of the paraoccipital muscular bundles as a laterally directed manual stretch is instituted, using the leverage of the arms, as though attempting to 'open out' the occiput.
• The thumbs are then drawn laterally across the fibers of muscular insertion into the skull, in a series of strokes culminating at the occipitoparietal junction.
• The finger tips which act as a fulcrum to these movements should by now rest on the mastoid area of the temporal bone.
• Several very light but searching strokes are then performed by one thumb or the other running caudad directly over the spinous process from the base of the skull to the upper dorsal area. Pressure should be light (2–3 ounces at most) and very slow.
• Wherever localized tissue changes are perceived and especially if these evoke a painful response, they should be carefully palpated to ascertain whether they are active trigger points.

Box 11.13 PRT (strain-counterstrain) for any painful areas located in the posterior cervical musculature

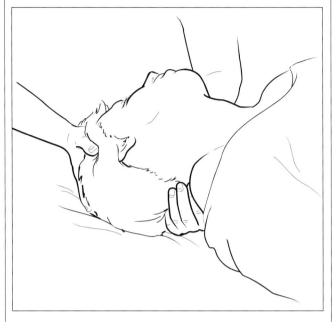

Figure 11.47 SCS position for posterior cervical dysfunction.

- With the patient supine an area of localized tenderness ('tender point') is identified on the posterolateral or posterior aspects of the neck.
- Compression is applied to the tender point, sufficient to elicit a degree of sensitivity or pain which the patient is told represents a score of '10'.
- The head/neck is then carefully eased into light extension until a reduction is achieved in the reported sensitivity.
- The pressure on the tender point can be constant or intermittent, with the latter being preferable if sensitivity is great.
- Once a position is found which reduces the pain 'score', fine-tuning maneuvers commence, with movement of the head/neck into rotation away from the side of palpated pain being the commonest beneficial direction.
- If this fails to reduce the pain score, variations should be attempted, slowly, one at a time, including sideflexion away from and toward the pain side, as well as rotation toward and/or translational movements.
- Any fine-tuning movement which either increases the pain 'score' or creates pain elsewhere indicates that the movement or position is not appropriate and alternative directions should be explored.
- Once a reduction in sensitivity of at least 70% is achieved, full inhalation and exhalation are monitored by the patient to see which phase of the breathing cycle reduces sensitivity more and this phase of the cycle is maintained for a comfortable period during which time the overall position of ease is maintained.
- If intermittent pressure on the point is being used, it needs to be applied periodically during the holding period in order to ensure that the position of ease has been maintained (by virtue of a non-return of palpation-induced pain).
- After 90 seconds, a very slow and deliberate return to neutral is performed and the patient is allowed to rest for several minutes.
- The tender point should be repalpated for sensitivity which should have reduced markedly, as should the degree of hypertonicity in the surrounding tissues.

Static pressure and friction are continued at 1″ intervals along the remainder of the suboccipital ridge to treat SCM, splenius capitis, longissimus capitis and obliquus capitis superior. Contralateral rotation of the head may be used with the caution above kept in mind. Pressure on the styloid process is avoided anterior to the SCM tendon where the styloid is located just inferior and slightly anterior to the earlobe.

Cranial to caudal friction may be used on the occipital tendon attachments as well which will have minor influence on suboccipital muscles but significant influence on the tissues overlying them.

The fingers are now placed caudally approximately ½″ and the steps repeated between C1 (atlas) and C2 (axis) to treat the inferior half of RCPMa and to include obliquus capitis inferior. If the spinous process of C2 is located, the fingers examine the space cephalad and slightly lateral to the process. This area influences rotation of the head. The center of the suboccipital triangle is avoided during the frictional techniques due to the location of the vertebral artery.

To influence and examine tissues caudal to the suboccipital muscles, this process may be continued throughout the posterior cervical muscles and is always repeated to the opposite side. Fibrotic bands or tendinous attachments may be treated with crossfiber friction and static pressure, as appropriate.

Platysma (Fig. 11.48)

Attachments: A broad sheet of muscular fibers arising from fascia of the upper chest which interlace medially with the contralateral muscle, below and behind the symphysis menti; intermediate fibers attach to the lower border of the mandibular body while posterior fibers cross the mandible and the anterolateral part of the masseter and attach to subcutaneous tissue and skin of the lower face

Innervation: Facial nerve (cranial nerve VII)

Muscle type: Not established

Function: May assist in depressing the mandible or draw the lower lip and corners of the mouth inferiorly, especially when the jaw is already open wide; produces skin ridges in the neck which may release pressure on underlying veins (Moore 1980)

Synergists: *To mandibular depression*: lateral pterygoid, mylohyoid, digastric, geniohyoid, gravity

Antagonists: Masseter, medial pterygoid, temporalis

Indications for treatment

- Prickling pain to the lower face and mandible or over the front of chest
- Presence of sternocleidomastoid trigger points.

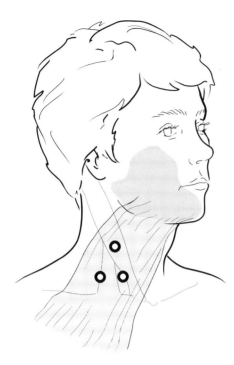

Figure 11.48 The prickling pain pattern of platysma is distinct from the pattern of the underlying SCM (see Fig. 11.51).

Special notes

While the platysma does not seem to have an important function, its referral pattern and potential influence on muscles located in its target zone may lead to indirect influences and perpetuation of trigger points in those tissues. The muscles of mastication (masseter especially) might be thus influenced. Since somatic-visceral referrals are known to occur in other body areas (see p. 31), it would be logical that tissues overlying the thyroid gland might have influence on glandular function. Platysma (as well as sternocleidomastoid, infrahyoids and scalenes) should be examined when glandular dysfunctions are noted.

Studies indicate activity during sudden deep inspiration and vigorous contraction during sudden, violent effort (*Gray's anatomy* 1995).

CAUTION: While spray and stretch techniques for treatment of trigger points are excellent applications for the anterior neck muscles, sustained hot or cold applications over the carotid artery and thyroid gland are not recommended. Clear warnings should be given to *avoid standing under a hot shower with the neck stretched in extension in order to allow a hot spray on the anterior neck*, as the patient may experience a rapid fluctuation in blood pressure accompanied by dizziness which could result in loss of balance and injury. A loosely wrapped hydrocolator pack which focuses its heat primarily onto the posterior cervical and filters somewhat onto the anterior neck can be applied with the patient reclined

or seated. Adequate time should be given after application before the patient is asked to stand.

 ## NMT for platysma

The skin of the anterior neck is fairly elastic and therefore usually lifts easily to be rolled. To address the fibers of platysma, the skin of the anterior neck is gently and slowly rolled between the thumb and fingers in an attempt to distinguish tender points or trigger points. When tender tissue is encountered, gentle static pressure can be applied to assess for referral patterns and taut fibers which feel as though they are 'glued' to the internal surface of the skin.

CAUTION: Aggressive techniques of tractioning the skin, tugging it or stretching it away from the neck or continuously rolling the tissues over and over should not be used, to avoid damaging its attachments to the underlying tissues. The skin over the anterior neck tends to loosen with aging. The elastic and collagen fibers are fragile and should be treated with special care to avoid inducing a 'saggy neck'.

General anterior neck muscle stretch utilizing MET

- For involvement of rectus capitis anterior, suprahyoids, infrahyoids, platysma, suprathyroids and infrathyroids the two procedures described immediately below are performed with the *mouth closed*.
- For involvement of longus colli and longus capitis, the mouth is held *slightly opened*.

Note: Sternocleidomastoid and scalene stretches described elsewhere in this chapter will automatically produce stretching of many of these anterior neck muscles.

CAUTION: Avoid traction or sidebend, especially with rotation of the neck, if disc damage is suspected or immediately after an accident until extent of injuries is known.

Variations

1. Supine

- This is a general non-specific stretching procedure (Fig. 11.49). It would not be used if anterior displacement of the articular disc is suspected as even mild mandibular condyle pressure into the articular fossa may create intense discomfort.
- The use of an open or closed mouth to involve different structures as explained above should be noted.
- The practitioner places his forearm (left in this example) in a position which allows the mid-cervical spine to rest on it and with the right hand cups the patient's jaw (which should be relaxed throughout the procedure,

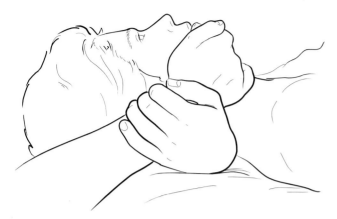

Figure 11.49   General cervical stretch, supine, following isometric contraction.

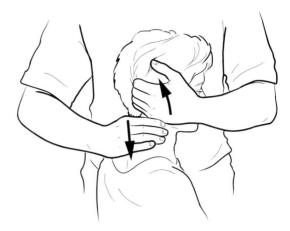

Figure 11.50   General cervical stretch, seated, following isometric contraction.

whether open for longus colli and longus capitis, or closed for other anterior hyoid-related muscles).

• The practitioner grasps his own right distal forearm with the left hand, so forming a stable contact.

• When the practitioner gently leans backward a degree of mild traction is introduced into the patient's cervical spine, to remove slack.

• The patient is asked to lightly move the head into flexion against the resistance of the contact hand on the (relaxed) jaw. This isometric contraction position is held for 7–10 seconds.

• Following release of the effort, a mild amount of extension (10°) is introduced to effectively stretch the anterior muscles of the neck.

• The practitioner gently leans backward so that a degree of mild traction is introduced into the patient's cervical spine. This traction is released extremely slowly.

• The procedure is stopped if pain or dizziness is reported.

2. Seated. A general MET stretch involving most of the deep and shallow muscles attaching to the anterior cervical spine, skull and hyoid bone is performed as follows (Fig. 11.50).

• The patient is seated and the practitioner stands at the side facing (in this example) the left side of the head.

• The practitioner's left hand wraps around the right side of the patient's head, palm of hand cupping the ear and mastoid, stabilizing the head firmly against the practitioner's chest or upper abdominal region.

• Female practitioners should introduce a shallow cushion between the patient's head and their own torso, in order to avoid inappropriate contact.

• The use of an open or closed mouth to involve different structures as explained above should be noted.

• The practitioner's left hand small finger is at the level of the patient's axis (C2).

• The practitioner's right hand stabilizes the posterior

aspect of the neck in order to support it below the level of C3.

• Traction is gently initiated as a slow movement is made into pure extension of the head and neck of about 10° *at most*.

• The patient is asked to gently (20% of strength) take the head and neck forward into flexion, as the practitioner resists this effort, mainly with the left-hand contact.

• The contraction is held for 7–10 seconds after which, with traction still being maintained, a further 5° of extension is initiated and held for not less than 10 seconds.

• To introduce stretch into muscles attaching more distal than C3, the contact hand on the posterior neck can be lowered, one segment at a time, for subsequent isometric contractions and stretches.

• A slight movement (5°) toward the neutral position should be produced before each contraction and subsequent stretch.

• Immediately discontinue stretching if any dizziness is reported.

• To produce greater emphasis on stretching of one side or the other, a moderate degree of sidebend (about 20°) away from that side should be introduced prior to the extension.

Sternocleidomastoid (Fig. 11.51)

Attachments: *Sternal head*: Anterior surface of the sternum to the mastoid process and occipital bone (lateral half of superior nuchal line)
   Clavicular head: from the superior surface of the medial 1/3 of the clavicle to blend with the tendon of the sternal head and attach with it to the mastoid process and occipital bone

Innervation: Accessory nerve (cranial nerve XI) and branches of ventral rami of C2–4 cervical spinal nerves. May also include motor fibers from vagus nerve which join at the jugular foramen (Simons et al 1998)

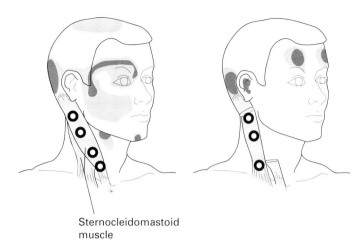

Figure 11.51 Composite referral patterns of SCM muscle.

Muscle type: Postural (type 1), shortens when stressed

Function: *Unilaterally*: rotates the head contralaterally (and tilts it upward) and sidebends the head and neck ipsilaterally

Bilaterally: flexes or extends the head, depending on the position of the cervical vertebrae (see below), lifts the head from the pillow when the patient is supine, may assist in forced inspiration (especially when the intercostals are paralyzed)

Synergists: *For rotation*: trapezius of the same side, contralateral splenius capitis and cervicis, obliquus capitis inferior and levator scapula

For lateral flexion: scalenes, trapezius

For flexion of cervical column (see below): longus colli

Antagonists: *For rotation*: contralateral SCM and trapezius, ipsilateral splenius capitis, splenius cervicis, levator scapula and obliquus capitis inferior

For lateral flexion: contralateral SCM, scalenes, trapezius

Indications for treatment

- A diagnosis of atypical facial neuralgia, tension headaches or cervicocephalangia
- Persistent dry cough or sore throat
- Mimics trigeminal neuralgia and produces facial pain or scalp tenderness
- Blurred vision, perception of dimmed intensity of light
- Visual disturbances, eye pain, excessive lacrimation and difficulty raising the eyelid
- Inflamed or congested sinuses
- Hearing loss
- Disturbances in orientation including postural dizziness, vertigo, disequilibrium, ataxia, sudden falls and nausea

Special notes

Sternocleidomastoid (SCM) is a prominent muscle of the anterior neck and is closely associated with the trapezius.

Box 11.14 Balancing of the head on the cervical column

The head is in equilibrium when the eyes look horizontally. In this position the plane of the bite, shown here by a piece of cardboard held tightly between the teeth, is also horizontal, as is the auriculo-nasal plane (AN), which passes through the nasal spine and the superior border of the external auditory meatus.

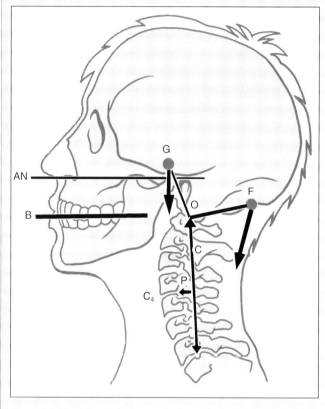

Figure 11.52 The posterior cervical muscles counterbalance the anteriorly placed center of gravity of the cranium (reproduced, with permission, from Kapandji (1998)).

The head taken as a whole constitutes a lever system:

- *B is the plane of the bite*
- *C is the cord subtending the arc*
- *P is the perpendicular*
- *the fulcrum O lies at the level of the occipital condyles*
- *the force G is produced by the weight of the head applied through its centre of gravity lying near the sella turcica*
- *the force F is produced by the posterior neck muscles which constantly counterbalance the weight of the head, which tends to tilt it forwards.*

This anterior location of the centre of gravity of the head explains the strength of the posterior neck muscles relative to the flexor muscles of the neck. In fact, the extensor muscles counteract gravity whereas the flexors are helped by gravity. This also explains the constant tone in these posterior neck muscles preventing the head from tilting forwards. When one sleeps while sitting the tone of these muscles is reduced and the head falls ... [toward] the chest. (Kapandji 1974)

SCM often acts as postural compensator for head tilt associated with postural distortions found elsewhere (spinal, pelvic or lower extremity functional or structural inadequacies, for instance) although it seldom causes restriction of neck movement.

SCM is synergistic with anterior neck muscles for flexion of the head and flexion of the cervical column on the thoracic column, when the cervical column is already flattened by the prevertebral muscles. However, when the head is placed in extension and SCM contracts, it accentuates lordosis of the cervical column, flexes the cervical column on the thoracic column and adds to extension of the head. In this way, SCM is both synergist and antagonist to the prevertebral muscles (Kapandji 1974).

SCM trigger points are activated by forward head positioning, 'whiplash' injury, positioning of the head to look upward for extended periods of time and structural compensations. The two heads of SCM each have their own patterns of trigger point referral which include (among others) into the ear, top of head, into the temporo-mandibular joint, over the brow, into the throat and those which cause proprioceptive disturbances, disequilibrium, nausea and dizziness. Tenderness in SCM may be associated with trigger points in the digastric muscle and digastric trigger points may be satellites of SCM trigger points (Simons et al 1998).

Simons et al (1998) report:

When objects of equal weight are held in the hands, the patient with unilateral TrP involvement of the clavicular division [of SCM] may exhibit an abnormal weight test. When asked to judge which is heaviest of two objects of the same weight that look alike but may not be the same weight (two vapocoolant dispensers, one of which may have been used) the patient will [give] evidence [of] dysmetria by underestimating the weight of the object held in the hand on the same side as the affected sternocleidomastoid muscle. Inactivation of the responsible sternocleidomastoid TrPs promptly restores weight appreciation by this test. Apparently, the afferent discharges from these TrPs disturb central processing of proprioceptive information from the upper limb muscles as well as vestibular function related to neck muscles.

Lymph nodes lie superficially along the medial aspect of the SCM and may be palpated, especially when enlarged. These nodes may be indicative of chronic cranial infections stemming from a throat infection, dental abscess, sinusitis or tumor. Likewise, trigger points in SCM may be perpetuated by some of these conditions (Simons et al 1998).

Lewit (1999) points out that tenderness noted at the medial end of the clavicle is often an indication of SCM hypertonicity. This will commonly accompany a forward head position and/or tendency to upper chest breathing and will almost inevitably be associated with hypertonicity, shortening and trigger point evolution in associated musculature, including scalenes, upper trapezius and levator scapula (see crossed syndrome notes on p. 55).

NMT for SCM

The patient is supine and the practitioner is seated cephalad to the head and positioned slightly away from mid-line on the side to be treated. The patient's head is rotated approximately 45° ipsilaterally and passively sidebent to shorten the SCM so it may be lifted while also moved somewhat away from the carotid artery. There still remains an area where the artery lies vertically deep to the now diagonally overlying SCM. Orienting the head and neck in this manner avoids positioning the SCM to overlie the entire length of the artery and decreases the chance of disturbance of the artery. However, caution is exercised to avoid compression of the artery in all circumstances.

The SCM is compressed in a broad general release between the flattened fingers and opposing thumb of the same treating hand. The finger pads provide more effective compression against the opposing thumb pad than the finger joints do. As thickened bands or nodules are located in the sternal head of SCM, the cranium may be placed in varying positions which stretch the fibers slightly while still allowing the muscle to be lifted and held in flat compression. The muscle fibers may be rolled between the fingers and thumb gently to reveal more localized contractures. The bands are examined through their entire length for thickenings associated with trigger point formation or for exquisitely tender spots. When

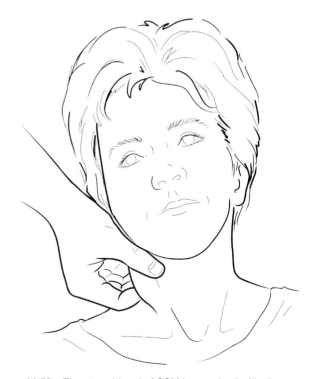

Figure 11.53 The sternal head of SCM is examined with pincer compression at thumb-width intervals from the mastoid process to the sternal attachment.

active loci are found, pressure is applied into the suspected myofascial tissue to meet and match the tension of the contracture. The patient should report a mid-range on the discomfort scale and may describe referral patterns for active (recognized pattern) or latent (unfamiliar pattern) trigger points. The finger tips (rather than finger pads) often provide a more precise compression against the thumb once bands have been identified.

Duplication of the patient's symptoms, particularly those which agree with known referral patterns for that muscle, indicate a trigger point has been located and local twitch responses, when seen or felt, serve as confirmation. Trigger point pressure release is applied to any trigger points found. The tissue can be gently taken into stretch as compression is applied, if appropriate.

The compression techniques can be applied in thumb-width intervals from the upper portion of the belly of the sternomastoid head to the sternal attachment site. The treating hand may need to be pronated as it nears the thorax to better reposition the fingers for grasping near the attachment. The sternal attachment may be frictioned if not too tender but it is often the site of exquisite tenderness. (Fig. 11.54)

The occipitomastoid attachment of both heads of the SCM can often be grasped between the thumb and first two fingers close to the cranial attachment. Sometimes separation of the clavicular and sternal heads is distinct; however, often the tissue will feel thick, indistinct, fibrotic or otherwise undefined. Short gliding strokes applied with the thumb (or fingers) may be used to soften the

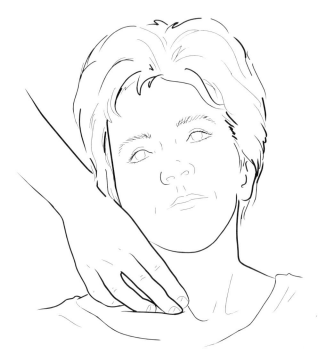

Figure 11.54 Sternal and clavicular attachments of SCM are gently frictioned.

tendons and uppermost portions of muscle fibers so that they may eventually be lifted and grasped. The gliding strokes must be kept short since the carotid artery is relatively exposed a few inches inferomedial to the attachment. Additionally, lubrication used for gliding will need to be removed or a thin cloth or paper tissue laid over the tendon so that grasping fingers do not slip when the subsequent compressions are applied.

The clavicular head of SCM can sometimes be distinguished from the overlying sternal head if they are allowed to gently (intentionally) slip between the grasping fingers. Once isolated, the full length of the clavicular head may sometimes be addressed in the same grasping, compressional manner used for the sternal head. However, the deeper head is often difficult to grasp, even when the cranium is repositioned to shorten it. If it cannot be isolated for compression without intrusion into the underlying tissues, stretching techniques may be used to elongate its fibers and to soften them. They may eventually be distinguished, either at the end of the session or at subsequent sessions. The clavicular attachment is often very tender when friction is applied. Static pressure may be substituted or ice applications used until central trigger points are deactivated and stress on the attachment is reduced.

Longissimus capitis and splenius capitis attachments may sometimes be influenced on the mastoid process deep to the SCM attachment. The head lies on a bolster or wedge to bring it into supported flexion of around 45° which passively shortens the SCM. The patient must completely relax the SCM and can therefore offer no assistance in maintaining head position. The head is rotated contralaterally to access the posterior (medial) aspect of the occipital attachment of SCM. If the SCM tendon has been softened, the practitioner's thumb or finger tips may be able to displace the most posterior fibers and slide slightly under the SCM's most posterior (medial) edge. This step may also be applied with the head in ipsilateral rotation (without elevation), which utilizes the weight of the cranium to create pressure on the attachment site. The fingers displace the most medial fibers while also applying pressure on as much of the cranial attachments as possible under the edge of the SCM. Static pressure or light friction may be used with either head position.

Treatment of shortened SCM using MET (Fig. 11.55)

The patient is supine with the head supported in a neutral position by one of the practitioner's hands. The shoulders rest on a cushion, so that when the head is placed on the table it will be in slight extension. The patient's contralateral hand rests on the upper aspect of the sternum to act as a cushion when pressure is applied during the stretch phase of the operation.

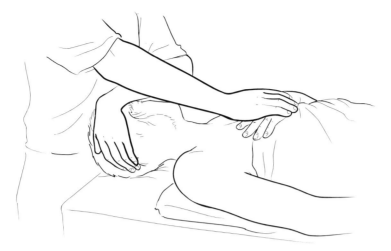

Figure 11.55 MET treatment of sternocleidomastoid.

• The patient's head is fully but comfortably rotated contralaterally.

• The patient is asked to lift the fully rotated head a small degree toward the ceiling and to hold the breath.

• When the head is raised there is no need for the practitioner to apply resistance as gravity effectively provides this.

• After 7–10 seconds of isometric contraction with breath held, the patient is asked to slowly release the effort (and the breath) and to allow the head/neck (still in rotation) to be placed on the table, so that a small degree of extension is allowed.

• The practitioner's hand covers the patient's 'cushion' hand (which rests on the sternum) in order to apply oblique pressure/stretch to the sternum to take it away from the head and toward the feet.

• The hand not involved in stretching the sternum caudally should gently restrain the tendency the head will have to follow this stretch, but should *not* apply pressure under any circumstances to stretch the head/neck while it is in this vulnerable position of rotation and slight extension.

• The degree of extension of the neck should be slight, 10–15° at most.

• This stretch, which is applied as the patient exhales, is maintained for not less than 20 seconds to achieve release/stretch of hypertonic and fibrotic structures.

• The other side should then be treated in the same manner

CAUTION: Care is required, especially with middle-aged and elderly patients, in applying this useful stretching procedure. Appropriate tests should be carried out to evaluate cerebral circulation problems (p. 172) which, if present, suggest that this particular MET method be avoided.

Suprahyoid muscles

The suprahyoid muscles attach the hyoid bone to the mandible (and to the cranium) while also positioning it in relationship to the cervical spine. The positioning of the hyoid bone, trachea and larynx/pharynx is critical since the air passageway lies between the hyoid and the cervical spine (approximately C3–4) as well as between the trachea and the lower cervical spine.

The suprahyoid muscles should be treated with the infrahyoids in cases of reduced cervical lordosis as together they contribute to flexion of the neck, acting as the long arm of a lever. When the mandible is fixed by the mandibular elevators, the supra- and infrahyoid muscles flex the head on the cervical column, as well as the cervical column on the thorax. Positioning in this way will also produce a flattening (reduction) of cervical curvature (Kapandji 1974).

The suprahyoid muscles are discussed in detail in Chapter 12 together with the cranium and craniomandibular muscles due to their obvious role in hyoid and mandibular positioning as well as their physical contribution to the floor of the mouth. The suprahyoid muscles are easily palpable from an intraoral aspect which especially addresses the bellies of the muscles. If attachments along the inferior surface of the mandible are tender to palpation, the intraoral treatment described on p. 290 is suggested.

Infrahyoid muscles (Fig. 11.56)

The infrahyoid muscle group consists of the sternohyoid, sternothyroid, thyrohyoid and omohyoid muscles. This group stabilizes and depresses the hyoid bone and, acting with the suprahyoid muscles, contributes to flexion of the cervical column when the mouth is closed.

Since somaticovisceral referrals are known to occur

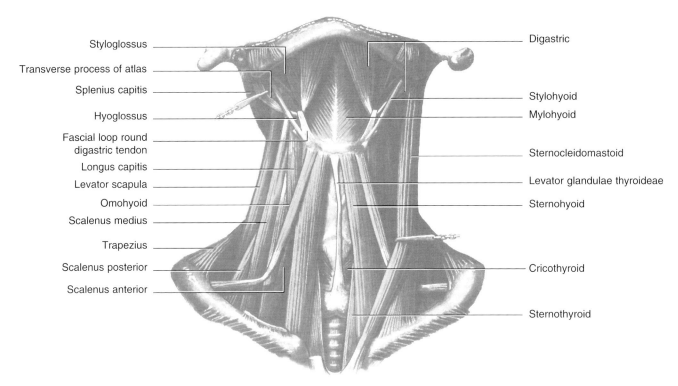

Styloglossus

Transverse process of atlas

Splenius capitis

Hyoglossus

Fascial loop round
digastric tendon

Longus capitis

Levator scapula

Omohyoid

Scalenus medius

Trapezius

Scalenus posterior

Scalenus anterior

Digastric

Stylohyoid

Mylohyoid

Sternocleidomastoid

Levator glandulae thyroideae

Sternohyoid

Cricothyroid

Sternothyroid

Figure 11.56 Supra- and infrahyoid muscles control positioning of the hyoid bone which, among other functions, assists in maintaining an adequate air passageway (reproduced, with permission, from *Gray's anatomy* (1995)).

in other body areas (see p. 31), it would be logical that tissues overlying the thyroid gland might have influence on glandular function. Infrahyoid muscles, sternocleidomastoid and scalenes should be examined when glandular dysfunctions are noted due to their proximity to the thyroid and parathyroid glands.

Sternohyoid

Attachments: Posterior surface of the manubrium sternum, the medial clavicle and the sternoclavicular ligament to attach to the inferior border and inner surface of the body of the hyoid bone, its fibers merging with the contralateral sternohyoid near the mid-belly

Innervation: Ansa cervalis (C1–3)

Muscle type: Phasic (type 2), weakens when stressed

Function: Depresses the hyoid bone (especially from an elevated position during swallowing); functions with the infrahyoid group to flex the cervical column with the mouth closed

Synergists: *For hyoid movement*: sternothyroid/thyrohyoid unit, omohyoid
For hyoid stabilization: suprahyoids and remaining infrahyoids
For flexion of cervical column: longus colli, longus capitis, sternocleidomastoid, scalene group, rectus capitis anterior and lateralis, suprahyoids and remaining infrahyoids

Antagonists: *To hyoid movement*: suprahyoid muscles
To flexion of cervical column: posterior cervical muscles

Indications for treatment

- Dysfunction in hyoid bone movement during swallowing
- Preparation for prevertebral treatment (longus colli, longus capitis)
- Difficulties in swallowing

Sternothyroid

Attachments: Posterior surface of the manubrium sternum and from the 1st rib cartilage to the thyroid cartilage

Innervation: Ansa cervalis (C1–3)

Muscle type: Phasic (type 2), weakens when stressed

Function: Depression of larynx, depression of hyoid bone when acting as a unit with thyrohyoid; functions with the infrahyoid group to flex the cervical column with the mouth closed

Synergists: *For hyoid movement*: sternohyoid, thyrohyoid, omohyoid
For hyoid stabilization: suprahyoids and remaining infrahyoids
For flexion of cervical column: longus colli, longus capitis, sternocleidomastoid, scalene group, suprahyoids and remaining infrahyoids

Antagonists: *To depression of larynx*: thyrohyoid
To hyoid movement: suprahyoid muscles
To flexion of cervical column: posterior cervical muscles

Indications for treatment

- Dysfunction in hyoid bone movement during swallowing
- Preparation for prevertebral treatment (longus colli, longus capitis)
- Changes in voice range (larynx positioning)
- Difficulties in swallowing

Special notes

Sternothyroid draws the larynx downwards during swallowing and speech and during the singing of low notes, for example. The linkage between the sternum and the hyoid allows this muscle to influence cranial mechanics.

The fibers of sternothyroid lie in direct contact with the anterolateral surface of the thyroid gland and should be examined and treated with all glandular dysfunctions. However, caution should be exercised to avoid frictioning where the gland lies. Further studies are needed to assess the trigger point referral patterns of the infrahyoid muscles and their possible role in neck, throat, thyroid, voice and TMJ dysfunctions.

Thyrohyoid

Attachments: Anterior surface of thyroid cartilage to the lower portion of the greater horn and body of hyoid bone
Innervation: Hypoglossal nerve
Muscle type: Phasic (type 2), weakens when stressed
Function: Depresses the hyoid bone; elevates the larynx; functions with the infrahyoid group to flex the cervical column with the mouth closed
Synergists: *For hyoid movement*: sternohyoid, sternothyroid, omohyoid
For hyoid stabilization: suprahyoids and remaining infrahyoids
For flexion of cervical column: longus colli, longus capitis, sternocleidomastoid, scalene group, suprahyroids and remaining infrahyoids
Antagonists: *To hyoid movement*: suprahyoid muscles
To flexion of cervical column: posterior cervical muscles
To elevation of the larynx: sternothyroid

Indications for treatment

- Dysfunction in hyoid bone movement during swallowing
- Preparation for prevertebral treatment (longus colli, longus capitis)
- Changes in voice or voice range (larynx positioning)

Omohyoid

Attachments: The inferior belly of this two-bellied muscle arises from the upper margin of the scapula near the scapular notch and its superior belly from the lower border of the hyoid bone lateral to the insertion of sternohyoid. The two bellies are joined by a central tendon which is ensheathed by a fibrous loop which may extend to the deep cervical fascia and attaches to the clavicle and 1st rib
Innervation: Ansa cervicalis profunda (C1–3)
Muscle type: Phasic (type 2), weakens when stressed
Function: Depresses the hyoid bone; tenses deep cervical fascia which reduces the possibility of soft tissue being sucked inwardly during respiration; dilates the internal jugular vein; functions with the infrahyoid group to flex the cervical column with the mouth closed
Synergists: *For hyoid movement*: sternohyoid, sternothyroid, thyrohyoid
For hyoid stabilization: suprahyoids and remaining infrahyoids
For flexion of cervical column: longus colli, longus capitis, sternocleidomastoid, scalene group, suprahyroids and remaining infrahyoids
Antagonists: *To hyoid movement*: suprahyoid muscles
To flexion of cervical column: posterior cervical muscles

Indications for treatment

- Dysfunction in hyoid bone movement during swallowing
- Preparation for prevertebral treatment (longus colli, longus capitis)

The extraordinary connections of this muscle, linking as it does the scapula, clavicle and hyoid bone (which via other attachments links it indirectly to the mandible), give some idea of the potential for cranial problems arising from numerous influences on these structures, including respiratory and postural dysfunctions. Omohyoid may arise from the clavicle instead of the scapula and, if so, would be referred to as the cleidohyoid muscle.

NMT for infrahyoid muscles

CAUTION: The treatment protocols of the superficial and deep anterior cervical muscles are some of the most delicate and precise used in NMT. They are to be approached with extreme caution due to the proximity of the carotid artery and the thyroid gland. Training (with hands-on supervision) is strongly recommended prior to practice of any anterior neck techniques.

The practitioner stands at shoulder or chest level of the supine patient and faces the throat. The hyoid bone is stabilized with the index finger of the practitioner's most caudal hand by reaching across the patient to the opposite greater horn of the hyoid bone and carefully placing the index finger on its outer surface. Caution must be exercised to stay in contact with the hyoid bone and not allow the stabilizing finger or its posteriorly oriented finger tip to venture off the lateral edge of the hyoid bone where the carotid artery resides. Additionally, the hyoid bone must not be pressed posteriorly but only stabilized enough to discourage its movement when frictional techniques are used.

With the index finger of the practitioner's cephalad hand, gentle friction may be applied to the supra- and infrahyoid muscles on the superior, anterior and inferior aspect of the hyoid bone. Caution must be exercised to keep the treating finger in contact with the hyoid bone and not allow it to slide or be accidentally placed lateral to the edge of the hyoid bone or thyroid cartilage due to the location of the carotid artery (see Fig. 11.57A).

The stabilizing finger is relocated to the thyroid cartilage on the contralateral side. The treating finger is placed on the uppermost medial aspect of the anterior surface of the thyroid cartilage and is used to press the overlying infrahyoid muscles onto the thyroid cartilage where static pressure or gentle transverse friction is used to assess their fibers. When the proper pressure is used, the vertical fibers may be distinctly felt as they are captured against the underlying cartilaginous surface or as the treating finger is slid across them in gentle frictional movements. If too little pressure is used, the skin will merely slide over the muscles and benefit of treatment will be significantly reduced. Too much pressure might press the entire structure posteriorly into the esophagus, longus colli, longus capitis and the anterior surface of the cervical vertebrae. The right amount of pressure will meet and match the tension found in the tissues and elicit a mid-range response on the patient's discomfort scale if tension exists in the tissues.

The treating finger is moved laterally one finger tip width and the frictional work repeated. It may be moved laterally once more in most cases, depending upon the size of the practitioner's hands and the width of the patient's cartilage (see Fig. 11.57B).

The anterior surface of the stabilized thyroid cartilage is treated in this compressional or frictional manner until the cricoid cartilage (first cartilaginous ring of the trachea) is reached at approximately mid-way between the hyoid bone and the sternal notch. Extreme care is used at the most lateral aspects of the hyoid bone and the thyroid cartilage along their full length to avoid allowing the treating finger to go laterally beyond the edge of the cartilage (even mildly during friction) as the carotid artery runs vertically the entire length of these structures. Friction applied near the lateral edge should be unidirectional toward the mid-line which adequately transverses the muscular fibers while avoiding contact with the artery.

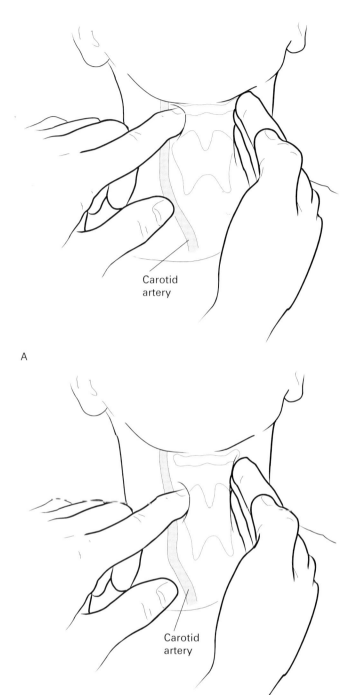

A

B

Figure 11.57 The infrahyoid group is examined at finger-tip intervals from the hyoid bone (A) to the cricoid cartilage (B). Extreme **CAUTION** is exercised to avoid the carotid artery (immediately lateral to the edge of the hyoid bone and thyroid cartilage) and the thyroid gland (caudal to the cricoid cartilage). See text for **CAUTIONS**.

Caudal to the cricoid cartilage, the thyroid gland lies relatively exposed, covered only by the skin, cervical fascia and the thin infrahyoid muscles. Frictional or compressional techniques (either flat or pincer) are not used caudal to (below) the cricoid cartilage since the thyroid gland would most likely be intruded upon. These lower portions of the fibers are easily stretched (in most cases) by extension of the head and neck with the mouth closed.

The patient's head is supported with a wedge or pillow in passive flexion at approximately 45° (chin toward chest). The practitioner's treating finger tip is placed on the posterior surface of the sternal notch. As the patient takes in and holds a deep breath, the sternum will lift away from the thorax and (sometimes dramatically) allow the finger to penetrate further (Fig. 11.58). The finger is swept first to one side and then the other while maintaining a firm contact onto the posterior surface of the sternum where the sternohyoid and sternothyroid muscles attach. Static pressure may be used if the attachments are too tender for frictional techniques.

〰️ 〰️ Soft tissue technique derived from osteopathic methodology

Simone Ross (1999), in discussing osteopathic approaches to dysphonia, describes the following safe soft tissue treatment technique.

Pitch control is primarily controlled by the thyrohyoid muscles. To treat these muscles, the patient lies supine and the [practitioner] fixes on the thyroid cartilage with the forefinger and thumb of one hand whilst the other hand fixes on the inferior border of the hyoid with a finger and thumb. The cartilages are then held apart for 20 seconds by fixing on one and moving the other. This stretch should be given in an inferior, superior direction and a lateral direction.

It is essential to treat the cricothyroid visor, if it is locked in position due to a restricted cricothyroid muscle for function of the vocal cords. These muscles are of particular importance as they affect the vocal folds directly. If the cricothyroid muscles are short and the visor mechanism locked they create an

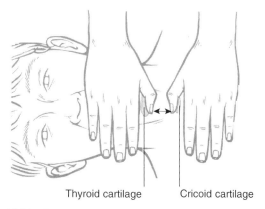

Thyroid cartilage   Cricoid cartilage

Figure 11.59 Technique for opening the thyrocricoid visor (reproduced, with permission, from the *Journal of Bodywork and Movement Therapies* 1999; **3**(3):141).

unhealthy stretching and elongation of the vocal folds. To open the visor, the thumb tip of one hand is placed on the anterior surface of the cricoid, whilst the other thumb tip is placed on the inferior aspect of the thyroid cartilage, gentle pressure is applied to both cartilages to open the visor.

Among the posttreatment effects, the patient might note a drop in pitch and increased resonance of voice, decrease in pain and discomfort, decreased tenderness in musculature and decreased hoarseness when these associated symptoms have been present. Spray and stretch applications for the anterior neck, as discussed by Simons et al (1998), could also be isolated to these tissues and the myofascial release described above used (Fig. 11.59).

Longus colli (Fig. 11.60)

Attachments: *Superior oblique portion*: anterior tubercles of transverse processes of C3–6 to the anterior tubercle of the atlas
Inferior oblique portion: from the first three thoracic vertebral bodies to the anterior tubercles of transverse processes of C4–7 (varies)
Vertical portion: from the vertebral bodies of C5–T3 to the vertebral bodies of C2–4

Innervation: Ventral rami (C2–6)

Muscle type: Not established

Function: Unilaterally, sidebends and contralaterally rotates the neck; bilaterally, flexes the cervical spine

Synergists: *For lateral flexion and rotation*: ipsilateral scalenes, SCM, longus capitis, levator scapula (Warfel 1985)
For flexion: longus capitis, suprahyoids, infrahyoids, rectus capitis anterior, SCM (when the neck is already flexed)

Antagonists: *To lateral flexion and rotation*: contralateral scalenes, contralateral levator scapula, SCM, longus capitis, longus colli
To cervical flexion: posterior cervical muscles, SCM (when the neck is already extended)

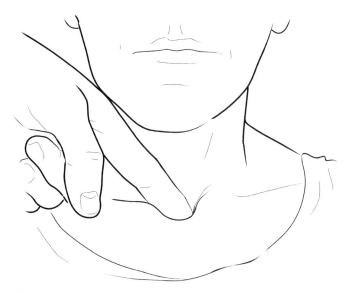

Figure 11.58 With the head passively elevated and the patient holding a deep breath, attachment of the sternohyoid and sternothyroid may be reached (on some patients) on the posterior aspect of the sternum.

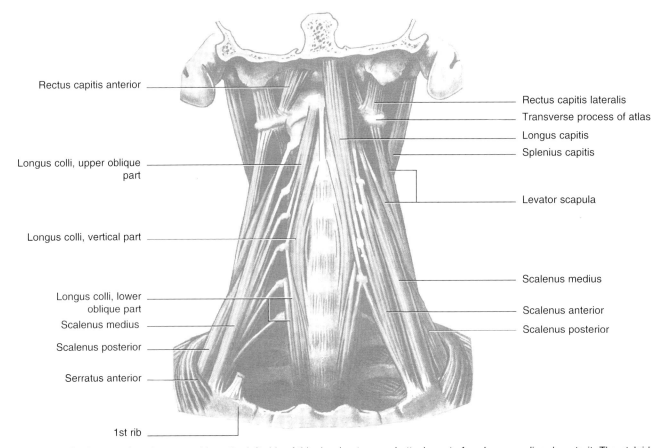

Figure 11.60 Scalenus anticus is removed from the left side of this drawing to reveal attachment of scalenus medius deep to it. The styloid process has also been removed anterior to rectus capitis lateralis (reproduced, with permission, from *Gray's anatomy* (1995)).

Longus capitis

Attachments: Anterior tubercles of the transverse processes of C3–6 to the basilar part of the occipital bone

Innervation: Ventral rami of C1–3

Muscle type: Phasic (type 2), weakens when stressed

Function: Unilaterally, rotates the neck contralaterally and flexes the head to the same side; bilaterally, flexes the head and neck

Synergists: *For lateral flexion and contralateral rotation*: scalenes, SCM, longus colli, levator scapula (Warfel 1985)

For cervical flexion: longus colli, suprahyoids, infrahyoids, rectus capitis anterior, SCM (when the neck is already flexed)

Antagonists: *To lateral flexion and rotation*: contralateral scalenes, SCM, longus capitis, longus colli, contralateral levator scapula

To cervical flexion: posterior suboccipitals, posterior cervical muscles, SCM (when the neck is already extended)

Indication for treatment of prevertebral muscles

- Difficulty swallowing

- Diagnosis of loss of cervical lordosis or 'military neck'
- Unstable cervical column
- Unstable atlas
- Chronic posterior cervical myofascial dysfunction
- Chronic dysfunctions elsewhere in the spinal column (compensatory)
- Loss of vertical dimension of cervical discs
- Posterior protrusion of cervical discs.

Special notes

Longus colli and longus capitis lie on the anterior surface of the vertebral bodies of the cervical spine. Superficial to them lie the hyoid bone, thyroid cartilage, larynx, pharynx, esophagus and trachea. Immediately lateral to these structures, the carotid arteries run vertically as they pass through the cervical region to serve the cranium. All of these surrounding structures require that extreme caution be exercised in the assessment and treatment of the prevertebral muscles. Fingernails of the treating fingers should be cut short and filed smooth.

Hoppenfeld (1976) notes: 'Difficulty or pain upon swallowing may be caused by cervical spine pathology such as bony protuberances, bony osteophytes, or by soft tissue swelling due to hematomas, infection, or tumor in the anterior portion of the cervical spine'. If the patient reports difficulty swallowing or if the practitioner encounters suspicious tissue, it is important to rule out these (as well as esophageal) pathologies prior to treatment of the deep cervical muscles.

The deep anterior cervical muscles produce flexion of the head and neck and therefore reduce the cervical curvature. When shortened, they can increase anterior pressure on the discs and can contribute to posterior protrusion of the disc into the spinal cord. Unilaterally, they also sidebend and rotate the column and therefore may be involved in scoliotic and other compensatory postural dysfunctions originating in other aspects of the spinal column or elsewhere in the body. The number of muscle slips for each varies greatly as do their individual attachments.

The superficial muscles of the anterior neck should always be treated before the longus colli and capitis to help release tension of the muscles covering the thyroid cartilage. The superficial structures must all be displaced in order to reach the prevertebral muscles. Tension in the overlying 'strapping' muscles may prevent the structures from being moved sufficiently to allow room for manual treatment to be applied.

Specific referral patterns for most of the deep anterior cervical muscles have not been established. Simons et al (1998) note they can refer to the anterior neck, laryngeal region and mouth. The anterior neck region is in clear need of research regarding many areas of myofascial pain and dysfunction.

CAUTION: The treatment protocols of the deep anterior cervical muscles are among the most delicate and precise used in NMT. They are to be approached with extreme caution due to the proximity of the carotid artery, vocal cords and the thyroid gland. Training (with hands-on supervision) is STRONGLY recommended prior to practice of these techniques.

 ## NMT for longus colli and capitis

The supine patient is facing toward the ceiling (head in neutral position) and the practitioner is standing at the level of the upper chest and facing the cervical region. The thumb of the practitioner's caudal hand is used to displace the hyoid bone, thyroid cartilage, esophagus and trachea away from the side being treated. All movements of these structures should be performed slowly, gently and with extreme regard for the carotid arteries, as directed below.

It may be necessary to create 'extra skin' to avoid stretching the superficial tissues which creates a taut, inflexible surface through which it is difficult to feel the underlying tissues. To assure a softer skin surface, 'extra

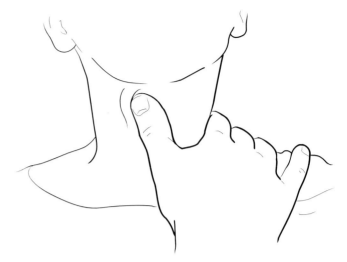

Figure 11.61 Skin is first displaced toward the side to be treated to create excess in order to provide a more flexible surface through which to palpate after the more superficial structures are displaced. See text for details and important cautions.

skin' is first displaced toward the side being treated by starting with the pad of the practitioner's caudal thumb past the mid-line of the thyroid cartilage and hyoid bone (Fig. 11.61). The thumb is moved laterally along with the underlying skin toward the side being treated. Without releasing the displaced skin, the underlying structures are then contacted by pressing through the skin and onto the ipsilateral edge of the thyroid cartilage. The cartilage is lifted slightly away from the underlying muscles (toward the ceiling) as all the superficial structures are moved contralaterally so that their lateral edge lies just past the mid-line. All downward (toward the cervical vertebrae) pressure is avoided as this would cause the superficial structures to scrape across the muscles as they are being displaced.

Once the structures are displaced to the mid-line or further, the carotid artery must be precisely located to ensure that there is enough room for one finger to be placed on the anterior surface of the cervical column. An index finger is placed gently onto the carotid artery and the pulse located. Extreme caution must be exercised *not* to friction the palpating finger, nor to disturb the artery in any way. At the bifurcation of the artery is the carotid sinus which contains pressure receptor nerve endings (baroreceptors) associated with blood pressure (Leonhardt 1986, *Stedman's medical dictionary* 1998). Disturbance of this area might cause a slowing of the heart or an uncontrolled fall in blood pressure. Additionally, the carotid glomus, a small organ whose chemoreceptors are sensitive to the partial pressure of oxygen in the blood, is also housed in the same location.

If there is not sufficient room between the artery and the displaced thyroid cartilage for the treating finger to be placed, the structures are gently allowed to return to their original position. This displacement can be applied again to reevaluate the conditions for treatment. When there is not sufficient room to treat the tissues manually, positional release, muscle energy techniques or other stretching methods may be substituted. **Under no circumstances** should the treatment be applied if the arterial pulse is found to be too close to the mid-line to allow safe application.

If the space between the arterial pulse and the displaced thyroid cartilage is at least slightly wider than the treating finger, the finger may be placed onto the anterior surface of the vertebral bodies as high as the overlying tissues will allow. This placement is usually about the C3 level, which is approximately level with the hyoid bone. The finger is then gently pressed into the tissues (toward the treatment table) which captures the muscles gently against the anterior surface of the underlying vertebra. The fibers of the longus colli and longus capitis are usually palpable when taut and may also be moderately tender. Static pressure or gentle, very narrow transverse friction may be applied while being extremely careful not to disturb the carotid artery laterally. The palpating finger may discern the rounded surface of the discs between the vertebral bodies or the hard protrusions of anterior calcific 'spurs'. Caution must be exercised to avoid excessive pressure onto the discs or onto the spurs to avoid damaging the tissues. The disc should *never* be pressed posteriorly in any attempt to relocate it as its anterior fibers may well be weak due to anterior protrusion and possible associated weakness of the anterior longitudinal ligament.

The treating finger is placed one finger tip caudally

and static pressure or gentle friction applied again. This application may be continued caudally as far as possible as long as the displacement of the structures and the location of the artery allow it. In the lower cervical region (approximately C5 or the level of the cricoid cartilage), the patient may feel the urge to cough or feel a 'choking' feeling, regardless of how gently the practitioner is working. At this point, the treatment is discontinued and the structures allowed to rest in normal position.

The procedures are repeated to the other side and the entire protocol repeated after a short rest. These prevertebral muscles usually respond quickly to manual treatment and very often one or two treatments produce a profound change in the tissue tension. Stretching techniques (as directed below) may follow these steps and may be given as 'homework' unless contraindicated due to ligamentous or disc damage.

MET stretch of longus capitis

CAUTION: **Stretching with the head in extension can be dangerous if circulation to the cranium is in any way compromised (see p. 172).**

- To treat right longus capitis, the patient is supine and positioned so that the head extends beyond the edge of the table. The practitioner stands facing the left side of the head (which is clear of the end of the table) and firmly supports it.
- The practitioner's right hand grasps the right side of the patient's occiput while stabilizing the head against the practitioner's trunk with the head in a neutral position.
- The practitioner's left forearm and hand lie across

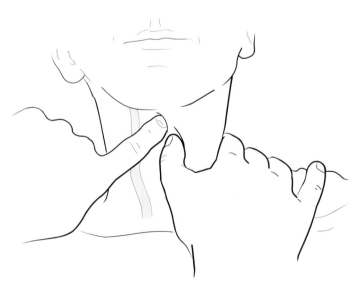

Figure 11.62 After the trachea, hyoid bone and thyroid cartilage are displaced, the carotid pulse is carefully located to assess if adequate space is available for palpation of longus colli and longus capitis (shown here). Extreme **CAUTION** is exercised to avoid any contact with the carotid artery as gentle friction or static pressure is applied. This technique is not recommended without prior hands-on, supervised

the patient's chest with the hand on the patient's right shoulder, pressing it onto the table.

- Using this hold, the practitioner applies gentle cephalad traction in order to take out slack and then introduces slight (10° maximum) extension, sidebending and rotation to the left (so stretching right-side longus capitis) by means of the firm occipital hold and body movement.
- When slack has been taken out the patient is asked to *gently* sideflex and turn the head back toward the right, against resistance, for 5–7 seconds.
- When this effort ceases the traction, extension, sidebending and rotation is then increased *slightly* by the practitioner and held for 10 seconds.
- This stretch effectively includes most of the anterior throat musculature including the various hyoid-related structures and platysma, as well as rectus capitis anterior.
- No force should be used and no pain produced by the procedure and the treatment should be stopped if dizziness is reported.
- Repeat on the opposite side.

Rectus capitis anterior

Attachments: Anterior aspect of the lateral mass of the atlas and the root of its transverse process to the inferior surface of the basilar portion of the occipital bone just anterior to the occipital condyles
Innervation: Ventral rami of C1–2 or C3
Muscle type: Phasic (type 2), weakens when stressed
Function: Flexes the head on the atlas
Synergists: Longus capitis, sternocleidomastoid (when the cervical spine is already in flexion)
Antagonists: Rectus capitis posterior major and minor, splenius capitis, semispinalis capitis, trapezius, SCM (when the cervical spine is already in extension)

Indications for treatment

- Loss of extension of cranium

Special notes

This muscle is sometimes called the rectus capitis anterior minor when the longus capitis is referred to as the rectus capitis anterior major. However, recently published texts refer to them as rectus capitis anterior and longus capitis. Trigger point referral patterns from or to these deep anterior cervical tissues have yet to be established.

According to Upledger & Vredevoogd (1983), bilateral hypertonicity of either longus capitis or rectus capitis anterior inhibits occipital flexion and unilateral hypertonicity would be likely to produce torsional forces at the cranial base (the sphenobasilar junction). The possibility of such a torsion occurring in an adult skull is remote once ossification has taken place.

Longus capitis may be reached behind the posterior pharyngeal wall through the open mouth (Simons et al 1998). If rectus capitis anterior can be palpated, it would be in a similar manner, through the longus capitis, deep to the uppermost portion of its fibers. However, this is a difficult technique and requires significant skill. It is doubtful whether it could be reached otherwise.

Muscle energy techniques and active stretches involving flexion and extension of the (isolated) altlanto-occipital joint will address rectus capitis anterior and lateralis, longus capitis and the upper posterior suboccipitals. Extension stretches should be sparingly and carefully applied due to the location of the vertebral artery in the suboccipital triangle.

Rectus capitis lateralis

Attachments: Upper surface of the transverse process of the atlas to the inferior surface of the jugular process of the occipital bone
Innervation: Ventral rami of C1–2
Muscle type: Phasic (type 2), weakens when stressed
Function: Unilaterally, slight lateral flexion of the cranium to the same side; bilaterally, flexes the head on the atlas
Synergists: *For head flexion*: suprahyoids and infrahyoids when the mouth is closed, rectus capitis anterior, SCM (when the neck is already flexed), longus capitis
For lateral flexion of the head: ipsilateral obliquus capitis superior, scalene medius when it attaches to the atlas, longissimus capitis, levator scapula
Antagonists: *To cervical flexion*: posterior cervical muscles (especially suboccipital muscles), SCM (when the neck is already extended)
For lateral flexion of the head: contralateral rectus capitis lateralis, longissimus capitis, obliquus capitis superior, contralateral levator scapula

Indications for treatment

- Unstable atlas or one locked in sidebend
- Tenderness or discomfort around the styloid process region

Special notes

The attachments on the styloid process should be addressed before beginning this work. They are presented in this text with the mandibular muscles on p. 280. Additionally, indiscriminate or accidental pressure onto the styloid process should be avoided when addressing the rectus capitis lateralis. The practitioner should be cautious with hand (finger) placement to avoid the styloid process as it is fragile as well as sharp. The fingernail of the treating finger should be cut short and filed smooth.

The external carotid artery and hypoglossal nerve course

near the styloid and transverse processes. Care must be taken not to occlude the neurovascular structures against the osseous elements.

 ### NMT for rectus capitis lateralis

CAUTION: **This NMT procedure should be carried out with extreme care**.

The patient is supine with the head rotated contralaterally approximately 45° away from the mid-line, which moves the styloid process slightly away from the transverse process and opens the space slightly into which the treating finger will be placed. The practitioner stands at the level of the upper chest and facing the patient's head.

To find the transverse process of the atlas (C1), the practitioner's index finger of either hand is placed *without any pressure* onto the anterior surface of the styloid process. From this position, the finger is moved one finger tip width posteriorly, then one finger tip width inferiorly, then one finger tip width medially. If the practitioner has large hands and the patient's structure is more petite, half finger widths should be applied or the smallest finger used as the treating tool. The order of movement is important to avoid the ligaments which course superficially to the mandible and to the hyoid bone and to ultimately place the treating finger onto the anterior surface of the transverse process of the atlas.

Gentle static pressure is applied directly onto the anterior surface of the transverse process of the atlas (Fig. 11.63). While rectus capitis lateralis attaches to the upper surface of the transverse process and very likely

will not be touched directly, connective tissue continuations may be influenced on the transverse process itself. If not too tender and if neurovascular structures are clear of the treatment finger, gentle medial/lateral friction may be applied as well. This area is often extremely tender and may require several applications of light pressure. The authors caution against the use of heavy, or even moderate, pressure on C1 when treating myofascial tissues. This upper cervical area is involved in major proprioceptive input as well as containing important and vulnerable neural structures and blood vessels and all manual approaches to it should be gentle.

Scalenes (Fig. 11.64)

Attachments: *Anticus*: C3–6 anterior tubercles of the transverse processes to the superior aspect of the 1st rib anterior to the subclavian artery
Medius: C2–7 posterior tubercles of the transverse processes to the superior surface of 1st rib posterior to the subclavian artery
Posticus: C4–6 posterior tubercles of the transverse processes to the 2nd rib
Minimus: C7 (C6) anterior tubercle to the suprapleural membrane and 1st rib
Innervation: Ventral rami – anterior: C4–6; medius: C3–8; posterior: C6–8; minimus: C8
Muscle type: Phasic (type 2), weakens when stressed, but modifies to type 1 (postural) if pattern of use demands this, as in asthmatic or habitual hyperventilation breathing (Lin 1994)

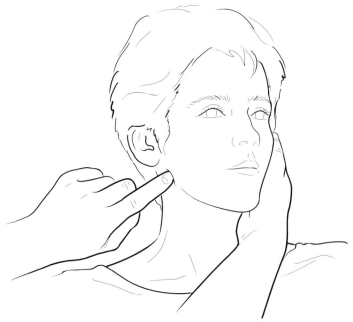

Figure 11.63 The styloid process is first located and pressure on it avoided when attempting to locate the anterior aspect of the transverse process.

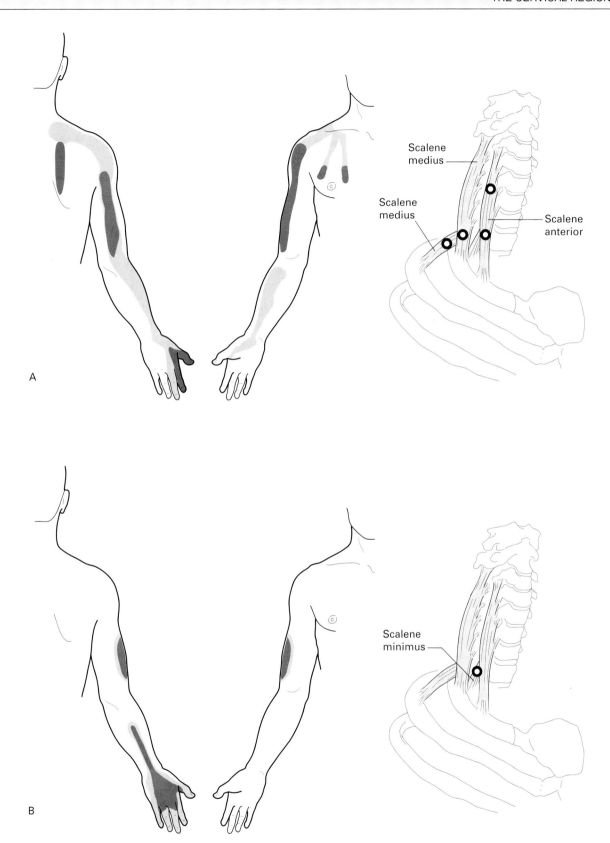

Figure 11.64   Scalene trigger points produce patterns of common complaint which may come from any of the scalene muscles.

Function: Unilaterally, the scalene group flexes the cervical spine laterally and rotates the spine contralaterally. Bilaterally, they flex the neck and assist in elevation of the 1st and 2nd rib (which assists inspiration)

Synergists: *For lateral flexion*: ipsilateral sternocleidomastoid, prevertebral muscles, posterior cervical muscles

For contralateral rotation: ipsilateral sternocleidomastoid, contralateral splenius cervicis, levator scapula, rotatores, multifidi

For flexion of the cervical spine: longus colli, longus capitis, suprahyoids, infrahyoids, platysma

Antagonists: *For lateral flexion*: contralateral scalenes, SCM, longus colli, posterior cervical muscles

For contralateral rotation: contralateral SCM, scalenes and ipsilateral splenius cervicis, levator scapula

For flexion of the cervical spine: posterior cervical muscles, SCM (when the neck is already extended)

Indications for treatment

- Arterial obstruction to arm
- Compression of brachial plexus
- Diagnosis of thoracic outlet syndrome or carpal tunnel syndrome
- Chest, back and arm pain (any or all of these)
- Tingling and numbness in hand associated with entrapment syndrome
- Whiplash syndrome, particularly if lateral flexion action was involved
- Cervical dysfunctions which are not responding to other modalities
- Sedentary lifestyle, leading to quiet breathing patterns as the norm
- Evidence of dysfunctional breathing patterns in general
- Loss of vertical dimension of cervical discs

Special notes

The attachment sites of the scalene muscles vary as does their presence. The scalene posterior is sometimes absent and sometimes blends with the fibers of medius. Scalene medius is noted to frequently attach to the atlas (*Gray's anatomy* 1995) and sometimes extend to the 2nd rib (Simons et al 1998). The scalene minimus (pleuralis), which attaches to the pleural dome, is present one-third (Platzer 1992) to three-quarters (Simons et al 1998) of the time on at least one side and, when absent, is replaced by a transverse cupular ligament (Platzer 1992).

The brachial plexus exits the cervical column between the scalenus anticus and medius. These two muscles, together with the 1st rib, form the scalene hiatus (also called the scalene opening or scalene posticus aperture) (Platzer 1992). It is through this opening that the brachial plexus and vascular structures for the upper extremity pass. When these muscle fibers are taut, they may directly entrap the nerves (scalene anticus syndrome) or may elevate the 1st rib against the overlying clavicle and indirectly entrap the vascular or neurologic structures (simultaneous compromise of both neural and vascular structures is rare) (*Stedman's medical dictionary* 1998). Any of these conditions may be diagnosed as thoracic outlet syndrome, which is 'a collective title for a number of conditions attributed to compromise of blood vessels or nerve fibers (brachial plexus) at any point between the base of the neck and the axilla' (*Stedman's medical dictionary* 1998).

During respiration, the scalenes assist by tractioning the upper two ribs and pleura cranially. This action increases the diameter of the thoracic cavity, thereby supporting inspiration. When diaphragmatic function is reduced, scalenes may become overloaded, especially in quiet breathing. See Chapter 14 for more detail of the important role these muscles play in respiration.

When longus colli holds the neck rigid and cervical lordosis is reduced, the bilateral scalenes flex the cervical column on the thoracic column (as in looking down at one's own chest). However, when the cervical column is not held rigid, bilateral contraction of the scalenes flexes the cervical column on the thoracic column *and accentuates cervical lordosis* (as if looking up) which, when dysfunctional, may contribute considerably to forward head posture when the eyes and ears are brought to horizontal level.

 NMT for scalenes

The treatment of the scalenes can be performed in either supine or sidelying posture (see Box 11.15). Both positions are discussed here.

The patient is supine with the head rotated contralaterally approximately 45°. The practitioner is seated cephalad to the patient's head and locates the sternal and clavicular attachments of the sternocleidomastoid muscle. The patient may need to lift the head slightly to make the SCM more obvious to palpation. Contralateral head rotation will move the SCM medially and allow a slightly better access to the scalene anticus, which often lies under SCM's lateral edge. Additionally, lateral flexion against resistance will assist the practitioner in locating the muscle bellies. One side is treated at a time.

The practitioner uses the first two fingers of the treating hand to locate the scalene anticus just lateral to or slightly under the edge of the clavicular head of SCM (Fig. 11.66A). It will feel similar to the clavicular SCM and will attach to the first rib. The subclavian artery is avoided by palpating its pulse and locating the fingers to avoid the artery which courses between the scalene anticus and medius.

Box 11.15   Sidelying position repose

It is frequently useful to place the patient in a sidelying position for treatment of particular muscles or when, due to the patient's physical condition (such as during pregnancy), she is unable to lie supine or prone. If a sidelying position is necessary for a particular treatment protocol but the person is unable to lie in that position, a supine or prone position can usually be substituted.

When the patient is placed in a sidelying position, the head is supported on a pillow or bolster so that the cervical spine is maintained straight in the mid-sagittal plane. The head should not remain unsupported during the session nor should the patient attempt to support the head with an arm, as cervical and upper extremity musculature might become stressed and uncomfortable. This potentially stressful position could activate trigger points as well as produce exacerbation of the current condition or discomfort in additional areas.

In a sidelying position, the lower leg (the one on the table) is kept fairly straight while the uppermost leg is flexed at the hip and knee which brings it forward, where it is laid on a bolster or thick support pillow to maintain the leg in a neutral sagittal plane. This positioning of the legs stabilizes the pelvis and discourages torsioning of the torso while also allowing access to the medial aspect of the thigh of the lower leg. Likewise, the lateral torso, uppermost lateral hip and upper extremity are more accessible in a sidelying posture. This is the preferred position described in this text for treatment of these areas.

When the upper extremity is addressed in the sidelying position, the patient's uppermost arm is often placed in a supported position (p. 346) so that the practitioner has both hands free. In the supported arm position, the patient's lower arm (tableside) is flexed to 90° at both the shoulder and the elbow and internally rotated to grasp the uppermost arm just above the elbow. The upper arm is also flexed to 90° with internal rotation and the forearm and hand passively hangs toward the floor (Fig. 11.65).

Chiropractor and certified Feldenkrais practitioner John Hannon (1999) has described a number of useful, supported positions which can enhance 'repose'. 'Repose embodies the state of quiet readiness. This represents more than peace of mind or muscular relaxation, although both may be featured prominently. Repose indicates as much stillness and restfulness as is consistent with the potential for instant action in any direction.'

Pillows and wedges are used to relieve inappropriate defensive

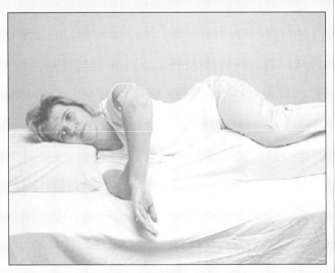

Figure 11.65   The lower body is comfortably bolstered in a sidelying position and the upper arm may be supported by the patient which allows the practitioner to use both hands when applying techniques.

muscular activity. Additionally, manual therapists may find Body Support Cushions™* to be a valuable tool in positioning the patient. Their design is intended to most ideally support the body in prone, supine or sidelying positions. Both authors encourage the principles on which the design of this system is based, offering as it does most of its support via bony prominences, allowing the soft tissues to release spontaneously during treatment. Additionally, the space built into the mid-portion of the body support system allows comfortable prone lying, even in advanced pregnancy.

*Body Support Systems Inc., PO Box 337, Ashland OR 97520 (800) 448–2400 or (541) 488–1172

The fingers apply unidirectional (laterally oriented) transverse friction in a gentle snapping manner, beginning near the 1st rib and working up toward the tubercle attachments. Uncontrolled aggressive snapping techniques are avoided and considerable caution must be exercised to avoid the artery and also the brachial plexus which exits the vertebrae between the first two scalene muscles. Entrapment of the nerves or irritation of them by the treating fingers should be avoided and the fingers repositioned if electrical-shock like referrals are provoked. Additionally, extreme caution is used to avoid pressing the nerves into the foraminal gutters which lie between the anterior and posterior tubercle. These gutters are sharp and could damage the nerves or myofascial tissues which attach nearby.

The treating fingers are moved posterolaterally and onto the scalene medius (Fig. 11.66B). This muscle is the longest and usually the largest of the scalene group. The treating fingers repeat the transverse frictional steps

while avoiding the brachial plexus which exits the spinal column between the first two scalene muscles. When taut bands are located in any of the scalene muscles, flat palpation against the underlying tubercles can be applied provided the nerves are not compressed or irritated by the treating fingers.

The fingers are moved again posterolaterally and onto the scalene posticus, which attaches to the 2nd rib and lies almost directly under the ear when the head is in neutral position and in proper coronal alignment (Fig. 11.66C). This muscle is often difficult to palpate. Transverse friction and static pressure techniques are again used to assess this short scalene muscle. Unidirectional finger movements oriented anteriorly will usually identify this muscle when it is present, if it can be palpated.

The tubercle attachments may be treated by flexing the fingers so that they arch around to the anterior aspect of the transverse processes and are placed directly onto

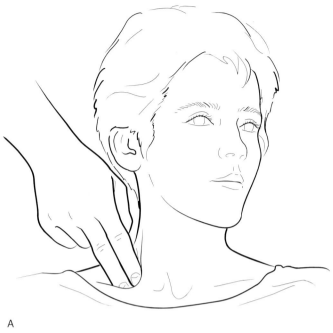

A

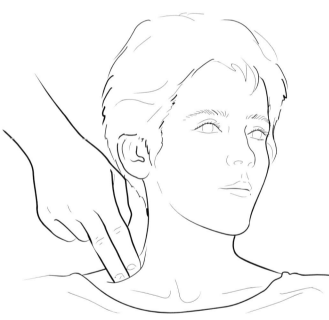

B

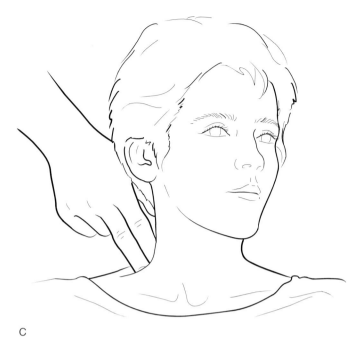

C

Figure 11.66 When the scalene muscles are treated, **CAUTION** must be exercised to avoid the brachial plexus which courses between the scalenus anterior and medius. A: Scalenus anterior. B: Scalenus medius. C: Scalenus posterior.

the anterior tubercles while taking care to avoid the nerves coursing immediately posterior to the tubercles (Fig. 11.67A). The posterior tubercles are found by sliding onto them from a posterior direction. The transverse processes are located and the fingers slide around their lateral tips and onto the posterior tubercles (Fig. 11.67B). Mild, minute frictional movements or light static pressure are used, while ensuring that the sharp foraminal gutters and cervical nerves are avoided.

Variation in sidelying position. The scalenes may also be treated with the patient in sidelying position and with the head rotated toward the table approximately 45°

(Fig. 11.68). The practitioner stands posterior to the head. The patient can simply begin to lift the head off the table with no resistance needed to activate the scalenes for verification of their location. The scalene anticus will be located just lateral to the SCM and will feel similar to the SCM clavicular head. The entire length of the anterior, middle and posterior scalenes are each separately assessed and treated in a manner similar to the supine description above. General gliding techniques on the lateral neck are *not* recommended due to the location of the brachial plexus and its close proximity to the sharp foraminal gutters.

 Treatment of short scalenes by MET

• The patient lies supine with a cushion or folded towel under the upper thoracic area so that, unless supported by the practitioner's contralateral hand, the head would fall into extension.

• The head is rotated contralaterally (away from the side to be treated).

• There are three positions of rotation required:

1. full contralateral rotation of the head/neck produces involvement of the more posterior fibers of the scalenes
2. a contralateral 45° rotation of the head/neck involves the middle fibers
3. a position of only slight contralateral rotation involves the more anterior fibers.

• The practitioner's free hand is placed on the side of

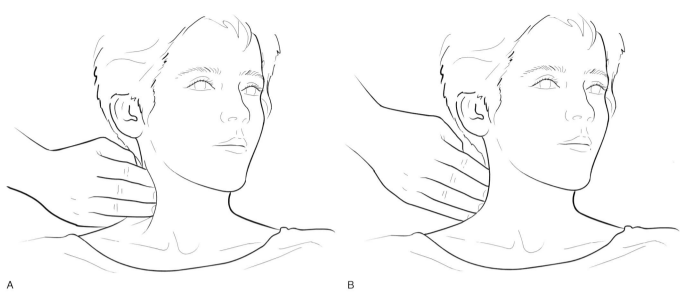

Figure 11.67 The anterior and posterior tubercles may be carefully palpated. **CAUTION** is exercised to avoid the sharp edges of the foraminal gutters and the brachial plaxus. A: Anterior tubercles. B: Posterior tubercles.

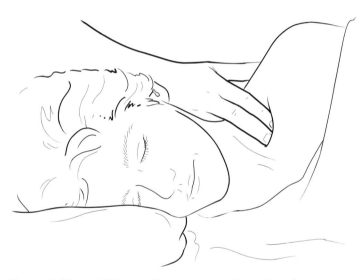

Figure 11.68 A sidelying position may be used to address the scalene muscles and their tubercle attachments.

the patient's head to restrain the isometric contraction which will be used to release the scalenes.

• With appropriate breathing cooperation ('Breathe in and hold your breath as you commence the effort, and exhale completely when ceasing the effort'), the patient is instructed to try to lift the forehead a fraction and to attempt to turn the head toward the affected side while resistance is applied by the practitioner's hand to prevent both movements ('lift and turn').

• Both the effort and the counterpressure should be modest and painless at all times.

• After a 7–10-second contraction the head is allowed to ease into extension.

• The patient's contralateral hand is placed (palm down) just inferior to the lateral end of the clavicle on the affected side.

• The practitioner's hand (which was acting to produce resistance to the isometric contraction) is now placed onto the dorsum of the patient's hand.

• As the patient slowly exhales, the contact hand, resting on the patient's hand, which is itself resting on the 2nd rib and upper thorax, pushes obliquely away and toward the foot on that same side, stretching the attached musculature and fascia.

• This stretch is held for at least 20 seconds after each isometric contraction.

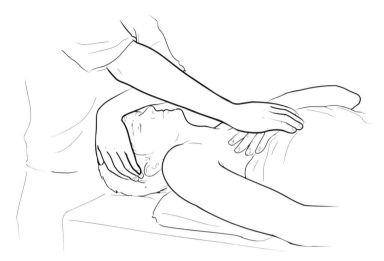

Figure 11.69 MET treatment of scalene anticus.

- The process is then repeated at least once more.
- The head is rotated 45° contralaterally and the hand contact which applies the stretch of the scalene medius is placed just inferior to the middle aspect of the clavicle (practitioner's hand on patient's hand which acts as a 'cushion').
- When the head is in neutral position for the scalene anticus stretch, the hand contact is on the upper sternum itself (again with the patient's contralateral hand as a cushion) (Fig. 11.69).
- In all other ways the methodology is as described for the first position above.

Note: It is important not to allow heroic degrees of neck extension during any phase of this treatment. There should be some extension but it should be appropriate to the age and condition of the individual.

- A degree of eye movement can assist scalene treatment.
- If the patient makes the eyes look caudally (toward the feet) and toward the affected side during the isometric contraction, she will increase the degree of contraction in the muscles.
- If during the resting phase when stretch is being introduced, she looks away from the treated side, toward the top of the head, this will enhance the stretch of the muscle.
- This whole procedure should be performed bilaterally several times in each of the three head positions.

Scalene stretches, with all their variable positions, clearly also influence many of the anterior neck structures.

Cervical lamina – prone

The muscles of the posterior cervical region may also be addressed in a prone position. This body position often reveals taut fibers which were not distinct in the supine position. The practitioner should listen carefully for communications from the patient as the face cradle may obscure the voice in a prone position. Additionally, hand signals may be needed for the patient to quickly communicate if pressure is too heavy or if trigger point referrals are experienced.

During the gliding strokes, osseous structures may be encountered in the lamina groove. These dense calcific protuberances may be bifid (split) spinous processes, a spinous process of a dysfunctional (rotated) vertebra or the effects of enthesitis on the multitude of myofascial tissues attaching in the lamina groove. When osseous tissue is found, the contralateral side is examined for similar structures. The soft tissues of the area should be examined and treated and osseous manipulations applied, if needed. However, the practitioner is strongly advised to practice within the scope of his or her professional license. Referral to the appropriate health-care practitioner for osseous assessment and manipulation may be necessary if the segments do not respond to soft tissue applications.

NMT for posterior cervical lamina – prone position

The prone patient's chin is tucked toward the chest. The practitioner stands at the level of the shoulder or chest and faces the head as he treats one side at a time. One or both of the practitioner's thumbs begin at the level of C7 and glide superiorly from C7 to the occiput, while maintaining contact against the lateral surface of the spinous processes and the lamina. The fingers provide stability for the thumbs as they repeat the gliding stroke 6–8 times (Fig. 11.70).

The thumbs are moved laterally about 1″ and the

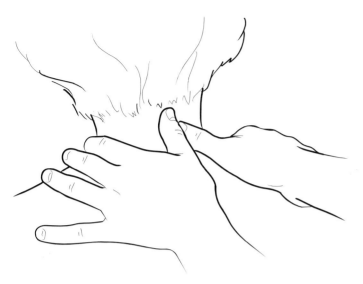

Figure 11.70   The fingers help to stabilize the thumbs when gliding cranially in the lamina groove.

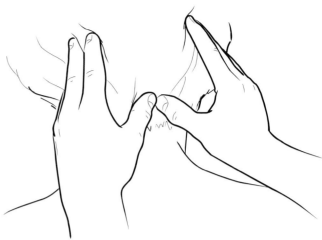

Figure 11.71   Multiple attachments on the posterior cranium may be assessed as the thumbs contact the occipital bone.

gliding strokes repeated 6–8 times. The gliding strokes are continued in strips in the lamina through the postero-lateral aspect of the transverse processes. The strokes are *not* continued further anteriorly due to the position of the brachial plexus and the sharp edges of the foraminal gutters on the anterolateral surface of the transverse processes.

Unidirectional or bidirectional transverse friction may be applied to the attachments of the levator scapula, splenius cervicis and other posterior cervical muscles unless contraindicated due to inflammation. Detailed protocols for assessing and treating the trapezius (p. 320) and the levator scapula (p. 329) are also offered in the prone position.

🖐️ 🖐️ NMT for posterior cranial attachments

The prone patient's chin is tucked slightly, in order to gently open the suboccipital space between the occiput and C1 (atlas). The practitioner remains at the level of the shoulder or chest, facing the head to treat the ipsilateral side. Excessive stretching into flexion is not recommended for these procedures which treat the soft tissues of the posterior suboccipital region, due to the position of the vertebral artery in the lateral aspect of the sub-occipital space between C1 and the occiput. Caution is exercised to avoid the vertebral artery which lies relatively exposed in the suboccipital triangle.

The fingers provide stability and support for the movements of the thumbs. The thumbs are touching end to end and are placed just caudal to the inferior nuchal line where the rectus capitis posterior major and minor attach and between the inferior and superior nuchal lines

where the obliquus capitis superior attaches (Fig. 11.71). Transverse (medial/lateral) friction is applied to the cranial attachments of posterior cervical muscles and mid-belly region of the suboccipital muscles. Static pressure may also be applied when trigger points are located in the suboccipital muscles or posterior cervical muscles lying superficial to them, or when tissues are too tender to be frictioned. The attachments of trapezius, semi-spinalis capitis, splenius capitis, longissimus capitis and sternocleidomastoid may be included in this examination of posterior cranial attachments. Cranial-to-caudal friction may also be used as long as the vertebral artery is avoided (see p. 206).

The frictional techniques are repeated between C1 (atlas) and C2 (axis) to address the inferior half of rectus capitis posterior major and obliquus capitis inferior through the overlying tissues. Lighter pressure may be needed and may only penetrate into the superficial tissues if they are too tender to be pressed through.

The attachments on the transverse process of C1 of obliquus capitis superior and inferior, levator scapula and splenius cervicis muscles are carefully examined. The SCM may need to be displaced anterolaterally in order to palpate the muscles attaching to the transverse process of C1. Caution is exercised to maintain contact with the posterolateral tip of the transverse process and not allow the thumbs to intrude into the suboccipital triangle due to the vertebral artery's location within the triangle (Fig. 11.72).

The thumbs are placed on the occipitalis muscle which lies approximately 1–2″ lateral to the occipital protuberance (Fig. 11.73). Transverse friction or static pressure can be used to examine the occipitalis muscle. This thin, flat muscle attaches to the superior nuchal line of the occipital bone and to the galea aponeurotica (epicranial aponeurosis), which attaches to the skin over the cranium

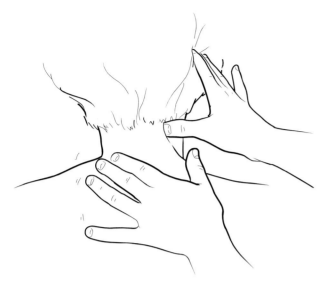

Figure 11.72 The transverse process of the atlas is the attachment site of several muscles which may be treated with carefully applied unidirectional (lateral) friction.

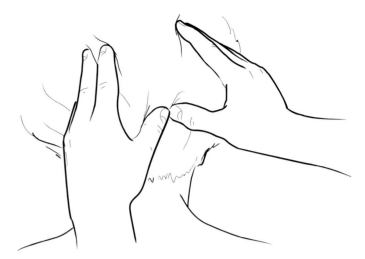

Figure 11.73 The thin, flat occipitalis muscle is part of the epicranius and refers strongly into the eye region.

and slides it over the bony surface of the cranium as the brows are lifted.

Occipitalis' fibers are often *not* distinct and the practitioner must rely on anatomy knowledge rather than palpation skills when locating it. When occipitalis' fibers are taut, they may be vaguely palpable but their tenderness and trigger point referrals will be apparent to the patient when they are involved. Movement of this muscle may be palpable on some individuals when the eyebrows

are raised repeatedly, since it merges with the cranial aponeurosis and connects with the frontalis muscle. However, with the patient prone, the face cradle may inhibit the movement of the cranial fascia and prevent palpation of distinct movement of the occipitals.

Trigger point referrals from occipitalis often produce strong patterns of pain, pressure and headache into and around the orbit of the ipsilateral eye. The weight of the head on a solid foam pillow may irritate occipitalis trigger points and cause the patient to awaken in the night with the headache (eyeache) pattern. See further discussion with the cranium in the following chapter.

REFERENCES

Allen M E (ed) 1996 The new whiplash. Musculoskeletal pain emanating from the head and neck. Haworth Press, New York

Buskila D, Neumann L 1997 Increased rates of fibromyalgia following cervical spine injury. Arthritis and Rheumatism 40(3):446–452

Cailliet R 1991 Neck and arm pain, 3rd edn. F A Davis, Philadelphia

Calais-Germain B 1993 Anatomy of movement. Eastland Press, Seattle

Cassidy 1996 Quebec Task Force on Whiplash Associated Disorders. Journal of Musculoskeletal Pain 4(4):5–9

Chaitow L 1991 Modified strain counterstrain. In: Soft tissue manipulation. Healing Arts Press, Rochester, Vermont

Chaitow L 1996a Modern neuromuscular techniques. Churchill Livingstone, New York

Chaitow L 1996b Muscle energy techniques. Churchill Livingstone, Edinburgh

Chaitow L 1999 Cranial manipulation: theory and practice. Churchill Livingstone, Edinburgh

Daniels L, Worthingham C 1980 Muscle testing techniques, 4th edn. W B Saunders, Philadelphia

Evjenth O, Hamburg J 1984 Muscle stretching in manual therapy. Alfta Rehab, Alfta, Sweden

Gough P 1996 Human occupant dynamics in low-speed rear-end collisions. In: Allen M (ed) The new whiplash. Musculoskeletal pain emanating from the head and neck. Haworth Press, New York

Gray's anatomy 1973 35th edn. Longman, London

Gray's anatomy 1995 (Williams P. ed), 38th edn. Churchill Livingstone, Edinburgh

Greenman P 1989 Principles of manual medicine. Williams and Wilkins, Baltimore

Greenman P 1997 Personal communication

Hack G, Koritzer R, Robinson W 1995 Anatomic relation between the rectus capitis posterior minor muscle and the dura mater. Spine 20:2484–2486

Hallgren R, Greenman P, Rechtien J 1993 MRI of normal and atrophic muscles of the upper cervical spine. Journal of Clinical Engineering 18(5): 433–439

Hallgren R, Greenman P, Rechtien J 1994 Atrophy of suboccipital muscles in patients with chronic pain. Journal of the American Osteopathic Association 94(12):1032–1038

Hannon J 1999 Pillow talk: the use of props to encourage repose. Journal of Bodywork and Movement Therapies 3(1):55–64

Harakal J 1975 An osteopathically integrated approach to whiplash complex. Journal of the American Osteopathic Association 74:941–956

Hendrickson T 1995 Manual of orthopedic massage. Privately published, Oakland, California

Hoppenfeld S 1976 Physical examination of the spine and extremities. Appleton and Lange, Norwalk

Hosono N 1991 Cineradiographic motion analysis of atlantoaxial instability at os odontoideum. Spine 16 (suppl 10):S480–482

Hu J, Vernon H, Tantourian I 1995 Changes in neck EMG associated with meningeal noxious stimulation. Journal of Manipulative and Physiological Therapeutics 18:577–581

Jacob B, McKenzie R 1996 Spinal therapeutics based on responses to loading. In: Liebenson C (ed) Rehabilitation of the spine. Williams and Wilkins, Baltimore

Janda V 1988 In: Grant R (ed) Physical therapy of the cervical and thoracic spine. Churchill Livingstone, New York

Janda V 1996 In: Liebenson C (ed) Rehabilitation of the spine. Williams and Wilkins, Baltimore

Johnston W 1985 Inter-rater reliability. In: Burrger A, Greenman P (eds) Empirical approaches to the validation of manipulative therapy. Charles C Thomas, Springfield, Illinois

Juhan D 1987 Job's body: a handbook for bodywork. Station Hill Press, Barrytown, NY

Kaltenborn F 1985 Mobilization of the extremity joints. Olaf Norlis Bokhandel, Oslo, Norway

Kapandji IA 1974 The physiology of the joints, vol. III, 2nd edn. Churchill Livingstone, Edinburgh

Kapandji IA 1982 The physiology of the joints, vol. I, 5th edn. Churchill Livingstone, Edinburgh

Kapandji IA 1998 The physiology of the joints, vol 3. The trunk and the vertebral column. Churchill Livingstone, Edinburgh

Kappler R 1997 Cervical spine. In: Ward R (ed) Foundations of osteopathic medicine. Williams and Wilkins, Baltimore

Kimmel D 1961 Innervation of the spinal dura mater and the dura mater of the posterior cranial fossa. Neurology 10:800–809

Kuchera W, Kuchera M 1994 Osteopathic principles in practice. Greyden Press, Columbus, Ohio

Leonhardt H 1986 Color atlas and textbook of human anatomy, vol 2, 3rd edn. Georg Thieme Verlag, Stuttgart

Lewit K 1985 Manipulative therapy in rehabilitation of the locomotor system. Butterworths, London

Lewit K 1992 Manipulative therapy in rehabilitation of the motor system, 2nd edn. Butterworths, London

Lewit K 1999 Manipulative therapy in rehabilitation of the motor system, 3rd edn. Butterworths, London

Liebenson C 1996 Rehabilitation of the spine. Williams and Wilkins, Baltimore

Lin J-P 1994 Physiological maturation of muscles in childhood. Lancet June 4:1386–1389

Mauraudas A, Stockwell R 1975 Factors involved in the nutrition of the human lumbar intervertebral disc: cellularity and diffusion of glucose in vitro. Journal of Anatomy 120:113

Mayer T, Brady S, Bovasso E 1994 Noninvasive measurement of cervical tri-planer motion in normal subjects. Spine 18:2191

McAtee R, Charland J 1999 Facilitated stretching. Human Kinetics, Champaign, Illinois

McKenzie R 1990 The cervical and thoracic spine: mechanical diagnosis and therapy. Spinal Publications, Waikanae, New Zealand

McPartland J, Brodeur R 1999 Rectus capitis posterior minor. Journal of Bodywork and Movement Therapies 3(1):30–35

McPartland J, Goodridge J 1997 Osteopathic examination of the cervical spine. Journal of Bodywork and Movement Therapies 1(3):173–178

Melzack R, Wall P 1989 Textbook of pain, 2nd edn. Churchill Livingstone, London

Mitchell B 1998 Attachments of ligamentum nuchae to cervical posterior dura and lateral occipital bone. Journal of Manipulation and Physiological Therapeutics 21(3):145–148

Mitchell F, Moran P, Pruzzo N 1979 Evaluation and treatment manual of osteopathic muscle energy techniques. MMP Associates, Valley Park, Missouri

Moore K 1980 Clinically oriented anatomy. Williams and Wilkins, Baltimore

Mulligan B 1992 Manual therapy. Plane View Services, Wellington, New Zealand

Myers T 1999 Kinesthetic dystonia. Journal of Bodywork and Movement Therapies 3(2):107–117

Norkin P, Levangie C 1992 Joint structure and function: a comprehensive analysis, 2nd edn. F A Davis, Philadelphia

Northfield D 1938 Some observations of headache. Brain 61:133–162

Oschman J 1997 Gravity structure and emotions. Journal of Bodywork and Movement Therapies 1(5):297–304

Peck D, Buxton D, Nitz A 1984 A comparison of spindle concentrations in large and small muscles acting in parallel combinations. Journal of Morphology 180:243–252

Penfield W, McNaughton F 1940 Dural headache and the innervation of the dura mater. Archives of Neurology and Psychiatry 44:43–75

Platzer W 1992 Color atlas text of human anatomy: vol I, locomotor system, 4th edn. Thieme, Stuttgart

Radanov B 1994 Relationship between early somatic, radiological, cognitive, psychological findings and outcome during one-year follow-up in 117 whiplash patients. British Journal of Rheumatology 33:442–448

Robbie D 1977 Tensional forces in the human body. Orthopaedic Review VI (11):46

Ross S 1999 Dysphonia: osteopathic treatment. Journal of Bodywork and Movement Therapies 3(3):133–142

Schafer R 1987 Clinical biomechanics. Williams and Wilkins, Baltimore

Simons D, Travell J, Simons L 1998 Myofascial pain and dysfunction: the trigger point manual, vol 1, 2nd edn. Williams and Wilkins, Baltimore

Spitzer W, Skovrom M, Salmi L 1995 Scientific monograph of the Quebec Task Force on Whiplash Associated Disorders. Spine 20:8S

Stedman's electronic medical dictionary 1998 version 4.0. Williams and Wilkins, Baltimore

Steiner C 1994 Osteopathic manipulative treatment – what does it really do? Louisa Burns Memorial Lecture October 12 1993. Journal of the American Osteopathic Association 94(1):85–87

Stiles E 1984 Manipulation – a tool for your practice. Patient Care 45:699–704

Taylor J 1994 Pathology of neck sprain. International Journal of Pain Therapy 4:91–99

Taylor J, Taylor M 1996 Cervical spine injuries. In: Allen M (ed) The new whiplash. Musculoskeletal pain emanating from the head and neck. Haworth Press, New York

Upledger J, Vredevoogd J 1983 Craniosacral therapy. Eastland Press, Seattle

Van Mamaren H 1992 Cervical spine motion in the sagittal plane II. Spine 17(5):467–474

Ward R (ed) 1997 Foundations of osteopathic medicine. Williams and Wilkins, Baltimore

Warfel J 1985 The extremities, 5th edn. Lea and Febiger, Philadelphia

Zink G, Lawson W 1979 An osteopathic structural examination and functional interpretation of the soma. Osteopathic Annals 12(7):433–440

12

The cranium

The head is so central to human function that reemphasis of its importance may seem unnecessary. However, aspects of its role may usefully be restated. Most important human functions are expressed by, through, in and on the cranium, whether this involves thinking, neurological processing, speaking, eating, seeing, listening, expressing or breathing. The cranium not only houses four of the five senses but is also a major element in a remarkable balancing act which allows normal function of these (e.g. breathing, hearing, sight, speech) and also helps create a state of equilibrium in the face of major challenges imposed by gravity and human behavior. Where the head is held in space helps determine muscle tone and critically influences the efficiency with which all bodily tasks are performed (Alexander 1957).

Craniosacral and sacrooccipital concepts have emerged which place dysfunction of the bones of the skull, its sutures and internal fascial structures (dura, reciprocal tension membranes, etc.), as well as the circulation of blood, lymph and cerebrospinal fluid through it, at the center of many health problems. In this chapter we will examine aspects of this vast range of cranial activities, from the perspective of the influences which can be modified by neuromuscular and associated techniques.

CRANIAL STRUCTURE

Before treating apparent cranial dysfunction, attention should be given to soft tissue changes, muscle and fascia, which could, for example, be impacting upon cranial suture mobility. The descriptions which follow will use the following format.

- Named bone and constituent parts
- Bones with which it articulates and named junctions (sutures) (*Gray's anatomy* 35th edn, 1973). This information will be provided either as text or as a detailed figure
- Reciprocal tension membrane relationships with named bone (if any)

- Muscular attachments (if any)
- Range and direction of motion to be anticipated if normal (using traditional cranial osteopathic and craniosacral terminology) (Box 12.1)
- Other associations and influences
- Dysfunctional patterns and consequences
- Palpation exercises (for some key bones)

The palpation exercises which are included derive from traditional cranial osteopathic methods (Brookes 1981). Additionally some of the methods described are taken from the teachings of acknowledged cranial experts to whom credit is offered in the text (Kingston 1996, Milne 1995, Wilson & Waugh 1996). In many of these exercises the phrase 'wait for release' or 'when you sense a release' will be found. Box 12.2 explains what this phrase means.

Single (central) cranial bones:

- occiput
- sphenoid
- ethmoid
- vomer
- mandible
- frontal.

Paired bones:

- parietals

Box 12.1 Cranial terminology and associated motion patterns based on traditional osteopathic methodology

During cranial **flexion** (also known as the *inhalation phase*), the paired bones of the skull *rotate externally*. This part of the cranial cycle is associated with the following.

- The occipital base is said to move anteriorly/superiorly.
- The sacral base moves posteriorly/superiorly ('sacral flexion').
- The mid-line bones of the skull 'flex'.
- The paired bones of the skull externally rotate.
- The effect of these movements is to flatten and widen the skull (transverse diameter increases while anteroposterior diameter decreases, vertex becomes flattened).
- The tentorium cerebelli flattens and falx cerebri shortens from front to back.
- The spinal column straightens as a whole.
- The ventricles fill.

During cranial **extension** (also known as the *exhalation phase*), the paired bones of the skull *rotate internally* as they return to their neutral starting position.

- All cranial motions in this phase involve a return to neutral.
- The occipital base is said to move posteroinferiorly.
- The sacral base moves anteroinferiorly (sacral 'extension').
- The mid-line bones 'extend' to their starting positions.
- The paired bones internally rotate to their starting positions.
- The effect of this is for the skull to become longer and narrower (transverse diameter decreases while anteroposterior diameter increases, vertex becomes more elevated).
- The tentorium cerebelli domes and the falx cerebri is restored to its normal position.
- The spinal curves are restored to normal.
- The ventricles empty.

Box 12.2 The meaning of 'release'

Holding tissues, sutures or joints in a position of relative comfort or ease or applying specific techniques may result in a 'release' of the dysfunctional pattern, either completely or partially. How is the practitioner to recognize when this occurs?

There are certain guidelines based on the clinical experience of many experts which can indicate a local tissue release.

- A sense of steady and strong pulsation, or of greater warmth, enters the area.
- A very definite change (reduction) in palpated tone is noted.
- A sense of the tissues 'lengthening' or 'freeing up' is perceived.

On a wider, whole-body level, such release phenomena may also involve deeper emotional release, sometimes called 'emotional discharge'. This may be accompanied by all or any of the following.

- The patient becomes flushed and a change in skin color is observed, from pale to ruddy perhaps.
- A light perspiration appears on the patient's upper lip or brow.
- The breathing pattern may alter and may become slow and deep or, in contrast, may become quicker and be accompanied by rapid eye movement and restlessness.
- Observation of the diaphragm region may provide useful information of such a change being imminent or current.
- Fasciculation may be observed, with trembling and twitching intermittently or constantly.
- The patient may express a wish to vomit or cry or may simply begin crying or laughing.

How should such changes be handled? If a local release is noted this can be held and gently released with nothing more being done to the particular area at that session apart from some soothing massage strokes. Alternatively, the holding pattern can continue at the new 'barrier', as the tissues are offered the opportunity to continue to release, perhaps in the form of an unwinding process. The skills appropriate for such technique application need to be learned in suitably detailed instructional forums.

The 'emotional release' phenomenon is discussed in detail in Chapter 4.

- temporals
- zygomae
- maxillae
- palatines.

Associated within the text but not discussed in detail:

- lacrimals (paired)
- inferior conchae (paired)
- nasal (single)
- sacral (single).

See Box 12.3 for anatomical groupings of these bones.

Occiput

- The squama, the main body of the bone which forms the posterior border of the foramen magnum
- The basiocciput, which forms the anterior border of the foramen magnum and which possesses a rostrum joining it to the sphenoid at the synchondrosis

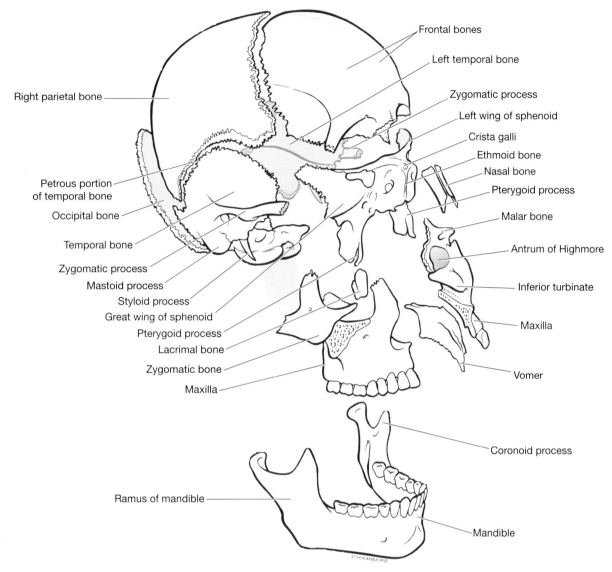

Figure 12.1 Disarticulated skull showing major bony components (reproduced, with permission, from Chaitow (1999)).

- The condyles, which form the lateral borders of the foramen magnum

Articulations

- With the atlas at the condyles.
- With the sphenoid at the synchondrosis – this is potentially mobile up to age 20 or so (*Gray's anatomy* 1973, p. 311).
- With the parietal bones at the lambdoidal suture.
- With the temporal bones. The jugular notch of the occiput and the jugular fossa of the temporal bone meet to form an articulation.
- Posterior to this notch there is a beveled articulation which is partially internally (anterior aspect of articulation) and partially externally (posterior aspect

of articulation) beveled, with a point of transition known as the condylosquamomastoid pivot which allows an easily achieved rocking potential in clinical evaluation and treatment.
- Anterior to the notch the basiocciput has a tongue-and-groove articulation with the petrous portion of the temporal bone.

Reciprocal tension membrane relationships with the occiput

- Both the falx cerebri and tentorium cerebelli attach to the occiput.
- The bifurcated falx cerebri attachment is above the internal protuberance and houses the superior sagittal sinus.

Box 12.3 Cranial bone groupings

Vault bones

- Two parietal bones
- Occipital squama
- Those portions of the temporal bone which develop from membrane

Cranial base

- Body of sphenoid
- Petrous and mastoid portions of temporal bones
- Basilar and condylar portions of the occiput (formed from cartilage)

Facial bones

- Malar
- Lacrimal
- Palatine
- Nasal
- Turbinate
- Ethmoid
- Maxillae
- Mandible
- Frontal
- Vomer

Bones of the ear

- Incus
- Stapes
- Malleus

Unpaired (mid-line) bones

- Occiput
- Sphenoid
- Ethmoid
- Vomer
- Mandible

Paired bones

- Parietals
- Temporals
- Frontals
- Zygomae
- Maxillae
- Palatines
- Lacrimals
- Inferior conchae
- Nasal
- Incus
- Stapes
- Malleus

- Below the internal protuberance is the attachment of the falx cerebelli.
- Lateral to the internal protuberance are double ridges formed by the bifurcated tentorium cerebelli attachments, with the transverse sinuses located within the bifurcations.

Muscular attachments (Fig. 12.2)

- Occipitofrontalis, which is really two muscles which cross many sutures:
  1. occipitalis which attaches to the occiput and temporal bones (via tendinous fibers to the mastoid), crossing the suture on the lateral aspects of the superior nuchal line
  2. frontalis which has no bony attachments but merges with the superficial fascia of the eyebrow area with some fibers continuous with fibers of corrugator supercilii and orbicularis oculi, attaching to the zygomatic process of the frontal bone and further linkage to the epicranial aponeurosis anterior to the coronal suture.
- Trapezius (upper) attaches to the superior nuchal line and external occipital protuberance as well as the ligamentum nuchae.
- Longus capitis attaches to the inferior surface of the basiocciput.
- Rectus capitis anterior attaches to the inferior basiocciput, anterior to the condyle and to the lateral mass and root of the transverse process of C1 (atlas).
- Splenius capitis attaches to the superior nuchal line and mastoid process, crossing the suture, and the spinous processes of the lower half of the cervical spine (Platzer 1992, Simons et al 1998) to T3 and the lower part of the ligamentum nuchae. *Gray's anatomy* (1973, 1999) notes that this muscle attaches to the ligamentum nuchae and spinous processes of C7 through T3 and their supraspinous ligaments.
- Semispinalis capitis and spinalis capitis attach to the superior and inferior nuchal lines and the transverse processes of C7, T1–7 and the articular processes of C4–6.
- Rectus capitis lateralis attaches to the jugular process of the occiput as well as the transverse process of the atlas.
- Rectus capitis posterior major is one of the suboccipital muscles which lie deep and attaches to the lateral aspect of the inferior nuchal line as well as to the spinous process of the axis.
- Rectus capitis posterior minor is one of the suboccipital muscles which lie deep and attaches to the medial aspect of the nuchal line and to the posterior arch of the atlas, commonly described as acting to bilaterally extend the head and maintain its postural integrity. This unusual muscle has been shown to attach to the posterior atlantooccipital membrane via dense connective tissue and to be fused to the dura by numerous connective tissue elements (only recently identified – see more detailed notes on pp. 34, 240) (Hack et al 1995).
- Obliquus capitis superior is one of the suboccipital muscles which lie deep and attaches between the inferior and superior nuchal lines as well as to the transverse process of the atlas.

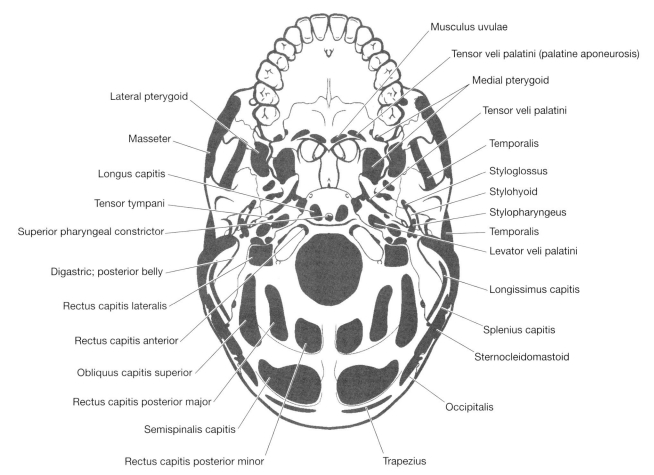

Musculus uvulae
Tensor veli palatini (palatine aponeurosis)
Medial pterygoid
Tensor veli palatini
Temporalis
Styloglossus
Stylohyoid
Stylopharyngeus
Temporalis
Levator veli palatini
Longissimus capitis
Splenius capitis
Sternocleidomastoid
Occipitalis
Trapezius

Lateral pterygoid
Masseter
Longus capitis
Tensor tympani
Superior pharyngeal constrictor
Digastric; posterior belly
Rectus capitis lateralis
Rectus capitis anterior
Obliquus capitis superior
Rectus capitis posterior major
Semispinalis capitis
Rectus capitis posterior minor

Figure 12.2 Inferior view of skull, without mandible, showing muscular attachments (reproduced, with permission, from Chaitow (1999)).

Restrictions and hypertonicity in any of these muscles, uni- or bilaterally, will strongly influence occipital function.

Range and direction of motion

The concept of any flexion potential in the adult occipitosphenoidal junction remains questionable. There is, however, an undoubted degree of pliability at the occiput's sutural junctions with the parietals. A powerful pivot point also exists between the occiput and the temporal bone which allows the temporals to 'externally rotate' when mobility is normal.

When palpating the occiput, the motion of this bone, easing anteriorly on inhalation and returning to its start position on exhalation, raises the question as to what drives it. Various hypotheses exist – respiratory influences; the reciprocal tension membrane responding to intrinsic forces (CSF, for example); direct response to muscular influences, and others. When palpating the bone, it is suggested that the slight degree of motion that may be noted is assessed with no preconceptions as to what may be driving it (Chaitow 1999).

Dysfunctional patterns

- Any injury affecting the atlantooccipital joint is likely to negatively influence occipital motion.
- Blows to the occiput from behind can cause a crowding or distortion pattern of the occipital base with the sphenoid, prior to ossification.
- Any injuries or strains affecting the temporal or parietal bones will influence the occiput, and sutural restrictions relating to parietal or temporal articulations may then evolve.
- Muscular dysfunction in the suboccipital region can directly influence dural status and thereby cerebrospinal fluid fluctuations (see notes on rectus capitis posterior minor above and in Chapters 3 and 11).
- Internal drainage of the cranium can be directly influenced by changes affecting the reciprocal tension membranes which attach to the occiput and which house both the superior sagittal and the lateral sinuses.

Palpation exercises

Palpation of sphenobasilar synchondrosis. This exercise is performed using two different holds.

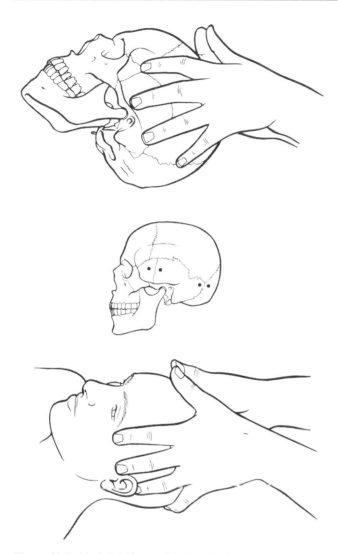

Figure 12.3 Vault hold for cranial palpation (reproduced, with permission, from Chaitow (1999)).

Vault hold (Fig. 12.3). Patient is supine, the practitioner is seated at her head with forearms resting on the table. Fingers are placed in a relaxed manner so that:

- small finger is on the squamous portion of the occiput
- ring finger rests behind the ear near the asterion so that the distal portion of finger is just on the mastoid
- middle finger is anterior to the ear to rest on the pterion with the tip touching the zygomatic process
- index finger rests on the great wing of sphenoid
- thumbs rest, touching each other or crossed, without touching the head if possible, allowing pressure between them to form a base for the flexor muscles of the hand to operate.

The practitioner sits quietly for at least 2 minutes or until cranial motion is noted (a sense of intermittent

'fullness' in the palms of the hands may be all that is noted initially).

As the flexion phase (also known as the inhalation external rotation phase) of the cranial cycle commences (manifested by noting of a sense of fullness, slight tingling, minute pressure in palms of hands or in wrists/forearms, by proprioceptors) the following *might* be noted:

- ring and middle fingers seem to be carried caudally and laterally
- index finger seems to be carried anteriorly and caudally.

These real or apparent motions are all passive with no effort on the part of the practitioner.

As sphenobasilar extension commences (exhalation/internal rotation phase) a sense *might* be noted of the palpated bones returning toward their starting position (index finger moves cephalad and posteriorly, while ring and middle fingers move cephalad and medially).

Frontooccipital hold (Fig. 12.4). Patient is supine and the practitioner sits to right or left near the head of the table.

- The caudad hand rests on the table cradling the occipital area so that the occipital squama closest to the practitioner rests on the hypothenar eminence, while the tips of the fingers support the opposite occipital angle.
- The practitioner's cephalad hand (closest to the head) rests over the frontal bone so that the thumb lies on one great wing of the sphenoid and the tips of the fingers on the other great wing, with as little contact as possible on the frontal bone.
- If the practitioner's hand is small, contacts are made on the lateral angles of the frontal bone. It may be some minutes before cranial motion is noted.

As sphenobasilar flexion (inhalation/external rotation phase) commences (sensation in the hands of fullness, tingling, etc.), the practitioner *might* feel:

- occipital movement which is caudad and anterior, while simultaneously
- the great wings seem to rotate anteriorly and caudally around their transverse axis.

If these motions are sensed they may be encouraged, in order to assess any restriction, by using very light pressure (grams only) in the appropriate directions to impede the movement described.

During sphenobasilar extension (exhalation/internal rotation phase) a return to neutral may be noted, as the lower hand goes cephalad and the upper hand goes cephalad and posteriorly.

These two palpation exercises offer an opportunity to assess the disputed mid-line motion functions, flexion

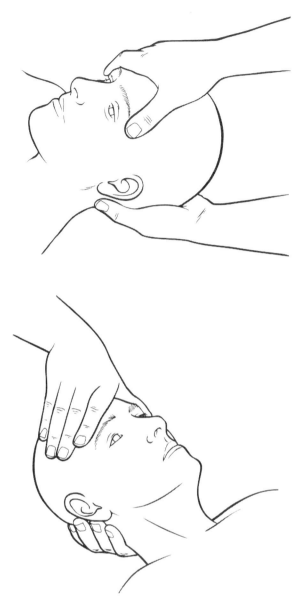

Figure 12.4 Frontooccipital hold for cranial palpation (reproduced, with permission, from Chaitow (1999)).

and extension, of the cranial mechanism, that of the sphenobasilar synchondrosis and all that flows from it.

- Can these motions of the occiput and/or the sphenoid be sensed?
- If movement is felt, what is actually moving?
- Does the movement continue when the patient holds the breath?
- Is the movement accentuated by deep inhalation and/or exhalation?

There are no definitive answers at present as to what is actually happening, with opinions varying from orthopedic to subtle energy hypotheses. Aspects of some of these concepts are included in this chapter – see in particular the 'liquid electric' hypothesis in descriptions of

sphenoidal function, immediately below (Chaitow 1999, Ettlinger & Gintis 1991, Greenman 1989, Upledger & Vredevoogd 1983).

Sphenoid

- The body, situated at the center of the cranium – a hollow structure enclosing an air sinus
- Two great wings, the lateral surfaces of which form the only aspect palpable from outside the head, the temples, and the anterior surfaces of which form part of the eye socket
- Two lesser wings, the anterior surfaces of which form part of the eye socket
- Two pterygoid processes which hang down from the great wings and which are palpable intraorally posteromedial to the 8th upper tooth
- The pterygoid plates which form part of the pterygoid processes and are important muscular attachment sites
- The sella turcica ('Turkish saddle') which houses the pituitary gland
- The sphenobasilar junction with the occiput, a synchondrosis which fuses in adult life (*Gray's anatomy* 1973)

Articulations

- With the occiput at the synchondrosis
- With the temporal bones at the petrous portion and posterolaterally with the squama
- With the parietal bones at the pterion
- Anteriorly with the ethmoid
- Inferiorly with the palatine bones
- Anteriorly both greater and lesser wings articulate with the frontal bone bilaterally
- Inferiorly with the vomer
- Anterolaterally with the zygomae

Reciprocal tension membrane relationships with the sphenoid

Both falx cerebri and tentorium cerebelli attach to the sphenoid.

Muscular attachments

- The temporalis muscle attaches to the great wing and the frontal, parietal and temporal bones, crossing important sutures such as the coronal, squamous and the frontosphenoidal.
- Specifically the attachments of temporalis are to the temporal bone and to the coronoid process and the anterior border of the ramus of the mandible.
- Attaching to the internal pterygoid plate are buccinator as well as a number of small palate-related muscles.
- Medial pterygoid attaches to the lateral pterygoid

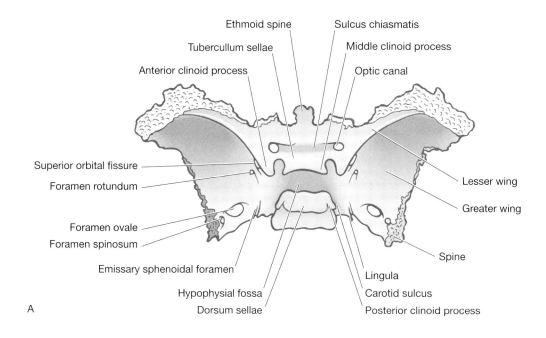

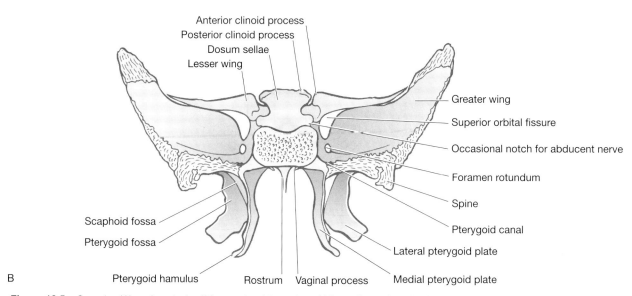

Figure 12.5 Superior (A) and posterior (B) aspects of the sphenoid bone (reproduced, with permission, from Chaitow (1999)).

plate and palatine bones running to the medial ramus and angle of the mandible.

- Lateral pterygoid attaches to the great wing of the sphenoid, the lateral pterygoid plate and the anterior neck of the mandible and its articular disc.

- Various small muscles relating to movement of the eye, as well as levator palpebrae which help raise the eyebrows, attach to those parts of the great wings of the sphenoid which form part of the eye socket.

Range and direction of motion

- In traditional osteopathic thinking the sphenoid rotates anteriorly on flexion and returns to a neutral position

during the extension phase of the cranial respiratory cycle (Fig. 12.7).

- In the adult skull, it is suggested that this motion is impossible (due to fusion of the sphenobasilar synchondrosis) but it remains a central part of the belief system of most craniosacral therapists.

- Models other than the original osteopathic one exist for explaining the influence of cranial function and dysfunction, including what is termed the 'liquid electric model' which hypothesizes that cranial bones move in response to motion of the brain, which is itself responding to the rhythmic pulls imparted by the spinal dura and a variety of muscular influences.

- In this model the cranial bones 'float' and move in

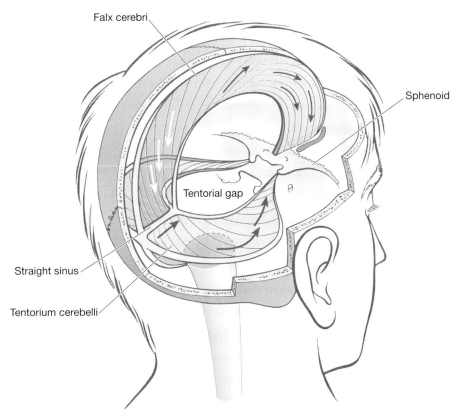

Figure 12.6 The reciprocal tension membranes of the cranium (reproduced, with permission, from Chaitow (1999)).

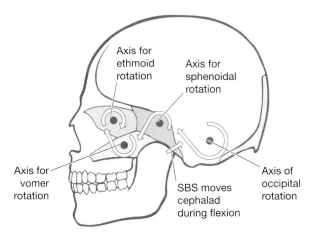

Figure 12.7 Schematic representation of hypothesized cranial motion features (SBS = sphenobasilar synchondrosis) (reproduced, with permission, from Chaitow (1999)).

relation to a central focal point at the center of the brain. There are in this concept no fixed axes or pivot points, with all movement responding to tissue changes elsewhere. Milne (1995) explains, 'Neurocranial bones float, as if they had neutral buoyancy and were suspended in water, and are pushed or pulled by tidal electrical, muscular, and osseous forces'.

• This model envisions a mechanism which is open to multiple forces and avoids the physiological denial inherent in the 'bending joint' of the classic osteopathic model.

Other associations and influences

• The first six cranial nerves have direct associations with the sphenoid, with the 2nd (optic), 3rd (part of oculo-motor), 4th (trochlear), 5th (nasociliary, frontal, lacrimal, mandibular and maxillary branches of trigeminus) and 6th (abducens) all passing through the bone into the eye socket (the 1st, the olfactory nerve, runs superior to the lesser wings).

• The intimate relationship with the pituitary gland suggests that endocrine function can be strongly influenced via dysfunction of the sphenoid which creates circulatory or other stresses on the gland.

• The muscular links with the mandible create a connection between temporomandibular dysfunction and sphenoidal dysfunction, with the influences being possible from either direction.

Dysfunctional patterns

• Because of the intimate linkage with neural structures, sphenoid dysfunction can be directly associated with optical, trigeminal and acoustic disturbances.

• Because of the proximity to the pituitary gland, endocrine disturbances may be an outcome of sphenoidal dysfunction.

• According to the structural/mechanical model a range of possible 'lesion' patterns may exist between the sphenoid and any of its articulating neighbors, deriving from trauma (possibly including forceps delivery or stressful birth trauma), which can be evaluated and treated by a process of testing (see palpation exercises below).

• If the 'energetic' or 'fluid' model is accepted, a different, more intuitive, unstructured approach to palpation is suggested, as discussed in the exercises section below.

Palpation exercises

General sphenoidal release (also known as 'sphenoid lift'). Since, in the mechanical/structural model of cranial therapy, it is considered that six possible dysfunction patterns can exist at the sphenobasilar junction, these are tested and treated while the occiput and sphenoid are lightly palpated.

• The patient's head is cradled in the hands so that the fingers enfold the occiput and the thumbs rest lightly on the great wings of the sphenoid.

• By lightly (ounces at most) drawing the thumbs

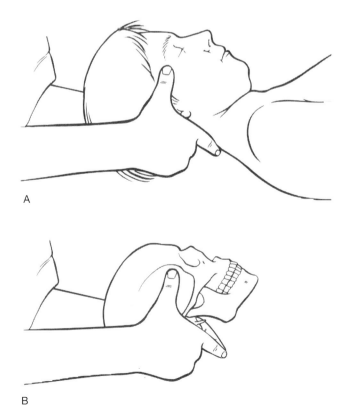

A

B

Figure 12.8 Hand positions for contact with the great wings of sphenoid (reproduced, with permission, from Chaitow (1999)).

toward the hands, the sphenoid is 'crowded toward the occiput'.

• This crowding is held for several seconds at which time the thumbs alter their direction of push and are lightly drawn directly toward the ceiling, so (theoretically) decompressing the sphenobasilar junction and applying traction to the tentorium cerebelli as the weight of the cranium drags onto the practitioner's palms and fingers.

• With the hold as described, the ease of movement of the sphenoid is very lightly, individually assessed. These methods will not be described as they require a degree of training for safe application.

In order to evaluate this approach through other eyes, a quotation from Hugh Milne's (1995) insightful text *The heart of listening* will be useful (p. 277). Milne suggests 1/5 of an ounce contact pressure which is approximately 5.5 grams, much the same as is recommended by Upledger & Vredevoogd (1983).

To introduce decompression of the sphenobasilar joint, first take out all the skin slack under your thumbs so that you have a firm purchase over the wings themselves – not on the supraorbital ridges or the orbital portions of the zygomae. Then gradually increase thumb pressure on the greater wings, monitoring the status of the sphenoid, the occiput and the sphenobasilar joint as you gently and fluidly introduce decompression.

Milne suggests that it is possible to distinguish six levels of tissue separation from first contact to final completion.

1. Skin, scalp and fascia
2. Slower muscular release (occipitofrontalis and temporalis mainly)
3. Sutural separation ('akin to prising apart a magnet from a piece of metal')
4. Dural release (like 'elastic bands reluctantly giving way')
5. Freeing of the cerebrospinal fluid circulation ('the whole head suddenly feels oceanic, tidal, expansive … this is the domain of optimized cerebrospinal fluid')
6. Finally energetic release ('a tactile sensation of chemical electrical fire unrolling and spreading outwards in waves under your fingers')

In this poetic language we can sense the nature of the debate between those who wish to understand what is happening in orthopedic terms and those who embrace 'fluid/electric' and energetic concepts.

Ethmoid

• A tissue paper-thin construction comprising a central horizontal plate (cribriform) which contains tiny openings for the passage of neural structures, surrounded by
• Shell-shaped air sinuses forming a honeycomb

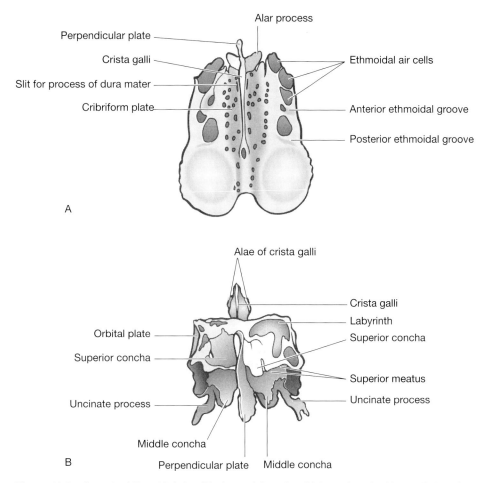

Perpendicular plate
Crista galli
Slit for process of dura mater
Cribriform plate

Alar process
Ethmoidal air cells
Anterior ethmoidal groove
Posterior ethmoidal groove

A

Alae of crista galli

Orbital plate
Superior concha
Uncinate process
Middle concha

Crista galli
Labyrinth
Superior concha
Superior meatus
Uncinate process

B
Perpendicular plate   Middle concha

Figure 12.9 Superior (A) and inferior (B) views of the ethmoid (reproduced, with permission, from Chaitow (1999)).

framework to each side of the plate which is crowned by

- A thin crest (crista galli) formed by the dragging attachment of the falx cerebri
- Thin bony plate-like structures which form the medial eye socket
- Additional projections and plates, one forming part of the nasal septum, with the perpendicular plate being a virtual continuation of the vomer (see below)

Articulations

There are interdigitated sutures with the sphenoid and non-digitated sutures with the vomer, nasal bones, palatines, maxillae and the frontal bone.

Reciprocal tension membrane relationships

- The falx cerebri attaches directly to the crista galli.
- The inferior border connects with the nasal cartilage.

There are no direct muscular attachments to the ethmoid.

Range and direction of motion

The traction of the falx on the crista galli pulls it superiorly and slightly anteriorly. Pulling of the falx must determine major aspects of the ethmoid's motion potential. The presumed axis of rotation suggests that the ethmoid rotates in an opposite direction to the supposed sphenoid rotational axis, as though they were geared together.

Air passing through the shell-like ethmoid air cells is warmed before reaching the lungs and the alternation of pressures as air enters and leaves the ethmoid must influence minor degrees of motion between it and its neighboring structures. Because in life its tissue paper-like delicacy has a sponge-like consistency it is presumed that the structure acts as a local shock absorber.

Other associations and influences

The 1st cranial (olfactory) nerve lies superior to the cribriform plate and from this derive numerous neural penetrations of it which innervate mucous membranes which provide us with olfactory sense.

Dysfunctional patterns

When sinus inflammation exists the ethmoid is likely to be swollen and painful. Because of its role as a shock absorber it is potentially vulnerable to blows of a direct nature and to soaking up stresses from any of its neighbors.

There is no direct way of contacting the ethmoid but it can be easily influenced via contacts on the frontal bone or the vomer.

Palpation exercises

Nasal release technique

- The patient's forehead (frontal bone) is gently cupped by the practitioner's caudad hand as he stands to the side and faces the supine patient.
- The practitioner's cephalad hand is crossed over the caudad hand so that the index finger and thumb can gently grasp the superior aspects of the maxillae, inferior to the frontomaxillary suture.
- The unused fingers of the previously cephalad and now caudad hand should be folded and resting on the dorsum of the other hand.
- A slow, rhythmical separation of the two contacts is introduced so that the hand on the forehead is applying gentle pressure toward the floor, so pushing the falx cerebri away from the ethmoid and dragging on it, while the finger and thumb of the now caudad hand are easing the maxillae anteriorly.
- The 'pumping', repetitive separation and release applications continue for at least a minute to achieve a local drainage effect, enhanced air and blood flow through the ethmoid and release of the sutural restrictions.

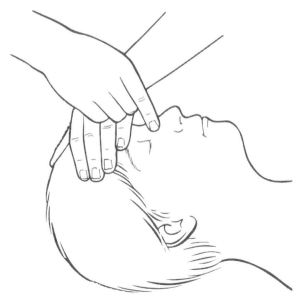

Figure 12.10 Treatment of the ethmoid using pincer contact (reproduced, with permission, from Chaitow (1999)).

- This method is thought to be more effective if this dual action coincides with what is perceived to be the flexion stage of the cranial cycle.
- Alternatively, the separation hold can be maintained until release (see Box 12.2) is noted.
- The separation action (pulsed or constant) eases sutural impaction which may exist between the ethmoid as it is taken away from the frontal, nasal and maxillary bones into its presumed external rotation position (flexion phase of the cycle).

Vomer

- This is a plough-shaped sandwich of thin bony tissue which houses a cartilaginous membrane, which forms the nasal cartilage.
- It separates and acts as a junction point between the ethmoid, maxillae, palatines and sphenoid.

Articulations

- Superiorly, it articulates with the sphenoid as a tongue-and-groove joint of spectacular beauty.
- On the inferior aspect of the sphenoid the vomer also has minor articulation contacts with the palatine bones at the rostrum.
- There is a direct, plain (not interdigitated) suture with the ethmoid at its anterosuperior aspect. The vomer is a virtual continuation of the ethmoid's perpendicular plate.
- The inferior aspect of the vomer articulates with the maxillae and the palatines.
- There is a cartilaginous articulation with the nasal septum.

There are no direct associations with the reciprocal tension membranes and there are no direct muscular attachments.

Range and direction of motion

The vomer's range of motion is identical to the ethmoid and opposite to the sphenoid.

Other associations and influences

- As with the ethmoid, this is a pliable shock-absorbing structure which conforms and deforms dependent upon the demands made on it by surrounding structures.
- The mucous membrane covering the vomer assists in warming air in nasal breathing.

Dysfunctional patterns

- In rare cases, the vomer can penetrate the palatine suture, producing an enlargement/swelling of the central portion of the roof of the hard palate, a condition known as torus palatinus.

- As with the ethmoid, inflammation of the vomer is probable in association with sinusitis.
- Direct trauma can cause deviation of the vomer and so interfere with normal nasal breathing.

Mandible

- A body, which is the horizontal portion which meets at the central jaw protuberance with the body of the other side, at the symphysis menti.
- Attached to the posterior aspect of the bodies are the rami, the vertical portions of the mandible.
- Each ramus forms two projections, the posterior of which becomes the articular condyle, via a slender neck, for its articulation with the temporal bone while the anterior forms the coronoid process to which attach the temporals.

Articulations

The only osseous articulation of the mandible is with the temporal bone via the disc at the temporomandibular joint. It also articulates with its teeth, which articulate (occlude) with the upper teeth set in the maxillae.

There are no reciprocal tension membrane connections.

Major muscular attachments

- Temporalis, which attaches to the temporal fossae, running and converging medial to the zygomatic arch with insertion on the coronoid process and the ramus of the mandible. The anterior/superior fibers occlude the teeth as the mandible is elevated while the posterior fibers assist in retraction of the jaw as well as lateral chewing movements.
- Masseter attaches via its superficial fibers to the zygomatic process and arch while the deeper fibers arise from the deeper surface of the zygomatic arch. Superficially, it inserts into the lateral ramus while the deeper fibers attach to the upper ramus and to the coronoid process. Its functions are to occlude the jaw during chewing and (by means of fibers running in different directions) to alternately retract and protrude the mandible during chewing. This is considered to be the most powerful muscle in the body.
- Lateral pterygoid attaches to the greater wing of the sphenoid as well as to the lateral pterygoid plate, both heads inserting via a tendon to the anterior aspect of the neck of the mandible and the articular disc of the temporomandibular joint. The various actions in which the muscle is involved include depression and protrusion of the mandible as well as offering stability to the temporomandibular joint when the mandible is closing.

- Medial pterygoid arises superficially from the tuberosity of the maxilla as well as from the palatine bone. A deeper origin is from the medial pterygoid plate and the palatine bone. Superficial and deeper fibers merge to attach to the medial ramus of the mandible close to the angle. The functions of the muscle are to elevate and protrude the mandible (acting with the lateral pterygoid and the masseter) and contralateral deviation of the mandible.
- Digastric arises from two sites: the posterior belly from the mastoid notch of the temporal bone and the anterior belly from the digastric fossa on the internal surface of the anterior aspect of the mandible. The two parts of the muscle link via a tendon which is attached to the hyoid bone by a fibrous connection. Its actions are to depress the mandible, elevate the hyoid bone and assist in retraction of the mandible.
- Platysma's anterior fibers interlace with the contralateral muscle, across the mid-line, below and behind the symphysis menti. Intermediate fibers attach to the lower border of the mandibular body while the posterior fibers cross the mandible and the anterolateral part of the masseter and attach to subcutaneous tissue and skin of the lower face. The actions of platysma involve reducing the concavity between the jaw and the side of the neck. Anteriorly, it may assist in depressing the mandible or draw the lower lip and corners of the mouth inferiorly, especially when the jaw is already open wide.
- Mylohyoid arises from the inner surface of the mandible and attaches to the hyoid bone. Its function is to depress the mandible and to elevate the hyoid during swallowing.
- Geniohyoid attaches at the symphysis menti and runs to the anterior surface of the hyoid bone, acting in much the same manner as mylohyoid.

Minor muscular attachments (not described here)

- Buccinator
- Depressor angularis oris
- Orbicularis oris
- Depressor labii inferioris
- Hyoglossus
- Mentalis
- Superior pharyngeal constrictor
- Genioglossus

Range and direction of motion

Involuntary motion of the mandible relates to motion of the temporal bones with which it articulates. This will be modified by the degree of muscular contraction at their junction.

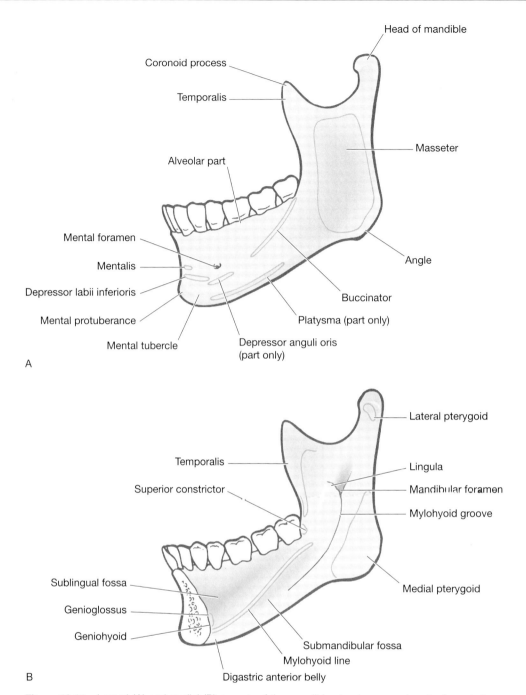

Figure 12.11 Lateral (A) and medial (B) aspects of the mandible showing muscular attachment sites (reproduced, with permission, from Chaitow (1999)).

There is some disagreement as to the 'normal' active range of motion of the mandible which in various texts is considered to be between 42 mm and 52 mm (Rocobado 1985, Tally 1990). Skaggs (1997) reports:

Rocobado (1985) states maximum mandibular opening to be 50 mm, thereby taking the periarticular connective tissue to 112% stretch. He qualifies that the stretch of the periarticular connective tissue should not exceed 70–80%, thus making functional mandibular range of motion approximately 40 mm. Okeson's recent (1996) guidelines cite normal minimum

interincisal distance and active ranges of motion to be 36 to 44 mm and less in women.

There is more to the range of motion of the mandible than mechanics, as Milne (1995) points out.

The mandible is more open to psychological input than any other bone in the head ... unexpressed aggression, determination, or fear of speaking out, cause changes in mandibular motion that range from subtle to dramatic. For instance, in states of rage the mandible is so muscularly tense that almost all movement is lost.

Dysfunctional patterns

Both physical and emotional injuries and stresses can result in dysfunctional temporomandibular joint behavior. The effects are demonstrated in pain, clicking and variations on the theme of restriction and abnormal opening and closing patterns (see Box 12.4, p. 271). We believe that in almost all instances of TMJ dysfunction, soft tissue considerations should be primary.

It is suggested that the soft tissues associated with the joint receive appropriate attention before joint corrections are attempted and that this be combined with home exercise strategies for rehabilitation, as well as with attention to underlying causes whether these lie in habits (bruxism, gum chewing, etc.) or emotional turmoil and stress coping abilities.

Palpation exercises

TMJ compression and decompression (Fig. 12.12).

CAUTION: Patients with anterior articular disc displacement may find the compression techniques too uncomfortable but they may receive benefit and relief with the decompression techniques. If the patient reports considerable discomfort with compression, discontinue immediately.

- The patient is supine and the practitioner is seated at the head.
- The palms of the hands are placed onto the side of the patient's face so that they follow the contours, the thenar eminences are placed over the TMJ and the fingers curve around the jaw. No lubricant is used at this stage.
- The hands are gently drawn cephalad so that traction is applied to the skin and fascia of the cheeks, until all the slack has been removed. The temporomandibular joint will in this way be overapproximated/crowded.
- This is held for not less than a minute and longer if it is not uncomfortable for the patient.
- The direction of traction is then reversed so that a distraction occurs as the skin and fascia is taken to its elastic limits and the underlying structures are eased away from the TM joint. This is held for at least one and ideally several minutes.
- A sense of 'unwinding' may be noted as the tissues release, in which case the motion is followed without any direction being superimposed.

MET method 1 (Fig. 12.13)

- If the mandible cannot open fully or adequately, reciprocal inhibition may be utilized.
- The patient is seated close to and facing the treatment table.
- The mouth is open to its comfortable limit and, following the isometric contraction (described below), it

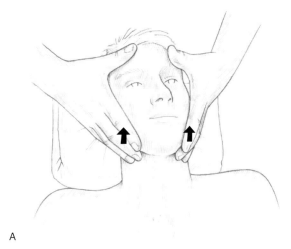

A

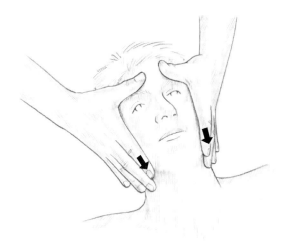

B

Figure 12.12 Crowding (A) and decompression (B) stages of temporomandibular treatment (reproduced, with permission, from Chaitow (1999)).

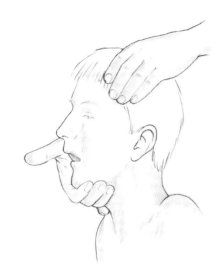

Figure 12.13 MET treatment of temporomandibular joint involving restricted opening (reproduced, with permission, from Chaitow (1999)).

is opened further (by the patient and/or the practitioner) to its new barrier, before repeating.

• The patient is asked to open the already open mouth further, against resistance applied by the practitioner's or the patient's own hand (in self-treatment the patient places her elbow on the table, chin in hand and attempts to open her mouth against her own resistance for 10 seconds or so), thus inhibiting the muscles which act to close the mouth.

• This MET method has a relaxing effect on those muscles which may be shortened or tight and which are acting to restrict opening of the mandible.

MET method 2 (Fig. 12.14)

• Lewit (1992) suggests the following method for TMJ problems, maintaining that laterolateral (lateral excursion) movements of the mandible are particularly important.

• The patient sits with the head turned to one side (say toward the left, in this example).

• The practitioner stands behind her and stabilizes the patient's head against his chest with his right hand.

• The patient opens her mouth, allowing the chin to drop, and the practitioner cradles the mandible with his left hand, so that the fingers are curled under the jaw.

• The practitioner draws the mandible gently toward his chest and when the slack has been taken up, the patient offers a degree of resistance to it being taken further laterally.

• After a few seconds of gentle isometric contraction, the practitioner and patient slowly relax simultaneously and the jaw will usually have an increased lateral excursion.

• This is repeated three times.

• This method should be performed so that the lateral pull is away from the side to which the jaw deviates on opening.

Self-treatment exercise

• Gelb (1977) suggests a retrusive exercise be used, as follows.

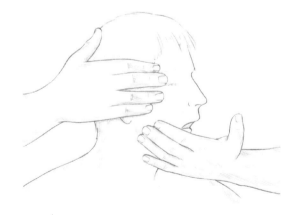

Figure 12.14 MET treatment of temporomandibular joint involving lateral deviation (reproduced, with permission, from Chaitow (1999)).

• The patient curls the tongue upwards, placing the tip as far back on the roof of the mouth as possible.

• While this is maintained in position, the patient slowly opens and closes the mouth (gently), to activate the suprahyoid, posterior temporalis and posterior digastric muscles (the retrusive group).

Frontal

• A central metopic suture which is usually fused but sometimes (rarely) interdigitated, on the inside of which lie the attachments for the bifurcated falx cerebri
• Bilateral concave domed bosses which house the frontal lobes of the brain as well as air sinuses at the inferior medial corner
• Superciliary arches, a nasal spine and the medial aspects of the eye socket

Articulations

• With the parietals at the interdigitated coronal suture.
• With the ethmoid at the ethmoidal notch.
• With the sphenoid at the greater and lesser wings.
• With the zygomae via the interdigitated zygomatic process at the dentate suture.
• With the maxillae via the frontal process.
• With the temporals (not always).
• With the lacrimal bones and the nasal bones.

Reciprocal tension membrane relationships

The falx cerebri attaches strongly to the inner aspect of the mid-line of the frontal bone at a double crest formed by its bifurcated attachments, which creates a space which becomes the superior sagittal sinus.

Muscular attachments (see Fig. 12.24, p. 265)

• Temporalis arises from the temporal fossa and its fibers converge to attach on the coronoid process and ramus of the mandible, medial to the zygomatic arch. The origin of temporalis crosses the coronal suture between the frontal and parietal bone as well as the suture between the temporal bone and the parietal.

• Occipitofrontalis covers the entire dome of the skull from the superior nuchal line to the eyebrows, completely enveloping the parietal suture. The muscle also spans the lambdoidal and coronal sutures, attaching via direct or indirect linkages with the frontal, temporal, parietal and occipital bones. Frontalis merges with the superficial fascia of the eyebrow area while some fibers are continuous with fibers of corrugator supercilii and orbicularis oculi attaching to the zygomatic process of the frontal bone,

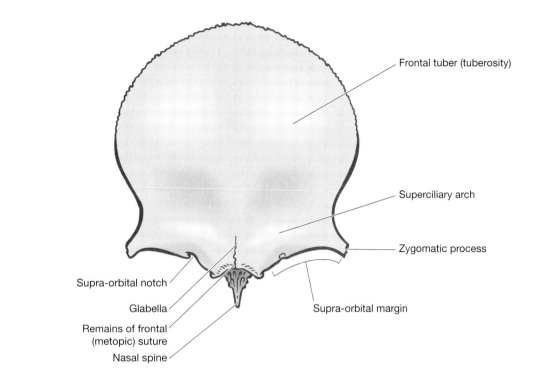

Frontal tuber (tuberosity)

Superciliary arch

Zygomatic process

Supra-orbital notch

Glabella

Remains of frontal
(metopic) suture

Nasal spine

Supra-orbital margin

A

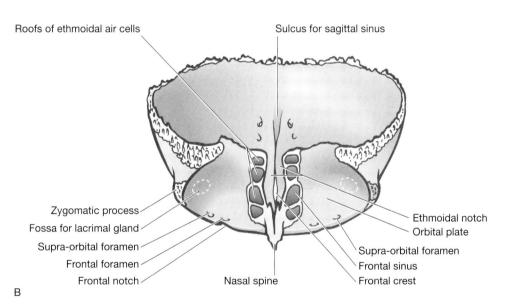

Roofs of ethmoidal air cells

Sulcus for sagittal sinus

Zygomatic process

Fossa for lacrimal gland

Supra-orbital foramen

Frontal foramen

Frontal notch

Nasal spine

Ethmoidal notch

Orbital plate

Supra-orbital foramen

Frontal sinus

Frontal crest

B

Figure 12.15   Frontal (A) and inferior (B) aspects of the frontal bone (reproduced, with permission, from Chaitow (1999)).

with further linkage to the epicranial aponeurosis anterior to the coronal suture.

• Corrugator supercilii lies medial to the eyebrow and comprises a small pyramid-shaped structure lying deeper than occipitofrontalis and orbicularis oculi.

• Orbicularis oculi is a broad flat muscle which forms part of the eyelids, surrounds the eye and runs into the cheeks and temporal region. Parts are continuous with occipitofrontalis.

• Procerus is a slip of nasal muscle which is continuous with the medial side of the frontal part of occipito-frontalis.

Range and direction of motion

During flexion the frontal bone is said to be:

...carried by the sphenoid wings and, held by the falx cerebri, and so rotates about an oblique axis through the squama so that the glabella moves posterior, the ethmoid notch widens, the orbital plate's posterior border moves slightly inferior and lateral, the zygomatic processes move anterior and lateral and the squama 'bend' and recede at the midline. (Brookes 1981)

It is the combined effect of sphenoidal flexion and the backwards pull of the falx during the flexion phase of the cycle which is thought to produce the mid-line frontal bone flexion, which would be conceivable if a true suture were present but clearly could not occur if the bones had fused, as happens in most cases.

Other associations and influences

Associations with problems of the eyes and sinuses are clear from the geography of the region alone and congestion and discomfort in this area can at times be related to frontal bone compression or lack of freedom of motion. The connection with the falx cerebri offers other possible linkages, in particular to cranial circulation and drainage.

Dysfunctional patterns

Apart from direct blows to the forehead, few problems seem to arise as a direct result of frontal dysfunction. However, as with the parietals (see below), problems may arise as a result of the accommodation of the bone to influences on it, temporal, parietal, sphenoidal or from the facial bones.

Palpation exercises

Hypothenar eminence application for frontal lift (Fig. 12.16)

- The patient is supine and the practitioner sits at the head of the table, elbows fully supported and fingers interlaced so that the hypothenar eminences rest on the lateral angles of the frontal bones with the fingers covering the metopic suture.

- As the patient exhales the interlaced hands exert light compressive force to take out slack (grams only) via the hypothenar eminences (bringing them toward each other) utilizing a very slight contraction of the extensor muscles of the lower arm (particularly extensor carpi radialis longus and brevis, extensor digitorum and extensor carpi ulnaris). By utilizing the forearm extensors in this way and avoiding flexor contraction, the contacts on the frontal bone avoid 'squeezing' it, while effectively increasing gentle compression.

- At the same time a slight upwards (slightly cephalad and toward the ceiling) lift is introduced bilaterally to release the frontal bone from its articulations with the parietals, sphenoid, ethmoid, maxillae and zygomae.

- This lift is held during several cycles of inhalation and exhalation after which the frontal bone is allowed to settle back into its resting position.

Parietals

- The simplest of cranial structures – two four-sided, curved, half-domes.

Articulations

See Figure 12.17.

Reciprocal tension membrane relationships

The falx cerebri attaches strongly into a groove on each side of the sagittal suture forming a space which is the

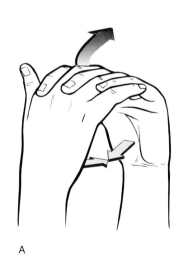
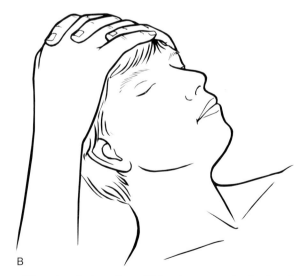

A   B

Figure 12.16 Hand actions and directions of force (A) and contact positions (B) for decompression treatment of frontal bone (reproduced, with permission, from Chaitow (1999)).

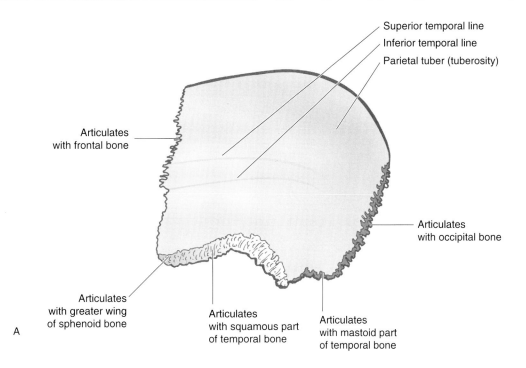

Superior temporal line
Inferior temporal line
Parietal tuber (tuberosity)

Articulates
with frontal bone

Articulates
with occipital bone

Articulates
with greater wing
of sphenoid bone

Articulates
with squamous part
of temporal bone

Articulates
with mastoid part
of temporal bone

A

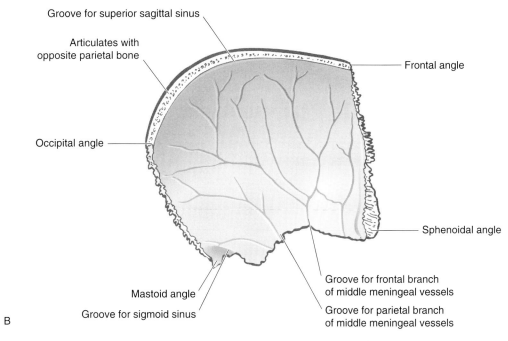

Groove for superior sagittal sinus

Articulates with
opposite parietal bone

Frontal angle

Occipital angle

Mastoid angle

Groove for sigmoid sinus

Sphenoidal angle

Groove for frontal branch
of middle meningeal vessels

Groove for parietal branch
of middle meningeal vessels

B

Figure 12.17   External (A) and internal (B) surfaces of the left parietal bone (reproduced, with permission, from Chaitow (1999)).

superior sagittal sinus. Any restriction of the sagittal suture's normal pliability (approximately 250 microns of rhythmic movement in normal subjects, 8–14 times per minute) (Lewandowski & Drasby 1996) might therefore be expected to negatively influence the status of both the attaching reciprocal tension membrane (the falx) as well as drainage via this important sinus.

Muscular attachments

• Temporalis arises from the temporal fossa and its fibers converge to attach on the coronoid process and ramus of the mandible, medial to the zygomatic arch. The origin of temporalis crosses the coronal suture as well as that between the temporal bone and the parietal.

- Auricularis superior is a thin fan-shaped muscle which arises from the epicranial aponeurosis, converging to insert by a flat tendon into the upper surface of the auricle.
- Occipitofrontalis does not attach directly to the parietals although its aponeurosis covers them.

Range and direction of motion

- Human studies indicate that approximately 250 microns of movement is available at the sagittal suture (Lewandoski & Drasby 1996). There is a greater degree of interdigitation on the posterior aspect of the sagittal suture where motion potential is therefore greatest.
- Osteopathic cranial concepts have the parietals flexing inferiorly ('flattening') at the sagittal suture.
- A more pragmatic view is that the pliability of the suture helps to absorb stresses imposed on the structure via either internal or external forces (Chaitow 1999).
- Other models (liquid/electric, energetic, etc.) offer different interpretations as to the motion potentials of these bones (Milne 1995).

Other associations and influences

The connection with the falx cerebri is one of the most important links the parietals have with the inner circulation and drainage of the cranium.

The temporal bone articulation is a key area for evidence of cranial dysfunction and for treatment, usually by means of temporal contact.

Dysfunctional patterns

Dysfunctional patterns in the parietals are rare apart from when they receive direct blows or when the resilient sutures lose their free articulation 'shock-absorbing' potential. The bones which articulate with the parietals are more likely to produce problems and when they do, the parietals are obliged to accommodate to the resulting stresses.

Palpation exercises

Parietal lift (Fig. 12.18)

- The patient is supine and the practitioner is seated at the head of the table.
- His fingers are placed so that the small finger tip rests close to the asterion anterior to the lambdoidal suture.
- The other finger pads rest on the parietal bone just above the temporoparietal suture so that the middle finger is approximately a finger width above the helix of the ear, on the parietal bone (not the temporal).
- The thumbs act as a fulcrum, bracing against each other or crossed above the sagittal suture without any direct contact.

- Gentle pressure is applied – approximately 10 grams – medially with the finger pads to crowd the sagittal suture and to disengage their temporal articulation.
- This pressure should be introduced by means of contraction of the wrist flexors rather than by hand action.
- The thumbs stabilize the hands as the pressure is maintained and a light but persistent lifting of the parietals directly cephalad is introduced from the finger pads (while the medial compression is maintained) for between 2 and 5 minutes, during which time a sensation might be noted of the parietals 'spreading' and lifting superiorly.
- During this procedure the other restricting influence, apart from the temporal suture contact, is that offered by the falx cerebri and sensitivity should be maintained to any resistance it is offering.
- Successful application of this parietal lift will enhance drainage via the superior sagittal sinus formed by the falx cerebri's attachments to the parietals.
- Contact with the temporals should be avoided during this procedure.

Temporals

A complex arrangement of different bone formats.

- A slim fan-shaped upper portion – the squama – with an internal bevel for articulation with the parietal.
- A long projecting column – the zygomatic process – which reaches forward to articulate with the zygoma.
- An anchorage point for the sternocleidomastoid – the mastoid process.
- A rock-like petrous portion the apex of which links to the sphenoid via a ligament.

Articulations

See Figure 12.19.

Reciprocal tension membrane relationships

On the petrous portion of the bone, a groove is apparent where the tentorium cerebelli attaches, forming the petrosal sinus.

Muscular attachments

- Sternocleidomastoid arises from heads on the manubrium sternum and the clavicle and powerfully attaches to the mastoid process (clavicular fibers) as well as to the superior nuchal line (sternal fibers). This muscular influence allows enormous forces to be exerted onto one of the most vulnerable and important of the cranial bones.
- Temporalis arises from the temporal fossae. The posterior aspect of the origin of the muscle lies on the

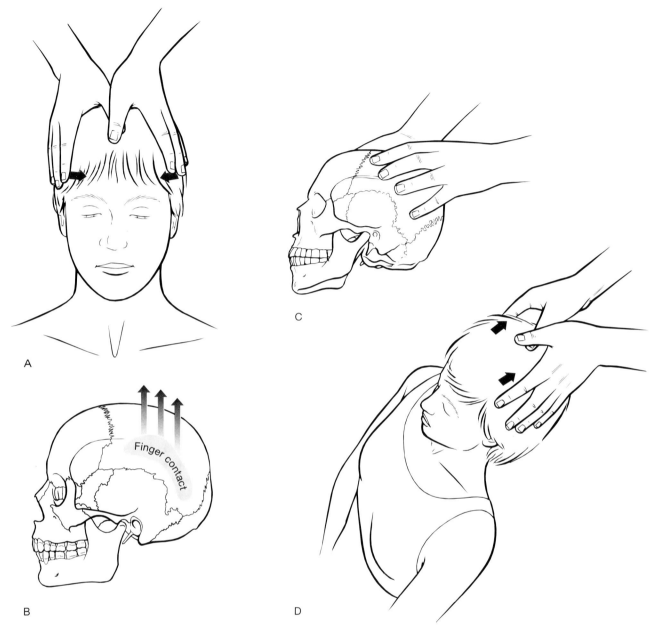

Figure 12.18 Parietal lift technique showing (A) hand positions, (B) finger contact sites, (C) contact sites avoiding sutures and (D) directions of applied light traction force (reproduced, with permission, from Chaitow (1999)).

temporal bone. The inferior attachment is to the coronoid process.

• Longissimus capitis arises from the transverse processes of T1–5 and the articular processes of C4–7 attaching to the mastoid process. This is also a powerful postural muscle which will shorten under prolonged mechanical stress and therefore is capable of producing sustained, virtually permanent drag on the mastoid in an inferior/posterior direction. If such traction were combined with a similar drag anteroinferiorly by sterno-cleidomastoid, the temporal bone's ability to move freely would be severely compromised.

• Splenius capitis arises from the spinous processes of C7–T3 as well as the lower half of the ligamentum nuchae and attaches to the mastoid process and the lateral aspect of the superior nuchal line. Any sustained traction from this would crowd the suture between the occiput and the temporal bone, reducing its potential for free motion.

Range and direction of motion

The motion during flexion can be visualized as a flaring outwards of the squama (as it pivots at its beveled

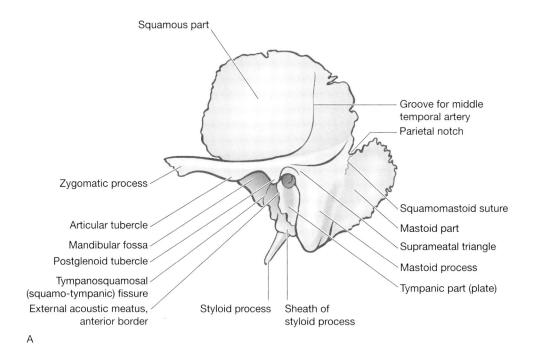

A

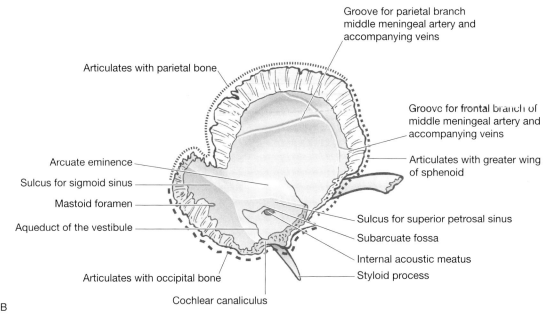

B

Figure 12.19 External (A) and internal (B) aspects of the left temporal bone (reproduced, with permission, from Chaitow (1999)).

junction with the parietal) while the mastoid tip moves posteromedially. These all return to neutral during the extension (internal rotation) phase of the cycle.

Other associations and influences

- The auditory canal passes through the temporal bone, while the internal auditory meatus carries the 7th and 8th cranial nerves.

- The trigeminal ganglion is in direct contact with the petrous portion.
- The jugular vein passes through the jugular foramen, part of which is formed by the temporal bone's inferior surface.
- The stylomastoid foramen allows passage of the 7th cranial (facial) nerve.
- The mandibular fossa forms part of the temporomandibular joint.

This is arguably the most complex (possibly excluding the sphenoid) bone in the cranium, which is subject to a variety of influences including thoracic and cervical stresses via sternocleidomastoid and longus capitis, as well as from dental influences via the temporomandibular joint and the temporalis muscle. The potential for direct negative influences on temporal mechanics, emerging from emotionally induced habits such as bruxism or upper chest breathing patterns, is clear.

Because of its direct linkage with the tentorium cerebelli, any dysfunctional pattern of a temporal bone automatically influences the other bones with which tentorium is connected, the other temporal as well as the occiput and the sphenoid.

Dysfunctional patterns

A wide range of symptoms may be associated with temporal dysfunction, often following trauma such as whiplash or a blow to the head. Among the commonest reported in osteopathic literature are:

- loss of balance, vertigo
- nausea
- chronic headaches
- hearing difficulties and recurrent ear infections in children
- tinnitus
- optical difficulties
- personality and emotional fluctuations ('mood swings')
- Bell's palsy
- trigeminal neuralgia.

Bitemporal rolling exercise (Fig. 12.20)

- The practitioner sits at the head of the supine patient with one hand cupped into the other, so that the head is cradled, thumbs on and parallel with the anterior surfaces of the mastoid processes, while the thenar eminences support the mastoid portion of the bone. The index fingers should cross each other (not shown in Fig. 12.20).
- An alternating rocking motion is introduced (one side going into flexion as the other goes into extension) at the thumb contact by pivoting the middle joints of the index fingers against each other.
- The amount of pressure introduced at the mastoid should be in grams only and should initially maintain and enhance the current rhythm of cranial motion.
- Following bitemporal rolling, synchronous rolling should be performed (next exercise).

Synchronous temporal rolling exercise

- The hand hold and general positioning is as in the exercise described above.
- The deep flexors of the fingers are employed to exert gentle pressure via the thumbs onto the mastoid processes during the inhalation (external rotation/flexion) phase of the cycle.
- This takes the mastoids posterior and medial and encourages normal flexion motion of the temporal bones.
- As exhalation (internal rotation/extension) occurs, the forearm muscles are released to prevent inhibition of a return to neutral.
- As this return to neutral occurs, a very slight (grams only) pressure can be introduced via the thenar eminences resting on the mastoid portion of the temporal bone, taking this slightly medial and posterior, encouraging a slight exaggeration of the extension phase.
- Repeating these motions will achieve an overall increase of the amplitude of both phases of the cranial motion cycle.
- A gradual acceleration of the rate is possible which is thought to encourage greater cerebrospinal fluid fluctuation.
- A slowing down of the rate is also possible, producing a relaxing effect.

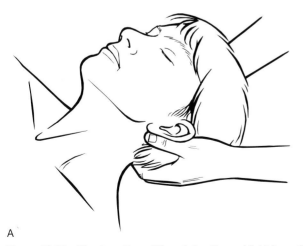
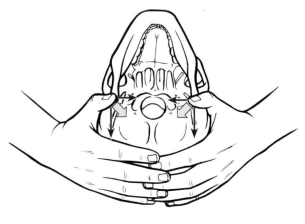

A   B

Figure 12.20   Hand positions (A) and directions of light force (B) in application of the bitemporal roll technique (reproduced, with permission, from Chaitow (1999)).

• This synchronous rolling should always be used to complete the treatment if alternate rolling has been used (see previous exercise).

• Always complete contact with the temporals during the neutral phase between the extremes of motion.

Zygomae

• A central broad curved malar surface
• A concave corner making up most of the lateral and half of the inferior border of the orbit
• An anteroinferior border articulating with the maxilla
• A superior process articulating superiorly with the temporal portion of the frontal bone (via interdigitations) and posteriorly with the great wing of sphenoid
• A posteromedial border articulating via interdigitations with the greater wing above and the orbital surface of the maxilla below

Articulations

See Figure 12.21.
There are no direct reciprocal tension membrane relationships.

Muscular attachments

See Figure 12.21.

Range and direction of motion

The orbital border is said to 'roll antero-laterally, and the tuberosity rolls inferior' in the classic osteopathic description of flexion motion (Brookes 1981).

Other associations and influences

The zygomae offer protection to the temporal region and the eye and are, as with the ethmoid and vomer, shock absorbers which spread the shock of blows to the face. Milne (1995) suggests that 'they act as speed reducers between the markedly eccentric movements of the temporals and the relative inertia of the maxillae'. The zygomaticofacial and the zygomaticotemporal foramina offer passage to branches of the 5th cranial nerve (maxillary branch of trigeminal).

Dysfunctional patterns

Sinus problems can often benefit from increased freedom of the zygomae. They should always receive attention after dental trauma, especially upper tooth extractions, as well as trauma to the face of any sort, as they are likely to have absorbed the effects of the forces involved.

Habits such as supporting the face/cheekbone on a hand when writing (for example) should be discouraged as the persistent pressure modifies the position of not just the maxillae but all associated bones and structures. They should be assessed and treated in relation to problems involving the temporals, maxillae and sphenoid.

Maxillae

See Figure 12.22.

Articulations

As described above, the maxillae articulate at numerous complex sutures, with each other, with the teeth they house, as well as with the ethmoid and vomer, the palatines and the zygomae, the inferior conchae and the nasal bones, the frontal bone and the mandible (by tooth contact) and sometimes with the sphenoid.

There are no direct reciprocal tension membrane relationships.

Muscular attachments

See Figure 12.22.

Range and direction of motion

These follow the palatines (which follow the pterygoid processes of the sphenoid) so that during the flexion phase of the cranial cycle 'the nasal crest moves inferior and posterior, the tuberosity moves lateral and slightly posterior, the frontal process posterior border moves lateral and the alveolar arch widens posteriorly' (Brookes 1981).

Other associations and influences

Because of the involvement of both the teeth and the air sinuses, the cause of pain in this region is not easy to diagnose. These connections (teeth and sinuses) as well as the neural structures which pass through the bone plus its multiple associations with other bones and its vulnerability to trauma make it one of the key areas for cranial therapeutic attention.

Dysfunctional patterns

Headaches, facial pain and sinus problems plus a host of mouth and throat connections with emotion (especially 'unspoken' ones) mean that purely structural and largely mind–body problems meet here, just as they do in dysfunctional breathing patterns.

Palatines

See Figure 12.23.

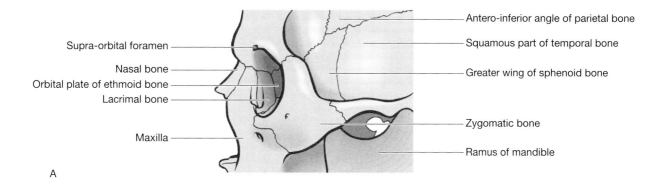

Supra-orbital foramen

Nasal bone

Orbital plate of ethmoid bone

Lacrimal bone

Maxilla

Antero-inferior angle of parietal bone

Squamous part of temporal bone

Greater wing of sphenoid bone

Zygomatic bone

Ramus of mandible

A

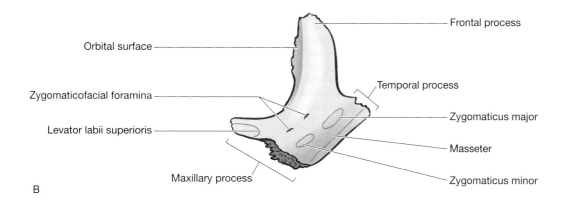

Orbital surface

Zygomaticofacial foramina

Levator labii superioris

Maxillary process

Frontal process

Temporal process

Zygomaticus major

Masseter

Zygomaticus minor

B

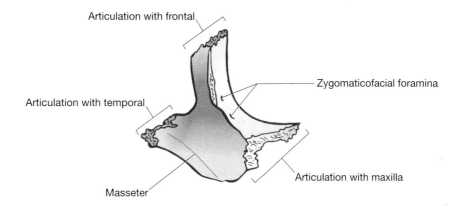

Articulation with frontal

Articulation with temporal

Zygomaticofacial foramina

Articulation with maxilla

Masseter

C

Figure 12.21 A: Left zygomatic bone and associated structures. B: Lateral aspect showing muscular attachments and articulations. C: Medial aspect (reproduced, with permission, from Chaitow (1999)).

Articulations

- The conchal crest for articulation with the inferior nasal concha.
- The ethmoidal crest for articulation with the middle nasal concha.
- The maxillary surface has a roughened and irregular surface for articulation with the maxillae.
- The anterior border has an articulation with the inferior nasal concha.

- The posterior border is serrated for articulation with the medial pterygoid plate of the sphenoid.
- The superior border has an anterior orbital process (which articulates with the maxilla and the sphenoid concha) and a sphenoidal process posteriorly (which articulates with the sphenoidal concha and the medial pterygoid plate, as well as the vomer).
- The median palatine suture joins the two palatines.

There are no direct reciprocal tension attachments.

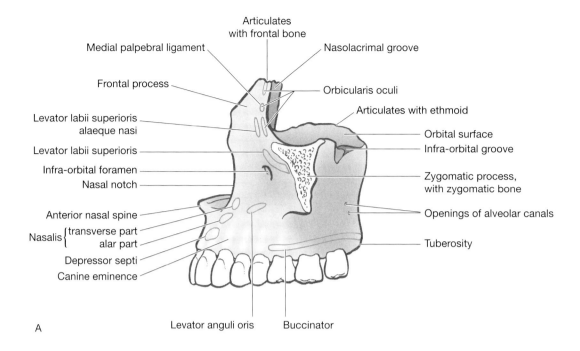

Medial palpebral ligament

Articulates
with frontal bone

Nasolacrimal groove

Frontal process

Orbicularis oculi

Levator labii superioris
alaeque nasi

Articulates with ethmoid

Orbital surface

Levator labii superioris

Infra-orbital groove

Infra-orbital foramen

Zygomatic process,
with zygomatic bone

Nasal notch

Anterior nasal spine

Openings of alveolar canals

Nasalis { transverse part
alar part

Tuberosity

Depressor septi

Canine eminence

A

Levator anguli oris   Buccinator

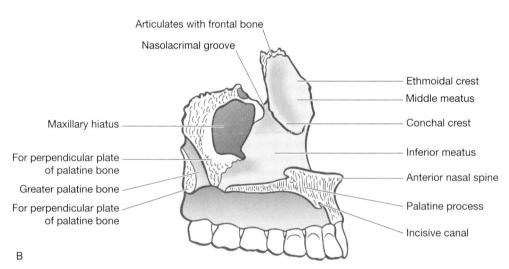

Articulates with frontal bone

Nasolacrimal groove

Ethmoidal crest

Middle meatus

Maxillary hiatus

Conchal crest

For perpendicular plate
of palatine bone

Inferior meatus

Greater palatine bone

Anterior nasal spine

For perpendicular plate
of palatine bone

Palatine process

Incisive canal

B

Figure 12.22 Lateral (A) and medial (B) aspects of the left maxilla showing attachments and articulations (reproduced, with permission, from Chaitow (1999)).

Muscular attachments

The medial pterygoid is the only important muscular attachment. It attaches to the lateral pterygoid plate and palatine bones running to the medial ramus and angle of the mandible.

Range and direction of motion

The palatines move, during flexion, to follow the pterygoid processes of the sphenoid with the nasal crest moving inferior and slightly posterior and the perpendicular part moving lateral and posterior.

Other associations and influences

These delicate shock-absorbing structures, with their multiple sutural articulations, spread force in many directions when any is exerted on them. They are capable of deformation and stress transmission and their imbalances and deformities usually reflect what has happened to the structures with which they are articulating.

Great care needs to be exercised in any direct contact on the palatines (especially cephalad pressure) because of their extreme fragility and proximity to the sphenoid in particular, as well as to the nerves and blood vessels which pass through them.

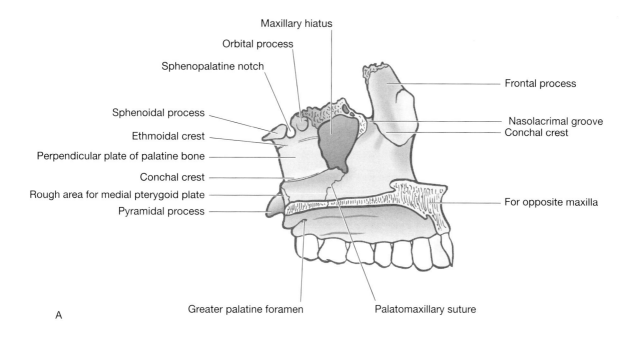

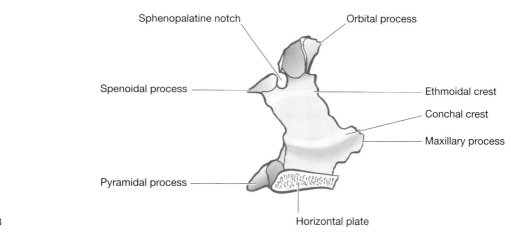

Figure 12.23 A: Medial aspect of left palatine bone articulating with the maxilla. B: Major features of the palatine bone (reproduced, with permission, from Chaitow (1999)).

CAUTION: In a report on iatrogenic effects arising from inappropriately applied cranial treatment, Professor John McPartland (1996) presented nine illustrative cases, two of which involved intraoral treatment. All cases seemed to involve excessive force being used but these cases highlight the need for care, especially when working inside the mouth.

CRANIAL TREATMENT TECHNIQUES

Muscles of expression

Mimetic muscles attach skin to skin, skin to underlying fascia or skin to bone and contribute to a wide variety of facial expressions. Youthful skin is highly elastic while aging skin does not recoil as well. Hence, wrinkles and folds of the skin commonly expressed by the contraction of these underlying muscles may remain etched on the aged face or on a younger face when the muscles are overused, such as a vertical furrow between the brows associated with eyestrain or frowning.

Mimetic muscles are easily divided into four regions (*Gray's anatomy* 1999, Platzer 1992), those being the scalp (epicranial), eyelids (circumorbital and palpebral), nose (nasal) and mouth (buccolabial). These regions work together in endless combinations to produce vast and often unconscious muscular movements which represent a physical expression of the wide variety of emotions experienced in daily life. These muscles, like those of postures which express general moods and feelings, are often used unconsciously by the person and frequently at chronic levels.

While not all of these muscles are discussed in detail within this text, most are offered in the following overview of the region. Those which are the most involved in head and facial pain are covered within this chapter. Orthodontic and cranial influences of the muscles of expression have yet to be fully established. Consider, for example, the influences which a tight, closed-lips smile of someone self-consciously covering the teeth could have on positioning of the anterior teeth and mandible. One has simply to produce that type of smile to feel the potential effect on the mandible. Consider also the insightful observations of Philip Latey (1996) who points out that during a lengthy osteopathic career he has seldom seen anyone suffering from migraine headaches who has a normal range of facial expression.

Mimetic muscles of the epicranium

The scalp itself is composed of five layers. The first three (skin, subcutaneous tissue and epicranius with its aponeurosis) are best considered together as a single layer since they remain connected to each other when torn or surgically reflected.

The deeper subaponeurotic areolar tissue allows the scalp to glide readily on the deepest layer, the pericranium.

Epicranial muscles express surprise, astonishment, attention, horror and fright and are used when glancing upwards. When pulling from below, the frontalis can draw the scalp forward as in worry, grief or profound sadness, especially in combination with other brow muscles.

Occipitofrontalis (Fig. 12.24)

Attachments: *Occipitalis portion*: highest nuchal line of occipital and temporal bones to the cranial aponeurosis (galea aponeurotica)
Frontalis portion: cranial aponeurosis (galea aponeurotica) anterior to the coronal suture to the skin and superficial fascia of the eyebrows, with fibers merging with procerus, corrugator supercilii and orbicularis oculi
Innervation: Facial nerve (cranial nerve VII)
Muscle type: Not established
Function: To elevate the eyebrows during expression, hence wrinkling the forehead
Synergists: None
Antagonists: Procerus, corrugator supercilii, orbicularis oculi

Indications for treatment

- Deep aching occipital pain
- Intense deep pain in the orbit and eye
- Frontal headaches
- Frontal sinus pain

Temporoparietalis and auricular muscles

Attachments: Epicranial aponeurosis to the anterior, superior or posterior ear
Innervation: Facial nerve
Muscle type: Not established
Function: To move the ear in various directions
Synergists: Occipitofrontalis, indirectly
Antagonists: None

Indications for treatment

- Tenderness anterior, superior and posterior to the attachment of the ear

Special notes

The occipitofrontalis is a broad, thin, musculofibrous layer which completely envelops the parietal suture. It additionally spans the lambdoidal and coronal sutures, attaching via direct or indirect linkages with the frontal, temporal, parietal and occipital bones, with the potential to significantly influence mobility and function of cranial structures.

Restrictions and tension in either the frontalis or occipitalis muscles will produce a 'tightening' of the scalp, which can be diagnostic. Lewit (1996) states, 'The scalp should move easily in all directions in relation to the skull. Examination of scalp mobility is warranted for patients with headache and/or vertigo'. Tension in the occipitofrontalis, or the epicranial aponeurosis, can also be seen to potentially interfere with the minute degree of mobility which exists between the occipital, parietal and frontal bones.

Flat palpation is used to locate and treat trigger points in the occipitofrontalis. Trigger points from the frontalis belly of this structure refer to the forehead while trigger points in the occipital fibers refer to the back of the cranium and to the area behind the eyes. Kellgren notes referral patterns of occipitalis giving rise to earache (Kellgren 1938, Simons et al 1998).

Temporoparietalis and auricular muscles lie superficial to the temporalis muscle and may be tender associated with trigger points in the underlying temporalis. While these muscles have significant use in most animals, they have very little obvious influence in most humans. However, *Gray's anatomy* (1999) notes that auditory

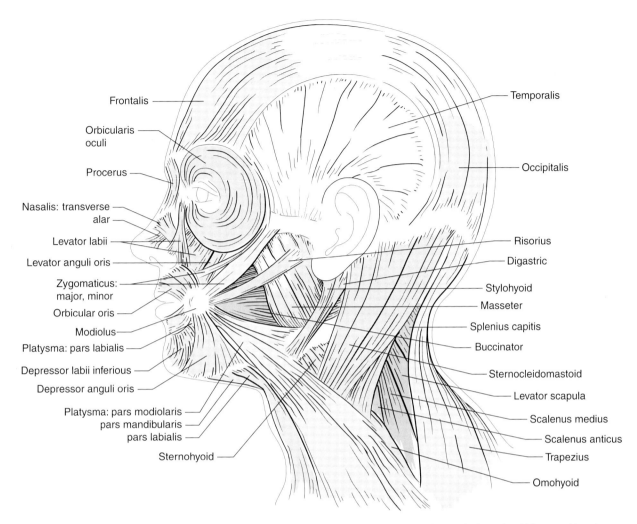

Frontalis

Orbicularis oculi

Procerus

Nasalis: transverse
alar

Levator labii

Levator anguli oris

Zygomaticus:
major, minor

Orbicular oris

Modiolus

Platysma: pars labialis

Depressor labii inferious

Depressor anguli oris

Platysma: pars modiolaris
pars mandibularis
pars labialis

Sternohyoid

Temporalis

Occipitalis

Risorius

Digastric

Stylohyoid

Masseter

Splenius capitis

Buccinator

Sternocleidomastoid

Levator scapula

Scalenus medius

Scalenus anticus

Trapezius

Omohyoid

Figure 12.24 Intense deep pain into the orbit and eye may be referred from occipitalis. Eye pathology should be considered, even when trigger points are found to reproduce the pain complaint. Note that the modiolus, a fibromuscular mass which is highly mobile and immensely complex, is shown here.

stimuli evoke patterned responses in these muscles. They may be irritated by ill-fitting glasses or telephone headsets.

The following techniques may be applied to assess the epicranial tissues. Frictional or hair traction techniques should be avoided where hair loss is occurring, where hair transplants have been embedded or if segmental neuropathy (shingles virus) is suspected, present or has occurred in the last 6 months. If the hair is missing completely, myofascial release may be used as needed. If the hair is too short to grasp, the frictional applications may still be used.

If the patient reports a current headache, the hair traction method may be applied and will sometimes relieve the headache. However, the frictional techniques usually prove too uncomfortable during active headache. Additionally, both techniques may be given to the patient for home care as they are easily self-applied.

 ## NMT for epicranium

The practitioner is seated cephalad to the supine patient. A pillow or bolster is placed under the patient's knees and in the case of an extreme forward head position, may also need to be placed under the head. Otherwise, the head rests on the table in neutral position. Rotation of the head will be necessary to reach the posterior aspect.

Transverse friction and small, circular massage techniques may be applied to the entire cranial surface to soften the superficial fascia and to begin therapy of the muscles of the cranium. Brisk frictional scalp massage will create heat, which may allow the external connective tissue to soften. Any tender areas found may be treated with combination friction or static pressure. Special attention should be given to cranial suture lines, which may be more tender than other areas and may indicate a need for further cranial attention.

Light to moderate hair traction may now be applied at palm-width intervals over the entire cranium, one handful at a time, if the hair is long enough to be grasped. The hair is gently lifted away from the scalp by the non-treating hand and the fingers of the treating hand slide into place close to the scalp with segments of hair lying between the fingers. As the fingers close into flexion, they also wrap around the hair shafts so that they grasp the hair close to the scalp (Fig. 12.25). The non-treating hand stabilizes the cranium while the grasping hand gently pulls the hair away from the cranium until slack is taken out and tension produced. The hair traction is sustained for 30 seconds to 2 minutes. If brisk friction has been applied immediately before hair traction, the fascial tissues will usually quickly loosen and soften. When friction is not applied first, the release of the tissues is delayed a minute or two.

The entire procedure may be repeated, although single applications are often adequate. If craniosacral therapy is to be applied, the cranial techniques may precede or follow hair traction or frictional massage.

The auricularis muscles may sometimes be manually stretched by pulling the ear into various positions by grasping the ear cartilage at its attachment to the head and tractioning it posteriorly, inferiorly and anteriorly. This technique may also have effects on the position of the temporal plate and should not be applied without concern for the cranial system. The practitioner who is unfamiliar with cranial therapy but uses ear traction for these tissues should end the treatment by pulling the ear gently directly laterally and holding for 30–60 seconds.

Manual treatment of occipitofrontalis. Direct manual release of the fascial restrictions in occipitofrontalis are recommended. Tension in the scalp interferes with cranial

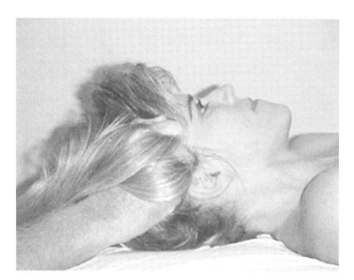

Figure 12.25 The fingers wrap around the hair shafts as they are gently pulled away from the cranium while stretching and releasing the cranial fascia.

motion, just as gross restriction in the thoracolumbar fascia can drag on the sacrum.

The methods which will achieve release of such structures can involve NMT, massage methods, myofascial release and positional release approaches. If NMT is employed, as outlined above, this can be assisted by an isometric contraction of the muscle prior to NMT. A strongly held frown, for 7–10 seconds, will reduce hypertonicity and allow easier manual applications to the soft tissues.

Positional release method for occipitofrontalis

- With the pads of two or three fingers the practitioner applies light compression, less than half an ounce, onto the skin overlying those parts of the muscle which appear most tightly adherent to the skull, identified by light to-and-fro gliding assessments of skin on the underlying fascia.
- The point of initial contact is the starting, 'neutral' point.
- From this contact assess the relative freedom of movement of the skin on underlying fascia in two opposite directions, say moving laterally one way, then back to neutral and then in the opposite direction.
- Decide which direction of movement is 'easiest' and glide the skin on the fascia toward that direction.
- Next, from this first position of ease, assess the relative freedom of glide in another pair of directions, say moving anteriorly and posteriorly.
- Which of these offers least resistance?
- Ease the tissues toward the direction, so achieving a combination of two positions of ease.
- From this second position of ease assess whether light rotational motion is easiest in a clockwise or a counterclockwise direction. Take the tissues toward this and hold it there for 20–30 seconds.
- After this allow the tissues to return to the starting position and reevaluate freedom of skin glide motion; it should have improved markedly compared with the commencing assessment.
- Repeat this approach wherever there appears to be a degree of restriction in free motion of the skin of the scalp over the underlying fascia.

Mimetic muscles of the circumorbital and palpebral region

Orbicularis oculi and corrugator supercilii comprise the mimetic muscles of the eye region (palpebral fissure). These two muscles are important not only for facial expression but also in ocular reflexes. Like all mimetic muscles, they are innervated by the facial nerve.

Orbicularis oculi is divided into three parts: orbital, palpebral and lacrimal. The orbital portion of orbicularis oculi encircles the eye and lies on the body orbit while the palpebral portion lies directly on the upper and lower eyelids. The short, small fibers of the lacrimal portion cross the lacrimal sac and attach to lacrimal crest. Its trigger points may refer to the nose or create 'jumpy print' when reading.

As a sphincter muscle, orbicularis oculi is responsible for closing the eye voluntarily or reflexively, as in blinking. It also aids in reducing the amount of light entering the eye and hence is involved with squinting. Levator palpebrae superioris antagonizes eye closure by elevating the upper eyelid.

Corrugator supercilii blends with the frontalis muscle and the orbicularis oculi and radiates into the skin of the eyebrows. It draws the brows toward the mid-line.

These two muscles are responsible for bunching the brows to shield the eye from intense light or when eyestrain produces a similar 'squinting' movement. They create vertical furrows between the brows which, over time, may become deeply entrenched lines. Additionally, orbicularis oculi produces radiating lateral lines commonly called 'crow's feet' and expresses worry or concern while corrugator supercilii is called the muscle of pathetic pain and also produces the expression associated with thinking hard.

 ### NMT for palpebral region

The eye region contains the most delicate tissues of the face which are treated with the most gentle touch. Extreme care must be exercised to avoid stretching the skin of the eye region. Spray and stretch techniques are not recommended near the eyes while injections into the eye region may result in ecchymosis, 'a black eye' (Simons et al 1998).

Flat palpation is used to press finger tip portions of the orbicularis oculi against the underlying bony orbit (Fig. 12.26). Gentle static pressure or an extremely gentle transverse movement may help assess the underlying muscle. However, frictional movements, gliding techniques or skin rolling, which may be effective to locate trigger points, may also be too aggressive for this delicate tissue. Use of 'skin drag' palpation (as described in Chapter 6, p. 71) is, however, gentle, safe and effective in localizing underlying trigger point activity.

The corrugator supercilii is easily picked up near the mid-line between the brows and compressed between the thumb and side of the index finger (Fig. 12.27). It can also be rolled gently between the palpating digits. This compression and rolling technique is applied at thumb-width intervals the width of the brow and may also include fibers of the procerus, frontalis and orbicularis oculi as well as corrugator supercilii.

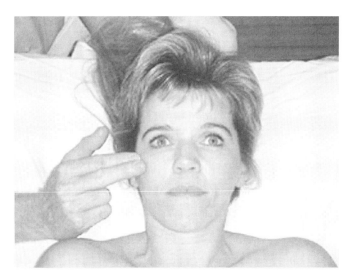

Figure 12.26 Any techniques applied to the eye region should be gentle and carefully placed as the connective tissue of this region is extremely delicate.

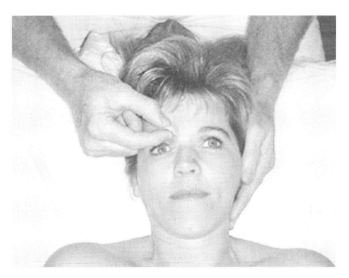

Figure 12.27 Compression and precise myofascial release may soften deep vertical furrows between the brows.

Mimetic muscles of the nasal region

Procerus arises from the facial aponeurosis over the lower nasal bone and nasal cartilage and attaches into the skin of the forehead between the eyebrows. It reduces glare from excess light and produces transverse wrinkles at the bridge of the nose. Expressions associated with procerus include menacing looks, frowns and deep concentration.

Nasalis consists of a transverse (compressor naris) portion which attaches the maxilla to the bridge of the nose and an alar (dilator naris) portion which attaches the maxilla to the skin on the nasal wing. The transverse portion compresses the nasal aperture while the alar portion widens it, reducing the size of the nostril and producing a look of desiring, demanding and sensuousness.

Depressor septi attaches the mobile portion of the nasal septum to the maxilla above the central incisor tooth. It depresses the septum during constriction and movement of the nostrils.

Levator labii superioris alaeque nasi attaches the skin of the upper lip and nasal wing to the infraorbital margin. When it contracts, it enlarges the nostrils and elevates the nasal wing, producing transverse folds in the skin on each side of the nose and a look of displeasure and discontent, especially noted when sniffing an unpleasant odor.

 ## NMT for nasal region

Procerus is easily grasped between the fingers and thumb at the bridge of the nose. Since this is an action people often perform when experiencing a headache or eye-strain, its association with those patterns of dysfunction may be implied.

Flat palpation and light friction may be used along the sides of the nose and spreading slightly laterally onto the cheeks to treat the remaining nasal muscles. The two index fingers, very lightly placed, may provide precise myofascial release but the practitioner is reminded that the facial tissues are very delicate and anything other than exceptionally light pressure is contraindicated. Strong tension of the tissues is also not recommended.

Trigger point locations and patterns of referral in this region have not yet been established but we suggest that these muscles be assessed when nose, lips and eye problems are encountered or facial pain or sensations are experienced near or into these tissues. Wrinkled skin may suggest underlying muscular tensions possibly involving chronic overuse.

Mimetic muscles of the buccolabial region

The movements of the lips are derived from a complex three-dimensional system which postures the lips and controls the shape of the orifice. Structure of the lips and their limits of motion are well discussed in *Gray's anatomy* (1995), as are details of the muscles listed below.

- *Elevators, retractors and evertors of the upper lip*: levator labii superioris alaeque nasi, levator labii superioris, zygomaticus major and minor, levator anguli oris and risorius
- *Depressors, retractors and evertors of the lower lip*: depressor labii inferioris, depressor anguli oris and mentalis
- *Compound sphincter*: orbicularis oris, incisivus superior and inferior
- Buccinator

The muscles of the buccolabial region function in eating, drinking and speech as well as emotional expression. A multitude of expressions, including reserve, laughing, crying, satisfaction, pleasure, self-confidence, sadness,

perseverance, seriousness, doubt, indecision, disdain, irony and a variety of other feelings, are displayed in the lower face by the action and combined actions of these muscles. The movements as well as individual expressions are covered in detail in both *Gray's anatomy* (1999) and *Color atlas/text of human anatomy, vol 1, locomotor system* (Platzer 1992).

A number of muscles of the buccolabial region converge into the *modiolus* just lateral to the buccal angle of the mouth. The modiolus can be palpated in an intraoral examination and is usually felt as a dense, mobile fibro-muscular mass which may or may not be tender. This fan-shaped radiation of muscular fibers allows the three-dimensional mobility of the modiolus to integrate facial activities of the lips and oral fissure, cheeks and jaws, such as chewing, drinking, sucking, swallowing and modulations of various vocal tones.

 ## NMT for buccolabial region

An intraoral examination including the labial area will address the muscles in this region. The practitioner should wear protective gloves – see precautions for intraoral examination on p. 280. Additionally, some of the attachments of buccolabial muscles can be treated when applying the masseter's external examination by continuing medially along the inferior surface of the zygomatic arch to near the nasal region.

The index finger of the gloved treatment hand is placed inside the mouth and the thumb is placed on the outside (facial) surface. The tissue is compressed between the two digits as the internal finger is slid against the external thumb while manipulating the tissue held between them (Fig. 12.28). The treating digits progress at thumb-width

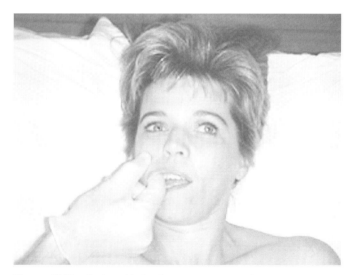

Figure 12.28 A gloved index finger compresses the buccolabial muscles against the external thumb at small intervals around the entire mouth.

intervals around the mouth until all the tissues have been examined. Tender spots or trigger points may be treated with static pressure or spray and stretch techniques, as described by Simons et al (1998), may be used with precautions as noted in their text.

The buccolabial muscles may also be treated from an external perspective by pressing them against the underlying maxilla, mandible or teeth and flat palpation can be used to assess and treat them. If the teeth or gums are obviously not healthy or are tender or painful, pressure against them should be avoided and referral to a dental health practitioner strongly encouraged. Infections of the teeth have been noted to be associated with TM joint pain and dysfunction (Simons et al 1998).

Muscles of mastication

The actions of fracturing food, blending it with saliva and preparing it for swallowing is a complex process collectively called mastication. Compressional forces are placed upon the food by the tooth surfaces due to the applied loads of the muscles which cross the temporomandibular (TM) joint. The process of mastication is a complex, coordinated interaction of numerous muscles and glands and is tremendously dependent upon the integrity of the TM joint and health of the associated myofascial tissues. Trigger points within these tissues, intrajoint dysfunctions or dental factors which inhibit normal occlusion of the teeth (such as the inability to chew on a particular side which, in turn, overloads the contralateral side) are only a few of the many conditions which interrupt and affect the synchronized action of eating. Since these muscles are also responsible for many of the activities needed for speaking, the dysfunctions associated with TM joint and tongue movements can have a far-reaching impact on our daily lives.

The suprahyoid muscles form the floor of the mouth and are involved in opening the mouth and deviating the mandible laterally. These muscles are discussed and addressed with the intraoral treatment following the external palpation. The muscles of the soft palate and tongue are also included in the intraoral approach.

The muscles which directly cross the TM joint include temporalis, masseter, lateral pterygoid and medial pterygoid. These muscles most powerfully move the mandible while others influence its quality of movement directly (as in digastric) or indirectly (as in those which position the head in space). In assessing the muscles associated with primary movement of the mandible, an external palpation and an intraoral treatment of the muscles can be used. While most of the external palpation is intended as assessment (with some benefit of treatment), the external palpation of temporalis is primary rather than secondary since it lies almost entirely exterior to the oral cavity. Only its tendon attachment to the coronoid

process is palpable from inside the mouth. Conversely, the internal applications to the remainder of the four muscles are considered their primary treatment.

External palpation and treatment of craniomandibular muscles

The therapist is seated cephalad to the supine patient's head. The ipsilateral hand is used throughout the external palpation. Each procedure is performed to both sides.

Since this joint is a bilateral joint (the mandible spans the cranium) dysfunctions affecting one side also affect the contralateral side. When techniques are applied to both sides which release the hypertonic, shortened muscles and/or assist in toning any inhibited (weakened or lax) muscles, a balanced state can be achieved which allows more normal joint function. However, if techniques are applied unilaterally imbalance of the musculature is probable with predictably undesirable consequences.

Although the treatment procedures (as described below) could conceivably be performed by applying the entire routine (first on one side and then the other), it is suggested that only one or two steps be performed before those same steps are repeated on the contralateral side, before continuing with the protocol. In this way, the practitioner can immediately compare the two sides while maintaining a more even balance of the musculature.

 ## NMT for temporalis

Caution: The following treatments should NOT be performed if temporal arteritis is suspected. See Box 12.5 regarding temporal arteritis.

The practitioner uses the first two fingers to apply transverse friction to the entire temporal fossa, a small portion at a time. The fingers begin cephalad to the zygomatic arch and on the most anterior aspect of the rather large tendon of temporalis (Fig. 12.36). The fingers are then moved cephalad to address the most anterior fibers of temporalis. Transverse friction is applied while pressing with enough pressure to feel the vertical fibers or to produce a mid-range discomfort level. The fibers are examined their entire length to the upper edge of the temporal fossa. Taut fibers are assessed for central and attachment trigger points and are treated with static pressure.

The fingers are moved posteriorly a finger tip width and placed once again on the tendon just above the zygomatic arch. The examination now addresses the next group of fibers in a similar manner. This process is continued throughout the temporal fossa. Since the muscle is shaped somewhat like a fan, the middle fibers lie on a diagonal while the most posterior fibers are oriented anteroposteriorly over the ear.

Box 12.4   Temporomandibular joint structure, function and dysfunction

The temporomandibular (TM) joint, located bilaterally just anterior to the tragus of the ear, is a compound (hinge-sliding) synovial joint, whose fibrocartilaginous surfaces and interposed articular disc allow for a tremendous variety of movements in response to the demands of eating, speaking and facial expression. The multiple movements of the mandible include protraction, retraction, lateral rotation, a degree of circumduction, depression and elevation. These motions are often in combination with each other as well as coordinated with the contralateral TM joint.

Synovial articulations, like that of the temporomandibular joint, are noted by *Gray's anatomy* (1999) to have:

- a fibrous capsule, usually having intrinsic ligamentous thickenings (often by internal or external accessory ligaments)
- osseous surfaces which are covered by articular cartilage (hyaline or fibrocartilage) and are not in continuity with each other
- synovial membranes, which cover all non-articular surfaces including non-articular osseous surfaces, tendons and ligaments partly or wholly within the fibrous capsule
- synovial membrane which usually covers and projects outwardly together with any tendon that attaches into the joint and issues from it
- an articular disc or meniscus (composed of fibrocartilage with the fibrous element usually predominant) which may occur between articular surfaces where congruity (conformity of the bones to each other) is low
- a viscous synovial fluid (synovia) which provides a liquid environment with a small pH range, lubrication, reduction of erosion and which is concerned with maintenance of living cells in the articular cartilages, disc or meniscus.

A disc may extend across a synovial joint, dividing it structurally and functionally into two synovial cavities in series, with the advantage of combined ranges for the two joints.

The function of the disc is uncertain and may include shock absorption, improvement of fit between surfaces, facilitation of combined movements, checking of translation at joints (such as the knee), deployment of weight over larger surfaces, protection of articular margins, facilitation of rolling movements and spread of lubrication.

Discs are connected peripherally to fibrous capsules, usually by vascularized connective tissue (vessels and afferent and motor (sympathetic) nerves).

The term 'meniscus' should be reserved for incomplete discs. Discs may be complete or perforated.

Where menisci are usual, complete discs may occur or may be slightly perforated.

The articular disc of the TM joint, composed of dense non-vascular fibrous tissue (Simons et al 1998), is bound tightly to the condyle, its inferior concave surface fitting the condyle like a cap while its concavoconvex upper surface corresponds to the mandibular fossa and glides against the articular tubercle. The joint surfaces as well as the interposed disc are designed to remodel in response to stress, changing its shape to accommodate forces imposed, such as oral mechanics, head positioning or from postural or structural compensations.

The disc is firmly attached at the medial and lateral condylar poles by strong bands and is attached anteriorly to the joint capsule, as well as to fibers of the upper head of lateral pterygoid. The upper head of lateral pterygoid also attaches to the condyle and pulls the disc and condyle forward as a unit during opening of the mouth (Cailliet 1992, Simons et al 1998). Posteriorly is the fibrovascular bilaminar zone where the thick fibers separate into two layers, the inferior one made of non-elastic fibrous tissue attaching to the back of condyle while the upper fibroelastic layer attaches to the posterior margin of the fossa. The area between the two layers is loose connective tissue that is highly vascularized and richly supplied with nerve endings.

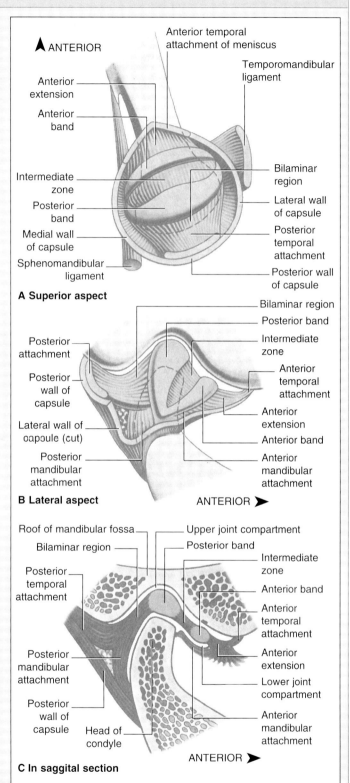

A Superior aspect

B Lateral aspect

C In saggital section

Figure 12.29   The temporomandibular intraarticular disc (reproduced, with permission, from *Gray's anatomy* (1999)).

Box 12.4   (*cont'd*)

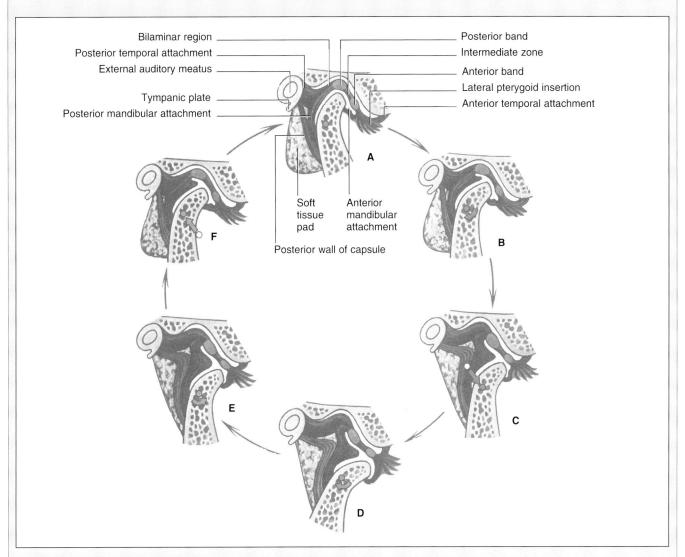

Bilaminar region
Posterior temporal attachment
External auditory meatus
Tympanic plate
Posterior mandibular attachment

Posterior band
Intermediate zone
Anterior band
Lateral pterygoid insertion
Anterior temporal attachment

Soft
tissue
pad

Anterior
mandibular
attachment

Posterior wall of capsule

A   B   C   D   E   F

Figure 12.30   Opening range and motion of the mandibular condyle and disc (reproduced, with permission, from *Gray's anatomy* (1999)).

The interposed disc is a deformable pad which is thicker anteriorly (pes) and posteriorly (pars posterior) and thinner in the center (pars gracilis). Increasing its load thickens its annulus (see below) (*Gray's anatomy* 1999). Its job is to allow considerable movement of roll, spin and glide of the condylar head (often performed with full loading) while reducing the possibility of trauma.

As the condyle hinges into place, in preparation for translation against the articular tubercle, it engages the central (thinner) portion of the disc, 'thereby "squeezing out" material to form a thickened zone, the annulus of Osborn, which surrounds the thin area – a recess for the mandibular condyle' (*Gray's anatomy* 1999). The lateral pterygoid engages the disc and the condyle to slide down the articular tubercle (by virtue of its incline) until the posterior fibroelastic elements are stretched to their limit. The condylar head may further hinge and glide against the inferior surface of the disc to articulate with its most anterior parts. During closure movements, the condylar head is seated in the central recess as it glides back up the incline and rests in the mandibular fossa.

Gray's anatomy (1999) points out that:

...while the disc is self-stabilizing its other principal role is to destabilize the mandibular condyle and allow complex free movement under load. The elastic tissues may act to withdraw tissues and thus prevent entrapment between the articular surfaces during mouth closure.

- *In protrusion the teeth are parallel to the occlusal plane but variably separated, the lower carried forwards by both lateral pterygoids.*
- *In retraction the mandible is returned to the position of rest (teeth slightly apart).*
- *In rotatory movements of mastication (in occlusal plane but clearly not in occlusion), one head with its disc glides forwards, rotating around a vertical axis immediately behind the opposite head, then glides backwards rotating in the opposite direction, as the opposite head comes forward in turn. This alternation swings the mandible from side to side.*

Box 12.4 (contd)

Ideally, the temporomandibular joint, enhanced by its design, should function normally as numerous daily demands are imposed upon it. Conditions which improve the chances for healthy joint function include the following.

- The disc stays firmly attached to the condyle and rests on it in an ideal position to load and transport the mandible in a variety of directions.
- The disc deforms during these motions and reforms after termination of motion (Cailliet 1992).
- The internal joint surfaces are well nourished and lubricated by healthy synovia.
- The musculature overlying the joint is free of contractures, trismus, trigger points and myofascial pain and allows full range of motion in all directions.
- The musculature whose trigger point target zones include the temporomandibular joint or any of the TM joint muscles are free of trigger points.
- The person's posture reflects symmetrical balance and coronal alignment with head and pelvis in neutral position when standing or seated.
- No significant traumas have been suffered by the joint or by the cervical region.
- Occlusion is harmonious.

Real-life situations seldom offer all of the above simultaneously. More often, various combinations to the contrary are observed and, in some cases, what is presented by the patient is contrary to all of the above and with nutritional, emotional and structural stresses imposed as well. The causes and effects of temporomandibular joint dysfunctions often require the efforts of a team of clinicians, each influencing the body and its healing process while interfacing with each other. Understanding the role the other team members play will assist in a well-formulated overall plan to remove the causes as well as some of the results of long-term dysfunction. Much of what is seen in the jaw may be the result of structural, habitual, postural, nutritional, hormonal or emotional stresses rather than the localized TM joint syndromes so often described. Likewise, reduction of occlusal interferences, splint therapy and reduction of infection might remove considerable stress, not only from the TM joint but also from the cervical region. The combined efforts in the areas of dental, musculoskeletal (especially postural) and emotional well-being may offer substantial and often immediate pain relief while recovery and restoration to functional stability progress.

A diagnosis of TM joint dysfunction (TMD) might include one or more of the following biomechanically faulted internal derangements of the disc. These may be due to gross trauma, such as that incurred in acceleration-deceleration injuries, or to strain imposed on the joint by faulty muscles, occlusal interferences, damaging oral habits or postural positioning.

Anterior displacement with reduction

The disc may be torn from the underlying condyle which may allow the lateral pterygoid fibers to dislocate it anteriorly (Cailliet 1992). When this occurs, the condylar head will need to overcome the thick posterior rim, producing a 'click' as it seats itself onto the disc (often with pain). If a reduction has occurred (condylar position recaptured), the condyle may translate (if not otherwise prohibited) and the jaw will open. When the disc is not reducible, the range of motion will abruptly end as the condylar head encounters the posterior aspect of the anteriorly displaced disc. Range of motion is usually significantly lessened with a non-reducible anterior displacement.

Rene Cailliet (1992) comments: 'In the presence of a click, indicating the possibility of a disc impingement syndrome, there are factors that influence the prognosis and even the preferred treatment. Pain or no pain with the click is a prognostic factor with the presence of pain being more ominous'.

Cailliet states that the response to conservative treatment is more favorable if the history of clicking is brief, if the click occurs early in the opening phase of jaw motion and if the click is reduced by repositioning the mandible (with orthosis), especially when little distance is required. The prognosis is less favorable if more than 3–5 mm of repositioning is needed to abolish the click.

Cailliet notes:

The earlier the placement of the orthosis from which the patient receives relief, the better is the long-range prognosis. If clicking is not painful, treatment is deferred unless the clicking is considered unacceptable to the patient. The implication is that clicking, per se, is usually reasonably innocuous. However, there is a prevalent opinion that clicking forebodes ultimate degeneration of the disc and/or the cartilage of the joint.

The click (as well as crepitation) produced during translation of the mandible may well be the first indication of a progressive TM joint problem. Often the patient issues no complaint until pain is experienced or until 'Suddenly one day I noticed I could not open my mouth to bite a sandwich'.

When the disc is anteriorly displaced, the posterior bilaminar zone (if still attached) is stretched and positioned to lie directly above the condylar head. Damage to the fibers, irritation to the neurovascular tissues and resultant excitation of the overlying muscles are some of the perils which may result the moment the disc displaces. Recapture of the disc (if possible) by orthotic intervention may reduce pressure on the elastic fibers by repositioning the condylar head forward and onto the disc in ideal position. By reducing pressure on the neurovascular tissues by both removal of the condylar head's presence as well as reduction of muscular tension and its often resultant intrajoint pressure, a quieting of the musculature may result, due to the effects of Hilton's law.

Hilton's law

The nerve supplying a joint supplies also the muscles which move the joint and the skin covering the articular insertion of those muscles.

Anterior displacement without reduction

A closed lock is a more serious condition. The process is similar to a displaced disc with reduction, except the disc is unable to reposition over the condyle and instead, impacts the condyle against the posterior aspect of the disc and is unable to translate further. This condition results in limitation of opening, often to 25 mm or less. This condition is a locked displacement without reduction and is a difficult one to correct with conservative measures.

Cailliet (1992) comments:

When there have been repeated dislocations with or without reduction, the cartilage of the glenoid and the condyle undergo damage and degeneration with resultant degenerative arthritis. In the presence of degenerative arthritic changes, there is a persistent crepitation, pain, joint range-of-motion limitation, and concurrent spasm of the muscles of mastication. In systemic inflammatory arthritis (rheumatoid, psoriatic, ankylosing, gouty, etc.), the TMJ frequently becomes involved. In these etiological conditions there is painful crepitation, limited opening, protrusion, and lateral and rotatory jaw movement, and concurrent masticatory muscle spasm with muscle pain and tenderness.

TM joint pain and associated factors

Forward head posture often accompanies TM joint pain and this should be a primary focus in rehabilitation of TM joint dysfunction.

Box 12.4 *(cont'd)*

Forward head posture and its related myofascial dysfunctions, including the evolution of nests and chains of trigger points, emphasize the important role these alarm mechanisms play in alerting the body (and the practitioner) to emerging problems, when strain, overuse, misuse or abuse of a tissue is occurring.

Examining for forward head posture (anterior head position) is noted by Simons et al (1998) to be 'the single most useful postural parameter' regarding head and neck pain. They note that a forward head position:

- occurs with rounded shoulders
- results in suboccipital, posterior cervical, upper trapezius and splenius capitis shortening to allow the eyes to gaze forward
- most often presents with a loss of cervical lordosis (flattening of cervical curve)
- overloads SCM and splenius cervicis
- places extra strain on the occipitoatlantal joint (places it in extension)
- increases the change of compression pathologies
- places the supra- and infrahyoids on stretch and places downward tension on the mandible, hyoid bone and tongue
- induces reflexive contraction of the mandibular elevators to counteract downward traction of the mandible (which then)
- results in increased intraarticular pressure in the TM joints which could give rise to the development of clicking, especially in a posteriorly thinned disc (see also crossed syndrome patterns in Chapter 5).

DeLany (1997) notes:

TMD is characterized by many symptoms that could arise from other ailments, and it therefore has a reputation as an elusive, baffling condition. These symptoms include headache, toothache, burning or tingling sensations in the face, tenderness and swelling on the sides of the face, clicking or popping of the jaw when opening or closing the mouth, reduced range of motion of the mandible, ear pain without infection, hearing changes, dizziness, sinus-type responses, overt pain behaviors and postures, as well as major losses in self-esteem and social support caused by decreases in normal social and occupational activities.

Larry Tilley DMD (1997) notes:

Even after finding a knowledgeable dentist we must remember that some patients are very 'straightforward' and respond to the most basic treatment. Others, however, require the most comprehensive, holistic and multidisciplinary approach. By the time many of these long-suffering patients have been diagnosed as having a TMD problem they have often become very serious pain and/or dysfunction cases. These patients require the practitioner to have the broadest possible knowledge or at least the understanding of many disciplines so that proper referrals can be made.

Tilley (1997) maintains that whatever the mode of treatment, active and thorough self-care is important.

The following should be considered:

- *avoid gum and other sticky, chewy foods*
- *avoid apples and thick sandwiches requiring excessive opening*
- *improve nutrition through a better diet and supplementation*
- *exercise: stretching (especially cervical and shoulders), strengthening, endurance*
- *avoid long-term use of analgesics, which can result in rebound headaches*
- *learn to use self-applied acupressure or neuromuscular techniques*
- *learn relaxation techniques*
- *avoid activities that aggravate the condition (lifting, sweeping, driving)*

- *evaluate work station for possible postural irritants – keyboard too high, cradling phone with shoulder*
- *keep headache diary*
- *elimination diet to identify and cut out offending substances*
- *avoid caffeine*
- *evaluate sleep posture – on back with cervical pillow and pillow under knees or on side with pillow between legs*
- *moist heat or cold compresses for temporal and cervical area*
- *herbal therapy might be considered*
- *continue to be active in family and church activities.*

While it is outside the scope of this text to discuss the dental factors which may be involved in TM joint dysfunctions, it is recommended that the clinician thoroughly understand the dental diagnosis and treatment plan as well as the case history, including history of head and neck pain, significant falls, direct traumas, motor vehicle accidents, habits such as nail biting and gum chewing, pertinent dental history, indications of habitual mouth breathing, stressful life situations, signs of hormonal changes (such as menopause or thyroid imbalance), known and suspected food allergies, use of over-the-counter and prescription medications and expected family (or other) support or resistance. Often a trail of clues is uncovered when questions are asked regarding what induces and what seems to relieve the pain. Modifications in physical and emotional environments may both be needed and may be synergistic with each other.

Examination of the soft tissues of the neck and cranium may reveal trigger points, postural tension, reduced range of motion and hypertonic myofascia. Release of the soft tissue elements, restoration of active range of motion to the cervical spine, shoulders and TM joints as well as steps toward assessing and enhancing whole-body postural balance are warranted from the onset of TM joint therapy. The dental orthosis (splint) or occlusion may need more frequent assessment if changes in pelvic, spinal or cranial positioning alter the position of the mandible and, therefore, the teeth or appliances.

Assessment of associated structures

The following assessments performed before and after applications of therapy will give basic information as to possible involved tissues as well as assisting in assessment of response to treatment.

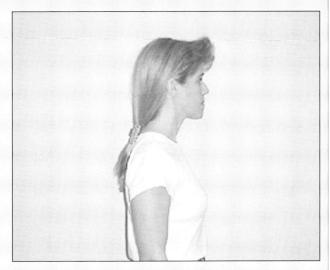

Figure 12.31 'Forward head' causes significant postural consequences.

Box 12.4 *(cont'd)*

Elimination of trigger points in TM joint muscles and associated cervical muscles, postural repositioning of head and neck and rebalance of the agonist and antagonist muscles of the TM joint may alter measurements, movement and tension in musculature of the TM joint. Charting of dietary, overuse and abuse habits as well as patterns and frequency of pain may offer insight as to areas of necessary modification. Education, counseling, lifestyle and nutritional changes, exercise and stretching coupled with myofascial modalities will supplement the efforts of the dental team (Cailliet 1992). Assessment and correction of forward head posture is of primary importance as noted by Simons et al (1998). 'Anterior head positioning with reflex elevator muscle activity also causes increased intraarticular pressure in the TMJs and can precipitate mild internal derangements in joints with compromised discs.' They also note that mandibular positioning, such as occurs in forward head position, can activate temporalis and/or its trigger points.

Forward head position may be associated with habitual mouth breathing or other breathing dysfunctions (overactive scalenes, for instance), which either directly or indirectly displace the head anteriorly. The additional stress placed upon the mandibular elevators and the occlusal alignment in response to the forward head is illustrated and discussed by Cailliet (1992) and is likely to be applicable to chronic shortness of the suprahyoids due to mouth breathing. Whole-body posture and steps toward symmetrical balance should be one concern when developing a treatment plan.

This text offers treatment options for the cervical region which should be included with the myofascial elements of temporomandibular joint dysfunction. The practitioner should include the upper trapezius, SCM, posterior cervical lamina gliding, suboccipital region, supra- and infrahyoids and, if indicated, anterior deep cervical muscles due to their postural influences as well as associated trigger point referral patterns. Trigger points from as far away as the soleus have been noted to refer into the temporomandibular region (Travell & Simons 1992).

Assessment of TM joint

• The practitioner's palpating fingers can be placed over the bilateral temporomandibular joints to assess local tenderness in response to mild or moderate pressure on the joint capsule.
• The angle of the mandible may be pressed gently toward the top of the head to assess for intrajoint tenderness. This step may

be omitted if anterior displacement of the disc is present as it may produce extreme discomfort within the joint.
• The condylar heads may be externally palpated during translation in all directions and compared for symmetry of movement.
• A simple millimeter ruler, dental gauge or Therabite® range of motion scale can compare pretreatment and posttreatment opening ranges to each other as well as to normal ranges. The adult incisal opening may measure 50–60 mm (*Gray's anatomy* 1999) with minimal normal opening being 36–44 mm (Simons et al 1998) and with 5–10 mm of range allowed in protrusion and lateral displacement in each direction, with much individual variation (*Gray's anatomy* 1999).
• A simpler, self-applied assessment of two (minimum) and three (maximum) knuckles (Simons et al 1998) placed vertically between the upper and lower incisors is a test readily usable by the patient to assess the need for self-applied or practitioner-applied neuromuscular therapy.

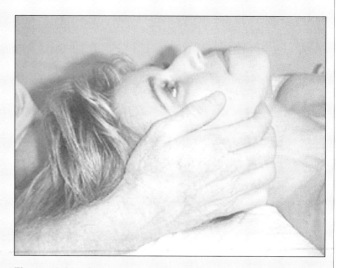

Figure 12.33 Gentle compression of the TM joint. This step is omitted if anterior disc displacement is present.

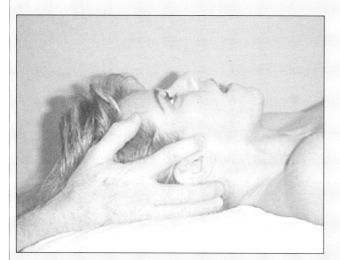

Figure 12.32 Movement of the TM joints may be bilaterally assessed for symmetry during opening and closing of the mouth.

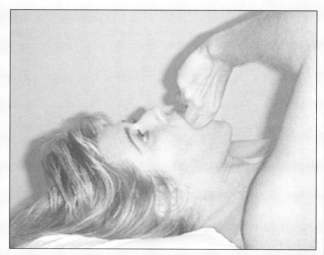

Figure 12.34 A minimal two-knuckle or maximal three-knuckle opening range of motion is an easy assessment the patient can perform on herself.

Box 12.4   (*cont'd*)

- An opening range greater than three knuckles (over 60 mm) may indicate ligamentous laxity and is a cautionary sign when applying intraoral work. Excessive opening may result in an open dislocation which is painful and frightening and can usually be avoided with special care.
- As the mandible is depressed during opening of the mouth, the practitioner may observe the lower central incisor path to note deviations or unusual movements during tracking. Such deviations may be the result of trigger points or shortened fibers within the musculature (deviation will usually be towards the side of shortening), internal derangement of the disc or other internal pathologies.
- A hard end-feel to opening, especially when the range is significantly reduced, may indicate anterior displacement without reduction or onset or presence of degenerative arthritis.
- Referral to a dental specialist for evaluation (or for a second opinion) can be of significant value and a necessary part of the course of treatment when soft tissue applications are successfully used due to their ability to significantly alter the position of the head and mandible and therefore the occlusion of the teeth.

Rehabilitation self-treatment method

- The patient gently wedges a wooden toothpick between the middle upper central incisors and another between the lower central incisors.
- The patient is seated in front of a mirror with lips retracted so that the two toothpicks protrude from between the lips.
- The patient *very slowly* opens and closes the mouth and in doing so concentrates on maintaining the tips of the toothpicks in line, one with the other.
- Repetition of this 5–10 times several times daily helps 'retrain' dysfunctional muscle patterns.

Several of the myofascial treatments offered in this section may be applied by the patient at home including masseter, temporalis, lateral pterygoid, tongue and floor of the mouth. Applications to the soft palate structures are best performed by a trained clinician due to the delicacy of the palatine bones, vomer and hamulus and possible (probable in seated position) stimulation of the gag reflexes.

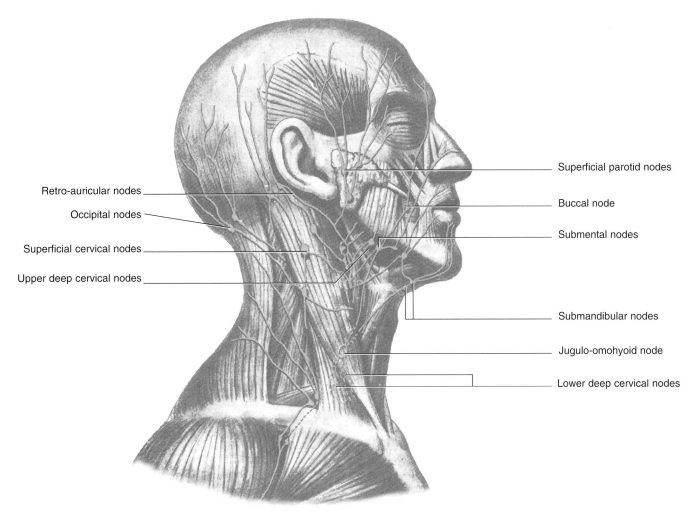

Retro-auricular nodes

Occipital nodes

Superficial cervical nodes

Upper deep cervical nodes

Superficial parotid nodes

Buccal node

Submental nodes

Submandibular nodes

Jugulo-omohyoid node

Lower deep cervical nodes

Figure 12.35   Superficial lymph flow of the head and neck region (reproduced, with permission, from *Gray's anatomy* (1999)).

Temporalis

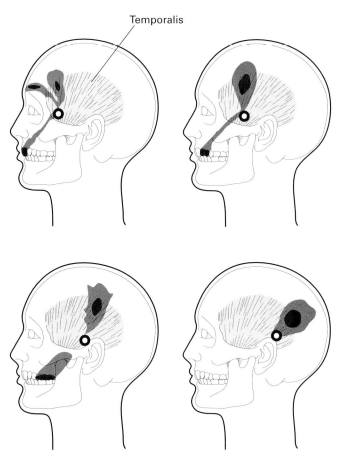

Figure 12.36 The temporalis fibers are vertically oriented anteriorly and horizontally oriented posteriorly, with varying diagonal fibers in between.

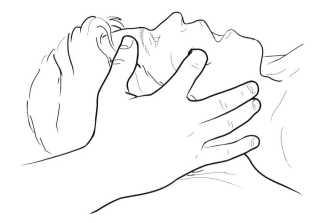

Figure 12.37 The patient's mouth must be widely open and the treating finger precisely placed to avoid the parotid duct while accessing the small portion of temporalis tendon available at the coronoid process.

The portion of the tendon which lies above the zygomatic arch can be assessed by using transverse friction while the mouth is either open or closed. An open mouth treatment stretches the tendon and requires less pressure than when the mouth is closed. The tendon may also be pressed as the patient actively and slowly shortens and lengthens the tissues under pressure.

With the mouth still open, the practitioner locates the coronoid process which is the first bone encountered (besides teeth) when moving the finger from the corner of the mouth toward the top of the ear. The mouth is opened as far as possible which will lower the coronoid process to below the zygomatic arch (unless depression of the mandible is restricted) and make the temporalis tendon available to palpation. Caution must be exercised along the anterior aspect of the coronoid process to avoid compressing the parotid duct against the anterior aspect of the bony surface. The duct may be palpated on most people by using a light cranial/caudal friction approximately mid-way along the anterior aspect of the coronoid process. Once located, the palpating finger is placed cephalad to the duct and avoids contact with it during treatment.

The palpating finger needs to be placed so that it is completely anterior to masseter and does not press through masseter fibers as this could be wrongly interpreted as temporalis tenderness. Additionally, the practitioner's index finger rests below the zygomatic arch with its lateral edge touching the arch and the palpating finger pad 'hooked' onto the anterior surface of the coronoid process. The fingernail faces toward the ceiling when the finger is properly placed on the supine patient's face (Fig. 12.37). When the tendon attachment is located, it is often found to be exquisitely tender and pressure may need to be reduced significantly. Static pressure may be used or, if not too tender, light friction may be applied.

 NMT for masseter

The masseter attachments to the zygomatic arch and the anterior portion of the attachment at the lateral surface of the lower angle of the mandible can be assessed with due caution applied to the parotid gland on the lateral face and to the TM joint itself just anterior to the auditory meatus. The mandible is supported on the contralateral side by the practitioner when any pressure is applied to avoid lateral displacement of the mandible during the procedure. One side is addressed at a time.

CAUTION: If there is evidence of inflammation or infection in the parotid (salivary) gland or the teeth, referral to a dentist or physician is suggested before applying any techniques to the face or internal musculature. If redness, edema, heat, extreme tenderness or other signs of infection are present, the procedure is delayed until a diagnosis reveals the extent of the condition. Salivary gland stones commonly occur within the glands and should be ruled out as a source of pain and infection. Applications of heat are contraindicated when edema or infections are present (or suspected).

Box 12.5 Temporal arteritis (Cailliet 1992)

This necrotizing arteritis condition is characterized by inflammation of medium- and small-sized blood vessels and is often initially manifested with fever, anorexia, weight loss, headache, fatigue and myalgia and progresses to head pain over the temporal artery or over the face, cranium and jaws. Examination may reveal tender, painful nodules in scalp tissues and the tender temporal artery may be devoid of pulse. Infiltration of polymorphonuclear leukocytes and eosinophils within the walls of the involved arteries may result in thrombosis and segmental fibrinoid necrosis (Cailliet 1992).

Rene Cailliet says:

This condition may be accompanied by ocular motor palsy with blindness from an optic neuropathy, occurring rapidly and usually irreversibly. Loss of vision is the most feared sequela of this condition, especially in patients not diagnosed and appropriately treated. Vision can be lost in the other eye within a week of the initial affliction. Gradual blindness rather than abrupt visual loss is rare.

Kappler & Ramey (1997) report:

This ... is usually seen in patients over age 50. The artery is swollen and tender. The associated headache is severe, throbbing, or stabbing and is localized over one temple. The pain is worse when the patient stoops or lies flat. The pain decreases when pressure is applied over the common carotid artery. Visual disturbances may develop secondary to ischemic optic neuropathy. The diagnosis is confirmed by biopsy.

Early treatment is critical. When the patient presents with the above symptoms, friction of the temporal area should be avoided until diagnosis rules out temporal arteritis. If it has been diagnosed, treatment of this area is avoided until the attending physician recommends that it is safe to perform it.

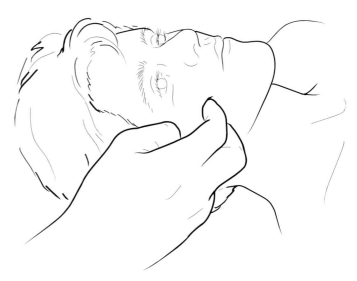

Figure 12.38 Light friction applied to the inferior surface of the zygomatic arch where masseter attaches.

The practitioner lightly lubricates the external face from the zygomatic arch to the lower angle of the mandible. The thumb pad is placed on the most anterior fibers of masseter just under the zygomatic arch. This muscular edge is easily palpated as the patient clenches the teeth but the muscle should be treated with the jaw relaxed and the teeth very slightly apart, lips together.

The thumb glides caudally 6–8 times and then is moved posteriorly onto the next segment of masseter fibers. The gliding techniques are repeated in segments until the entire masseter muscle has been treated. Since the parotid gland covers the posterior half of the masseter, care is taken to avoid excess pressure over the gland as well as the TM joint itself. Though skin care specialists usually advise people to glide superiorly on facial tissues, in this particular protocol which addresses craniomandibular dysfunctions, an exception is made and caudal glides are used to avoid pressing the mandible superiorly into the temporal fossa and against the articular disc or its posterior fibers.

The practitioner places the pad or tip of the index finger onto the face just lateral to the nose and presses onto the inferior aspect of the zygomatic arch or onto the maxilla and applies static pressure or friction (Fig. 12.38). The finger is moved one finger tip width laterally and the frictional techniques or static pressure are again applied. The first two or three finger placements may assess levator labii superioris, levator anguli oris, nasalis, zygomaticus or orbicularis oris, depending upon finger placement. The masseter will fill the remainder of the inferior surface of the zygomatic arch to just anterior to the TM joint. Avoid frictioning the TM joint.

The attachment of masseter on the lower lateral surface of the mandible can be assessed using flat palpation against the bony surface deep to it. Taut bands found in the anterior half of the muscle may be 'strummed' with snapping palpation or the practitioner may reassess them with the intraoral techniques offered later. Friction is not used on the posterior half of the masseter due to the overlying parotid gland (Fig. 12.39).

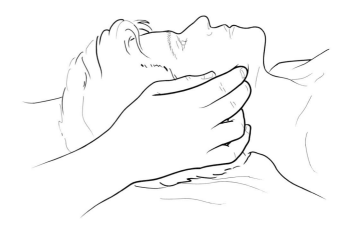

Figure 12.39 Pressure on the parotid gland is avoided when friction is applied to the lower attachment of masseter.

Massage/myofascial stretch treatment of masseter

- A very gentle myofascial release approach is achieved by sitting at the head of the supine patient and placing the pads of the three middle fingers onto the tissues just inferior to the zygomatic process. The contact should be 'skin on skin' with no perceptible pressure. The amount of force applied in an inferior/posterior direction should be minimal, barely a half ounce (14 grams). This is held for up to 3 minutes during which a sense of release or 'unwinding' may be noted.
- Immediately following this the thenar eminences are placed onto the tissues overlying the masseters with the fingers resting on the face, following its contours. A slightly increased degree of pressure should be applied, up to 4 ounces (112 grams), as the wrists gently move into and out of extension so that a slow repetitive stroking/kneading effect, in an inferior/posterior direction, is achieved along the long axis of the muscle. A light lubricant may be used.
- Goodheart (Walther 1988) recommends application of a 'scissor-like' manipulation across the muscle by the thumbs (or fingers) which form an 'S' bend – one thumb pushing superiorly across the fibers while the other pushes inferiorly (Fig. 12.40). The fibers which lie between the thumbs are thereby effectively stretched and held for some 10–15 seconds. A series of such stretches, starting close to the ramus of the jaw and finishing at the zygomatic arch, can be applied. The buccinator muscle is also effectively being treated at the same time.

 ## Positional release for masseter

Scariati (1991) describes a counterstrain method for treating tenderness in the masseter muscle.

- The patient is supine and the operator sits at the head of the table.
- One finger monitors the tender point in the masseter muscle, below the zygomatic process.
- The patient is asked to relax the jaw and with the free hand the operator eases the jaw toward the affected side until the tender point is no longer painful.
- This is held for 90 seconds before a return is allowed to neutral and the point repalpated.

 ## NMT for lateral pterygoid

With the patient's mouth open as far as possible without inducing pain, the practitioner locates the coronoid process. The index finger is placed just posterior to the coronoid process while remaining anterior to the mandibular condyle. As the patient closes the mouth slowly, the overlying tissues will soften and an indentation will

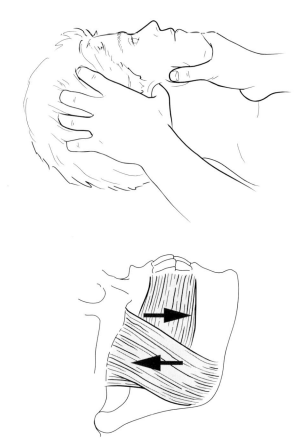

Figure 12.40 'S' bend myofascial release of masseter muscle.

be felt at the location of the mandibular notch. The mouth is open approximately half way (Fig. 12.41).

The index finger presses into the indentation (through the masseter muscle) and onto the lateral pterygoid muscle belly. Static pressure is applied to one side at a time while the mandible is supported on the opposite side of the face. This step most likely encounters the

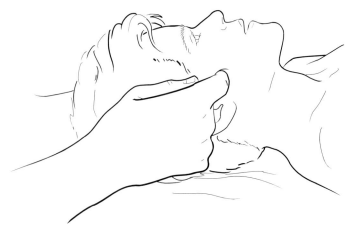

Figure 12.41 A small portion of lateral pterygoid may be influenced externally by pressing through the masseter with the patient's mouth half open.

upper head of lateral pterygoid and the posterior portion of the lower head (Simons et al 1998). Note that in pressing through masseter to reach lateral pterygoid, masseter tenderness may be mistaken for lateral pterygoid tenderness. The overlying masseter may need to be treated intraorally to reduce its involvement.

 ## NMT for medial pterygoid

With the patient's mouth closed, two fingers are placed onto the (external) interior aspect of the lower angle of the mandible, where the medial pterygoid muscle attaches (Fig. 12.42). Ipsilateral head rotation usually allows more room for the fingers to slide into place. Friction or static pressure is used on the medial aspect of the lower angle of the mandible while care is taken not to press the mandibular condyle toward the fossa and also to avoid pressing onto the styloid process.

Stylohyoid (see Fig. 12.52)

Attachments: Posterior surface of the styloid process to

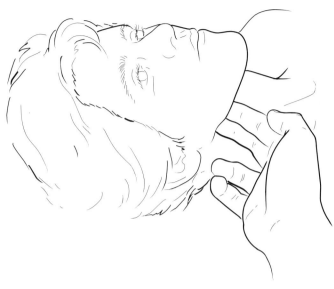

Figure 12.42 Medial pterygoid's lower attachment may be accessed externally when the head is rotated ipsilaterally.

the body of the hyoid bone at the junction of the greater horn (just above omohyoid)
Innervation: Facial nerve
Muscle type: Not established

Box 12.6 Notes on the ear

- The ear serves two major purposes: hearing and maintenance of equilibrium.
- The temporal bone houses most of the structures of the ear which suggests that temporal bone dysfunction may contribute to vertigo or hearing problems.
- This further suggests that imbalances in the muscles attaching to the temporal bone might also be implicated in hearing dysfunction or vertigo, notably:
  1. sternocleidomastoid which arises as two heads on the manubrium sternum and the clavicle and powerfully attaches to the mastoid process (clavicular fibers) as well as to the superior nuchal line (sternal fibers)
  2. temporalis which arises from the temporal fossae. The posterior aspect of the origin of the muscle lies on the temporal bone itself, while the inferior attachment is to the coronoid process of the mandible
  3. longissimus capitis, which arises from the transverse processes of T1–5 and the articular processes of C4–7, attaches to the mastoid process
  4. splenius capitis arises from the spinous processes of C7–T3 as well as the lower half of the ligamentum nuchae and attaches to the mastoid process and the lateral aspect of the superior nuchal line.
- The eustachian tube connects the nasopharynx and the middle ear and is designed to equalize middle ear and atmospheric pressure.
- Kappler (1997) states, 'Eustachian tube dysfunction is the most common cause of otitis media and benefits from … treatment to the cranium, medial pterygoid and cervical fascias'.
- Travell & Simons (1983) report that ear pain can result from trigger points in the lateral or medial pterygoids, sternocleidomastoid (clavicular) or masseter (deep).
- Tensor palatini appears to open the entrance to the auditory tube to equalize air pressure during swallowing and hypertonicity of this muscle has important clinical meaning as the auditory tube, when open, may provide an easy passageway for ororespiratory tract infections to reach the middle ear (Clemente 1987).

Box 12.7 How do we maintain equilibrium? (Gagey 1991, Gagey & Gentaz 1996)

Information which the brain integrates to maintain orthostatic posture derives from the following sources.

- retinal
- otolithic (vestibular)
- plantar exteroceptive
- proprioceptive sources in the 12 oculomotor muscles
- paraspinal muscles
- muscles of the legs and feet

Loss of balance may therefore result from failure of sensory information, including that from the vestibular mechanisms in the ears, or faulty integration of information received by the brain.

Labyrinthine test

- The patient is standing with eyes closed.
- The patient is asked to hold the head in various positions, flexed or extended with rotation in one direction or the other.
- Changes of direction of swaying are interpreted as the result of labyrinth imbalance.
- The patient sways in the direction of the affected labyrinth.

Rehabilitation choices

Standing and walking with eyes closed, with the floor covered in thick foam to reduce normal stimulation of receptors in the foot, retrains the vestibular and somatosensory systems.
Retraining of vestibular mechanisms may also involve use of hammocks and gym balls.

Function: Elevates the hyoid bone and pulls it posteriorly, which may indirectly influence opening of the mouth when the hyoid bone is stabilized by the infrahyoid muscles

Synergists: Suprahyoid muscles, especially digastric

Antagonists: *To elevation of hyoid bone*: infrahyoid muscles
To posterior positioning: geniohyoid
To opening of mouth: mandibular elevators

Indications for treatment

- Tenderness at styloid process
- Swallowing difficulties
- Posterior positioning of the hyoid bone
- Diagnosis of Eagle's syndrome – see below

Special notes

The stylohyoid muscle arises via a tendon from the posterior surface of the styloid process and attaches onto the hyoid bone, having been perforated by the tendon which joins the two bellies of the digastric muscle. Its action is to elevate the hyoid bone, drawing it backwards and elongating the floor of the mouth, thus influencing speech, chewing and swallowing.

Stylohyoid muscle fibers lie in close relationship to digastric, which sometimes also attaches to the styloid process (partially or wholly) (*Gray's anatomy* 1999). The fibers of stylohyoid and the posterior fibers of digastric are difficult to distinguish by palpation alone (Simons et al 1998). The digastric trigger point target zone includes the area of the stylohyoid muscle, whose pain pattern is not yet clearly established but is presumed to be similar (Simons et al 1998). Additionally, this referral pattern includes the superior portion of the sternocleidomastoid muscles and contributes to the expression 'pseudo-sternocleidomastoid pain' used by some practitioners.

Myofascial and ligamentous tension on the styloid process may result in elongation of the process due to calcium deposition which may, in turn, cause pressure or irritation to surrounding structures, including the carotid artery. Regardless of its etiology, the abnormal elongation of the styloid process resulting in facial pain is termed Eagle's syndrome (*Stedman's medical dictionary* 1998). Panoramic and frontal radiographs may confirm calcification of the styloid ligament or intraoral palpation of the process near the tonsillar fossa may reveal elongation of the process itself (Grossmann & Paiano 1998).

Grossmann & Paiano (1998) note: 'diffuse oral pain; the feeling of a foreign body in the throat; dysphagia; dysphonia and discomfort are all symptoms that have been associated with Eagle's syndrome'. They later conclude, 'In patients with mild symptoms, it is often possible to control it with conservative therapy. However, severe cases should be treated surgically'.

Simons et al (1998) cite trigger points in posterior digastric and stylohyoid as a factor in Eagle's syndrome.

The patient with this syndrome complains of pain in the angle of the jaw on the side of involvement, and also may have symptoms of dizziness and visual blurring with 'decreased' vision on the same side ... Active TrPs in these muscles can result in sustained elevation of the hyoid. The tenderness at the styloid process and calcification of the styloid ligament can represent enthesitis and subsequent calcification due to the sustained tension caused by TrP taut bands. The dizziness and blurred vision can be caused by associated TrPs in the adjacent sternocleidomastoid muscle.

Examination of the hyoid bone would also be warranted due to simultaneous tension which would be placed on it through the digastric central tendon attachment by fascial loop.

External palpation and treatment of styloid and mastoid processes

The head is rotated slightly contralaterally and a small amount of lubrication is applied to the styloid process. The index finger is placed just under the earlobe and posterior to the mandible with the pad of the finger placed directly on the styloid process (Fig. 12.43A). With a light to mild pressure, the finger slides caudally along the anterior surface of the styloid process to treat the styloglossus, stylopharyngeus and stylohyoid muscles and the stylohyoid and stylomandibular ligaments. The styloid process can be very fragile and only light pressure is used on this structure.

The index finger is moved posteriorly and onto the mastoid process. With light lubrication, gliding strokes are applied to the upper 2″ of the SCM muscle 8–10 times. The head is rotated further contralaterally and passively angled toward the ipsilateral shoulder to further relax

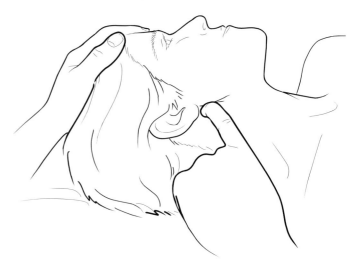

Figure 12.43 Three muscles and two ligaments attach to the fragile styloid process. Digastric attaches to the anterior surface of the mastoid process just posterior to the styloid process.

Box 12.8 Muscles producing movements of mandible (*Gray's anatomy* 1995)

Protrusion: medial and lateral pterygoid
Retraction: temporalis (posterior fibers), masseter (middle and deep fibers), digastric, geniohyoid
Elevation: temporalis, masseter, medial pterygoid, lateral pterygoid
Depression: lateral pterygoids, digastric, geniohyoid, mylohyoid, gravity
Lateral translation: medial and lateral pterygoid
Maintains position of rest: temporalis

Box 12.9 Latex allergy alert

Defensive reactions by the immune system against normally inoffensive substances often produce allergic responses. As with most allergic and sensitivity reactions, great variations exist in the degree of severity displayed, ranging from no apparent reaction to mild or severe skin eruptions, respiratory complications and, rarely, death.

Since universal precautions were initiated in the late 1980s to prevent communication of diseases, such as HIV and hepatitis, exposure to latex products (which provide barriers to these and other viruses) has increased significantly, especially for health-care providers. Latex, derived from the milky sap of the rubber tree and other plants from the Euphorbiaces family, is used in the production of medical supplies (including gloves), paints, adhesives, balloons and numerous other common products. It has only been recognized within the last 15 years as a cause of serious allergic reactions.

Latex is composed of proteins, lipids, nucleotides and cofactors. The protein element is thought to be the cause of allergic response, while the powders, which are often used to coat the gloves to make them easier to get on and off, provide the protein with additional airborne capabilities. Increased exposure to latex is apparently associated with increased sensitivity and onset of allergic reaction often appears insidiously. Although the exact connection is not fully understood, those people who are allergic to avocado, banana, kiwi and chestnut are often also latex sensitive.

Allergic responses may include hives, dermatitis, allergic conjunctivitis, swelling or burning around the mouth or airway following dental procedures or after blowing up a balloon, genital burning after exposure to latex condoms, coughing, wheezing, shortness of breath and occupational asthma with latex exposure. Extreme cases may result in anaphylactic shock which may prove fatal.

Avoidance of exposure is certainly recommended for those people who are already latex sensitive and may also be the best course of action to avoid future development of sensitivity. Additionally, the National Institute for Occupational Safety and Health (NIOSH) has published a 1997 alert titled *Preventing allergic reactions to natural rubber latex in the workplace* (NIOSH publication #97–135) which may be obtained by calling (800) 356–4674. At the time of publication of this text, numerous websites are available, including some which list latex-free alternative barriers, and may be found with a website search for the topic 'latex allergies'.

---

the SCM. The SCM is displaced posteriorly (if needed) and an index finger placed onto the anterior aspect of the mastoid process. Static pressure or mild friction is applied to the digastric attachment at the digastric notch of the mastoid process. Friction may be used if the area is not too tender. The treating finger remains posterior to the styloid process and pressure on the styloid process is avoided due to its fragility.

Intraoral palpation and treatment of craniomandibular muscles

Prior to the intraoral examination, it is recommended that the practitioner takes a full case history, including dental, medical, traumas or chronic conditions especially related to the oral cavity, face, jaw, cranium or neck. Allergies to latex should be noted and exposure avoided by using non-latex barriers. The practitioner should take all precautions to prevent latex overexposure for both the patient and himself, while also providing adequate barriers to direct intraoral contact. The fingernail of the index finger (or other treating finger) should be well trimmed.

Protective gloves are always worn when examining the intraoral cavity. Unpowdered gloves are recommended since allergy or sensitivity to the powder may not be known prior to its use. The used gloves are properly disposed of immediately after treatment. The practitioner who chooses to use latex gloves (see Box 12.9) should keep in mind that oil dissolves latex. The hands and any surfaces the gloves touch, including the patient's face, should be oil free.

Before beginning intraoral work, the practitioner should note any removable partial dentures, orthodontic appliances or any other structures which might tear the glove. In the case of orthodontic appliances, wax may be applied over sharp surfaces to avoid tearing the barrier.

A glance inside the mouth might also reveal bony excretions (mandibular or palatine torus), fleshy growths or discolorations of the gums or internal cheek. Reference to a dentist or oral specialist is recommended if diagnosis has not previously been made. Whereas the tori are usually of concern only if they interfere with dentures, partials or speech, suspicious intraoral tissues should be checked, especially if the patient does not frequent the dental office. Additionally, wearing patterns noted on the occlusal surfaces of the teeth might offer clues that the patient is bruxing, inappropriately translating the teeth on each other or otherwise abusing the dentition.

Intraoral NMT applications

The patient is supine throughout the intraoral examination and treatment. The practitioner stands at the level of the patient's shoulder for most of the steps and may reposition freely to avoid straining the wrist. While most of these steps are performed ipsilaterally, some of the muscles are best treated by reaching across the body to the contralateral side and are noted as such in the text. The practitioner should experience all the techniques as non-straining and should reposition the hands, switch hands or otherwise make adjustments to avoid strain and gain the best access to the muscle.

Temporalis

Attachments: Temporal fossa and deep surface of the temporal fascia which covers it to the medial, apex, anterior and posterior borders of the coronoid process and to the anterior border of the ramus of the mandible

Innervation: Temporal nerves from mandibular branch of trigeminal (cranial nerve V)

Muscle type: Not established

Function: Elevation and retraction of the mandible, lateral excursion

Synergists: *For elevation*: contralateral temporalis and bilateral masseters, medial pterygoids, lateral pterygoids (upper head)
For retraction: deep head of masseter

Antagonists: *To elevation*: suprahyoids, infrahyoids (stabilize hyoid bone), lateral pterygoid (lower head)
To retraction: lateral pterygoids

Indications for treatment

• Lateral headache
• Maxillary toothache or tooth sensitivity

Special notes

This fan-shaped structure covers a large part of the side of the skull. It passes deep to the zygomatic arch with anterior fibers coursing vertically, posterior fibers orienting horizontally and the intermediate fibers varying obliquely.

All fibers contribute to the major function of closing the mandible with the posterior fibers involved in retrusion and lateral deviation of the mandible toward the same side while the anterior fibers are largely involved in elevation (closure) and positioning of the anterior middle incisors. Temporalis is responsible for postural positioning and balancing the jaw. Masseter, on the other hand, is involved primarily with chewing, clenching and strong closure of the jaws.

The two temporalis muscles are directly connected to the temporal bones (fossa and squama), the parietals (squama), the great wings of the sphenoid and the postero-lateral aspects of the frontal bones, crossing the coronal sutures, the sphenosquamous sutures and the temporo-parietal sutures. It is hard to imagine muscles with greater direct mechanical influence on cranial function than these thick and powerful structures.

Upledger & Vredevoogd (1983) point out that when the teeth are tightly clenched, contraction of the temporalis draws the parietal bone down. Because of the architecture of the squamous suture between the temporal bone

(internal bevel) and the parietal bone (external bevel), a degree of sliding is possible between them.

Prolonged crowding of this suture (resulting from dental malocclusion, anger, tension, trauma, etc.) can lead to ischemic changes as well as pain locally and at a distance.

Subsequent influences might involve the sagittal sinus and possibly CSF resorption. Upledger & Vredevoogd (1983) report that such a scenario can lead to mild to moderate cerebral ischemia which is reversible.

Trigger points from the temporalis muscle refer to the side and front of the head, eyebrows, behind the eye and upper teeth, as well as the TM joint. Temporalis lies in the reference zone of several cervical muscles, including trapezius and sternocleidomastoid, and its trigger points may be satellites of trigger points in these muscles (Simons et al 1998) (see Fig. 12.36).

CAUTION: A differential diagnosis with polymyalgia rheumatica is necessary if widespread pain is a feature (PR usually occurs in the over-50s and its pain distribution is usually greater than trigger point influences on the face/head. A blood test confirms PR). Temporal arteritis should also be ruled out, especially if particularly severe head pain is localized over the temporal artery or widespread over the cranium, face or jaws, as sometimes sudden unilateral blindness will result (see Box 12.5). Temporal arteritis shares many of the symptoms of polymyalgia rheumatica (*Stedman's medical dictionary* 1998).

 NMT for intraoral temporalis tendon

The practitioner treats the ipsilateral temporalis. The patient is asked to open the mouth as far as possible without inducing pain and to shift the mandible toward the side being treated to allow sufficient room for the treating finger to rest between the coronoid process and the teeth. The pad of the index finger touches the inside cheek surface and the finger glides posteriorly until it runs into the coronoid process, a bony surface embedded in the cheek.

The index finger slides onto the inside surface of the coronoid process and uses static pressure or gentle friction to examine the anterior, superior, interior and posterior aspects of the coronoid process (or what can be reached of them) where the temporalis tendon attaches (Fig. 12.44). The tendon is very hard and will feel like a continuation of the coronoid process. It is often very tender so light pressure is applied and increased only if appropriate to do so.

Masseter (Fig. 12.45)

Attachments: Three heads arise from the zygomatic process of the maxilla as well as from the inferior aspect

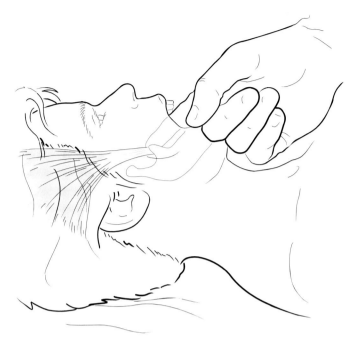

Figure 12.44   The mandible is shifted toward the side being treated to allow more room for the finger to reach the internal aspect of the coronoid process and the temporalis tendon attachment.

of the zygomatic arch inserting onto inferior, central and upper aspects of the lateral ramus of the mandible

Innervation: Masseteric nerve from mandibular branch of trigeminal (cranial nerve V)

Muscle type: Not established

Function: Elevates mandible; some influence in retraction, protraction and lateral deviation (*Gray's anatomy* 1999)

Synergists: *For elevation*: bilateral temporalis and medial pterygoid, contralateral masseter. Superior head of lateral pterygoid remains controversial (Simons et al 1998)

Antagonists: Suprahyoids and the inferior head of lateral pterygoid

Indications for treatment

- Pain in areas indicated in Fig. 12.45
- Restricted opening of the mouth
- Tinnitus, unilateral unless both masseters are involved
- Bruxism
- Repetitive habits, such as gum chewing, nail biting or clenching the teeth

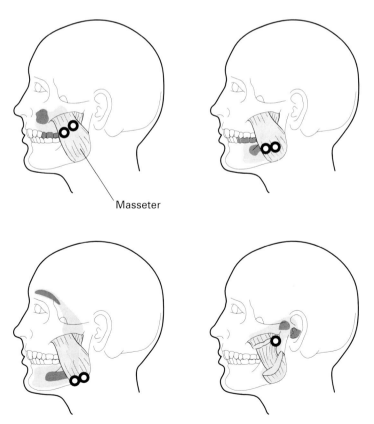

Masseter

Figure 12.45   Masseter and other masticatory muscles may refer directly into the teeth, creating pain or sensitivity.

Special notes

Masseter comprises three layers stacked onto each other. The deeper stratum of masseter, whose fibers lie vertically, is not as large as the diagonally oriented superficial portion. Its geographical position can result in disturbance of the temporal bone and TM joint and its sharing of considerable nociceptive neurons (Simons et al 1998) with the joint may explain its high tendency to be involved when TM joint pain is present.

Marked restriction in opening range is often associated with trigger points in the muscle. Deep triggers here can also cause unilateral tinnitus or bilateral tinnitus if both sides are involved. Emotional problems which lead to excessive jaw clenching can cause major problems in the muscle, which may also be involved in malocclusion. Similarly, the pain and dysfunctions associated with this and other TM joint muscles may contribute to emotional stress.

Masseter is involved primarily with chewing, clenching and strong closure of the jaws. Temporalis, on the other hand, is responsible for postural positioning and balancing the jaw. Advice should be given regarding irritant activity including mouth breathing, chewing gum, bruxism, clenching and grinding the teeth as well as possible dental involvement.

NMT for intraoral masseter

The outside surface of the face is supported with the dorsum of the external hand. The gloved index finger of the intraoral hand is placed inside the mouth and just inferior to the zygomatic arch with the pad of the finger facing toward the cheek. Gliding strokes are applied from the zygomatic arch to the lower edge of the mandible while compressing the masseter and buccinator muscles against the dorsum of the external hand. The strokes are repeated 8–10 times in strips until the entire masseter has been treated. The external hand's index finger is not allowed to touch the face since it will treat the opposite side intraorally.

With the finger still in place, the patient is asked to clench the teeth to contract the masseter's deep portion and then to relax the jaw. It may be necessary to have the patient shift the mandible toward the side being treated to allow room for the treatment finger.

Static pincer compression which matches the tension found in the tissues is applied at finger-width intervals beginning just caudal to the zygomatic arch and working down the muscle as far as possible, one finger tip at a time (Fig. 12.46). Pressure may be applied against an external finger of the opposite hand (except the index 'treating' finger) or between the external thumb and internal finger of the same hand. While most tissues respond to compression within 8–12 seconds, masseter

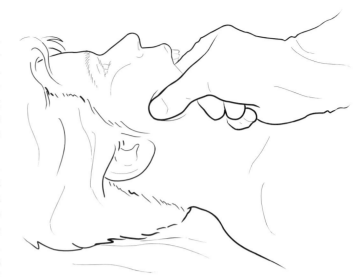

Figure 12.46 Compression is applied to the masseter in finger-width intervals down the muscle's belly and also along the inferior surface of the zygomatic arch.

may release quickly or may require a longer compression of 15–20 seconds.

Stretch of the muscle is achieved by a sustained but not forceful forward and downward pull, taking out all available slack and then holding to allow a 'creeping' release to evolve. Care must be taken to avoid the use of force when opening the mouth as the articular disc could be damaged. Manual treatment as listed above is best applied first, to release muscular restrictions so as to better determine if restriction of range of motion is due to myofascial or osseous (in this case disc) tissue.

There is often a profound change in the tension of masseter when a thorough (not aggressive) treatment has been applied. The patient will usually note an appreciable difference when comparing the side which has been treated with the other. Both sides are always treated to avoid unbalancing the mandible.

Lateral pterygoid

Attachments: Upper head arises from the infratemporal crest and lateral surface of the greater wing of sphenoid to insert onto the pterygoid fovea (on neck of mandible) and to the articular disc and capsule; lower head arises from lateral surface of lateral pterygoid plate to attach to the neck of the mandible

Innervation: Lateral pterygoid nerve from mandibular branch of trigeminal (cranial nerve V)

Muscle type: Not established

Function: Moves the condyle and disc complex as a unit; active during opening and closure of the jaw, protrusion of the mandible and contralateral deviation

Synergists: *Opening*: suprahyoid muscles
Closure: masseter, temporalis, medial pterygoid

Protrusion: superficial masseter, anterior temporalis, medial pterygoid

Contralateral deviation: ipsilateral medial pterygoid, contralateral masseter and contralateral temporalis

Antagonists: *To opening*: masseter, temporalis, medial pterygoid

To closure: suprahyoids

To protrusion: portions of temporalis, deep masseter

To deviation: contralateral medial and lateral pterygoids and ipsilateral masseter and temporalis

Indications for treatment

- Pain or clicking in TM joint
- Occlusal disharmony, premature contact
- Maxillary sinus pain, excessive secretion or sinusitis
- Tinnitus
- Bruxism
- Repetitive habits, such as gum chewing, nail biting or clenching the teeth
- Lateral deviation patterns when opening or closing the jaw

Special notes

The mandibular attachments of the two heads of the lateral pterygoid remain controversial although there is full agreement on their cranial attachment to the pterygoid plate and sphenoid bone (Simons et al 1998). There is general agreement that both heads attach to the neck of the condyle but disagreement as to the amount of attachment of the upper head to the disc and condyle. Simons et al (1998) report a review by Klineberg (1991) of studies examining the attachments. The results imply that, 'The traction that is applied by the superior pterygoid (superior division) during mouth closure affects the condyle and disk complex as a unit and does not affect the disk selectively'.

The actions of the lateral pterygoid are also confusing when one compares various texts, particularly if older texts are involved. The lateral pterygoids (collectively) are involved in all movements of the mandible except retraction.

Simons et al (1998) reports that reciprocal activity of the two heads as antagonists during vertical and horizontal mandibular movements may be indicated but later state:

Since it is now generally agreed that there is not always a separate attachment of the superior division to the disc, it is now thought that both divisions of the muscle affect the condyle and disc complex as a unit. Any tendency to reciprocal activity [of the two heads to each other] would most likely reflect mechanical advantage by one or the other division because of the difference in angulation of their fibers.

Adding to lateral pterygoid confusion is the use of various terms to identify the two heads of the lateral pterygoid or to distinguish lateral and medial pterygoid, which are sometimes called the external and internal pterygoids, respectively. In this text, the terms found in *Gray's anatomy* (1999) have been used, that being lateral and medial pterygoid muscles and, regarding lateral pterygoid, the two portions being called upper and lower heads, except where quoted from other texts.

TMJ dysfunction often involves lateral pterygoid which, due to its attachment sites, may also influence more widespread cranial dysfunction, most notably of the sphenoid. Travell & Simons (1983) state, 'The external (lateral) pterygoid muscle is frequently the key to understanding and managing TMJ dysfunction syndrome and related craniomandibular disorders'.

Upledger & Vredevoogd (1983) report that, 'It [lateral pterygoid] is a frequent cause of recurrent craniosacral and temporomandibular joint problems'. Along with other key muscles of the region, assessment and (if needed) therapeutic attention to the lateral pterygoid is an absolute prerequisite of craniosacral therapy.

Referred trigger point pain from this muscle focuses into the TMJ area and the maxilla. Because dysfunction of the upper head of lateral pterygoid may directly impact TM joint disc status (leading to clicking and possible condylar and/or disc displacement) it is important to treat associated trigger points in this muscle as well as those in other muscles which include this area in their target zone of referral.

Intraoral palpation requires great sensitivity as this muscle is often extremely tender. The intraoral technique described below most likely reaches only the anterior aspect of the lower head. The posterior aspect of the upper head of lateral pterygoid and the posterior portion of the lower head may possibly be influenced from an external perspective (Simons et al 1998), discussed on p. 278.

NMT for intraoral lateral pterygoid

The practitioner will reach across the face to treat the contralateral side. The patient's mouth is open and the jaw deviated toward the side being evaluated to allow room for the treating finger to be placed between the maxilla and coronoid process. The finger nail rests against the cheek while the finger pad rests against the maxilla.

A gloved index finger (pad facing medially) is slid on the maxilla above the gingival margin as far posteriorly as possible. Pressure is applied medially (toward the lateral pterygoid plate). If the tissue is not tender, the finger is moved slightly caudally and again pressed toward the mid-line. The finger may sometimes be moved another finger tip caudally and sometimes may be slid 'under' the muscle slightly to reach a small portion of its caudal aspect. At each location, mild pressure is used until the tissue tenderness is evaluated and pressure is increased only if appropriate to do so (see Fig. 12.48).

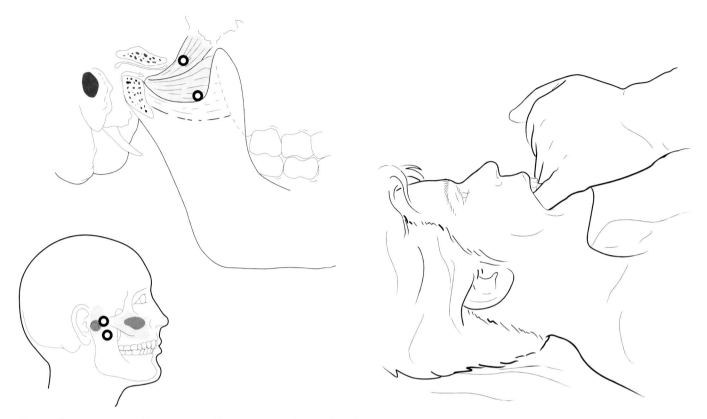

Figure 12.47 A portion of lateral pterygoid may be treated internally with the index finger or smallest digit (shown here) if the index finger is too large. The mandible is shifted ipsilaterally to create more room.

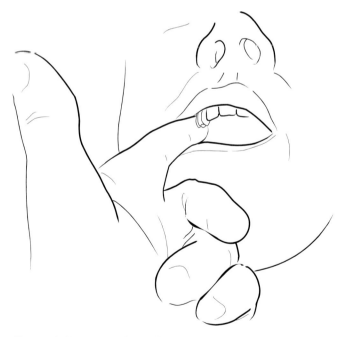

Figure 12.48 Finger position for intraoral access to lateral pterygoid.

If the treating finger continues medially, the medial pterygoid would be encountered as would the sharp pterygoid hamulus. Pressure on the hamulus is to be avoided during this and all other intraoral palpation

as the delicate overlying tissues may be damaged by indiscriminate or excessive pressure.

It is important to note that when the finger is placed correctly with the pad facing the maxilla, the lateral pterygoid is the muscle treated; however, if the finger is turned so that the pad faces the cheek and presses against the coronoid process, the temporalis tendon is addressed. It is important to differentiate and localize the tenderness the patient reports.

Medial pterygoid

Attachments: The palatine bone and the medial surface of the lateral pterygoid plate of the sphenoid bone to the pterygoid tuberosity on the posteroinferior part of the medial surface of the mandibular ramus and angle

Innervation: Medial pterygoid branch of the mandibular division of trigeminal (cranial nerve V)

Muscle type: Not established

Function: Elevates mandible; some influence in protraction, contralateral deviation and rotation about a vertical axis (*Gray's anatomy* 1999)

Synergists: *For elevation*: bilateral temporalis and masseter, contralateral medial pterygoid

For protrusion of mandible: lateral pterygoid

For contralateral deviation: same side lateral pterygoid

Antagonists: *To elevation*: digastric and lateral pterygoid
To contralateral deviation: contralateral medial and lateral pterygoids

Indications for treatment

- Pain in TM joint, especially if increased by chewing, clenching the teeth or opening of mouth
- Sore throat
- Painful swallowing
- Restricted range of mandibular opening

Special notes

Medial pterygoid's position on the medial aspect of the mandible mirrors the position of the masseter lateral to it and they form a mandibular sling for powerful elevation of the mandible. A hypertonic medial pterygoid can interfere with sphenoid function, with the maxilla and with normal motion of the palatines. It is commonly involved in TM joint problems.

Observation of opening and closing of the mouth will usually demonstrate contralateral deviation when medial pterygoid is hypertonic (usually in association with the lateral pterygoid). Trigger points in this muscle involve swallowing difficulties, sore throat and restriction in ability to fully open the jaw, as well as TM joint pain.

 NMT for intraoral medial pterygoid

These steps are best done on the same side on which the practitioner is standing. The gag reflex is easily activated in this region and may be temporarily inhibited by having the person exhale or inhale fully and hold the breath. This can be further inhibited by the patient forcing the tip of her tongue lateral and posterior, away from the palpated side, as strongly as possible during the palpation.

The index finger of the treating hand is placed between the upper and lower molars and moved posteriorly until it contacts the most anterior edge of the medial pterygoid muscle, which is posterior and medial to the last molar. Static pressure or short gliding strokes may be applied onto the belly of the medial pterygoid (Fig. 12.49). Extreme tenderness is likely if there is an active trigger in the muscle so pressure should be mild until tenderness is assessed.

The finger may be carefully slid up to the medial pterygoid's attachment on the medial pterygoid plate and the palatine bone as long as the hamulus is avoided due to its sharp tip and the overlying delicate tissues. Pressure on the palatine bones is also to be avoided. The palatoglossus and palatopharyngeus muscles may be treated at the same time.

The treating finger glides caudally as far as possible while attempting to reach the inferior attachment on the

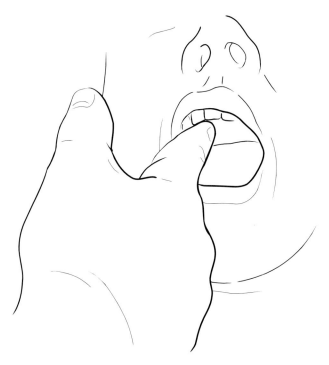

Figure 12.49 The finger is placed medial to the teeth to access medial pterygoid while lateral pterygoid is reached with the finger placed lateral to the teeth.

inside surface of the ramus of the mandible (Fig. 12.50). If gliding down the medial pterygoid causes too much discomfort or a gag reflex is provoked, the lower angle may be reached by gliding the index finger along the inside surface of the mandible until the internal surface of the lower angle is reached. Static pressure or gentle friction may be applied if appropriate.

Musculature of the soft palate (see Fig. 12.52)

The soft palate is a mobile muscular flap that hangs down from the hard palate with its posterior border free and, when elevated, closes the passageway between the nasopharynx and the oropharynx. The uvula hangs from the posterior border and, when relaxed, rests on the root of the tongue. The elevated uvula aids the tensor and levator veli palatini muscles in sealing off the nasopharynx. Nearby are the palatine tonsils and the sharp hamulus, around which the tensor veli palatini turns to radiate horizontally into the palatine aponeurosis.

The palatine musculature includes levator and tensor veli palatini, palatoglossus, palatopharyngeus and musculus uvula. Innervation to the soft palate musculature is controversial (*Gray's anatomy* 1999) and may include the vagus, trigeminal, mandibular, glossopharyngeal and facial nerves. These muscles are involved in swallowing and speech. Palatoglossus is discussed with the tongue and palatopharyngeus is considered with deglutition later in this section.

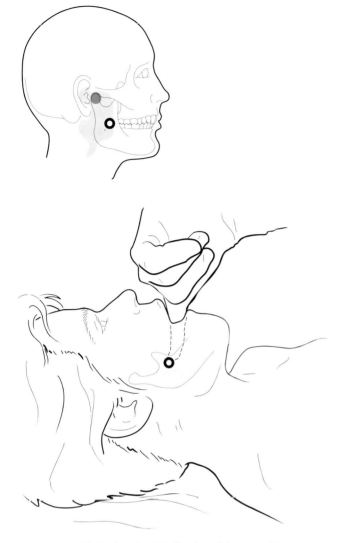

Figure 12.50 Palpation of mid-belly of medial pterygoid.

Levator veli palatini is a cylindrical muscle which courses from the petrous portion of the temporal bone, the carotid sheath and the inferior aspect of the cartilaginous part of the auditory tube to blend into the soft palate and palatine aponeurosis. This muscle pulls the soft palate upward and backward. It has little effect on the pharyngotympanic tube (*Gray's anatomy* 1999).

Tensor veli palatini is a thin, triangular muscle which attaches to the root of the pterygoid process, the spine of the sphenoid bone and the membranous wall of the pharyngotympanic (auditory) tube. It wraps around the hamulus before attaching to the palatine aponeurosis, which it elevates during swallowing. Its primary role, however, appears to be to open the entrance to the auditory tube to equalize air pressure during swallowing. Hypertonicity of this muscle has important clinical meaning as the auditory tube, when open, may provide an easy passageway for ororespiratory tract infections to reach the middle ear (Clemente 1987).

Ear infections in young children and their relationship with tensor veli palatini hypertonicity and trigger points is an area deserving of clinical research. Since these infections readily (and most often) occur in young children who are in a chronic sucking stage (thumbs, fingers, pacifiers, toys, nipple of the bottle or breast), the association of the tensor veli palatini seems obvious and deserves consideration. Kappler & Ramey (1997), however, suggest that 'Eustachian tube dysfunction is the most common cause of otitis media' and that this can be the result of fixation of the temporal bone (see discussion of temporal bone earlier in this chapter).

The paired uvulae muscles attach the uvula to the hard palate and soft palate. They radiate into the uvular mucosa, elevating and retracting to seal off the nasopharynx. The uvula may contain trigger points which induce hiccups (Simons et al 1998, Travell 1977).

NMT for soft palate (Fig. 12.51)

The patient tilts the head into extension and breathes through the mouth slowly or holds the breath on full inhalation or exhalation to inhibit the gag reflex. A confident but not aggressive pressure is used to avoid a tickling sensation which might cause gagging.

The index finger of the practitioner's treating hand is placed just lateral to the mid-line of the hard palate and glides posteriorly on the hard palate until it reaches the soft palate. No pressure is placed on the palatine bones or the vomer. The finger is hooked into a 'C' shape

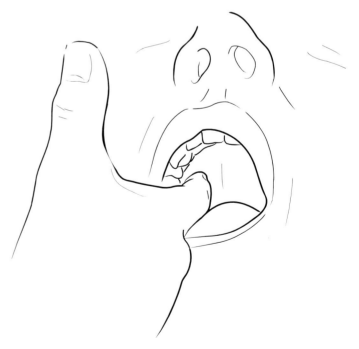

Figure 12.51 The soft palate musculature is carefully addressed to avoid the palatine bones, the sharp hamulus and the gag reflex mechanisms.

as it sinks into the soft palate posterior to the palatine bone and sweeps out to the lateral one-third of the soft palate. A back and forth medial/lateral movement of the finger or static pressure is applied into the lateral third of the soft palate while pressing through the superficial tissues of the soft palate and onto the palatini muscles.

Muscles of the tongue (Fig. 12.52)

Extrinsic tongue muscles arise from outside the tongue to act upon it, while intrinsic muscles arise wholly within it and have the primary task of changing the shape of the main body of the tongue (Leonhardt 1986). The tongue muscles are innervated by the hypoglossal nerve (cranial nerve XII).

Extrinsic muscles of the tongue include the following.

• *Hyoglossus* attaches the side of the tongue to the hyoid bone below by vertical fibers which serve to depress the tongue (as in saying *aahh*).

• *Genioglossus* courses from the geniotubercle (cephalad from geniohyoid) fanning posteriorly and upwardly to attach to the hyoid bone, blend with the middle pharyngeal constrictor, attach to the hyoglossal membrane

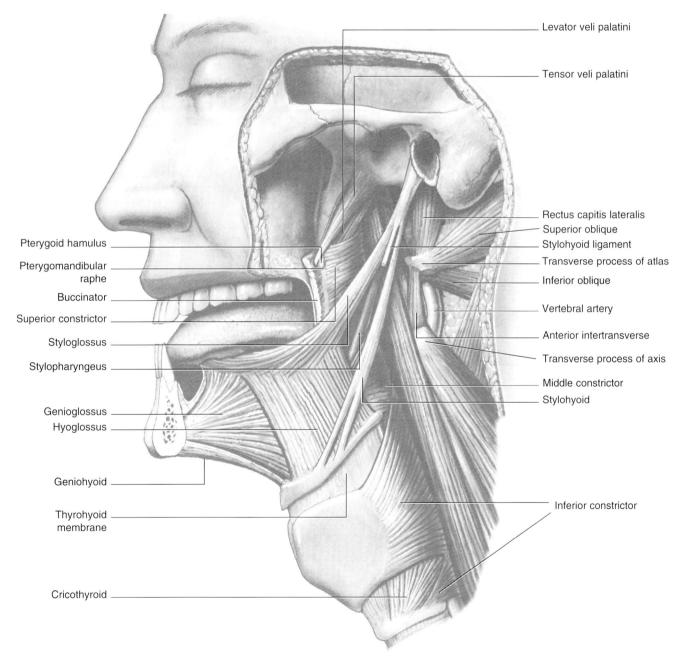

Figure 12.52 Muscles of the styloid process, tongue and soft palate (reproduced, with permission, from *Gray's anatomy* (1999)).

and the whole length of the ventral surface of the tongue from root to apex and intermingle with intrinsic lingual muscles. It tractions the tongue forward to protrude its tip from the mouth.

• *Styloglossus* anchors the tongue to the styloid process near its tip and to the styloid end of the stylomandibular ligament. Its fibers divide into a longitudinal portion, which merges with the inferior longitudinal muscle, and an oblique portion, which overlaps and crosses hyoglossus to decussate with it. It draws the tongue posteriorly and upwardly.

• *Chondroglossus* ascends from the hyoid bone to merge with the intrinsic musculature between the hyoglossus and genioglossus and assists the hyoglossus in depressing the tongue.

• *Palatoglossus* extends from the soft palate to the side of the tongue and the dorsal surface and intermingles with the transverse lingual muscle. It elevates the root of the tongue while approximating the palatoglossal arch, thus closing the oral cavity from the oropharynx.

Intrinsic muscles of the tongue include the following.

• *Superior longitudinal* bilaterally extends from submucous tissue near the epiglottis and from the median lingual septum to the lingual margins and apex of the tongue. It shortens the tongue and turns the tip and sides upward to make the dorsum concave.

• *Inferior longitudinal* extends from the lingual root and the hyoid bone to the tip of the tongue, blending with styloglossus. It shortens the tongue and turns the tip and sides downward to make the dorsum convex.

• *Transverse lingual* extends from the median fibrous septum to the submucous fibrous tissue at the tongue's lingual margin. It narrows and elongates the tongue.

• *Vertical lingual* extends from the dorsal to the ventral aspects in the borders of the anterior tongue. It makes the tongue flatter and wider.

The tongue muscles can act alone or in pairs and in endless combination. They provide the tongue with precise movements and tremendous mobility, which impacts not only the acts of chewing and swallowing but also speech. Though trigger point location and referral patterns are not yet established for these muscles, one author (JD) has observed trigger points in several of these muscles, most notably the most caudal, most posterior lateral aspect of the tongue in regard to chronic sore throat and the immediate relief of the condition with application of static pressure and gliding strokes as described below.

Myofascial tissues are known to produce trigger points and trigger points are known to produce patterns of referral as well as dysfunctions in coordinated movement of the muscles in which they are housed. It seems reasonable to assume that the tongue muscles might also contain trigger points and that they might produce pain in sur-

rounding tissues, as well as being involved in dysfunctional responses which interfere with swallowing or with normal speech patterns. The tongue should be examined and, if necessary, treated, in these conditions as well as in those involving voice dysfunction, elevated hyoid bone or sore throat.

 NMT for muscles of the tongue

These muscles are most easily addressed by reaching across the body to the opposite side of the tongue. The practitioner's gloved index finger is placed on the lateral surface of the tongue as far posteriorly as possible. The finger curls into a 'C' shape as it is slid forward the full length of the tongue. The curling action of the finger sinks it into the side of the tongue and penetrates the musculature more effectively than does sliding a straight finger (Fig. 12.53).

The gliding, curling movement is repeated 6–8 times. The finger is moved caudally at finger tip widths and the process repeated as far caudally as possible. Special attention should be given to the most caudal, most posterolateral aspect of the tongue, where the long gliding strokes previously applied may become shorter and more precisely applied or static pressure may be used.

The tongue may also be gently pulled forward and the muscles stretched by grasping it firmly through a clean cloth (Fig. 12.54). This stretch can be held for 30–60 seconds and the direction of tension changed by pulling the tongue to one side or the other.

Since these muscles are readily treated by the patient, self-care can be applied at home when indicated. Tongue stretching, as described, may usefully be combined with spray and stretch methods (applied to the anterior neck) as described by Simons et al (1998) for the suprahyoids.

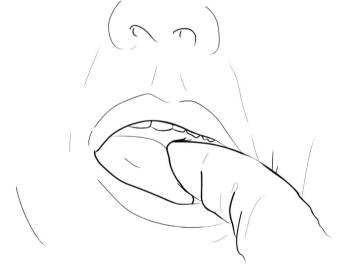

Figure 12.53 The treating finger is curled as it is dragged forward to penetrate the tongue muscles.

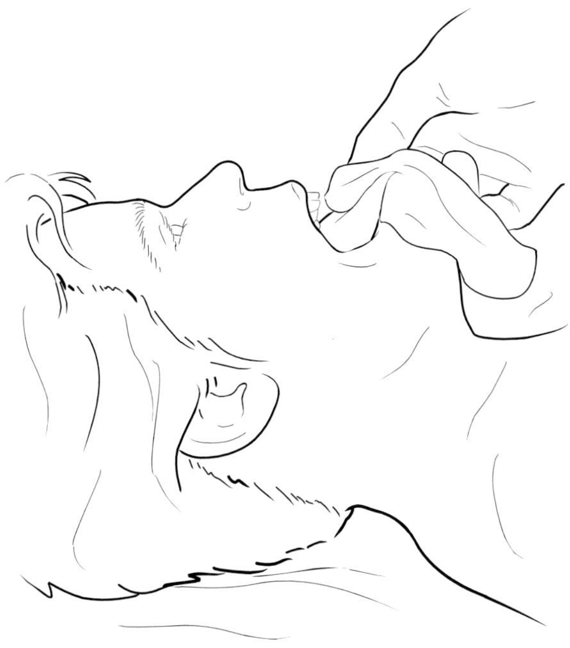

Figure 12.54 Tongue muscles may be gently stretched by pulling the tongue forward.

Suprahyoid muscles – the floor of the mouth

The suprahyoid group form the floor of the mouth and serve to position the hyoid bone and, when the hyoid bone is fixed by the infrahyoids, depress the mandible. The stylohyoid has been discussed previously with palpation of the external cranial muscles (p. 278). The remaining suprahyoids, which include digastric, mylohyoid and geniohyoid, are presented here and should be addressed with the treatment of the anterior neck, temporomandibular joint and the muscles of the tongue. They are innervated by the trigeminal and hypoglossal nerves.

- *Geniohyoid* extends from the hyoid bone to the symphysis menti on the inner surface of the mid-portion of the mandible where it serves to elevate the hyoid bone and draw it forward and to depress the mandible when the hyoid is fixed.
- *Mylohyoid* extends from the whole length of the mylohyoid line of the inner mandible to the front of the body of the hyoid bone. Its anterior and middle fibers decussate in a fibrous raphe which extends through the mid-line from the hyoid bone to the symphysis menti, allowing this muscle to form the floor of the mouth. It elevates the floor of the mouth as well as the hyoid bone and depresses the mandible when the hyoid is fixed.
- *Digastric* has two bellies joined by a central tendon. The posterior belly arises from the mastoid notch of the temporal bone while the anterior belly attaches to the digastric fossa of the mandible (near symphysis). They are joined together by a common tendon which passes through a fibrous sling that is attached to the hyoid bone and is sometimes lined by a synovial sheath. The tendon perforates stylohyoid. The fibers of stylohyoid and the posterior fibers of digastric are difficult to distinguish by palpation alone (Simons et al 1998). Digastric depresses

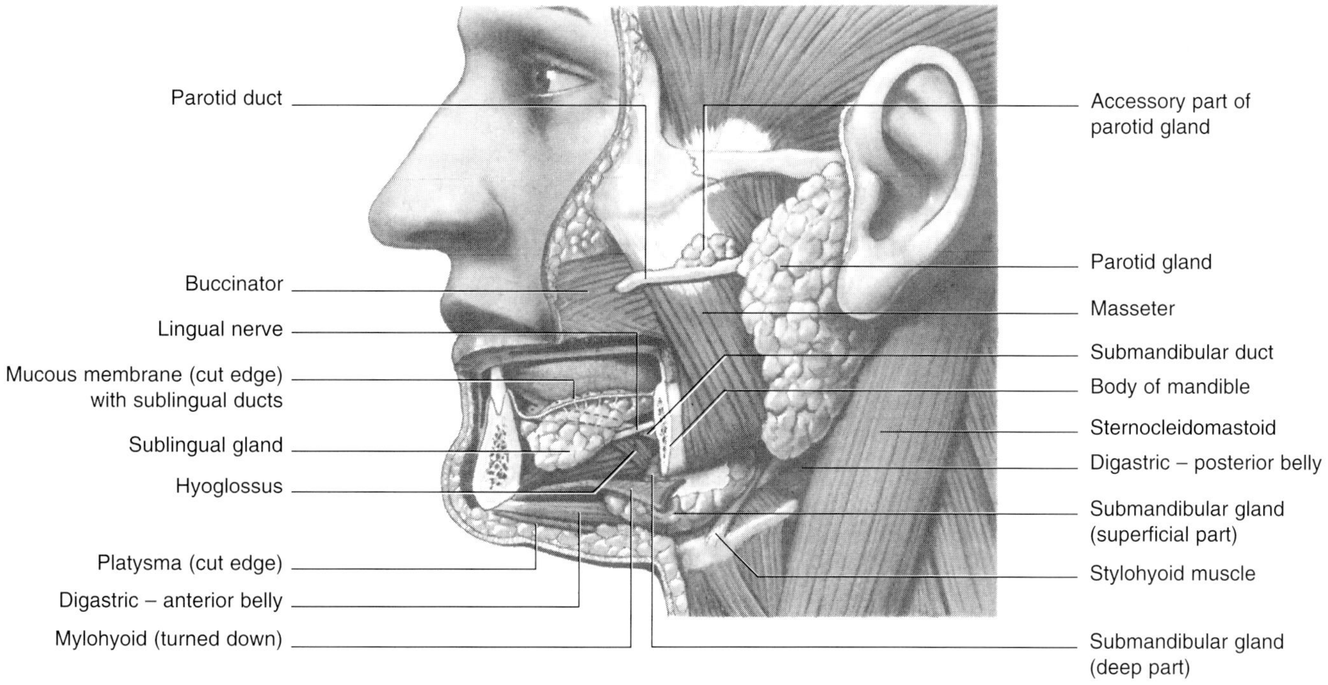

Figure 12.55 Compression of the salivary glands is avoided when addressing the suprahyoid muscles in the floor of the mouth (reproduced, with permission, from *Gray's anatomy* (1999)).

the mandible (secondary to lateral pterygoid), elevates the hyoid bone and, together with geniohyoid, can assist retraction of the mandible. When digastric is hypertonic it places a load onto the contralateral temporalis and masseter which attempt to balance the deviation which a taut digastric may produce.

The suprahyoid muscles usually function as a paired team in the movements described. Since the position of the hyoid bone is important to the maintenance of a clear air passageway, of consistent dimension, as well as a food passageway, its freedom of movement is critical in swallowing, normal breathing patterns and speech. When habitual mouth breathing is noted, these muscles, as well as any tendency to a forward head position, should be addressed, along with the causes of the mouth breathing (allergies, deviated septum, sinus infections, etc.). The upper abdominal area as well as the diaphragm should be evaluated (and treated if necessary) as well as the intercostals (see respiratory section, p. 429).

Submandibular salivary gland infections may incite dysfunction in surrounding muscular tissue which may, in turn, create dysfunctional movement patterns of the mandible, including lateral excursion during opening (producing a zig-zag pattern of tracking) and occlusal interferences. Glandular infections and stones within the salivary glands should be considered and ruled out, especially when the suprahyoid muscles are unilaterally tender to palpation.

Upledger & Vredevoogd (1983) point out that the mylohyoid can interfere with cranial mechanics because of its action in opening the mouth, when the hyoid is stabilized by the infrahyoid, an action which would be counteracted by muscles attaching to the maxillae and the zygomatic bones. The complex of stabilization and counterpressures can, they suggest, 'interfere with the function of the craniosacral system and contribute to temporomandibular dysfunction'.

Trigger points in the posterior belly of digastric can refer pain to the upper part of the sternocleidomastoid muscle as well as neck and head pain while triggers in the anterior belly refer to the lower incisors. If a trigger in digastric is referring into the lower incisors then a rapid tensing of the anterior neck muscles by the patient ('pull the corners of your mouth down vigorously') will activate the trigger and reproduce the pain. The digastric trigger point target zone includes the area of the stylohyoid muscle, whose pain pattern is not yet clearly established but is presumed to be similar (Simons et al 1998).

The posterior attachment of digastric as well as the stylohyoid have been previously discussed together with the mastoid and styloid processes (p. 280). The intraoral treatment of the anterior belly of digastric, as well as the mylohyoid and geniohyoid, is described here.

NMT for intraoral floor of mouth

These muscles may be treated either ipsilaterally or contralaterally depending upon the comfort of the practitioner and the angle of the jaw. While using no pressure to position the finger for treatment, the index finger of the practitioner's treating hand (usually the most caudal hand) is placed onto one side of the floor of the mouth and slid posterior as far as possible. A finger of the external hand opposes the internal finger to provide a

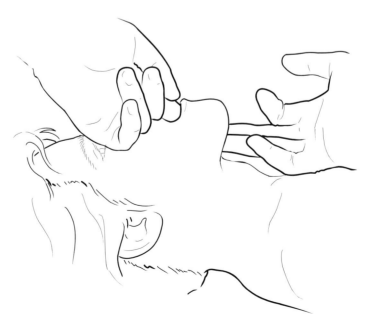

Figure 12.56 The entire floor of the mouth may be treated with one finger placed intraorally and opposing digits providing pressure externally.

Box 12.10 Deglutition (Fig. 12.57)

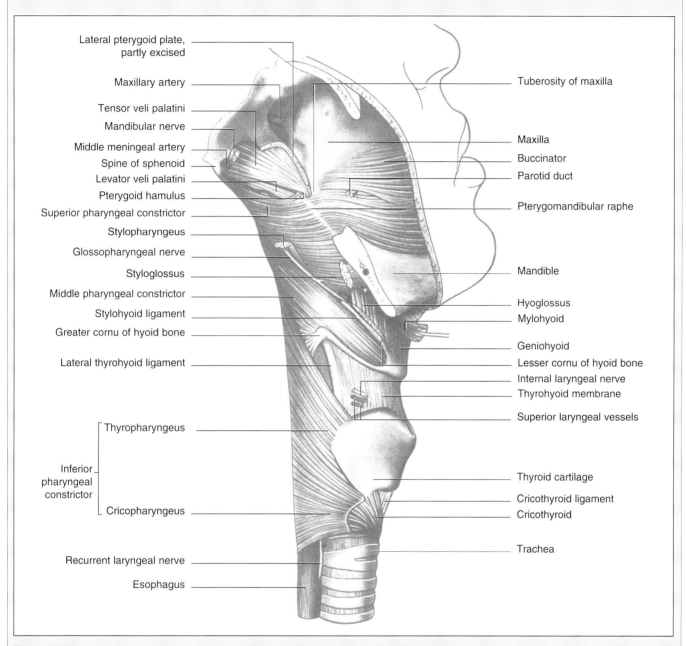

Lateral pterygoid plate, partly excised

Maxillary artery

Tensor veli palatini

Mandibular nerve

Middle meningeal artery

Spine of sphenoid

Levator veli palatini

Pterygoid hamulus

Superior pharyngeal constrictor

Stylopharyngeus

Glossopharyngeal nerve

Styloglossus

Middle pharyngeal constrictor

Stylohyoid ligament

Greater cornu of hyoid bone

Lateral thyrohyoid ligament

Thyropharyngeus

Inferior pharyngeal constrictor

Cricopharyngeus

Recurrent laryngeal nerve

Esophagus

Tuberosity of maxilla

Maxilla

Buccinator

Parotid duct

Pterygomandibular raphe

Mandible

Hyoglossus

Mylohyoid

Geniohyoid

Lesser cornu of hyoid bone

Internal laryngeal nerve

Thyrohyoid membrane

Superior laryngeal vessels

Thyroid cartilage

Cricothyroid ligament

Cricothyroid

Trachea

Figure 12.57 Buccinator and muscles of the pharynx (reproduced, with permission, from *Gray's anatomy* (1999)).

Helmut Leonhardt (1986) has summarized the processes of deglutition as follows.

Voluntary inception of swallowing

- The muscles of the floor of the mouth contract and the tongue, together with the bolus (of food), is pressed against the soft palate.
- Subsequent movements are due to stimulation of the receptors in the mucosa of the palate.

Safeguarding the airway by reflex action

- The palate is tensed and raised by the tensor and levator veli palatini muscles to press against the posterior wall of the pharynx.

- The latter protrudes like a torus due to superior pharyngeal constrictor contraction (Passavant's ring torus), separating food passage from the upper airways.
- If the palatal muscles are paralyzed, e.g. after diphtheria, food will enter the nose during deglutition.
- Mylohyoid, digastric and thyrohyoid muscles lift the floor of the mouth and assist in visible and palpable elevation of the hyoid bone and the larynx, while the entrance to the larynx and the entrance to the epiglottis approximate.
- The root of the tongue lowers the epiglottis with the help of the aryepiglottic muscles and the entrance to the larynx is (incompletely) closed.
- Simultaneously, breathing stops as the rima glottidis is closed.

Box 12.10 (cont'd)

- Thus, food passage is completely prevented from entering the lower airways.

Transport of the bolus through the pharynx and esophagus

Leonhardt explains further that:

The slit of the pharynx unfolds upward and forward when the larynx ascends. Then the tongue is pulled like a piston by the styloglossus

and hyoglossus muscles and pushes the bolus over the fauces into the pharynx. The bolus slides mainly through the piriform recesses primarily and partly over the epiglottis.

Pharyngeal constrictors can then push the bolus through the dilated esophagus 'right down to the cardia'.
Leonhardt concludes: 'The bolus can also be propelled into the stomach by continuous waves of contraction of circular muscle (peristalsis), even against gravity, if the subject adopts an appropriate posture'.

---

supporting surface against which to press the muscles (Fig. 12.56).

The treating finger is pressed toward the external finger, capturing a portion of the suprahyoid musculature between the two digits. The tissue may be compressed or frictioned between the two digits at finger-tip intervals until the entire floor of the mouth has been treated. The submandibular salivary glands should be avoided but the tissue surrounding them should be thoroughly examined.

The external finger may also be used as the treating finger with the internal finger offering stability. This reversal of roles particularly addresses the anterior belly of digastric.

REFERENCES

Brookes D 1981 Lectures on cranial osteopathy. Thorsons, Wellingborough
Cailliet R 1992 Head and face pain syndromes. F A Davis, Philadelphia
Chaitow L 1999 Cranial manipulation: theory and practice. Churchill Livingstone, Edinburgh
Clemente C 1987 Anatomy: a regional atlas of the human body, 3rd edn. Urban and Schwarzenberg, Baltimore
DeLany J 1997 Temporomandibular dysfunction. Journal of Bodywork and Movement Therapies 1(4):198–202
Ettlinger H, Gintis B 1991 Cranial osteopathy. In DiGiovanna E (ed) Osteopathic approaches to diagnosis and treatment. Lippincott, Philadelphia
Gagey P-M 1991 Non-vestibular dizziness and static posturography. Acta Otorhinolaryngolica Belgica 45:335
Gagey P-M, Gentaz R 1996 Postural disorders of the body. In: Liebenson C (ed) Rehabilitation of the spine. Williams and Wilkins, Baltimore
Gelb H 1977 Clinical management of head, neck and TMJ pain and dysfunction. W B Saunders, Philadelphia
Gray's anatomy 1973 35th edn. Churchill Livingstone, Edinburgh
Gray's anatomy 1999 (Williams P. ed) 39th edn. Churchill Livingstone, Edinburgh
Greenman P 1989 Modern manual medicine. Williams and Wilkins, Baltimore
Grossmann E, Paiano G 1998 Eagle's syndrome: a case report. Journal of Craniomandibular Practice 16(2):126–130
Hack G, Robinson W, Koritzer R 1995 Report at a meeting of the American Association of Neurological Surgeons and the Congress of Neurological Surgeons, Phoenix, Arizona, February 14–18
Kappler R, Ramey K 1997 Head: diagnosis and treatment. In: Ward R (ed) Fundamentals of osteopathic medicine. Williams and Wilkins, Baltimore
Kellgren J H 1938 Observations on referred pain arising from muscle. Clinical Science 3:175–190
Kingston B 1996 Understanding muscles. Bernard Kingston/ Chapman Hall, London
Klineberg I 1991 The lateral pterygoid muscle: some anatomical, physiological and clinical considerations. Annals of the Royal Australian College of Dental Surgeons 11:96–108
Latey P 1996 Feelings, muscles and movement. Journal of Bodywork and Movement Therapies 1(1):44–52
Leonhardt H 1986 Color atlas and textbook of human anatomy: vol 2, internal organs, 3rd edn. Georg Thieme, Stuttgart
Lewandowski M, Drasby E 1996 Kinematic system demonstrates

cranial bone movement about the cranial sutures. Journal of the American Osteopathic Association 96(9):551
Lewit K 1992 Manipulative therapy in rehabilitation of the motor system. Butterworths, London
Lewit K 1996 Role of manipulation in spinal rehabilitation. In: Liebenson C (ed) Rehabilitation of the spine: a practitioner's manual. Williams and Wilkins, Baltimore
McPartland J 1996 Craniosacral iatrogenesis. Journal of Bodywork and Movement Therapies 1(1):2–5
Milne H 1995 The heart of listening. North Atlantic Books, Berkeley
Okeson J 1996 Orofacial pain: guidelines for assessment, diagnosis and management. Quintessence Publishing, Chicago
Platzer W 1992 Color atlas/text of human anatomy: vol 1, locomotor system, 4th edn. Georg Thieme, Stuttgart
Rocobado M 1985 Arthrokinematics of the temporomandibular joint. In: Clinical management of head, neck and TMJ pain and dysfunction. W B Saunders, Philadelphia
Scariati P 1991 Strain and counterstrain. In: DiGiovanna E (ed) An osteopathic approach to diagnosis and treatment. Lippincott, London
Simons D, Travell J, Simons L 1998 Myofascial pain and dysfunction: the trigger point manual, vol 1, 2nd edn. Williams and Wilkins, Baltimore
Skaggs C 1997 Temporomandibular dysfunction: chiropractic rehabilitation. Journal of Bodywork and Movement Therapies 4(1):208–213
Stedman's electronic medical dictionary 1998 version 4.0. Williams and Wilkins, Baltimore
Tally R 1990 Standards of history, examination and diagnosis in treatment of TMD. Journal of Craniomandibular Practice 8:60–77
Tilley L 1997 Temporomandibular dysfunction: holistic dentistry. Journal of Bodywork and Movement Therapies 1(4):203–207
Travell J G 1977 A trigger point for hiccup. Journal of the American Osteopathic Association 77:308–312
Travell J, Simons D 1983 Myofascial pain and dysfunction: the trigger point manual, vol 1. Williams and Wilkins, Baltimore
Travell J, Simons D 1992 Myofascial pain and dysfunction: the trigger point manual, vol 2, the lower extremities. Williams and Wilkins, Baltimore
Upledger J, Vredevoogd J 1983 Craniosacral therapy. Eastland Press, Seattle
Walther D 1988 Applied kinesiology. SDC Systems, Pueblo, Colorado
Wilson K, Waugh A 1996 Anatomy and physiology in health and disease. Churchill Livingstone, New York

13

Shoulder, arm and hand

SHOULDER

STRUCTURE

The shoulder is an immensely complicated structure and it is easy to become confused by its complexity and the wide range of assessment protocols that are used during clinical evaluation. Evidence from tests involving range of motion, neurological reflex evaluation, muscle strength and weakness assessment, postural analysis, and palpation relating to altered tissue tone, pain patterns, and myofascial trigger points may all be usefully gathered and collated. A host of other 'functional pathologies' may also be discovered, not to mention actual pathology, including inflammatory processes, arthritic changes and other degenerative possibilities.

It is easy to see how, as a result of the availability of all these data 'information overload' might occur, with no clear indication of where to begin therapeutic intervention. Liebenson (1996) states the clinical conundrum as follows: 'So many structural and functional pathologies are present in asymptomatic individuals that they may not be clinically significant when seen in symptomatic patients'.

Liebenson's insightful statement leads us to question how it may be possible to find a way through the maze of information and to identify and extract the key elements in each particular case. This is most certainly not a recommendation for skimping on assessment; however, it does offer the opportunity for meaningful evaluation of functional patterns, which can often highlight what have been termed 'key stereotypic movement patterns' (Jull & Janda 1987, Lewit 1991). How is the area working? Is it behaving normally? Are firing patterns sequential and within normal parameters? Is the range of movement optimal? Functional assessment protocols are described (see p. 303) which may be used to highlight particular structures which may then receive primary attention. These concepts should be kept in mind as we work our way through the many essential aspects of shoulder function and dysfunction, the joints and soft tissue components and the tests associated with these.

Key joints affecting the shoulder

When considering shoulder movements, seven joints must be functional for ease and integrity of shoulder use. It is useful to think of the shoulder girdle as being made up of these seven separate joints, each interdependent on the integrity and function of the others.

In summary form, these seven joints are (more detailed discussion follows):

• glenohumeral joint (scapulohumeral) is a true joint in that it has two bones directly articulating (the head of the humerus with the glenoid fossa), is lined with hyaline cartilage, has a joint capsule and is filled with synovial fluid. The humeral head may glide up or down the fossa, anteriorly, posteriorly and with inversion or eversion

• suprahumeral joint (subdeltoid) is a false joint in that it does not have a direct apposition of two bones nor do they have an articulating surface, but instead is comprised

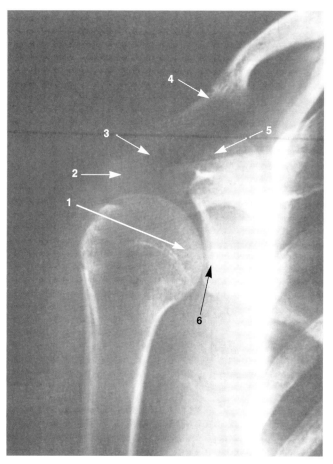

Figure 13.1 Anteroposterior radiography of an 18-year-old female showing 1. head of humerus, 2. acromion, 3. acromioclavicular joint, 4. clavicle, 5. coracoid process, 6. glenoid articular surface (reproduced, with permission, from *Gray's anatomy* (1999)).

of a bone (humeral head) moving in respect to another bone (acromioclavicular joint) and the overhanging coracoacromial ligament

• scapulothoracic (scapulocostal) joint is a false joint composed of the scapula and its gliding movements on the thoracic wall (thoracoscapular articulation)

• acromioclavicular joint is a true joint articulation of the acromial process of the scapula to the lateral end of the clavicle. This articulation forms an overhanging ledge which, while offering protection, also impinges on movement of the humeral head beneath the ledge. The only bony attachment of the scapula to the entire thorax is the acromioclavicular joint. All other attachments are muscular

• sternoclavicular joint is a true joint whose movement is often overlooked as part of the shoulder girdle. Since the distal end of the clavicle must elevate and rotate with the acromion during elevation of the arm, its sternal articulation and movement are vital as well

• sternocostal joint – true joint

• costovertebral joint – true joint.

Glenohumeral joint

The glenohumeral joint is arguably the most important joint of the shoulder girdle. With healthy movements of this joint, even though the others may be dysfunctional, the arm may be functional to some degree. When the glenohumeral joint is restricted, even if the other joints are free, there will be little or no use of the arm. When all tissues associated with the joint are functioning normally, this joint has a greater degree of movement than any other joint in the body.

The proximal end of the humerus is a convex ovoid which significantly exceeds the surface area of the glenoid fossa, with which it articulates. Therefore, only a small part of the surface of the humeral head articulates with the glenoid at any given time. Additional surface area is provided by the glenoid labrum, a fibrocartilaginous rim which extends the glenoid into a modified 'socket' which is further supported by the joint capsule.

The rotator cuff muscles (supraspinatus, infraspinatus, teres minor and subscapularis – SITS) blend their fibers with the joint capsule and offer muscular support. The SITS tendons are so closely approximated to the joint capsule that they are especially vulnerable to injury.

The head of the humerus is capable of many combinations of swing and spin, producing a highly mobile joint as well as relatively unstable one. However, it has basically three planes of movement (abduction/adduction, flexion/extension and medial/lateral rotation) which are most apparent when the scapula is fixed.

Accessory movements, such as translation of the humeral head in all directions on the glenoid face (joint play), should also be manually possible. Osseous, ligamentous and muscular dysfunctions can limit joint play, as well

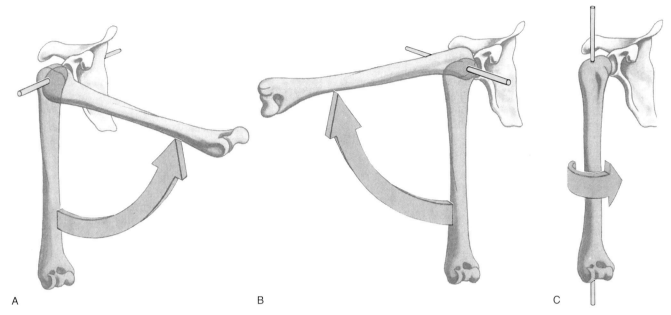

Figure 13.2 The three degrees of freedom of movement of the shoulder joint. A: Flexion-extension. B: Abduction-adduction. C: Medial-lateral rotation (reproduced, with permission, from *Gray's anatomy* (1995)).

as ranges of motion, and should be corrected when joint play has been lost.

Suprahumeral joint

Located directly cephalad to the humeral head is the overhanging acromioclavicular joint and the coracoacromial ligament. Even though their relationship does not constitute a true joint, the humeral head moves in relation to overhanging structures and therefore is vulnerable to the development of several pathological conditions affecting the acromion. The supraspinatus tendon, the humeral head itself, the inferior surface of the acromioclavicular joint or the coracoacromial ligament may be damaged (repetitively) when the suprahumeral joint space is compromised.

The suprahumeral joint space may be compromised:

- when tissue normally residing there becomes enlarged through overuse or inflammation
- by loss of normal position of the acromioclavicular joint due to muscular imbalance
- by repositioning of the acromioclavicular joint due to postural compensations
- by the existence of a subacromial osteoarthritic deposit.

When the joint space has been reduced and the humeral head is abducted beyond 90°, the supraspinatus tendon may be entrapped between the structures and damaged. Excessive abrasion of the tendon will lead to inflammation and eventually deposition of calcium into the tendon. This calcific deposit may then become a mechanical block to abduction and overhead elevation of the arm. Addi-

tionally, the subdeltoid bursa, which is located between the tendon and acromioclavicular joint, may become inflamed or infiltrated by calcium, resulting in adhesions and 'frozen shoulder' syndrome (or adhesive capsulitis).

To avoid impaction against the overhanging structures, the humeral head has one distinct advantage – its ability to rotate laterally. When the arm is elevated beyond 90° of abduction, lateral rotation will move the greater tuberosity and its attached supraspinatus tendon posteriorly, thereby avoiding the bony protuberances above. This rotation, coupled with adequate elevation of the acromioclavicular joint (achieved by upper and middle trapezius) and scapular rotation, will help insure correct movement (see p. 338).

Scapulothoracic joint

With movements of the scapulothoracic joint, the concave surface of the scapula translates and rotates against the convex surface of the thorax. The scapula may be abducted, adducted, elevated, depressed and rotated both laterally (so the glenoid faces superiorly) and medially (glenoid fossa faces inferiorly).

Movements of the scapulothoracic (scapulocostal) joint are not only critical to movement of the humerus but are precisely coordinated with it. During humeral abduction, there is a proportionate movement of both the humerus and scapula, called the *scapulohumeral rhythm*, at an approximate 2:1 ratio. That is, when the humerus has been elevated to 90°, the scapula has rotated 30° while the humerus has moved 60°, making the total movement 90°. The 2:1 ratio 'rule' may also be applied to full elevation (180° – scapula 60°, humerus 120°). If, however, the muscles of the region are dysfunctional, with weakness of the lower fixators (e.g. lower trapezius, serratus), there will be excessive scapula movement during the first 60° of abduction. During the first 60° of abduction movement should take place mainly at the glenohumeral joint, therefore the 2:1 ratio may not pertain at every degree of abduction (Cailliet 1991). This is the basis of the scapulo-humeral rhythm test (described on p. 303) which demonstrates whether there is undue scapula movement before 60° of abduction, indicating poor stabilization of the lower fixators and excessive tone in the upper fixators (levator scapula and upper trapezius). It is the coordinated movement of the arm with the scapula, coupled with proportional rotation of the humerus, that results in physiologic arm motion (Cailliet 1991).

The space between the scapula and the thorax is filled by two muscles (serratus anterior and subscapularis) and areolar tissue, which makes direct bony articulation impossible but nevertheless allows movement. This is why this joint is termed a 'false joint'.

Contractures and hypertonicity of serratus anterior and/or subscapularis may directly influence the scapula's ability to rotate. Scapular function may also be impaired due to adhesion of these muscles to each other. Scapular mobilization techniques, such as that discussed on p. 146, may be necessary to restore rotation and translation of the scapula.

Acromioclavicular joint

The acromion's articulation with the lateral end of the clavicle, forming the acromioclavicular joint, a true joint, is important not only because of the potential for impaction (as discussed above) but also because it is itself required to move in order for elevation of the upper extremity to occur. Movement of the clavicle against the acromion occurs in all directions and axial rotation of the clavicle allows further movement augmented by its crankshaft design.

An articular disc often exists between the surfaces of the clavicle and the acromion, having developed into a meniscoid from a fibrocartilaginous bridge at 2–3 years of age. Degenerative changes may occur in response to repetitious and/or rotatory traction forces imposed upon it.

Instability of this joint can occur if any of its supporting ligaments are damaged. Loss of joint integrity can then impede movement of the humeral head upon the glenoid fossa. Additionally, chronic inflammation caused by repetitive impactions against the acromioclavicular joint's inferior surface may lead to formation of a subacromial osteoarthritic deposit. While such calcification of the joint may offer stability and structural support, mobility will be impaired.

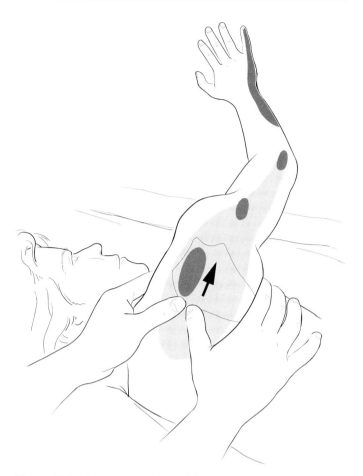

Figure 13.3 Adequate scapula mobility allows a 'hidden' trigger point for serratus posterior superior to be reached (see p. 446).

Sternoclavicular joint

The sternoclavicular joint is a true joint whose movement is often overlooked as part of the shoulder girdle. Since the distal end of the clavicle must rise with the acromion during elevation of the arm, its sternal articulation and movement are vital. Serving as the two ends of a crankshaft engineered for twisting, the sternoclavicular joint and the acromioclavicular joint are similarly designed. The sternal end of the clavicle articulates with the sternum through an articular disc and also directly with the first costal cartilage.

Compared with the acromioclavicular joint, few degenerative changes occur in the sternoclavicular joint. Its strength relies on its ligamentous support and its weakness is to fracture rather than dislocate, although its mobility can be restricted because of dysfunctional attaching musculature (subclavius, for example).

Sternocostal joint

Since the clavicle articulates with the sternocostal cartilage of the first rib, the health of this sternocostal joint is important. In extreme overhead positions, weight might be distributed onto the costal cartilage from the clavicle and transmitted onto the sternum. The first sternocostal joint is therefore considered to be part of the shoulder girdle and its mobility and integrity are important to shoulder care. Its integrity can be compromised by excessive force imposed by the scalenes, according to Lewit (1991), who states, 'Tension in pectoralis and pain points at the sternocostal junction of the upper ribs seems to be connected with tension in the scalenes'. He continues, 'Blockage of the first rib goes hand in hand with reflex spasm of the scalenus on the same side, which is abolished by treatment of the first rib'.

Costovertebral joint

As the rib translates structurally to the vertebral column, the costovertebral joint assumes the stress. The costovertebral joints throughout the thorax should be mobile and pain free. However, the health and position of the first two ribs are particularly important due to the attachments of the scalene muscles. The scalenes' influences on shoulder pain are numerous, including trigger point referral patterns and nerve entrapment possibilities. Their influence on upper rib fixation may therefore indirectly impact on shoulder function.

ASSESSMENT

Manual treatment is far more likely to be successful if its application is based on identifiable dysfunctional features. The practitioner needs a 'story' to work with, whether this is a possible connection between the patient's symptoms and a palpable feature (something that is tense, tight, restricted, etc.) or a demonstrable abnormality (restricted range, weakness, etc.) or symptoms which can be modified manually (increase or decrease of pain as evaluation is performed, for example).

In order for the 'story' to be clinically useful it needs to connect the patient's presenting symptoms with something which is identified by palpation and assessment as in some way causing, contributing to or maintaining the symptoms. Appropriate treatment choices flow naturally from such a sequence.

History + symptoms + 'dysfunctional features' = a 'story' which helps to determine treatment choices

In taking a history of a patient and her condition, important questions which we should ask include the following.

- How long have you had the symptoms?
- Are the symptoms constant?
- Are the symptoms intermittent and if so, is there any pattern?

- What is the location of the symptoms?
- Do they vary at all?
- If so, what do you think contributes to this?
- What, if anything, starts, aggravates and/or relieves the symptoms?
- Do any of the following movements improve or worsen the symptoms – for example, turning the head one way or the other; looking up or down; bending forward; standing, walking, sitting down or getting up again; lying down, turning over and getting up again; stretching out the arm, and so on?
- Has this happened before?
- And if so, what helped it last time?

It is very important to identify what eases symptoms as well as what worsens them, as this may reveal patterns which 'load' and 'unload' the biomechanical features out of which the symptoms emerge. The patient's own viewpoint as to what helps and what worsens symptoms, as well as the practitioner's evaluation as to where restrictions and abnormal tissue states exist and how dysfunction manifests during standard testing and palpation, should together form the basis, with the history, for making a tentative initial assessment.

Repetitions are important

In performing assessments (testing a shoulder for internal rotation, for example), if performing the action once produces no symptom, it may be useful to have the movement performed a number of times. As Jacob & McKenzie (1996) explain:

Standard range of motion examinations and orthopedic tests do not adequately explore how the particular patient's spinal [or other area of the body] mechanics and symptoms are affected by specific movements and/or positioning. Perhaps the greatest limitation of these examinations and tests is the supposition that each test movement needs to be performed only once to fathom how the patient's complaint responds. The effects of repetitive movements or positions maintained for prolonged periods of time are not explored, even though such loading strategies might better approximate what occurs in the 'real world'.

- Assessments should evaluate symptoms in relation to posture and position, as well as to function or movement.
- Function needs to be evaluated in relation to *quality*, as well as *symmetry* and *range of movement* involved.
- Any assessment needs to take account of the gender, age, body type and health status of the individual being assessed, as these factors can all influence a comparison with the 'norm'.

Attention should be paid to the effect of movement on symptoms (does it hurt more or less when a particular movement is performed?), as well as to the degree of functional normality revealed by the movement. In the

Box 13.1 Ligaments of the shoulder girdle

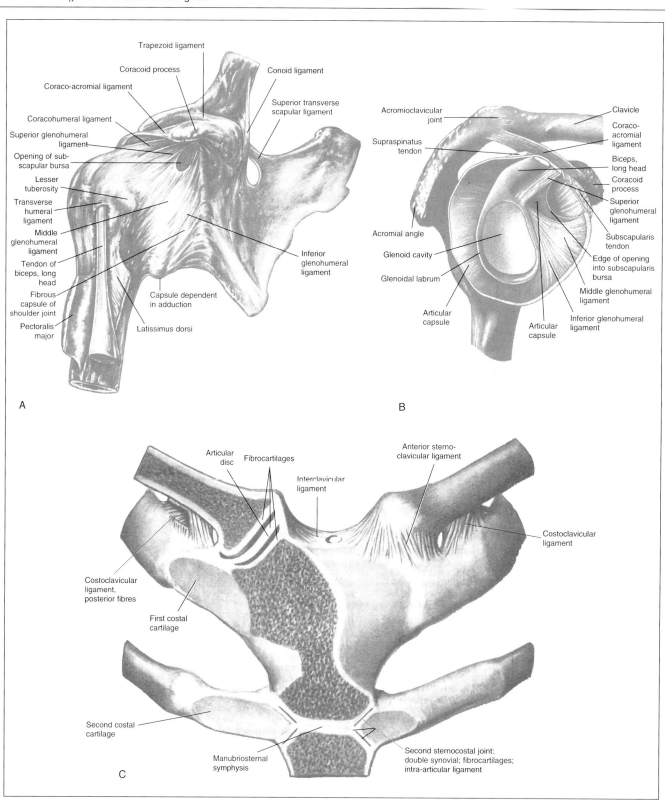

Figure 13.4 A–C: Various ligaments of the shoulder girdle (reproduced, with permission, from *Gray's anatomy* (1995)).

Box 13.1   (cont'd)

Most joints of the appendicular skeleton (apart from the pubis and the tibiofibular junction) are synovial. Synovial joints comprise a thick capsule which protects the joint and somewhat restricts excessive movement while allowing it a great degree of mobility.

The fibrous outer layer of the capsule merges with the periosteum of the bones which form the joint.

In the case of the shoulder the following characteristics apply to the *fibrous capsule* (1) and associated ligaments.

- The capsule attaches medially to the circumference of the *glenoid cavity* (2) beyond the *glenoid labrum* (3).
- Superiorly it attaches to the root of the *coracoid process* (4), enveloping the origin of the *long head of the biceps* (5).
- Laterally the capsule attaches to the *neck of the humerus* (6) close to the articular margin, apart from the medial aspect where the attachment is approximately 1 cm lower on the bone. The capsule is sufficiently lax to allow the remarkable degree of mobility at the joint.
- The joint's stability depends to a large extent on the muscles and the supporting ligaments (*glenohumeral ligaments* (7, 8, 9)) which merge with and surround the capsule.
- The capsule is reinforced by muscles:
  1. superiorly by supraspinatus
  2. inferiorly by the long head of triceps
  3. posteriorly by the tendons of infraspinatus and teres minor
  4. anteriorly by subscapularis.
- The tendons of subscapularis, supraspinatus, infraspinatus and teres minor all blend with the capsule, creating a cuff.
- The inferior aspect of the capsule (and joint), which during abduction has great strain imposed on it, is the least stable. This is because the long head of triceps does not have as close a relationship with the capsule as do the previously mentioned muscles, due to the presence of neural structures and blood vessels.
- Further stabilization of the capsule derives from the three *glenohumeral ligaments* (7,8,9) (superior, middle and inferior bands).
- These all attach at their scapular end to the superior aspect of the medial margin of the glenoid cavity, merging with the *glenoid labrum* (3) (a fibrocartilaginous rim attaching to the margin of the glenoid cavity).
- The *superior band of the glenohumeral ligament* (7) runs along the medial aspect of the biceps tendon before attaching above the lesser tubercle of the humerus.
- The *middle band of the glenohumeral ligament* (8) attaches to the inferior aspect of the lesser tubercle.
- The *inferior band of the glenohumeral ligament* (9) attaches to the lower aspect of the anatomical neck of the humerus.
- The tendons of pectoralis major and teres major further strengthen the anterior aspect of the capsule (and therefore the joint as a whole).

Additional ligamentous features of the shoulder joint include the following.

- The *acromioclavicular ligament* (10) which covers the superio

aspect and fibrous capsule of this joint before merging with the fibers of the aponeurosis of trapezius and the deltoid.
- The *coracoclavicular ligament* (11) attaches the clavicle to the coracoid process of the scapula, efficiently maintaining the clavicle's contact with the acromion. If the acromioclavicular joint dislocates, this ligament may tear which allows the scapula to drop away from the clavicle. This ligament has two parts, the trapezoid and the conoid portions.
  1. The *trapezoid ligament* (12) runs almost horizontally, attaching inferiorly to the upper surface of the coracoid process and superiorly to the inferior surface of the clavicle.
  2. The narrow end of the *conoid ligament* (13) attaches inferiorly to the posteromedial edge of the root of the coracoid process and superiorly, at its broader end, to the conoid tubercle on the inferior surface of the clavicle.
- The *coracoacromial ligament* (14) comprises a strong triangular band which links the coracoid process of the scapula with the acromion. In some instances pectoralis minor attaches into the shoulder capsule (rather than the usual attachment at the coracoid process) its tendon passes beneath the coracoacromial ligament.
- The *coracohumeral ligament* (15) is a broad structure which strengthens the superior aspect of the capsule (its lower and posterior borders merge with the capsule). The ligament attaches to the base of the coracoid process and travels obliquely inferiorly and laterally to the anterior aspect of the greater tubercle of the humerus where it blends with the supraspinatus tendon.
- The *transverse humeral ligament* (16) runs from the lesser to the greater tubercle of the humerus forming a canal for the retinaculum of the long head of the biceps.

At the sternal end of the clavicle additional ligamentous structures occur.

- At the sternoclavicular joint the surface of the sternal articulation is smaller than that of the surface of the clavicle, which is covered with a saddle-shaped fibrocartilage, and separated from the sternal notch by an articular disc.
- This articulation is, as in the case of the shoulder itself, surrounded by a fibrous capsule.
- The *anterior sternoclavicular ligament* (17) covers the anterior surface of the joint attaching superiorly to the clavicle and attaching inferomedially to the anterior aspect of the manubrium sternum and the first costal cartilage.
- The *posterior sternoclavicular ligament* (18) lies on the posterior aspect of the joint, attaching superiorly to the clavicle and inferiorly to the posterior aspect of the manubrium.
- The *interclavicular ligament* (19) merges with the deep cervical fascia superiorly and connects the superior aspects of the sternal ends of the clavicles. Some fibers also attach to the manubrium. In approximately 7% of the population small ossified structures are present in the ligament, the suprasternal ossicles. These usually pyramid-shaped structures are originally cartilaginous, ossifying in adolescence. They may be fused to, or articulate with, the manubrium.
- The *costoclavicular ligament* (20) attaches inferiorly to the first rib and its adjacent cartilage and superiorly to the clavicle.

case of a shoulder, for example, abduction of the arm may be achieved to its full range, with minimal symptoms, but:

- is this being achieved by the appropriate sequence of movements of the scapula, with hinging occurring at the acromion and the prime movers performing their actions efficiently?
- or is the arm hinging from the base of the neck with inappropriate muscular input from the synergists?

The *quality* of a movement, combined with its *range* and *effect on symptoms*, all need to be evaluated. Janda's functional tests are useful in achieving this (see p. 60).

In this section aspects of shoulder assessment will be detailed with descriptions of examination methods for discovery of:

- range of motion
- strength

- reflex information
- specific condition tests

CAUTION: AVOID TESTING (active or passive) for range of motion if there is a possibility of dislocation, fracture, advanced pathology or profound tissue damage (tear).

General comments

- The commonest limiting factors relating to loss of range of motion of the shoulder involve spasm, contracture, fracture and dislocation.
- Restrictions which have a hard end-feel during passive range of motion assessment are usually joint related.
- Restrictions which have a less hard end-feel, with slight springiness still available at the end of range, are usually due to extraarticular soft tissue dysfunction.
- Refer to the notes on 'tightness/looseness' in Chapter 8 (p. 96) which describe the concept of the 'tethering' of tissues, as well as their end-feel. Awareness of these features (end-feel, tight/loose, ease/bind) is important in making therapeutic decisions based on what is being palpated during examination (Ward 1997).
- If the cause of arm pain lies in the upper extremity then there is usually associated restriction of full range of motion.
- However, when pain is referred from elsewhere – viscera, perhaps, or from the cervical spine but not from trigger points – passive motion is seldom restricted (Simons et al 1998) and pain will usually be diffuse rather than localized and will commonly be worse at night. In such cases, other symptoms may offer a clue to the origin (digestive problem, neck pain, cough, etc.).
- Atrophy in a muscle is usually due to:
1. disuse (immobilization, disuse due to injury, handedness)
2. nerve or muscle disease (reflexes will be increased and paralysis may be obvious in upper motor neuron disease)
3. spinal dysfunction
4. trauma which denervates the structure, in which

case there will be no muscle strength or tendon reflex and a marked reduction in size as fatty tissue replaces muscle (see evidence regarding rectus capitis posterior minor in Chapter 3)
5. nerve entrapment by soft tissue structures at various sites along the nerve's path (such as scalenes, pectoralis minor, triceps or supinator entrapment of radial nerve) (see Neurological impingement and the upper extremity p. 369).

In discussing shoulder-arm syndrome, Lewit (1991) states:

Experience has shown that any type of pain originating in the cervical spine, even in its upper part as far down as the upper thoracic and upper ribs – and even the viscera, the heart, lungs, liver, gall bladder and stomach – may be the origin of pain referred to the dermatome C4.

Lewit notes that British and American charts usually show the shoulder region covered by the C5 dermatome. He disagrees:

The phrenic nerve, originating from the C4 segment, provides a much more credible explanation of this widespread irradiation than does the dermatome C5. This explains the somewhat vague term 'shoulder-arm' syndrome.

Janda's perspective

In Chapter 5 details were given of the research work of Czech researcher Vladimir Janda MD (1982, 1983). He has described the upper crossed syndrome in which the following postural muscles shorten and tighten (see p. 55):

- pectoralis major and minor
- upper trapezius
- levator scapula
- sternocleidomastoid

while at the same time:

- lower and middle trapezius
- serratus anterior and rhomboids

are inhibited and weaken.

As these changes take place the relative positions of the head, neck and shoulders modify, so that cervical stress develops while, more specifically, there is a change in shoulder biomechanics.

- The scapula abducts and rotates due to increased tone in upper trapezius and levator scapula, inhibiting serratus anterior and the lower trapezius.
- This produces an altered direction of the axis of the glenoid fossa so that the humerus demands additional levator scapula, upper trapezius and supraspinatus stabilization, further stressing these already compromised muscles.
- A part of the outcome of such changes will be the

evolution of trigger points in the stressed structures and referred pain to the chest, shoulders and arms.

• Pain mimicking angina may be noted plus a decline in respiratory efficiency.

Janda stresses the need to identify shortened structures and to stretch and relax them, after which proprioceptive reeducation is indicated. Whatever local treatment these trigger points receive, reeducation of posture and use is an essential aspect of rehabilitation.

Janda's scapulohumeral rhythm test

In order to obtain a rapid overview of the function of the postural muscles associated with shoulder and scapula behavior, Janda has devised a series of 'functional tests'. The reasoning is that if a normal action can be demonstrated to involve excessive activity of key postural (type 1, see Chapter 5) muscles, this implies that:

1. the postural muscle(s) so identified will be overactive, therefore by definition short
2. the phasic antagonists will therefore be inhibited and not performing their roles as prime movers, so that
3. synergists will probably become overactive in compensation
4. as a result most of these muscles will develop localized areas of distress and trigger points will evolve.

The method of the scapulohumeral rhythm test, which has direct implications for neck and shoulder dysfunction, is as follows.

• The patient is seated and the practitioner stands behind, observing.
• The patient is asked to let the arm on the tested side hang down and to flex the elbow to 90°, thumb upwards.
• The patient is asked to slowly abduct the arm toward the horizontal.
• A normal abduction will include elevation of the shoulder with rotation or superior movement of the scapula commencing only after 60° of abduction.
• Abnormal performance of this test occurs if elevation of the shoulder or rotation, superior movement or winging of the scapula occurs within the first 60° of shoulder abduction.
• This would indicate levator scapula and/or upper trapezius as being overactive and therefore shortened, with lower and middle trapezius and serratus anterior inhibited and weak.
• Objectively, the area about a third of the way between the angle of the neck and the lateral edge of the shoulder will 'mound' during this test if levator scapula is excessively overactive.
• Another way of viewing the test is to judge whether the 'hinge' of arm abduction is occurring at the acromioclavicular joint or at the base of the neck.

Variation

• The patient is seated or standing with the practitioner standing behind, a finger tip resting on the upper trapezius muscle of the side to be tested.
• The patient is asked to take the arm being tested into extension.
• If, at the very outset of this movement of the arm, there is discernible firing of upper trapezius, it is overactive and by implication shortened.
• By implication, this overactivity suggests that lower fixators are weak with the same sort of imbalance noted in the initial findings of the test described above.

It is always useful to confirm a functional test such as this with evidence of actual shortening. Tests to establish this evidence will be described later in this section.

Observation

Observe the person's shoulders simultaneously.

• Is there evidence of asymmetry (one shoulder high or deviation of the neck in a scoliotic curve, for example)?
• Is one or are both of the shoulders rounded? (postural placement)
• Is the upper crossed syndrome apparent?
• What, if any, are the influences of spinal curves (for example, is there increased thoracic kyphosis?)
• Is there altered skin color (blanching indicating ischemia or increased hyperemia suggesting inflammation, for example)?
• What evidence is there of muscle hypertrophy (accentuated development of upper trapezius, for example) or atrophy (extreme laxity and weakness of lower scapula fixators, for example)?
• Are there any tremors, suggesting neurological dysfunction?

Palpation of superficial soft tissues

• Assess skin and muscle tone and size.
• Test brachial and radial pulses (brachial is medial to biceps tendon, radial is on ventrolateral aspect of wrist) as well as assessment of general reflexes and range of motion. If there exists asymmetry of rate, rhythm, strength or wave form in the arterial pulses, circulatory dysfunction is probable.

Range of motion of shoulder structures

Controversy exists regarding the normal range of motion of the shoulder and which muscles are involved in particular movements. The following list will give some reference for the practitioner as to which muscles are

Box 13.3 Reflex tests (always compare both sides) (Schafer 1987)

• *Biceps reflex test.* Practitioner and patient are seated facing each other. Tested arm (say right side) rests (completely relaxed) on practitioner's left forearm; practitioner's left thumb rests in cubital fossa on biceps tendon. That thumbnail is tapped with a neurological hammer and if the reflex is normal the biceps should produce a slight jerk close to the tendon which will be both palpable and visible. This evaluates neurological integrity at C5.
• *Brachioradialis reflex test.* Same position as for previous test but this time the neurological tap is to the brachioradialis tendon at the distal end of the radius. There should be a slight 'jump' of the brachioradialis, indicating normal C6 integrity.
• *Triceps reflex test.* Same position but this time the tap is to the triceps tendon as it crosses the olecranon fossa. A 'jump' of the triceps close to the tendon indicates normal C7 integrity.

Note: These spinal levels are important to shoulder function since the main nerve supply to the key muscles of this region derive from C4–7.

Box 13.4 What is normal range of arms?

The normal range of movement of the arms is a matter of dispute. (Cyriax 1982)

synergistic in particular movements. By referring to the antagonistic movements, the practitioner might also discern which muscles might be restricting range of motion.

The list is not intended to add to the controversy but instead to be an aid in a thorough examination of tissues which might be involved. What is 'normal' will likely remain controversial, at least until latent trigger points (which restrict range of motion without pain symptoms) are assessed and deactivated in the 'normal' patients used in the studies of ranges of motion.

Flexion (anteversion) 0–180°

0–60° at glenohumeral joint – anterior fibers of deltoid, coracobrachialis, clavicular fibers of pectoralis major, biceps brachii, supraspinatus (possibly); 60–120° involves scapular rotation – the above plus trapezius, serratus anterior; 120–180° involves the spinal column – all the above plus lumbar muscles which extend the trunk and stabilize the torso.

Extension (retroversion) 0–50°

Teres major/minor, posterior fibers of deltoid, latissimus dorsi, long head of triceps, rhomboids, middle trapezius.

Adduction 0–45°

Pectoralis major, latissimus dorsi, teres major/minor,

triceps long head, clavicular and spinal fibers of deltoid, coracobrachialis (to neutral), biceps short head.

Abduction 0–90°

Deltoid, supraspinatus, infraspinatus, teres minor, biceps long head.

Elevation 90–180°

Deltoid, supraspinatus, infraspinatus, teres minor, biceps long head, trapezius, serratus anterior (at 120°, these plus contralateral lumbar muscles which laterally flex the trunk to the opposite side).

Lateral (external) rotation 0–80°

Infraspinatus, teres minor, posterior deltoid, supraspinatus (possibly).

Medial (internal) rotation 0–100°

Subscapularis, pectoralis major, latissimus dorsi, teres major, anterior deltoid.

Horizontal flexion 0–140°

Deltoid, subscapularis, pectoralis major/minor, serratus anterior, biceps short head, coracobrachialis.

Horizontal extension 0–40°

Deltoid, supraspinatus, infraspinatus, teres major/minor, rhomboids, trapezius, latissimus dorsi.

Circumduction

Combines the movements about the three cardinal axes.

• Sagittal plane – flexion and extension
• Frontal plane – adduction and abduction
• Horizontal plane – horizontal flexion and extension.

Scapular elevation

Upper trapezius, levator scapula, rhomboids major and minor.

Scapular depression

Lower trapezius (indirectly latissimus dorsi and pectoralis major through their humeral attachments). Lower fibers of serratus anterior are questionable for this function.

Scapular adduction

Trapezius, rhomboids major and minor.

Scapular abduction

Serratus anterior, pectoralis minor.

Active and passive tests for shoulder girdle motion (standing or seated)

Both active and passive range of motion tests may be used to assess:

- limits of movement of the glenohumeral joint
- scapular motion
- soft tissue involvement.

Bilateral comparison is possible by both sides performing the action simultaneously. If active testing shows normal range without pain or discomfort, passive tests are usually not necessary. However, remember McKenzie's suggestion (above) that repetition of an active movement a number of times, simulating 'real-life' behavior, offers a more accurate assessment than single movements.

These initial active tests offer a view of normal movement and symmetry.

- **Elevation** (lateral rotation of scapula) and **depression** (medial rotation of the scapula) – hunch (shrug) shoulders and return to normal.
- **External rotation and abduction** – reach up and over shoulder to touch the superior medial angle of contralateral scapula with one hand and then the other.
- **External rotation and abduction tested bilaterally** – place both hands behind neck (fingers interlocked) and move elbows laterally and posteriorly in an arc.
- **Internal rotation and adduction** – reach across the chest with elbow close to chest and touch opposite shoulder tip; or reach behind at waist level and touch inferior angle of opposite scapula.
- **Bilateral abduction** – abduct arms horizontally to 90° with elbows straight, palms upwards. Continue abduction (elevation) until hands meet in the center.

Impingement syndrome test

Patient is supine with arms at side.

- The elbow on the side to be tested is flexed to 90° and internally rotated so that the forearm rests on the patient's abdomen.
- The practitioner places one hand to cup the shoulder in order to stabilize this, while the other hand cups the flexed elbow.
- A firm compressive force is applied through the long axis of the humerus, forcing the humerus against the inferior aspect of the acromion process and glenohumeral fossa.
- If symptoms are reproduced or if pain is noted, supraspinatus and/or bicipital tendon dysfunction is indicated (see false-positive information below).

False-positive compression test (see also impingement syndrome test above)

An association has frequently been shown between thoracic outlet syndrome and first rib restriction (Nichols 1996, Tucker 1994). However, a connection between second rib restriction and shoulder pain has not been recorded in the literature until recently.

Boyle (1999) reports on two case histories in which symptoms were present which resembled, in all respects (diagnostic criteria, etc.), shoulder impingement syndrome or rotator cuff partial tear which responded rapidly to mobilization of the second rib. The patients both had positive tests for shoulder impingement, implicating supraspinatus and/or bicipital tendon dysfunction (see impingement test description above).

Boyle (1999) describes evidence to support the way(s) in which second rib restrictions (in particular) might produce false-positive test results and shoulder symptoms.

- The dorsal ramus of the 2nd thoracic nerve continues laterally to the acromion, providing a cutaneous distribution in the region of the posteriolateral shoulder (Maigne 1991).
- Rotational restrictions involving the cervicothoracic region have been shown to produce a variety of neck and shoulder symptoms. Since the 2nd rib articulates with the transverse process of T1 (costotransverse joint) and the superior border of T2 (costovertebral joint), rotational restriction of these vertebrae could produce rib dysfunction (Jirout 1969).
- Habitual overactivity involving scalenus posterior can produce 'chronic subluxation of the second rib at its vertebral articulation' (Boyle 1999). This could result in a superior glide of the tubercle of the 2nd rib at the costotransverse junction.
- Boyle reports that 'true' impingement syndrome is often related to overactivity of the rhomboids which would 'downwardly rotate the scapula', impeding elevation of the humerus at the glenohumeral joint.
- He suggests that rhomboid overactivity might also impact on the upper thoracic region as a whole (T1 to T4), locking these segments into an extension posture. If this situation were accompanied by overactivity of the posterior scalene, the second rib might 'subluxate superiorly on the fixed thoracic segment', leading to pain and dysfunction mimicking shoulder impingement syndrome.
- Boyle hypothesizes that mechanical interference might occur involving 'the dorsal cutaneous branch of the second thoracic nerve ... in its passage through the tunnel adjacent to the costotransverse joint'. This nerve might be 'drawn taut, due to the superior anterior subluxation of the second rib' leading to pain and associated restricted movement symptoms.
- The reason for a false-positive impingement test, Boyle suggests, relates to the internal rotation component

which adds to the mechanical stress of the dysfunctional rib area. This could also, through pain inhibition, result in rotator cuff muscles testing as weak, suggesting incorrectly that a partial tear had occurred.

• The possibility of a 2nd rib involvement should not disguise the possibility that this coexists with a true impingement lesion.

Strength tests for shoulder movements

In the absence of atrophy, weakness of a muscle may be due to:

• compensatory hypotonicity relative to increased tone in antagonist muscles
• palpable trigger points in affected (weak) muscle, notably those close to the attachments
• trigger point in remote muscles for which the tested muscle lies in the target referral zone.

Muscle strength is most usually graded as follows.

• Grade 5 is normal, demonstrating a complete (100%) range of movement against gravity, with firm resistance offered by the practitioner.
• Grade 4 is 75% efficiency in achieving range of motion against gravity with slight resistance.
• Grade 3 is 50% efficiency in achieving range of motion against gravity without resistance.
• Grade 2 is 25% efficiency in achieving range of motion with gravity eliminated.
• Grade 1 shows slight contractility without joint motion.
• Grade 0 shows no evidence of contractility.

For efficient muscle strength testing it is necessary to ensure that:

• the patient builds force slowly after engaging the barrier of resistance offered by the practitioner
• the patient uses maximum controlled effort to move in the prescribed direction
• the practitioner ensures that the point of muscle origin is efficiently stabilized
• care is taken to avoid use by the patient of 'tricks' in which synergists are recruited.

Muscular relationships (Janda 1983)

• The *prime mover* in any action (*agonist*) performs the greater part of the movement.
• The *assisting muscles* (*synergists*) assist the prime mover but do not carry out the actual movement unless the agonist is severely damaged or paralyzed.
• Movement in the opposite direction is performed by the *antagonist(s)* which are passively elongated during normal movement initiated by the agonist. Therefore, if

there is shortening of the antagonist(s), movement range will be limited.
• Muscles which stabilize parts of the body during movement of an area are *stabilizers*. These do not perform the movement but if they are inefficient in producing stabilization, it becomes more difficult for the agonist to perform its function and strength evaluations may be meaningless.
• Some muscles act as *neutralizers*. Based on its anatomical position each muscle operates in at least two directions. If a muscle can both flex and supinate (biceps for example) and if an action of pure flexion is required, a muscle (or group of muscles) which act as a pronator (pronator teres in this example) has to neutralize the supination potential of biceps.

Box 13.5 Neutralizers

Neutralizers are of great importance in daily life, but in muscle function testing they are a nuisance. Their action is greatly diminished by correct positioning of the extremities to allow accurate resistance and good fixation. (Janda 1983)

Janda (1983) states:

As a rule when testing a two-joint muscle good fixation is essential. The same applies to all muscles in children and in adults whose cooperation is poor and whose movements are incoordinated and weak. The better the extremity is steadied, the less the stabilizers are activated and the better and more accurate are the results of the muscle function test.

The authors highly recommend Janda's text and the other referenced texts mentioned in this chapter for further exploration of the art of assessment.

Shoulder flexion strength (Fig. 13.5A)

(Anterior deltoid and coracobrachialis with assistance from pectoralis major, clavicular head and biceps) Practitioner stands behind patient whose elbow is locked in flexion at 90°. Stabilizing hand is on shoulder (placed so that it can also palpate anterior deltoid during the test). The other hand holds anterior aspect of lower arm and patient is asked to flex shoulder. Strength is graded and compared with other side. If weakness is noted consider the nerve supply from C4 to C8, as well as trigger point input to the active muscles.

Extension strength (Fig. 13.5B)

(Latissimus dorsi, teres major, posterior deltoid with assistance from teres minor and long head of triceps) Stabilizing hand on shoulder palpating posterior deltoid, other hand holds posterior aspect of flexed lower arm (as in previous test) as patient is asked to extend shoulder.

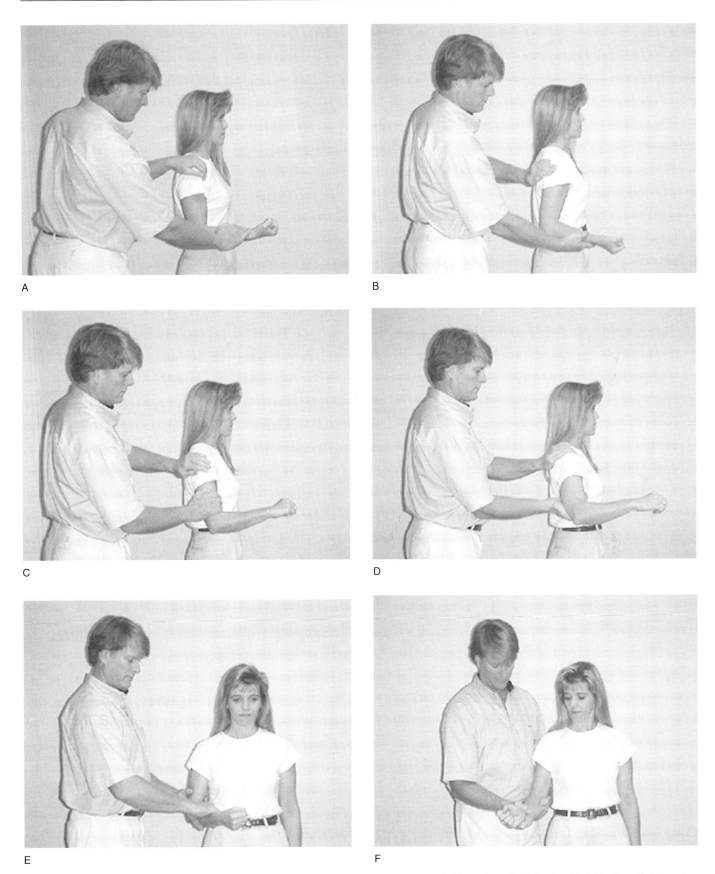

Figure 13.5 Strength tests for two-joint muscles of various arm movements. A: Flexion. B: Extension. C: Abduction. D: Adduction. E: Internal rotation. F: External rotation.

Strength should be recorded as suggested above. If weakness is noted consider the nerve supply from C4 to C8, as well as trigger point input to the active muscles.

Abduction strength (Fig. 13.5C)

(Middle deltoid, supraspinatus with assistance from serratus anterior plus anterior and posterior deltoid) Stabilizing hand is on shoulder palpating middle deltoid, increasing resistance is offered above flexed elbow as abduction is introduced. Strength should be recorded as suggested above. If weakness is noted consider the nerve supply from C4 to C8, as well as trigger point input to the active muscles.

Adduction (Fig. 13.5D)

(Pectoralis major, latissimus dorsi assisted by teres major, anterior deltoid and possibly posterior deltoid) Stabilizing hand is on shoulder tip, patient's flexed arm is abducted and resistance is offered from a position medial to and above the elbow as the patient attempts to adduct. Strength should be recorded as suggested above. If weakness is noted consider the nerve supply from C4 to C8, as well as trigger point input to the active muscles.

Internal rotation (Fig. 13.5E)

(Subscapularis, pectoralis major, latissimus dorsi, teres minor assisted by anterior deltoid) Arm at side, elbow flexed to 90° and with the elbow supported. Patient attempts to take the forearm medially across the trunk while resistance is offered. Strength should be recorded as suggested above. If weakness is noted consider the nerve supply from C4 to C8, as well as trigger point input to the active muscles.

External rotation (Fig. 13.5F)

(Infraspinatus, teres minor assisted by posterior deltoid) Flexed elbow rests in stabilizing hand (elbow remains at the side throughout) with practitioner's thumb at the elbow crease. The other hand holds the wrist and applies increasing resistance as the patient attempts to externally rotate the shoulder by moving the forearm laterally. Strength should be recorded as suggested above. If weakness is noted consider the nerve supply from C4 to C8, as well as trigger point input to the active muscles.

Elevation of the scapula

(Trapezius, levator scapulae assisted by rhomboids major and minor) Practitioner behind patient evaluates relative strength as the patient's attempt to shrug is resisted – this assesses spinal accessory nerve integrity. Strength should be recorded as suggested above. If weakness is noted consider the nerve supply from C2 to C8, as well as trigger point input to the active muscles.

Depression of the scapula

(Rhomboid major and minor, assisted by trapezius) Practitioner stands in front and places hands so that fingers cover shoulders over the upper deltoids and thumbs rest anteriorly below the clavicles. Patient is asked to take shoulders back and down as practitioner resists and assesses strength. Since C5 is the sole innervation of the primary muscles involved (although trapezius is innervated from C2) weakness may relate to its integrity. Strength should be recorded as suggested above. If weakness is noted consider the nerve supply from C2 to C8, as well as trigger point input to the active muscles.

Protraction of the scapula

(Serratus anterior) Examiner is behind, patient flexes arm so that it is parallel to the floor with elbow flexed and forearm at 90° to upper arm facing medially. Stabilization is offered by the practitioner in the mid-scapular region to prevent spinal movement while the other hand cups the flexed elbow, offering resistance, as the patient attempts to push the arm forwards, away from the body. If winging occurs during this, it implies weakness of lower fixators of the shoulder. If there is weakness in any of the movements described, but particularly scapular depression, C5 may be implicated (or C4 – see Lewit's views above). Strength should be recorded as suggested above. If weakness is noted consider the nerve supply from C4 to C8, as well as trigger point input to the active muscles.

Spinal and scapular effects of excessive tone

- Trapezius – pulls shoulder girdle medially, occiput posteroinferiorly, associated spinous processes laterally, elevates shoulder, rotates scapula laterally.
- Levator scapula – pulls scapula medially and superiorly, rotates scapula medially and associated transverse processes (C1–4) inferiorly, laterally and posteriorly.
- Rhomboid major and minor – pulls scapula medially and superiorly and associated spinous processes laterally and inferiorly, rotates scapula medially.

Shoulder pain and associated structures

Lewit summarizes some of the most common sources of shoulder dysfunction and pain and states that if shoulder pain exists, the following structures and their functions require evaluation and palpation.

- Cervical spine and craniocervical junction
- Cervicothoracic junction, upper ribs
- Scapulohumeral joint (including joint play with arm horizontal)
- Clavicular joints
- Abduction arc
- All available muscle insertions
- Potential trigger point sites
- Epicondyles
- Carpal bone joint play

Note: Not all Lewit's suggested evaluations are described in this section (shoulder) of the book.

Lewit (1991) also describes chain reactions which are relevant to shoulder dysfunction.

- Craniocervical junction restriction is often associated with upper rib restriction (most often the 3rd rib) and vice versa.
- Atlantooccipital restriction is often associated with suboccipital extensor dysfunction ('spasm').
- If C1 or C2 is restricted the lateral aspect of the spinous process of C2 is usually painful and trigger point activity is likely in sternocleidomastoid inferior to the mastoid process.
- If postural stress is evident (forward drawn head or persistent head anteflexion during work) or if shoulder upper fixators are excessively tight, C2 tenderness (spinous process) can be anticipated, along with cervical restrictions in this region. Levator scapula attachment on the scapula as well as the clavicular attachment of SCM are likely to house active trigger points at their attachment sites.
- A chain of interconnected dysfunction may exist between the subclavicular pectoralis and SCM. This may be associated with upper chest breathing patterns which would also involve the scalenes and the masseter muscles (with resultant trigger point activity likely in all or any of these muscles).
- Epicondylar pain may be linked with mid-cervical restriction, which is itself likely to relate to craniocervical junction dysfunction. More locally, 'Pain at the styloid process of the radius … may be the only sign of blocking of the elbow (radioulnar) joint'.
- Pain in the epicondyles, which usually involves overstrained forearm muscles, is likely to be related to increased muscle tension in the shoulder girdle, all of which require individual assessment.
- Carpal tunnel syndrome is commonly related to thoracic outlet dysfunction, involving the cervicothoracic junction, upper ribs, scalenes and probably a dysfunctional breathing pattern. An epicondyle connection is also probable.

- Disturbed muscle function. It is important when considering neck, shoulder and arm dysfunctions to recall discussion of the upper crossed syndrome earlier, as described by Lewit (1991) and Janda (1982, 1983). In this pattern of dysfunction, imbalances occur between:
  1. short tight pectorals and weak (inhibited) interscapular muscles
  2. short tight upper shoulder fixators (upper trapezius, levator scapula and possibly the scalenes) and weakened, inhibited, lower fixators (lower trapezius, serratus anterior)
  3. short tight neck extensors (cervical erector spinae, upper trapezius) and weak, inhibited deep neck flexors (longus cervicis, longus capitis, omo- and thyrohyoid)
  4. leading to an unbalanced situation which has, as key features, exaggerated cervical lordosis and consequent 'chin poking', dorsal kyphosis and a generally rounded shoulder posture, with winged scapulae which drift laterally, leading inevitably to excessive strain on the rotator cuff muscles as they struggle to maintain normal position and function of the humerus, which now meets the glenoid fossae in the wrong plane.

Therapeutic choices

If shoulder pain is accompanied by *muscular imbalances* (as described by Lewit and Janda in the upper crossed syndrome), the following elements are called for.

- Assessment of joint restrictions, shortened muscles and local myofascial trigger points.
- Elimination of active myofascial trigger points (NMT).
- Restoration of balance between hypertonic and inhibited muscles (MET).
- Mobilization of restricted joints (articulation and possibly manipulation).
- Rehabilitation tactics, postural and, possibly, breathing reeducation.

If shoulder pain radiates from *spinal structures* the symptoms will be aggravated by head or neck movement and some degree of joint blockage (restriction) will be noted. This requires normalization and among the choices available are:

- identification and treatment of active trigger points
- normalization of associated muscle and soft tissues (see Lewit's discussion of chain reactions above)
- use of MET to encourage normal joint function (p. 142)
- use of Ruddy's pulsed MET to encourage normal joint function (p. 137)
- use of positional release methods to encourage normal joint function (p. 147)

- high-velocity thrust techniques (if licensed to perform these).

If shoulder pain originates in the *upper ribs*, treatment may include:

- use of MET, PRT and/or NMT (especially to the intercostal musculature and all attaching muscles)
- positional release and MET methods for restoring normal function to elevated and depressed ribs, discussed on p. 435.

Note: Some of the signs of rib involvement with shoulder pain may include the following.

- If the first rib is dysfunctional shoulder pain is likely, with marked tenderness anteriorly when its attachment to the manubrium sternum is palpated.
- Scapula pain is noted, along with shoulder pain, in dysfunction involving ribs 2, 3 and 4, with marked tenderness on palpation of the medial scapula border.

Specific shoulder dysfunctions

The tests and evaluations described below are mainly derived from the following sources.

- Janda V 1983 Muscle function testing. Butterworths, London
- Lewit K 1991 Manipulative therapy in rehabilitation of the locomotor system. Butterworths, London
- Liebenson C 1996 Rehabilitation of the spine. Williams and Wilkins, Baltimore
- Schafer R 1987 Clinical biomechanics. Williams and Wilkins, Baltimore
- Ward R (ed) 1997 Foundations of osteopathic medicine. Williams and Wilkins, Baltimore

Capsulitis (aka scapulohumeral dysfunction, 'frozen shoulder')

Generalized rather than localized pain in the shoulder may suggest capsulitis or contracture of the joint capsule. Pain is usually apparent on active as well as passive movement. Pain is felt more at night and when the arm is hanging down, moving or when carrying. Cyriax (1982) suggests that there are three stages, each lasting 3–4 months. These are:

1. pain severe and worsening with some restriction
2. pain lessens but restriction remains
3. pain and restriction slowly vanish, with the whole process lasting around a year.

Capsulitis may follow bursitis or tendinitis or it may relate to chronic pulmonary disease, myocardial infarction or diabetes mellitus. When these more serious (potentially life-threatening) visceral conditions exist as the underlying cause of the shoulder pain and therapy reduces the pain to a manageable level without addressing the cause, the visceral condition(s) may progress unnoticed. A differential diagnosis from a physician is therefore essential.

The condition may relate to overuse or to a subluxation which has reduced spontaneously or via treatment. If adhesions form within the joint capsule, the head of the humerus may bond to the glenoid surface (adhesive capsulitis). The condition is most common in women between the ages of 45 and 65.

Pain is usually pronounced at the deltoid tendon attachment as well as in subscapularis. The deltoid, infra- and supraspinatus muscles may atrophy in severe cases and circulatory changes may be noted (involving cyanosis and/or edema). Methods of treatment are called for which do not irritate the inflammatory processes but which attempt to normalize associated joint and muscle dysfunction.

Lewit states, 'The usual mobilization and manipulation techniques are useless in dealing with the shoulder joint itself'. This highlights the critical importance of soft tissue evaluation and treatment in this joint in particular and in most joints of the body, in our opinion.

Supraspinatus tendinitis

This may be associated with subdeltoid or acromial bursitis or rotator cuff dysfunction (such as a sequel to supraspinatus strain). Symptoms include:

- ache at rest, especially when lying on affected side
- increased discomfort on abduction
- pain may refer toward deltoid insertion
- pain on activity is restricted to a painful arc (see tests below) due to effect of acromion process on tendon during excursion of arm
- localized tenderness on palpation will be noted over the inflamed tissues.

Abduction 'scratch' test

- Seated or standing patient raises arm overhead (abduction) and flexes elbow, placing fingers as far down contralateral scapula as possible.
- The arm is then taken back to the side and the patient attempts to place the arm behind the back to reach as far up the contralateral scapula as possible.
- If pain is noted on either movement, one of the rotator cuff tendons is probably inflamed, with supraspinatus the most likely.
- If there is limitation but no pain, soft tissue restriction or osteoarthritis is probable, without active inflammation.

'Drop arm' test. The patient fully abducts the arm and starts to slowly lower it toward the side of the body. If the arm drops to the side from around 90° of abduction, rotator cuff damage is likely with supraspinatus most probably involved.

Bicipital tendinitis

- There will be palpable tenderness over the inflamed portion of the tendon.
- Symptoms are similar to supraspinatus tendinitis but differ in location as referral is to biceps insertion.
- If bicipital rupture (long head) or subluxation of the tendon from the groove has occurred there will be pain noted on abduction and extension.
- Specific tests (below) help to localize the dysfunction.

Lippman's test (Fig. 13.6)

- Patient is seated with elbow passively flexed and relaxed on lap.
- The tendon of the long head of the biceps is palpated (approximately 8 cm below the glenohumeral joint on the lateral surface of the shoulder).
- Pressure is applied in an attempt to displace the tendon medially or laterally.
- If this can be achieved or if symptom pain is reproduced then an assessment of a unstable tendon and possible tenosynovitis is confirmed.
- Variation: Have the patient lift a 2 kg weight overhead and slowly lower it to the lateral horizontal position. If symptoms are reproduced by this (whether or not there is displacement of the tendon from the groove) a positive test result is noted.

Resistive supination test

- Seated patient's arm is flexed at the elbow, palm down.
- Resistance is offered to the forearm proximal to the wrist as the patient attempts to supinate the forearm.

- Pain localized to the proximal tendon attachment area indicates possible inflammation and instability (or displacement) of the long head of the tendon.

Yergason's (tendon stability) test (Fig. 13.7)

- The patient fully flexes the elbow while the practitioner grasps proximal to the wrist.
- The patient is asked to resist the attempt by the practitioner to supinate and extend the forearm.
- An unstable tendon will displace and pain will be noted.

Hueter's sign (aka Speed's test) (Fig. 13.8)

- Patient flexes the supinated forearm against resistance.
- If pain or symptom duplication is noted a partial rupture of the biceps is suggested.

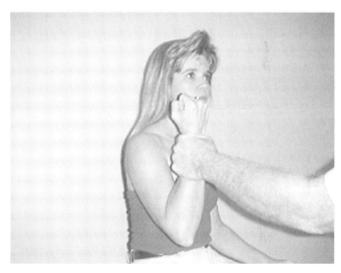

Figure 13.7   Yergason's test.

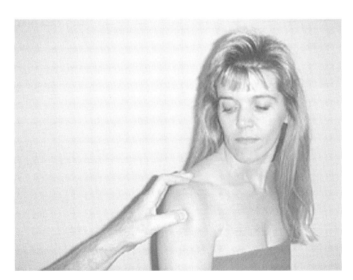

Figure 13.6   Bicipital tendinitis.

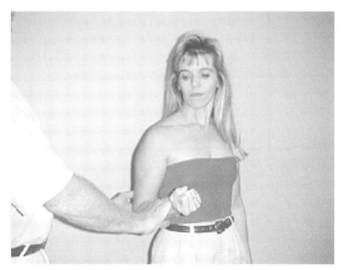

Figure 13.8   Hueter's sign.

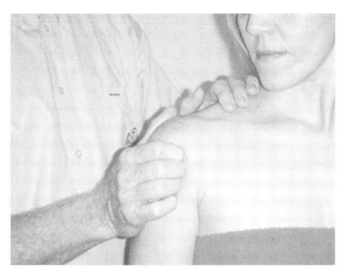

Figure 13.9 Subdeltoid bursitis.

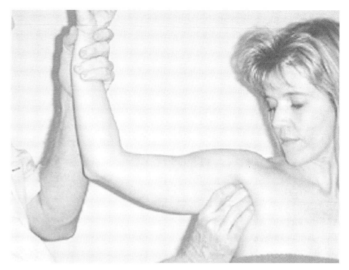

Figure 13.10 Subacromial bursitis.

● If pain increases in the area of the bicipital groove tendinitis is suggested.

Note: Flexion and extension strength will be limited by bicipital tendinitis.

Subdeltoid bursitis (Fig. 13.9)

● Inflammation produces severe, deep-seated, localized pain with general weakness but especially on abduction.
● Movements in rotation, flexion and extension may be limited.
● Palpation of the bursa and region around the tendon will reveal edema which greatly restricts the humeral tuberosity in its movement into abduction.
● Tendons which pass through the bursa will be affected (bicipital, rotator and subscapularis).
● When chronic, the condition moves from localized pain to one of severe limitation of movement, (particularly abduction and external rotation) as capsular adhesions form.
● The condition commonly follows degenerative changes in the rotator cuff at the base of the subdeltoid bursa, which result in calcification and associated inflammation.

Subacromial bursitis (Fig. 13.10)

● Abduction of the arm which is painful or limited may suggest subacromial bursitis.
● Schafer (1987) reports: 'A painful, faltering abduction arc is characteristic of subacromial bursitis. To differentiate, the coracoid process is palpated under pectoralis major. It is found by circumducting the humerus which is normally tender. Once the process

is found, the finger is slid slightly laterally and superiorly until it reaches a portion of the subacromial bursa. If the same palpation pressure here causes greater tenderness than at the process it is a positive sign of subacromial bursitis'.
● During this procedure care must be taken to avoid applying pressure onto the neurovascular bundle coursing through this region.
● The practitioner stands behind the patient and applies pressure to the subacromial bursa area (just below the coracoid process), producing some pain.
● The patient's arm just proximal to the wrist is grasped and is gently taken into abduction to approximately 100°.
● Digital pressure is maintained to patient tolerance and *if bursitis is present*, pain should lessen significantly as abduction proceeds. Particular attention is required to maintain constant palpation pressure as pain reduction might result from the practitioner losing good digital contact on the bursa as the deltoid tissue bunches.
● If pain induced by pressure remains the same, or increases, during abduction, bursitis is not likely.

Supraspinatus calcification

The tendon of supraspinatus inserts on the superior facet of the greater tuberosity, at which site calcification may occur. Symptoms are as follows.

● Severe pain (but not as severe as supraspinatus tendinitis), which is made worse by most shoulder movements, is localized to the region superficial to its insertion at the greater tuberosity of the humerus.
● Pain may be noted on abduction, especially in the early stages of arm abduction.

- Bursitis may also be present.
- X-ray evidence of calcification may be noted above the outer head of the humerus.
- Spontaneous reabsorption may occur, particularly when mechanical interference is removed.

Triceps brachii calcification

- Throwing injuries may aggravate and inflame posterior capsule structures leading to osteotendinous calcification in the infraglenoid area close to the attachment of the long head of triceps brachii.
- Throwing action, especially the follow-through, will be limited and painful.

Specific muscle evaluations

General tests for muscle weakness have been outlined earlier in this chapter. Excellent resources are easily available describing more specific testing procedures (see recommended book list on p. 310). There are also a number of assessment methods which can identify dysfunctional states of postural muscles. Some of these offer clear evidence of shortness, others suggest a tendency toward that state by virtue of the inappropriate activity of the muscle. In order to clarify the last statement it is worth repeating that when 'stressed' (overused, abused, misused, disused), muscles which have a greater stabilizing role (postural – type 1) will shorten over time whereas those with a more movement-oriented task (phasic – type 2) will weaken (see Chapter 2).

If inappropriate activity can be identified, as in the functional evaluation described earlier in this chapter (scapulohumeral rhythm test, p. 303), relating to the upper crossed syndrome in general and upper trapezius activity in particular, shortness can be assumed. If a muscle fires out of sequence and it is also a postural (type 1) muscle, it *is* short or *is going to become* short.

A simple extension of that knowledge tells us that the muscles which are antagonists to the overactive, hypertonic postural muscles are going to become inhibited (weak). The overactive muscle which is shortening *may* test as weak but it is certain that its antagonist *will* be weaker than it ought to be.

Trigger points can and do evolve in stressed soft tissues and whenever muscles are in a shortened state, there is a strong likelihood that they will house active trigger points. Weakened antagonists may also harbor trigger points, which leads to the conclusion that all muscles need to be searched for triggers which could be contributing to or be the result of dysfunctional muscular activity.

Tests for shortness of the following postural (type 1) muscles, which have a direct connection with shoulder function, are described below.

- Infraspinatus
- Levator scapula
- Latissimus dorsi
- Pectoralis major and minor
- Supraspinatus
- Subscapularis
- Upper trapezius

Infraspinatus

The patient is asked to reach backwards and across the back to touch the medial border of their opposite scapula (internal rotation of the humeral head). Pain is indicative of infraspinatus dysfunction/shortness.

An additional assessment involves the patient lying supine with upper arm abducted to 90° and elbow flexed to 90°, forearm pointing caudad, palm downwards (internal rotation of the humeral head). The forearm should be able to lie parallel to the floor without the shoulder lifting from the table surface. If the forearm is elevated, infraspinatus is short (Fig. 13.12).

Levator scapula

The practitioner is standing at the head of the table, supporting the supine patient's neck which he takes into full flexion and sidebend, away from the side to be tested. Rotation of the head is then introduced, also away from

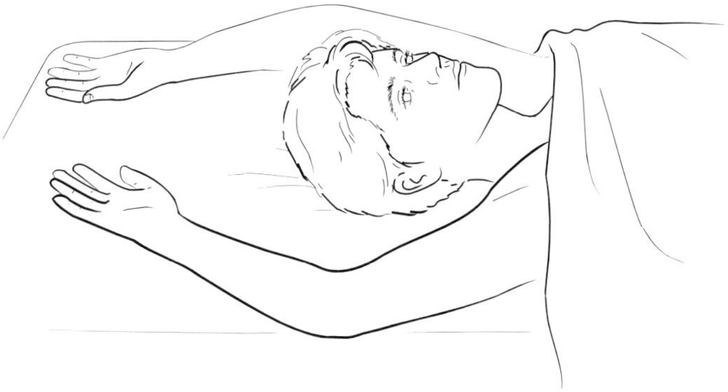

Figure 13.11 Test position for latissimus dorsi.

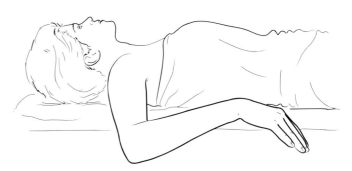

Figure 13.12 Test and MET treatment position for infraspinatus shortness.

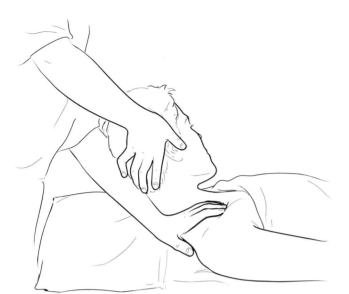

Figure 13.13 MET treatment position for shortness of levator scapula.

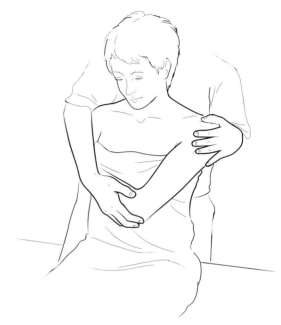

Figure 13.14 Assessment and MET treatment position for shortness of supraspinatus.

the side to be tested. The head and neck are stabilized in this position with one of the practitioner's hands, while the other hand contacts the top of the shoulder (tested side) to assess the ease with which it can be depressed (moved distally). There should be an easy springing sensation as the shoulder is pushed toward the feet with a soft end-feel to the movement. If there is a harsh, sudden end-feel, levator scapula is short (Fig. 13.13).

Latissimus dorsi

The patient lies supine with head 18 inches (45 cm) from the top end of the table and is asked to rest arms fully extended (elbows straight) above the head so that they lie on the treatment surface, palms upwards. The arms should be able to easily reach the horizontal while being directly above the shoulders, in contact with the surface for almost all of the length of the upper arms, with no arching of the back or twisting of the thorax. If an arm does not lie parallel to the other above the shoulder but is held laterally, elbow flexed and pulled outwards, then latissimus dorsi is probably short on that side.

Pectoralis major or minor

Using the same starting position as latissimus above, if an arm cannot rest with the dorsum of the upper arm in contact with the table surface without effort, then pectoralis major or minor fibers are almost certainly short.

Another way of evaluating pectoralis major is to have the patient lying supine close to the edge of the table on the side to be tested. It is important that the trunk be maintained in a stable position without any twisting (knees may be flexed to assist in this). The arm on the

tested side is taken into abduction and should easily reach a horizontal level. Any degree of elevation indicates shortness. Other positions of the arm may be introduced; for example, to evaluate the costal portion of the muscle, abduction together with approximately 45° of degree of elevation above shoulder level is introduced. The arm can then be allowed to hang loosely off the table. At this time the practitioner should apply light pressure to the anterior surface of the shoulder joint, toward the table, and a 'soft barrier' should be noted. If the costal portion of pectoralis major is short a firm, hard barrier will be noted.

Supraspinatus

The practitioner stands behind the seated patient, with one hand stabilizing the shoulder on the side to be assessed while the other hand reaches in front of the patient to support the forearm (elbow flexed). The patient's upper arm is adducted until an easy barrier is sensed (i.e. not forced) and the patient attempts to abduct the arm. If pain is noted in the posterior shoulder region this is diagnostic of supraspinatus dysfunction (Fig. 13.14).

Subscapularis

Patient is supine with upper arm abducted to 90° and elbow flexed to 90°, forearm pointing cephalad, palm upwards (external rotation of humeral head). The forearm should be able to lie parallel to the floor without the shoulder lifting from the table surface. If the forearm is elevated, subscapularis or pectoralis minor is short.

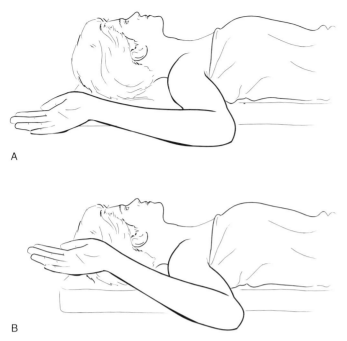

Figure 13.15 Assessment position for shortness of subscapularis or pectoralis minor. A: normal. B: short.

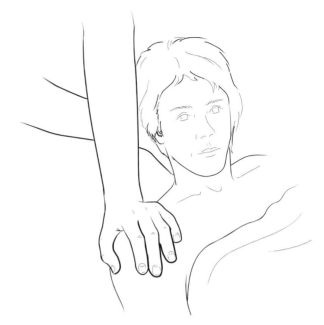

Figure 13.16 Hand positions for assessment and MET treatment of upper trapezius.

Upper trapezius

The patient is supine with the neck fully rotated and sidebent away from the side to be tested. At this point the practitioner, standing at the head of the table, uses a contact on the shoulder (tested side) to assess the ease with which it can be depressed (moved distally). There should be an easy springing sensation as the shoulder is pushed toward the feet, with a soft end-feel to the movement. If there is a harsh, sudden end-feel, the posterior fibers of upper trapezius are probably short. Rotation of the head *toward* the side being tested can be introduced to evaluate anterior fiber shortness in a similar manner (Fig. 13.16).

Is the patient's pain a soft tissue or a joint problem?

In Chapter 7 several simple screening tests devised by Professor Freddy Kaltenborn (1980) were listed. He suggested that we ask:

1. Does passive stretching (traction) of the painful area increase the level of pain? If so, it indicates extraarticular soft tissue involvement.

2. Does compression of the painful area increase the pain? If so, it indicates intraarticular dysfunction.

3. Are *active* movements (controlled by the patient) restricted or do they produce pain in one direction of movement, while *passive* movement (controlled by the practitioner) in precisely the opposite direction also produces pain (and/or is restricted)? If so, the contractile tissues of the area (muscle, ligament, etc.) are implicated. This can be confirmed by resisted tests.

4. Do active movement *and* passive movement in the same direction produce pain (and/or restriction)? If so, joint dysfunction is probable. This can be confirmed by use of traction, compression and gliding of the joint.

Resisted tests are used to assess both strength and painful responses to muscle contraction, either from the muscle or its tendinous attachment. These tests involve producing a maximal contraction of the suspected muscle while the joint is kept immobile somewhere near the middle of range position. No joint motion should be allowed to occur during such an assessment.

Resisted tests may usefully be performed after test 3 (above) to confirm a soft tissue dysfunction rather than a joint involvement. Kaltenborn suggests that before performing the resisted test, it is wise to perform the compression test (2 above) to clear any suspicion of joint involvement. These thoughts should also be kept in mind when the Spencer sequence, described in Box 13.6, is carried out.

The Spencer sequence

A traditional osteopathic assessment sequence is described in Box 13.6. This sequence is highly recommended as an addition to neuromuscular therapy since it offers precise evaluation of even minor restrictions in shoulder range and quality of motion, with the added advantage of allowing treatment from the test position (see p. 321).

Box 13.6 Spencer's assessment sequence (Patriquin 1992, Spencer 1916)

The Spencer sequence, which derives from osteopathic medicine in the early years of the 20th century, is taught at all osteopathic colleges in the USA. As the shoulder is put through its various ranges of motion, close attention is paid to any signs of restriction and these are noted. From what is palpated and observed in this sequence, clear indications can be derived as to which structures may be involved in creating any particular restriction.

For example, if restriction is noted in shoulder flexion, it is reasonable to assume that one or various soft tissues involved in shoulder extension are involved in whatever is restricting that movement. These soft tissue dysfunctions may be secondary to actual osseous dysfunction or soft tissue changes might be (indeed usually are) the main cause of restrictions in range of motion. The quality of end-feel helps to indicate whether restrictions are primarily the result of osseous or soft tissues.

Over the years the sequence of assessment has been modified to include treatment elements other than the original mobilization intent. Both muscle energy (MET) and positional release (PRT) treatment possibilities could be included and will be outlined in the shoulder treatment section (Box 13.9).

When this assessment sequence is being employed for assessment and treatment, the scapula should be held fixed firmly to the thoracic wall to isolate involvement of the glenohumeral joint. The patient remains in a sidelying position throughout, with the side to be assessed uppermost. The practitioner stands in front facing the patient at shoulder level.

1 Assessment of shoulder extension restriction (Fig. 13.17A)

• The practitioner's cephalad hand cups the shoulder, firmly compressing the scapula and clavicle to the thorax while the patient's flexed elbow is held by the practitioner's caudad hand as the arm is taken into extension toward the optimal 90°.
• Be aware of any restriction in range of motion, ceasing movement at the first indication of resistance to movement. If the movement is less than 90°, restriction may be a result of shoulder flexor shortness (possibly involving anterior deltoid, coracobrachialis or the clavicular head of pectoralis major).

2 Assessment of shoulder flexion restriction (Fig. 13.17B)

• The patient has same starting position as previous test.

• The practitioner stands at chest level, half facing cephalad.
• The non-tableside hand grasps patient's forearm while tableside hand holds the clavicle and scapula firmly to the chest wall.
• The practitioner slowly introduces shoulder flexion in a plane which is parallel to the floor as range of motion to 180° is assessed, by which time the elbow will be in extension.
• The position of very first indication of restriction in movement into shoulder flexion is noted and if this is less than 180°, dysfunction is assumed.
• If any restriction toward flexion is noted the soft tissues implicated in maintaining this dysfunction would be the shoulder extensors (posterior deltoid, teres major, latissimus dorsi, and possibly infraspinatus, teres minor and long head of triceps).

3a Assessment of circumduction capability with compression

• The patient is sidelying with elbow flexed (Fig. 13.17C).
• The practitioner's cephalad hand cups the shoulder while firmly compressing the scapula and clavicle to the thorax.
• His caudad hand grasps the elbow and takes the shoulder through a slow passive clockwise circumduction while adding compression through the long axis of the humerus.
• This is repeated several times in order to assess range, freedom and comfort of the circumducting motion, as the humeral head moves on the surface of the glenoid fossa.
• Any discomfort or restriction is noted.

3b Assessment of circumduction capability with traction (Fig. 13.17D)

• The patient is sidelying with arm straight.
• The practitioner's cephalad hand cups the shoulder firmly, compressing the scapula and clavicle to the thorax, while the caudad hand grasps immediately proximal to the wrist and introduces slight traction, before taking the arm through slow clockwise circumduction.
• This is assessing range of motion in circumduction, as well as the status of the capsule of the glenohumeral joint.
• The same process is repeated counterclockwise.
• Any restriction is noted.

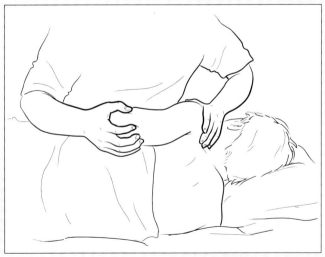

A

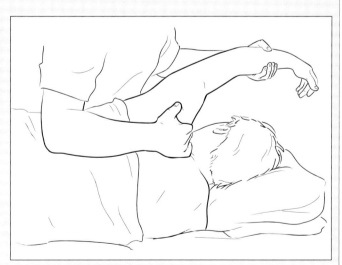

B

Figure 13.17A&B (see caption next page)

Box 13.6 (*cont'd*)

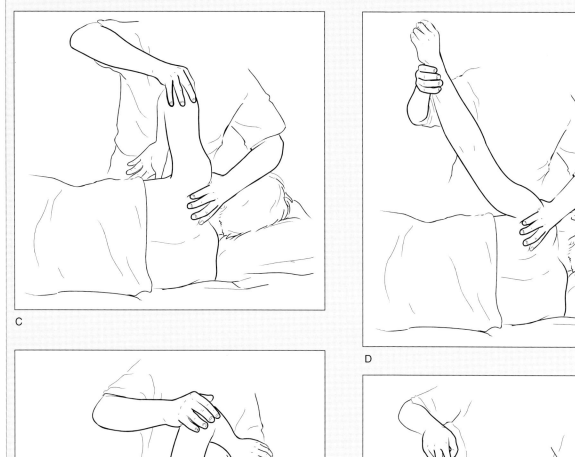

C

D

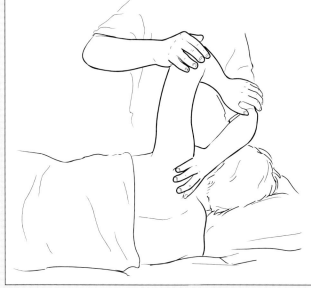

E

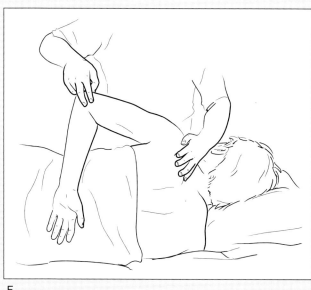

F

Figure 13.17   Spencer sequence positions. A: Shoulder extension. B: Shoulder flexion. C: Circumduction with compression. D: Circumduction with traction. E: Abduction with external rotation of shoulder. F: Internal rotation of shoulder (see p. 323).

Note: If restriction or pain is noted in either of the circumduction sequences (utilizing compression or traction), it is possible to evaluate which muscles would be active if precisely the opposite movement were undertaken and it is these which would be offering soft tissue restriction to the movement.

Obviously there are likely to be articular or capsular reasons for these restrictions and, if this is the case, soft tissue involvement would be secondary.

4 Assessment of shoulder abduction restriction (Fig. 13.17E)

- Patient is sidelying and the practitioner cups the shoulder and compresses the scapula and clavicle to the thorax with the cephalad hand, while cupping the flexed elbow with the caudad hand.
- The patient's hand is supported on the practitioner's cephalad forearm/wrist to stabilize the arm.
- The elbow is abducted toward the patient's head as range of motion is assessed.

Box 13.6 (cont'd)

- Some degree of external rotation is also involved in this abduction.
- Pain-free easy abduction should be close to 180°.
- If there is a restriction toward abduction the soft tissues implicated in maintaining this dysfunction would be the shoulder adductors (pectoralis major, teres major, latissimus dorsi and possibly the long head of triceps, coracobrachialis, short head of biceps brachii).
- As with all Spencer movements this is a passive activity.

5 Assessment of shoulder adduction restriction (not illustrated)

- With the patient sidelying, the practitioner cups the shoulder and compresses the scapula and clavicle to the thorax with the cephalad hand, while cupping the elbow with the caudad hand.
- The patient's hand is supported on the practitioner's cephalad forearm/wrist to stabilize the arm.

- The elbow is taken in an arc *forward of the chest* so that the elbow moves both cephalad and medially as the shoulder adducts and externally rotates.
- The action is performed slowly and any signs of resistance are noted.
- The degree of adduction which may be regarded as normal in this movement would be one which allowed the movement to progress, unrestricted, until the flexed elbow approached the mid-line of the thorax.
- If there is a restriction toward adduction, the soft tissues implicated in maintaining this dysfunction would be the shoulder abductors (deltoid and supraspinatus).
- Since external rotation is also involved, other muscles implicated in restriction or pain may include internal rotators (subscapularis, pectoralis major, latissimus dorsi and teres major).

Box 13.7 Clavicular assessment (Greenman 1989)

Note: In the author's experience these clavicular restrictions can usually be normalized using soft issue approaches. Appropriate treatment methods will be outlined in the text.

1 Assessment and treatment of restricted abduction sternoclavicular joint

As the clavicle is abducted it rotates posteriorly.

- The patient lies supine (or is seated) with arms at side.
- The practitioner places index fingers on *superior* aspect of medial clavicle.
- The patient is asked to shrug her shoulders while movement of the clavicle is palpated.
- Each clavicle should move slightly caudad (toward the feet).
- If either fails to do so, there is a restriction of the associated joint.

2 Assessment of restricted horizontal flexion of the upper arm (Fig. 13.18)

- The patient lies supine, the practitioner is at the side, at waist level facing cephalad, with index fingers lying on the anteromedial aspect of each clavicle.
- The patient is asked to bring her arms together in front of her face, arms extended, so that her hands are in a 'prayer' position pointing toward the ceiling, while clavicular movement is monitored as the patient pushes her hands toward the ceiling.
- If the joint is functioning normally there will be a 'dropping' of the clavicular head toward the floor (a posterior movement), on that side.
- If one or both clavicular heads fail to drop but remain static or actually rise (toward the ceiling), there is restriction.

3 Assessment for restricted acromioclavicular (AC) joint

Stiles (1984) suggests initial evaluation of AC dysfunction at the scapula, the mechanics of which closely relate to AC function.

- The patient sits erect and the spines of both scapula are palpated by the practitioner, who is standing behind.
- The hands are moved medially, until the medial borders of the scapulae are identified, at the level of the spine of the scapula.
- Using the palpating fingers as landmarks, the levels are checked to see whether they are the same. Inequality suggests AC dysfunction.

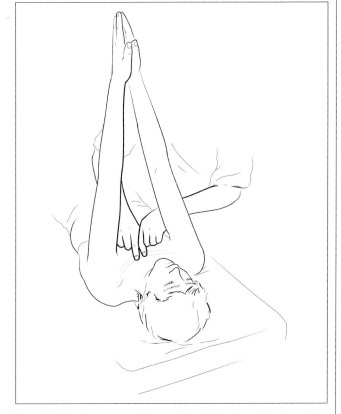

Figure 13.18 Assessment for restriction in horizontal flexion at the sternoclavicular joint.

- The side of dysfunction remains to be assessed (i.e. the scapula might be superior or inferior on the side of dysfunction, so that while inequality of scapula height suggests dysfunction, it is the specific assessment (below) that identifies which side is dysfunctional).
- Each side is then tested separately.
- To test the right AC joint, the practitioner is behind the patient

Box 13.7 (cont'd)

with the left hand fingers palpating over the joint. The right hand holds the patient's right elbow. The arm is lifted in a plane, 45° from the sagittal and frontal planes.
• As the arm approaches 90° elevation, the AC joint should be carefully palpated for hinge movement between the acromion and the clavicle.

• In normal movement, with no restriction, the palpating fingers should move slightly caudad, as the arm is abducted beyond 90°.
• If the AC is restricted, the palpating digit will move cephalad and little or no action will be noted at the joint itself, as the arm goes beyond 90°.

Box 13.8   Acromioclavicular and sternoclavicular MET approaches (Janda 1988, Kaltenborn 1985, Lewit 1985, Stiles 1984)

The test for AC restriction is to be found in clavicular assessment on p. 318.

 MET for restriction of AC joint

• Muscle energy technique is employed with the arm held at the restriction barrier, as for testing as described in Box 13.7, i.e. at the point just prior to a cephalad rise of the clavicle as the arm is elevated.
• If the scapula on the side of dysfunction (failure of AC joint to hinge appropriately) had been shown to be more proximal than that on the normal side, then before arm elevation commences the humerus is placed in external rotation, which takes the scapula caudad against the barrier.
• If, however, the scapula on the side of the AC dysfunction was more distal than the scapula on the normal side, then before arm elevation commences the arm is internally rotated, taking the scapula cephalad against the barrier before the isometric contraction commences.
• The left hand (we assume this to be a right-sided problem) stabilizes the lateral aspect of the clavicle, with light but firm caudad pressure being applied by the left thumb which rests on its superior surface.
• The arm, supported at the elbow by the practitioner (and internally or externally rotated at the shoulder, depending on indications gained from scapulae imbalance), is raised until the first sign of inappropriate movement at the AC joint is sensed (a feeling of 'bind'), identifying the barrier.
• It is important at this stage to ensure that all slack has been removed from the internal or the external rotation of the upper arm.
• An unyielding counterpressure is offered at the point of the patient's elbow by the right hand and the patient is asked to try to take that elbow towards the floor with less than full strength.
• After 7–10 seconds the patient and practitioner relax, greater internal or external rotation is introduced to take out any slack now available and the arm is elevated towards the barrier until 'bind' is sensed.
• Firm but not forceful pressure is sustained on the clavicle in a caudad direction as the slack is being removed from the tissues.
• A further mild isometric contraction is asked for and the procedure repeated several times, until no further improvement is noted in terms of range of motion or until it is sensed that the clavicle has resumed normal function.

The test for abduction restriction of the sternoclavicular joint is found in Box 13.7.

MET treatment of restricted abduction at the sternoclavicular (SC) joint

• The practitioner stands behind the seated patient with his thenar eminence on the superior margin of the medial end of the clavicle to be treated.
• To achieve this, the practitioner's arm needs to be passed

anterior to the patient's throat and care needs to be taken to avoid any pressure on this.
• The other hand cups the patient's flexed elbow and holds this at 90°, with the upper arm externally rotated and abducted.
• The patient is asked to adduct the upper arm for 5–7 seconds against resistance using about 20% of available strength.
• Following the effort and complete relaxation, the arm is abducted further and externally rotated further, until a new barrier is sensed ('bind' is sensed at the SC joint by the practitioner).
• As this is done, a firm caudad pressure is maintained on the medial end of the clavicle.
• The process is repeated until free movement of the medial clavicle is achieved.

The test for horizontal flexion restriction of the sternoclavicular joint is to be found in Box 13.7.

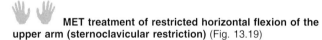 **MET treatment of restricted horizontal flexion of the upper arm (sternoclavicular restriction)** (Fig. 13.19)

• The patient lies supine and the practitioner stands on the side contralateral to that being treated.

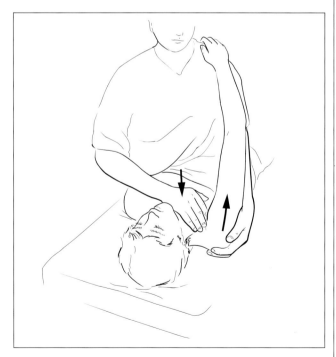

Figure 13.19   MET treatment for restriction in horizontal flexion at the sternoclavicular joint.

Box 13.8 (cont'd)

- The practitioner's non-tableside thenar eminence is placed over the medial end of the clavicle, holding it towards the floor.
- The tableside hand is placed, palm upwards, under the patient's ipsilateral shoulder so that it is in broad contact with the dorsal aspect of the scapula.
- The patient is asked to stretch out the arm on the side to be treated so that the hand can rest behind the practitioner's neck or tableside shoulder.
- The practitioner leans back slightly to take out all the slack from the patient's extended arm and shoulder, while at the same time lifting the scapula slightly from the table.

- The patient is then asked to attempt to pull the practitioner towards herself.
- Firm resistance is offered for 7–10 seconds.
- Following complete release of all the patient's efforts, the downwards thenar eminence pressure – to the floor – is maintained (painlessly) and more slack is taken out (practitioner leans back a little more).
- The process is repeated once or twice more or until the 'prayer' test proves negative.
- No pain should be noted during this procedure.

TREATMENT

Trapezius (see p. 188)

Attachments: *Upper fibers*: mid-third of nuchal line and ligamentum nuchae to the lateral third of the clavicle

Middle fibers: spinous processes and interspinous ligaments of C6–T3 to the acromion and spine of the scapula

Lower fibers: spinous processes and interspinous ligaments of T3–12 to the medial end of the spine of the scapula

Innervation: Accessory nerve (cranial nerve XI) supplies primarily motor while C2–4 supply mostly sensory

Muscle type: *Upper trapezius*: postural (type 1) shortens when stressed

Middle and lower trapezius: phasic (type 2) weakens when stressed (Janda 1996b)

Function: *Entire muscle*: assists extension of the cervical and thoracic spine when contracting bilaterally

Upper fibers: unilaterally extend and laterally flex the head and neck to the same side, aid in contralateral extreme head rotation, elevation of the scapula via rotation of the clavicle, assist in carrying the weighted upper limb, help to rotate the glenoid fossa upward

Middle fibers: assist in adduction of the scapula and in upwardly rotating the scapula after rotation has been initiated

Lower fibers: adduct the scapula, depress the scapula. Rotation of the scapula remains a controversial function of the lower fibers (Simons et al 1998); however, they may stabilize the scapula while other muscles rotate it (Johnson et al 1994)

Synergists: The trapezius pair are synergistic with each other for head, neck or thoracic extension

Upper fibers: SCM (head motions); supraspinatus, serratus anterior (Norkin & Levangie 1992) and deltoid (rotation of scapula during abduction)

Middle fibers: rhomboids (adduct scapula); deltoid, supraspinatus and long head of biceps brachii (elevation of the arm at the shoulder joint)

Lower fibers: serratus anterior (upward rotation of the

glenoid fossa); pectoralis minor (Norkin & Levangie 1992) and latissimus dorsi (Kendall et al 1993) (depression)

Antagonists: *Upper fibers*: levator scapula (scapular rotation) and lower fibers of trapezius

Middle fibers: pectoralis major, pectoralis minor (Kendall et al 1993)

Lower fibers: upper fibers of trapezius, levator scapula

Indications for treatment

Upper fibers

- Headache over or into the eye or into the temporal area
- Pain in the angle of the jaw, neck pain
- Stiff neck
- Pain with pressure of clothing, purse or luggage strapped across upper shoulder area

Middle fibers

- Burning interscapular pain
- Acromial pain
- Gooseflesh on the lateral upper arm

Lower fibers

- Neck, acromial, suprascapular or interscapular pain

Special notes

- In assessing and treating the trapezius, the muscle is divided into upper, middle and lower fibers in regards to nomenclature as well as function. The upper, middle and lower portions of the muscle often function independently (*Gray's anatomy* 1995).
- When the shoulder is fixed, trapezius extends and sidebends the head and neck.
- With shortening of the muscle, the occiput will be pulled inferolaterally via very powerful fibers. The potential negative influence of trapezius dysfunction is directly to occipital, parietal and temporal function in cranial therapy.

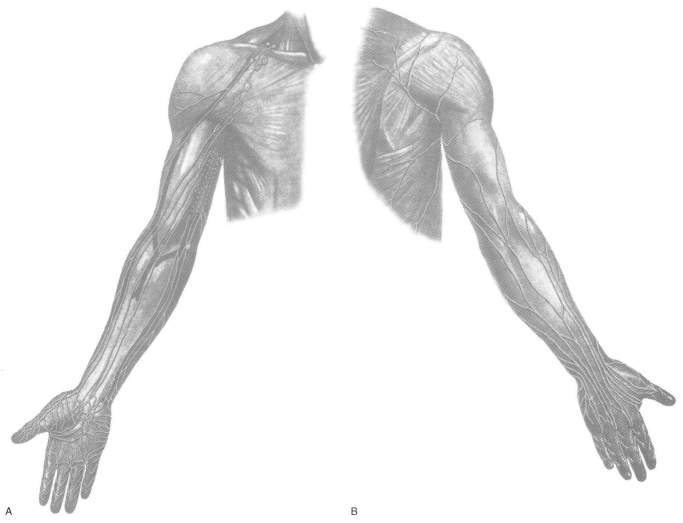

Figure 13.20 A&B: Lymph drainage pathways of upper extremity (reproduced, with permission, from *Gray's anatomy* (1995)).

Box 13.9 Spencer's assessment sequence including MET and PRT treatment

The Spencer sequence, which derives from osteopathic medicine in the early years of the 20th century, is taught at all osteopathic colleges in the USA. Over the years it has been modified to include treatment elements other than the original articulation intent. The sequences can be transformed from an assessment/articulatory technique into a muscle energy approach or into positional release. When used for assessment and treatment, the scapula is fixed firmly to the thoracic wall to focus on involvement of the glenohumeral joint. In all Spencer assessment and treatment sequences, the patient is sidelying, with the side to be assessed uppermost, arm lying at the side with the elbow (usually) flexed, with the practitioner facing slightly cephalad, at chest level (Patriquin 1992, Spencer 1916).

1a Assessment and MET treatment of shoulder extension restriction (Fig. 13.17A)

• The practitioner's cephalad hand cups the shoulder, firmly compressing the scapula and clavicle to the thorax while the patient's flexed elbow is held by the practitioner's caudad hand, as the arm is taken into passive extension toward the optimal 90°.

• Any restriction in range of motion is noted, ceasing movement at the first indication of resistance.

• At that barrier the patient is instructed to push her elbow toward her feet or anteriorly or to push further toward the direction of extension, utilizing no more than 20% of her strength, building up force slowly.

• This effort is firmly resisted and after 7–10 seconds, the patient is instructed to slowly cease the effort. (The direction in which the patient is asked to push is arbitrary, to investigate the benefit in terms of subsequent increased freedom of movement.)

• After completely relaxing and upon exhalation, the elbow is moved to take the shoulder further into extension, to the next restriction barrier, and the MET procedure is repeated (Liebenson 1990, Mitchell et al 1979).

• A degree of active patient participation in the movement toward the new barrier is usually helpful as it will create an inhibitory response in the tissue being stretched (Chaitow 1996a).

1b Alternatively – PRT (Goodheart 1984, Jones 1985)

• If restriction is noted during movement towards extension the soft tissues implicated in maintaining this dysfunction would be the shoulder flexors – anterior deltoid, coracobrachialis and the clavicular head of pectoralis major.

• Palpation of these should reveal areas of marked tenderness.

Box 13.9 (*cont'd*)

• The most painful tender point (painful to digital pressure) elicited by palpation is used as a monitoring point as the arm is moved into a position which will reduce that pain by not less than 70%.

• This position of ease usually involves some degree of flexion and fine tuning to slacken the muscle housing the tender point.

• This ease state should be held for anything from 30 to 90 seconds before a slow return to neutral and a subsequent reevaluation of the range of motion.

2a Assessment and MET treatment of shoulder flexion restriction (Fig. 13.17B)

• Patient and practitioner have the same starting position as in the previous test.

• The practitioner's non-tableside hand grasps the patient's forearm while the tableside hand holds the clavicle and scapula firmly to the chest wall.

• The practitioner slowly introduces passive shoulder flexion in the horizontal plane, as range of motion to 180° is assessed, by which time the elbow is fully extended.

• At the position of *very first indication* of restriction in movement, the patient is instructed to pull the elbow toward her feet or posteriorly or to push further toward the direction of flexion, utilizing no more than 20% of her strength, building up force slowly.

• The patient's effort is firmly resisted and after 7–10 seconds the patient is instructed to slowly cease the effort simultaneously with the practitioner.

• After the patient completely relaxes and upon exhalation, the elbow is moved to take the shoulder further into flexion to the next restriction barrier, where the MET procedure is repeated.

• A degree of active patient participation in the movement toward the new barrier is usually helpful as it will create an inhibitory response in the tissue being stretched.

2b Alternatively – PRT

• If there is a restriction toward flexion the soft tissues implicated in maintaining this dysfunction would be the shoulder extensors – posterior deltoid, teres major, latissimus dorsi, and possibly infraspinatus, teres minor and long head of triceps.

• Palpation of these should reveal areas of marked tenderness.

• The most painful tender point (painful to digital pressure) elicited by palpation should be used as a monitoring point, as the arm is moved into a position which will reduce that pain by not less than 70%.

• This position of ease will probably involve some degree of extension and fine tuning to slacken the muscle housing the tender point.

• This ease state should be held for anything from 30 to 90 seconds before a slow return to neutral and a subsequent reevaluation of range of motion.

3a Articulation and assessment of circumduction capability with compression (Fig. 13.17C)

• The patient is sidelying with elbow flexed while the practitioner's cephalad hand cups the shoulder firmly, compressing the scapula and clavicle to the thorax.

• The practitioner's caudad hand grasps the elbow and takes the shoulder through a slow clockwise circumduction, while adding compression through the long axis of the humerus.

• This is repeated several times in order to articulate the joint and assess range, freedom and comfort of the circumduction motion as the humeral head moves on the surface of the glenoid fossa.

• The same procedure is then performed anticlockwise. If any

restriction is noted Ruddy's 'pulsed MET' can be introduced, in which the patient attempts to execute a series of minute contractions toward the restriction barrier (20 times in a period of 10 seconds) at which time the articulation is continued (Ruddy 1962).

3b Articulation and assessment of circumduction capability with traction (Fig. 13.17D)

• The patient is sidelying with arm straight while the practitioner's cephalad hand cups the shoulder firmly, compressing scapula and clavicle to the thorax.

• The practitioner's caudad hand grasps the patient's arm above the elbow and introduces slight traction, before taking the arm through slow clockwise circumduction.

• This process articulates the joint while assessing range of motion in circumduction as well as the status of the capsule of the glenohumeral joint.

• The same process is repeated anticlockwise.

• If any restriction is noted, Ruddy's 'pulsed MET' can be introduced in which the patient attempts to execute a series of minute contractions toward the restriction barrier (20 times in a period of 10 seconds) before articulation is continued.

3c PRT for circumduction pain or restriction

• If restriction or pain is noted in either of the circumduction sequences (utilizing compression or traction), evaluate which muscles would be active if precisely the opposite movement were undertaken.

• For example, if on compression and clockwise rotation, a particular part of the circumduction range involves either restriction or discomfort/pain, cease the movement and evaluate which muscles would be required to contract in order to produce an active reversal of that movement (Chaitow 1996b, Goodheart 1984, Jones 1985).

• In these antagonist muscles, palpate for the most 'tender' point and use this as a monitoring point as the structures are taken to a position of ease which reduces the perceived pain by at least 70%.

• This is held for 30–90 seconds before a slow return to neutral and retesting.

4a Assessment and MET treatment of shoulder abduction restriction (Fig. 13.17E)

• The patient is sidelying as the practitioner cups the shoulder and compresses the scapula and clavicle to thorax with his cephalad hand, while cupping the flexed elbow with his caudad hand.

• The patient's hand is supported on the practitioner's cephalad forearm/wrist to stabilize the arm.

• The elbow is abducted toward the patient's head as range of motion is assessed.

• Some degree of external rotation is also involved in this abduction.

• Pain-free easy abduction should be close to 180°.

• Note any restriction in range of motion.

• At the position of *very first indication of resistance* to movement, the patient is instructed to pull the elbow toward her waist or to push further toward the direction of abduction, utilizing no more than 20% of her strength, building up force slowly.

• This effort is firmly resisted and after 7–10 seconds the patient is instructed to slowly cease the effort simultaneously with the practitioner.

• After completely relaxing and upon exhalation, the elbow is moved to take the shoulder further into abduction, to the next restriction barrier, where the MET procedure is repeated if necessary (i.e. if there is still restriction).

Box 13.9   (*cont'd*)

• A degree of active patient participation in the movement toward the new barrier is usually helpful.

 4b Alternatively – PRT

• If there is a restriction toward abduction the soft tissues implicated in maintaining this dysfunction would be the shoulder adductors – pectoralis major, teres major, latissimus dorsi, and possibly the long head of triceps, coracobrachialis, short head of biceps brachii.
• Since external rotation is also occurring in this movement there might be involvement of internal rotators in any restriction or pain.
• Palpation of these muscles should reveal areas of marked tenderness.
• The most painful tender point (painful to digital pressure) elicited by this palpation should be used as a monitoring point, as the arm is moved and fine tuned into a position which reduces that pain by not less than 70%.
• This position of ease will probably involve some degree of adduction and external rotation, to slacken the muscle housing the tender point.
• This ease state should be held for anything from 30 to 90 seconds, before a slow return to neutral and a subsequent reevaluation of range of motion.

 5a Assessment and MET treatment of shoulder adduction restriction (not illustrated)

• The patient is sidelying and the practitioner cups the shoulder and compresses the scapula and clavicle to the thorax with his cephalad hand, while cupping the elbow with his caudad hand.
• The patient's hand is supported on the practitioner's cephalad forearm/wrist to stabilize the arm.
• The elbow is taken in an arc forward of the chest so that the elbow moves both cephalad and medially as the shoulder adducts and externally rotates.
• The action is performed slowly and any signs of resistance are noted.
• At the position of the *very first indication of resistance* to movement, the patient is instructed to pull the elbow toward the ceiling or to push further toward the direction of adduction, utilizing no more than 20% of her strength, building up force slowly.
• This effort is firmly resisted and after 7–10 seconds the patient is instructed to slowly cease the effort.
• After completely relaxing and upon exhalation, the elbow is moved to take the shoulder further into adduction, to the next restriction barrier, where the MET procedure is repeated if restriction remains.
• A degree of active patient participation in the movement toward the new barrier is usually helpful.

 5b Alternatively – PRT

• If there is a restriction toward adduction the soft tissues implicated in maintaining this dysfunction would be the shoulder abductors – deltoid, supraspinatus.
• Since external rotation is also involved, other muscles implicated in restriction or pain may include internal rotators such as subscapularis, pectoralis major, latissimus dorsi and teres major.
• Palpation of these should reveal areas of marked tenderness.
• The most painful tender point (painful to digital pressure) elicited by palpation should be used as a monitoring point as the arm is moved into a position which will reduce that pain by not less than 70%.
• This position of ease will probably involve some degree of abduction together with fine tuning involving internal rotation, to slacken the muscle housing the tender point.

• This ease state should be held for anything from 30 to 90 seconds before a slow return to neutral and a subsequent reevaluation of range of motion.

 6a Assessment and MET treatment of internal rotation restriction (Fig. 13.17F)

• The patient is sidelying and her flexed arm is placed behind her back to evaluate whether the dorsum of the hand can be painlessly placed against the dorsal surface of the ipsilateral lumbar area.
• This arm position is maintained throughout the procedure.
• The practitioner cups the shoulder and compresses the scapula and clavicle to the thorax with his cephalad hand while cupping the flexed elbow with the caudad hand.
• The practitioner slowly brings the elbow (ventrally) toward his body and notes any sign of restriction as this movement, which increases internal rotation, proceeds.
• At the position of *very first indication of resistance* to this movement, the patient is instructed to pull her elbow away from the practitioner, either posteriorly or medially or both simultaneously, utilizing no more than 20% of her strength, building up force slowly.
• This effort is firmly resisted and after 7–10 seconds the patient is instructed to slowly cease the effort simultaneously with the practitioner.
• After completely relaxing and upon exhalation, the elbow is moved to take the shoulder further into abduction and internal rotation, to the next restriction barrier, where the MET procedure is repeated.

 6b Alternatively – PRT

• If there is a restriction toward internal rotation the soft tissues implicated in maintaining this dysfunction would be the shoulder external rotators – infraspinatus and teres minor, with posterior deltoid also possibly being involved.
• Palpation of these should reveal areas of marked tenderness.
• The most painful tender point (painful to digital pressure) elicited by palpation should be used as a monitoring point as the arm is moved into a position which will reduce that pain by not less than 70%.
• This position of ease will probably involve some degree of external rotation to slacken the muscle housing the tender point.
• This ease state should be held for anything from 30 to 90 seconds before a slow return to neutral and a subsequent reevaluation of range of motion.

 7 Spencer's general soft tissue release (and lymphatic pump)

• The patient is sidelying with the practitioner half facing cephalad at chest level.
• The patient's hand (elbow extended) rests on the practitioner's tableside shoulder. Both practitioner's hands enfold the patient's upper humerus.
• Traction is applied to the humerus, taking out the slack in periarticular soft tissues.
• The traction is slowly released.
• Compression is applied to the glenoid fossa by gently forcing the humerus into it. The cycle of compression and traction is rhythmically alternated until a sense of freedom is achieved.
• In addition, translatory motions can be introduced, for example anterior/posterior or cephalad/caudad, in combination with the alternating traction and compression.

Note: All Spencer movements are performed passively (apart from the MET isometric contraction element) in a controlled, slow and repetitive manner.

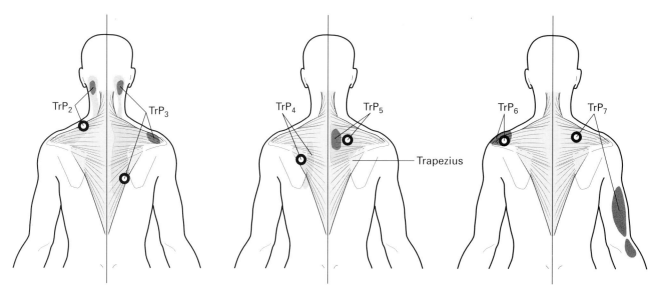

Figure 13.21 The combined patterns of common trapezius trigger points (see also Fig. 11.27, p. 190).

• In some people upper trapezius fibers merge with sternocleidomastoid, offering other possible areas of influence when dysfunctional (*Gray's anatomy* 1995).

• The motor innervation of trapezius is from the spinal portion of the XI cranial (spinal accessory) nerve. Arising within the spinal canal from ventral roots of the first five cervical segments (usually), it rises through the foramen magnum, exiting via the jugular foramen, where it supplies and sometimes penetrates sternocleidomastoid before reaching a plexus below trapezius (*Gray's anatomy* 1995).

• Upledger & Vredevoogd (1983) point out that hypertonicity of trapezius can produce dysfunction at the jugular foramen with implications for accessory nerve function, so increasing and perpetuating trapezius hypertonicity.

Fibers of upper trapezius initiate the rotation of the clavicle to prepare for elevation of the shoulder girdle. The middle fibers then join to lift the acromioclavicular joint off the humeral head and to elevate the entire shoulder. Since the overhanging ledge created by the acromioclavicular joint can occlude the supraspinatus tendon and the subacromial bursa and can impact the humeral head, the inability to fully lift it off the underlying structures is significant. Additionally, this action is often used to support a phone to the ear, to carry articles strapped across the shoulder (luggage, purses, backpacks) and when carrying weight in the dependent hand (bucket of water, luggage).

Any position which strains or places the trapezius in a shortened state for periods of time without rest may shorten the fibers and lead to the activation of trigger points. Lengthy telephone conversations, particularly when the shoulder is elevated to hold the phone, working from a chair set too low for the desk or computer terminal, elevation of the arm for painting, drawing, playing a musical instrument and computer processing, particularly for extended periods of time, can all shorten trapezius fibers. Overloading of fibers may activate or perpetuate trigger point activity or may make tissue more vulnerable to activation even when a minor trauma occurs, such as a simple fall, minor motor vehicle accident or when reaching (especially quickly) to catch something out of reach.

Trigger points in the upper trapezius (see pp. 190, 324) are some of the most prevalent and potent trigger points found in the body and are relatively easy to locate. They are also easily activated by day-to-day habits and abuses, such as repetitive use, sudden trauma, falls and acceleration/deceleration injuries ('whiplash'). They are often predisposed to activation by postural asymmetries, including pelvic tilt and torsion which require postural compensations by these and other muscles.

The upper trapezius helps maintain the head's position and serves as a 'postural corrector' for deviations originating further down the body (in the spine, pelvis or feet). Therefore, fibers of the upper trapezius may be working when the patient is sitting or standing, to make adaptive corrections for structural distortions or strained positions. Additional treatment of the cervical portion and occipital attachment of upper trapezius is discussed with the cervical region on p. 188.

The instructions given below, for a prone position, are usually the easiest for learning these palpation techniques. However, a sidelying position is also effective for examining the trapezius and in some cases advantageous. When the patient is sidelying with the upper arm lying on the (uppermost) lateral surface of the body, the upper, middle and lower trapezius may be easily palpated and lifted from the underlying tissues. Additionally, the fibers of each may be shortened or elongated simply by positioning the shoulder with the weight of the arm supported on the patient's body. A prone or sidelying position has an advantage over a seated assessment since the trapezius would not be supporting the shoulder girdle or the head during the examination (as it would be with an upright posture). A sidelying position is discussed with the cervical region on p. 229.

Assessment of upper trapezius for shortness

1. See scapulohumeral rhythm test (p. 303) which helps identify excessive activity or inappropriate tone in levator scapula and upper trapezius which, because they are postural muscles, indicates shortness.

2. Patient is seated and practitioner stands behind with one hand resting on the shoulder of the side to be tested. The other hand is placed on the side of the head which is being tested and the head/neck is taken into side bending away from that side without force while the shoulder is stabilized. The same procedure is performed on the other side with the opposite shoulder stabilized. A comparison is made as to which side-bending maneuver produced the greater range and whether the neck can easily reach a 45° angle from the vertical, which it should. If neither side can achieve this degree of side bend then both trapezius muscles may be short. The relative shortness of one, compared with the other, is evaluated.

3. The patient is seated and the practitioner stands behind with a hand resting over the muscle on the side to be assessed. The patient is asked to extend the shoulder, bringing the flexed arm/elbow backwards. If the upper trapezius is stressed/short on that side it will inappropriately activate during this movement. Since it is a postural muscle, shortness in it can then be assumed.

4. The patient is supine with the neck fully (but not forcefully) sidebent away from the side being assessed. The practitioner, standing at the head of the table, uses a cupped hand contact on the shoulder (tested side) to assess the ease with which it can be depressed (moved distally). There should be an easy 'springing' sensation as the shoulder is pushed toward the feet, with a soft end-feel to the movement. If depression of the shoulder is difficult or if there is a more wooden end-point, upper trapezius on that side is probably short (see p. 302).

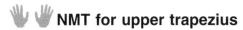 **NMT for upper trapezius**

Cervical portion. The most superficial layer of the posterior cervical region is the upper trapezius. Its fibers lie directly beside the spinous processes and orient verti-

cally at the higher levels and turn laterally near the base of the neck. With the patient supine, prone or sidelying, these fibers may be grasped between the thumbs and fingers and compressed (one side at a time or both sides simultaneously) against each other. The occipital attachment may be examined with light friction and should be differentiated from the thicker semispinalis capitus which lies deep to it.

Upper trapezius. The patient is prone with the arm hanging off the side of the table to reduce tension in the upper fibers of trapezius. This arm position will allow some slack in the muscle which makes it easier to grasp the fibers as they coil anteriorly in a slight spiral to their clavicular attachments. If appropriate and needed, the fibers may be slightly stretched by placing the patient's arm beside them on the massage table. This additional elongation may make the taut fibers more palpable and precise compression possible; however, it may also stretch taut fibers so much that they are difficult to palpate or it may aggravate trigger points due to the tension increased by the stretch. The practitioner's non-treating hand can rest gently on the person's back for 'comforting support'.

Flat compression near the center of the muscle belly (fibers held between thumb and several fingers – flattened like a clothes pin) will provide a general release and can be applied in 1–2″ segments along the upper fibers to examine their full length. Pincer compression (fingers and thumb held like a C-clamp) can then be used to more precisely examine and treat the remaining taut fibers.

The fibers of the outermost portion of the trapezius can be uncoiled by dragging 2–3 fingers on the anterior surface of the fibers while the thumb presses through the fibers (from the posterior aspect) and against the uncoiling fingers (Fig. 13.22). As the fingers uncoil directly across the hidden deep fibers, palpable bands, trigger point nodules and twitch responses may be felt. The wrist is kept low to avoid flipping over the most anterior fibers as snapping across them often produces extreme discomfort for the patient and elicits referred pain. While controlled and specific snapping techniques can be developed and used as a treatment modality or to elicit twitch responses for trigger point verification, they should not be accidentally applied to these vulnerable fibers. Static pincer compression should be applied to taut bands, trigger points or nodules found in the upper fibers of trapezius. Toothpick size strands of the outermost fibers of upper trapezius often have noxious referrals into the face and eyes and local twitch responses are readily felt in these easily palpable, often taut fibers.

The patient's arm is allowed to rest on the treatment table beside them to place the glenohumeral joint and the scapula in fairly neutral positions. The practitioner's thumb can be used to glide from the middle of the upper trapezius laterally to the acromioclavicular joint. The

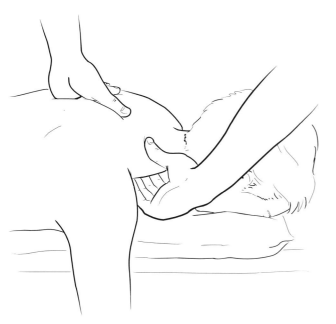

Figure 13.22 The fingers curl around the forward 'lip' of the anterior fibers of trapezius.

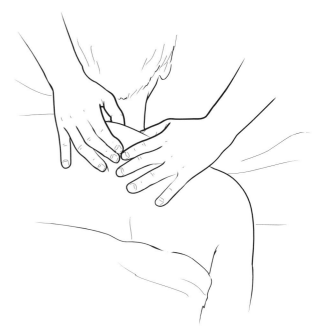

Figure 13.23 The middle trapezius fibers may be lifted away from underlying tissue, rolled between the thumb and fingers or compressed to release trigger points. When fibers are difficult to lift, the overlying skin may be tractioned in a similar manner to provide myofascial release.

thumb is then returned to the middle of the muscle belly and used again to glide medially toward C7 or T1. These alternating, gliding techniques are repeated to spread the sarcomeres and taut bands from the muscle's center toward its attachment sites (see p. 118). A double thumb glide applied by spreading the fibers from the center simultaneously toward the two ends will traction the shortened central sarcomeres and may produce a profound release. Full-length glides may reveal remaining thickness within the tissue which needs to be readdressed with compression or other techniques. Myofascial release may also be used to soften and elongate the upper fibers.

Central trigger points in these upper fibers refer strongly into the cranium and particularly into the eye. Attachment trigger points and tenderness may be associated with tension from central trigger points and may not respond well until central trigger points have been abolished.

 NMT for middle trapezius

This portion of the trapezius may be outlined by drawing parallel lines from each end of the spine of the scapula toward the vertebral column. The fibers lying between these two lines represent the middle trapezius. The central portion of most of these fibers lifts readily if the practitioner's hands are positioned correctly. If needed, the humeral head may be elevated 3–4" (by a rolled-up towel, wedge, etc.) to further approximate the fibers of both middle and lower trapezius which often allows them to be grasped and lifted.

While standing cephalad to the patient's shoulder, the practitioner grasps the middle fibers of the trapezius

with both hands (Fig. 13.23). Compression may then be applied to the mid-belly region of the upper half of middle trapezius, where its central trigger points are usually found. These tissues may also be manipulated by rolling them between the fingers and thumb. The lower fibers of the middle trapezius normally lie flat to the torso and are not easily lifted by the fingers. Those fibers are addressed with gliding strokes after the lower trapezius has been treated.

 NMT for lower trapezius

The diagonal fibers of lower trapezius traverse the mid-back from T12 to the inferior aspect of the medial third of the spine of the scapula. Occasionally the lower trapezius fibers will be more accessible without the towel (or wedge) elevation mentioned above.

The practitioner is repositioned to stand just cephalad to the patient's waist and faces toward the opposite shoulder. The practitioner should grasp and lift the outer (diagnoal) edge of the lower trapezius (Fig. 13.24). If appropriate, compression and manipulation as described above may be applied to the fibers to reveal taut bands and trigger points. Trigger point pressure on or gentle mid-belly (double-thumb) traction of the contractures will usually release trigger points found in these fibers.

When muscle fibers of the lower trapezius will not lift, flat palpation may be used against the ribs and underlying muscles. (The grasp may be tested by lifting the

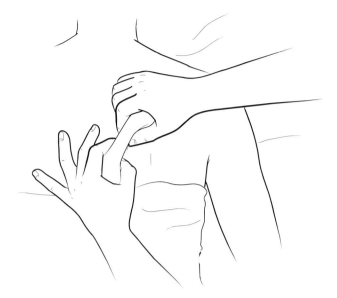

Figure 13.24   The lower trapezius fibers are treated in the same way.

fibers and allowing them to gently slip through the compressed fingers to be assured of holding more than just skin.) Additionally, the lower trapezius may be freed from fascial restrictions when the skin overlying its outer fibers is lifted toward the ceiling and held for 1–2 minutes. The skin should be stretched to its elastic barrier and then held, allowing the fascia to soften and elongate. As the skin becomes more mobile, the muscular fibers deep to it will demonstrate greater freedom of movement in relation to surrounding tissues.

 ## NMT for trapezius attachments

The humeral head is lowered and the arm allowed to rest comfortably. Lubricated gliding strokes may be applied to the lamina groove beside the spinous processes from C7 to L1 and on the scapula and acromion. Thumb glides applied to the lamina groove in progressively deeper strokes may release layers of tendinous tension and reveal locations of attachment trigger points and enthesitis in any of the layers attaching into the spinous and transverse processes (which form the 'walls' of the groove). Additionally, a beveled pressure bar (beveled rubber tip) may be used in the lamina groove (see p. 443) to assess and treat the numerous tendons which attach there.

Static pressure or friction applied with the finger, thumb or the beveled pressure bar can be used directly medial to and against the acromioclavicular joint for the upper fiber attachment of trapezius.

CAUTION: Friction or use of the pressure bar is contra-indicated when moderate to extreme tenderness is present or when other symptoms indicate inflammation.

Whether using the beveled pressure bar or digital friction, the pressure may be angled anteriorly against the trapezius attachment on the clavicle (see p. 191) where static pressure or transverse friction may be lightly applied with the pressure increasing only if appropriate. Extreme caution should be exercised when examining more than one or two finger tip widths medial to the acromioclavicular joint on the clavicle. Medial to this point (exact position varies based on width of trapezius attachment on the clavicle) lies the lateral edge of the supraclavicular fossa, an area in which the brachial plexus lies relatively exposed. Intrusion might damage the nerves and accompanying blood vessels in this area.

The beveled pressure bar or finger should be placed immediately medial to the acromioclavicular joint and pressed straight in (caudally, through the trapezius) to treat the tendon of supraspinatus and (possibly) the tendon of biceps (long head).

CAUTION: This step is contraindicated if a supraspinatus tear, subacromial bursitis or bicipital tendinitis is suspected as surrounding tissues may be inflamed (see assessments on p. 299 and impingement syndrome test, p. 305).

The beveled pressure bar is angled posteriorly against the superior aspect of the spine of the scapula and transverse friction is applied at ½" intervals to the superior aspect of the spine of the scapula to treat trapezius attachments. Additionally, the inferior aspect of the spine of the scapula may be addressed in the same manner.

Lubricated, gliding strokes in all directions may be used on all portions of the trapezius to soothe the tissues and increase blood flow. This is particularly important when more aggressive techniques, such as manipulation and pressure bar work, have been used. Gliding strokes along attachment sites may also reveal areas of enthesitis (inflammation of muscular or tendinous attachment to bone) and periosteal tension which may respond favorably to applications of ice rather than heat. Gliding is particularly applied to any aspects of the trapezius which have not been addressed during the previous steps.

If central trigger points are located, pincer compression may be used if the tissue can be lifted or flat compression against underlying structures may be applied. Additionally, gliding strokes may be applied from the center of the fibers (where most central trigger points will be found) toward the attachment sites. These techniques are intended to manually traction the actin and myosin elements and spread the tense central sarcomeres toward the periosteal tension at the attachment sites. If inflammation is suspected at the attachments, stripping should definitely be toward the attachments so as to avoid placing further tension on these already distressed connective tissues.

Lief's NMT for upper trapezius area
(see pp. 192 and 210)

• In Lief's NMT the practitioner begins by standing half-facing the head of the table on the left of the prone patient with his hips level with the mid-thoracic area.

• The first contact to the left side of the patient's head is a gliding, light-pressured movement of the medial tip of the right thumb, from the mastoid process along the nuchal line to the external occipital protuberance. This same stroke, or glide, is then repeated with deeper pressure. The practitioner's left hand rests on the upper thoracic or shoulder area as a stabilizing contact.

• The treating/assessing hand should be relaxed, molding itself to the contours of tissues. The finger tips offer balance to the hand.

• After the first two strokes of the right thumb – one shallow and diagnostic, the second deeper, imparting therapeutic effort – the next stroke is half a thumb width caudal to the first. A degree of overlap occurs as these strokes, starting on the belly of the sternocleidomastoid, glide across and through the trapezius, splenius capitis and posterior cervical muscles.

• A progressive series of strokes is applied in this way until the level of the cervicodorsal junction is reached. Unless serious underlying dysfunction is found, it is seldom necessary to repeat the two superimposed strokes at each level of the cervical region. If underlying fibrotic tissue appears unyielding, a third or fourth slow, deeper glide may be necessary.

• The practitioner now moves to the head of the table. The left thumb is placed on the right, lateral aspect of the first dorsal vertebra and a series of strokes are performed caudally and laterally as well as diagonally toward the scapula.

• A series of thumb strokes, shallow and then deep, is applied caudally from T1 to about T4 or 5 and laterally toward the scapula and along and across all the upper trapezius fibers and the rhomboids. The left hand treats the right side and vice versa with the non-operative hand stabilizing the neck or head.

• By repositioning himself to one side, it is possible for the practitioner to more easily apply a series of sensitively searching contacts into the area of the thoracic outlet. Thumb strokes which start in this triangular depression move toward the trapezius fibers and through them toward the upper margins of the scapula.

• Several light palpating strokes should also be applied directly over the spinous processes, caudally, toward the mid-dorsal area. Triggers sometimes lie on the attachments to the spinous processes or between them.

• Any trigger points located should be treated according to the protocol of integrated neuromuscular inhibition technique (INIT) – p. 10.

 MET treatment of upper trapezius

• The patient lies supine, head/neck side bent away from the side to be treated just short of the restriction barrier, with the practitioner stabilizing the shoulder with one hand and cupping the ear/mastoid area of the same side of the head with the other.

• In order to treat all the fibers of the muscle, MET needs to be applied sequentially. The neck should be placed into different positions of rotation, coupled with the side bending as described for different fibers.

• With the neck side bent and fully rotated, the posterior fibers of upper trapezius are involved in any contraction and stretch (as are levator scapulae fibers).

• With the neck fully side bent and half rotated, the middle fibers are involved.

• With the neck fully side bent and slightly turned toward the side from which it is side flexed, the anterior fibers are being treated.

• This maneuver can be performed with the practitioner's arms crossed, hands stabilizing the mastoid area and shoulder, or not crossed as comfort dictates, and with practitioner standing at the head or the side, also as comfort dictates (Fig. 13.16).

• The patient should be asked to introduce a light resisted effort (20% of available strength) to take the stabilized shoulder toward the ear (a shrug movement) and the ear toward the shoulder. The double movement (or effort toward movement) is important in order to introduce a contraction of the muscle from both ends. The degree of effort should be mild and no pain should be felt.

• After the 10 seconds (or so) of contraction and complete relaxation of effort, the practitioner gently eases the head/neck into an increased degree of side bending, before stretching the shoulder away from the ear while stabilizing the head, through the barrier of perceived resistance if chronic, as appropriate.

• The patient can usefully assist in the treatment by initiating, on instruction, the stretch of the muscle ('As you breathe out please slide your hand toward your feet'). No stretch is introduced from the head end of the muscle as this could stress the neck unduly.

 Myofascial release of upper trapezius (see p. 193)

• Patient is seated erect, feet separated to shoulder width and flat on the floor below the knees, arms hanging freely.

• The practitioner stands to the side and behind the patient with the proximal aspect of the forearm closest to the patient resting on the lateral aspect of the muscle to be treated. The forearm is allowed to glide slowly medially toward the scapula/base of the neck, all the while maintaining a firm but acceptable pressure toward the floor (Fig. 11.31, p. 193).

- By the time the contact arm is close to the medial aspect of the superior border of the scapula, the practitioner's treatment contact should be with the elbow itself.
- As this slow glide is taking place, the patient should equally deliberately be turning the head away from the side being treated, having been made aware of the need to maintain an erect sitting posture. The pressure being applied should be transferred through the upright spine to the ischial tuberosities and ultimately the feet. No slump should be allowed to occur.
- If areas of extreme tension are encountered by the moving arm, it is useful to maintain firm pressure to the restricted area, during which time the patient can be asked to slowly return the head to the neutral position and to make several slow rotations of the neck away from the treated side, altering the degree of neck flexion as appropriate to ensure maximal tolerable stretching of the compressed tissues.
- Separately or concurrently, the patient can be asked to stretch the finger tips of the open hand on the side being treated toward the floor, so adding to the fascial 'drag' which ultimately achieves a degree of lengthening and release.

Levator scapula (see p. 204)

Attachments: From the transverse processes of C1 and C2 and the dorsal tubercles of C3 and C4 to the medial scapular border between the superior angle and the medial end (root) of the spine of the scapula
Innervation: C3–4 spinal nerves and the dorsal scapular nerve (C5)
Muscle type: Postural (type 1), shortens when stressed
Function: Elevation of the scapula, resists downward movement of the scapula when the arm or shoulder is weighted, rotates the scapula medially to face the glenoid fossa downward, assists in rotation of the neck to the same side, bilaterally acts to assist extension of the neck and perhaps lateral flexion to the same side (Warfel 1985)
Synergists: *Elevation/medial rotation of the scapula*: rhomboids
Neck stabilization: splenius cervicis, scalenus medius
Antagonists: *To elevation*: serratus anterior, lower trapezius, latissimus dorsi
To rotation of scapula: serratus anterior, upper and lower trapezius
To neck extension: longus colli, longus capitis, rectus capitis anterior, rectus capitis lateralis (Norkin & Levangie 1992)

Indications for treatment

- Neck stiffness or loss of range of cervical rotation

- Torticollis
- Postural distortions including high shoulder and tilted head

Special notes

The levator scapula usually spirals as it descends the neck to attach to the upper angle of the scapula. It is known to split into two layers, one attaching to the posterior aspect of the upper angle while the other merges its fibers anteriorly onto the scapula and the fascial sheath of serratus anterior (*Gray's anatomy* 1995; Simons et al 1998). Between the two layers of the proximal attachment, a bursa is often found and may be the site of considerable tenderness for this region.

The transverse process attachments are joined by numerous other tissues attaching nearby, including scalene medius, splenius cervicis and intertransversarii, which may be addressed at the same time with lateral (unidirectional) transverse friction. Medial frictional strokes are avoided since they could bruise the tissue against the underlying transverse process. Caution must be exercised to avoid slippage of the treating fingers which could press the nerve roots against sharp foraminal gutters.

Levator scapula's attachment onto the posterior aspect of the upper angle of the scapula is often a site of crepitus, a sensation felt by the palpating finger when gas or air in the subcutaneous tissues is encountered. Whether accompanied by calcific deposits, scar tissue or inflammation, the 'crunchiness' or thickness felt by the finger is often tender and the site of frequent self-treatment. The anterior surface of the upper angle, while often the source of deep ache, is usually neglected during treatment unless special accessing positions are used. These buried fibers may be touched directly to address attachment trigger points and for relief of the often accompanying enthesitis.

Assessment for shortness of levator scapula

- The patient lies supine with the arm of the side to be tested stretched out with the hand and lower arm tucked under the buttocks, palm upwards, to help restrain movement of the shoulder/scapula.
- The practitioner's (contralateral to the side being tested) arm is passed across and under the neck to cup the shoulder of the side to be tested with the forearm supporting the neck (see p. 314, Fig. 13.13).
- The practitioner's other hand supports the head.
- With the forearm the neck is lifted into *full pain-free flexion* (aided by the other hand) and is turned *fully toward lateral flexion and rotation*, away from the side to be treated.
- With the shoulder held caudad and the head/neck in the position described, at its resistance barrier there is

a stretch on levator from both ends and if dysfunction exists and/or it is short, discomfort will be reported at the attachment on the upper medial border of the scapula and/or pain reported near the spinous process of C2.

- The hand on the shoulder should now gently 'spring' it caudally.

- If levator is short there will be a harsh, wooden feel to this action. If it is normal there will be a soft feel to the springing.

 ### NMT for levator scapula

The patient is prone with the arm lying on the table or hanging off the side. The practitioner stands at the level of the shoulder on the side to be treated.

The skin is lightly lubricated superficial to the portion of trapezius which lies directly over the levator scapula. The practitioner's thumbs glide 6–8 times from the upper angle of the scapula to the transverse processes of C1–4. This glide remains in the most lateral aspect of the lamina groove and on the posterior aspect of the transverse processes. Unidirectional (lateral) crossfiber strumming may be applied to the tendon attachments at the transverse processes. Only laterally oriented strokes are used to avoid bruising the tissue against the transverse processes (see p. 234).

The practitioner is repositioned to stand cephalad to the shoulder being treated. Gliding strokes are applied 6–8 times caudally superficial to the levator scapula, from the transverse process attachments to the upper angle of the scapula. Transverse friction may be applied to the upper angle attachment (through the trapezius) (Fig. 13.25) if fibrotic fibers are encountered. Frictional

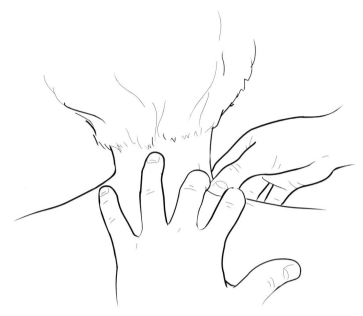

Figure 13.26 Levator scapula and surrounding muscles.

techniques are avoided if tissue is excessively tender or if inflammation is suspected.

The trapezius may be displaced medially to allow direct palpation of the central portion of the belly of levator scapula (Fig. 13.26) where central trigger points develop. To do so, the upper trapezius must be slackened by passive elevation of the shoulder so its fibers will be loose enough to be moved aside. Palpating fingers or thumb may isolate levator scapula and perhaps posterior scalene which lies nearby.

To address the anterior aspect of the upper angle of the scapula, the practitioner uses his most caudad hand to grasp the lower angle of the scapula and press it toward the patient's ear to elevate the upper angle of the scapula off the top of the shoulder and to secure this elevation while the tissue is addressed. It may be necessary to place the patient's hand behind the small of the back to access the scapula but this may be too uncomfortable for a patient with a shoulder injury.

The practitioner's cephalad hand fingers are wrapped completely around the anterior fibers of the trapezius and directly contact the anterior surface of the (elevated) upper angle of the scapula while the caudal hand continues to maintain the scapula's displaced position (Fig. 13.27). The fingers should wrap all the way around the anterior fibers of the trapezius since pressing through the trapezius will not achieve the same results and might irritate trigger points located in these fibers. Palpation of the anterior surface of the upper angle will assess fiber attachments of the levator scapula, serratus anterior and possibly a small portion of the subscapularis muscles. In some cases, angling the fingers medially and laterally may (rarely) contact the rhomboid minor and omohyoid,

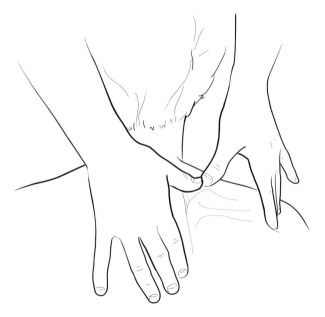

Figure 13.25 Levator scapula's attachment at the upper angle of the scapula often has a fibrotic quality.

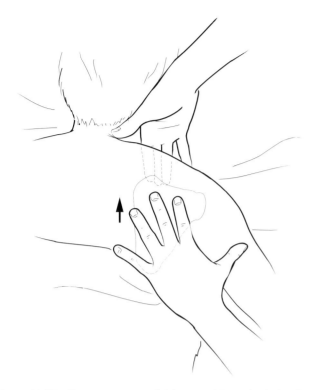

Figure 13.27 Fingers wrap completely around trapezius to touch directly on attachments at the anterior aspect of the upper angle of the scapula.

respectively. If tenderness is encountered, static pressure or gentle massage may be used to address these vulnerable tissues.

 MET treatment of levator scapula
(see p. 314)

The position described below is applied, just short of the easily reached end of range of motion, and should involve 20–30% of the patient's strength, not more. The duration of each contraction should be 7–10 seconds.

- The patient lies supine with the arm of the side to be tested relaxed at the side.
- The practitioner stands at the head of the table and passes his contralateral (to the side being treated) arm across and under the neck to cup the shoulder of the side to be treated while the forearm supports the neck.
- The practitioner's other hand supports the head at the occiput.
- The forearm eases the neck into *full pain-free flexion* (aided by the other hand) and the contact hand on the head guides it *fully toward lateral flexion and rotation* away from the side to be treated.
- With the shoulder held caudad and the head/neck in the position described, the patient is asked to bring her shoulder into a light 'shrug' against the practitioner's hand and simultaneously to take her neck and head

back toward the table, against the resistance of the practitioner's forearm and hand. This is maintained for 7–10 seconds.

- On release of the effort, the neck is taken to its new resistance barrier in flexion, side bending and rotation before the patient is asked to slide the hand toward her foot, through the resistance barrier and into stretch. The practitioner maintains this stretch for 20–30 seconds before repeating the procedure.

Rhomboid minor and major (Fig. 13.28)

Attachments: *Minor*: From the spinous processes of C7–T1 to the vertebral (medial) border of the scapula at the root of its spine
Major: From the spinous processes of T2–5 to the vertebral (medial) border of the scapula
Innervation: Dorsal scapular nerve (C4–5)
Muscle type: Phasic (type 2) weakens when stressed; however, rhomboids can modify their fiber type to postural (type 1) under conditions of prolonged misuse (Salmons 1985)
Function: Adducts and elevates the scapula; rotates the scapula medially to make the glenoid fossa face downward; stabilizes the scapula during arm movements
Synergists: *Adduction of scapula*: middle trapezius
Elevation of scapula: levator scapula, upper trapezius
Rotation of scapula: levator scapula, latissimus dorsi
Antagonists: *To adduction of scapula*: serratus anterior and, indirectly, pectoralis major
To elevation of scapula: serratus anterior, lower trapezius, latissimus dorsi
To rotation of scapula: upper trapezius, rhomboidii

Indications for treatment

- Itching or pain in the mid-thoracic region
- Posture reflecting retracted ('shoulders back') scapular position implies possible shortening involving overactivity/hypertonicity of rhomboids. Such overactivity may paradoxically actually be accompanied by relative weakness of these muscles. This highlights the fact that hypertonicity should not automatically be taken as a sign of strength.

Special notes

When the middle trapezius and rhomboid muscles are placed in strained positions, such as in computer processing, painting overhead or abducting and/or flexing the arm for prolonged periods of time, their trigger points may be activated or their fibers shortened to produce excess tension in the muscles. Since many trigger points refer into the area of rhomboid's scapular attachment, other muscles, including scalenes, serratus anterior, infra-

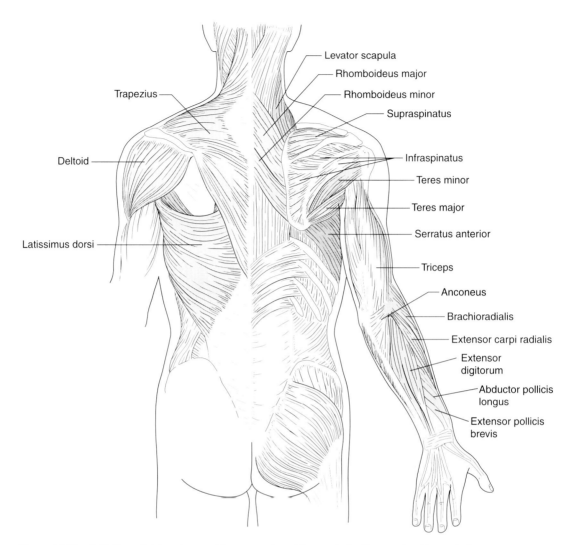

Figure 13.28 A-C: Superficial and second layer muscles of the posterior thorax, shoulder and elbow.

spinatus and latissim*us dorsi, should be examined as well. Other muscles attaching deep to the rhomboids, including iliocostalis thoracis (erector spinae), serratus posterior superior, multifidi and intercostals, may be the source of immediate as well as referred pain. Since each of the rhomboid's functions is also performed by stronger muscles, testing for their specific weakness is difficult. A 'winged scapula' may be an indicator of weakness in either rhomboids and/or serratus anterior, as their shared function is to flatten the scapula to the torso while they antagonize each other in adduction (retraction) and abduction (protraction), respectively.

Deep to the fibers of rhomboid minor lies a hidden trigger point in serratus posterior (see pp. 445–446). The scapula must be translated laterally to reach it, a position more easily achieved when the patient is sidelying.

Assessment for weakness of rhomboids

• The seated patient flexes the elbow to 90° while the

practitioner cups this with one hand and the shoulder with the other.

• The patient is asked to maintain the arm at the side as the practitioner attempts to abduct it using firm, increasing force. If the scapula moves away from the spine as the arm is forced into abduction, weakness of the rhomboids on that side can be assumed.

• In other words, if the arm abducts easily but the scapula remains relatively in place, the weakness demonstrated does not involve the rhomboids.

Assessment for shortness of rhomboids

• Direct palpation is the only way in which shortness and fibrotic changes can be evaluated (as in the NMT procedures described below).

• A useful alternative strategy for increasing localization of the rhomboids from the trapezius fibers is to have the prone patient place the dorsum of her hand onto her lower back.

- The practitioner places a flat hand against the patient's palm and requests the patient to push against his contact hand. This will cause rhomboids (and not trapezius) to stand out for easier palpation.
- In this way localized fibrotic, contracted tissues can be identified and palpated for trigger point activity.

 ## NMT for rhomboids

The patient is prone. The practitioner is standing at the level of the rhomboids and can move as needed to support gliding in all directions.

The broad, flat design of the rhomboids and the fibers of trapezius makes them difficult to lift. Flat palpation and gliding strips, which press against underlying muscles and rib cage, are best used here. The mid-thoracic area is lightly lubricated and the thumbs are used to glide in all directions between the vertebral border of each scapula and the spinous processes. Superficial glides may soften the overlying fibers of the trapezius and allow deeper penetration to the rhomboids. Still deeper pressure (through the trapezius and rhomboids) will influence the serratus posterior superior and erector spinae attachments. The spinous processes on tender or inflamed tissues are avoided, especially when deeper pressure is used.

The following steps may be performed more easily by the practitioner reaching across the body from the opposite side of the table. They may also be performed on the side on which the practitioner is standing or, if necessary, with the patient in a sitting position.

The patient's hand is placed behind the small of the back, if possible without pain in the shoulder, which will elevate the vertebral border of the scapula off the torso and allow palpation on the scapula's medial edge, medial aspect of its anterior surface and portions of the rib cage deep to its medial border. When the scapula's medial edge will not elevate, treatment of serratus anterior and scapular mobilization techniques may allow it to do so. Additionally, treatment of the infraspinatus and teres minor may be necessary to allow the hand to reach behind the back as these lateral rotators of the humerus, when taut, prevent the humerus from medial rotation, a movement necessary in order to reach behind the back.

- Lightly lubricated gliding strokes are applied directly to the vertebral border of the scapula where the rhomboids attach.
- Additionally, the pads of the thumbs or finger tips (with nails cut *very* short) may be placed under the anterior surface of the vertebral (medial) border of scapula with the pressure applied toward the scapula (Fig. 13.29A).
- Friction or gliding strokes may be used to examine the attachments of the serratus anterior and possibly a

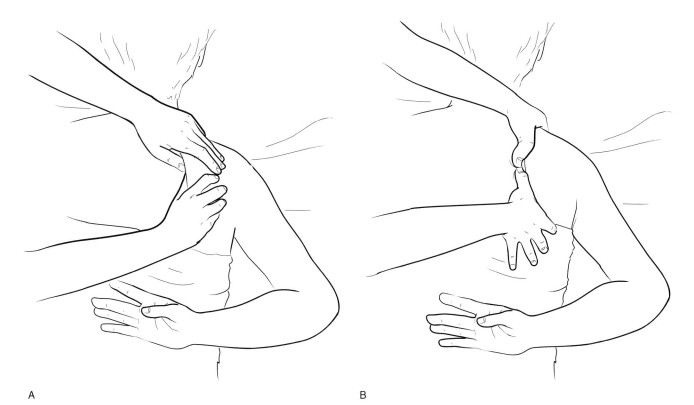

A   B

Figure 13.29   A&B: Applications to the anterior aspect of the medial scapula and the posterior thorax deep to the scapula.

small portion of subscapularis where they attach along the entire anterior vertebral border.

• With the medial edge of the scapula still elevated, the thumbs are placed deep to the vertebral border and pressure is applied down onto the rib cage to address the rib attachments of the serratus posterior superior (Fig. 13.29B), and its important 'hidden' trigger point.

• Static pressure release may be applied to trigger points and transverse friction may be applied to ischemic bands and mildly tender areas in the serratus posterior superior as well as other mid-thoracic muscles.

• The tissue deep to the medial edge of the scapula is more easily and effectively accessed with the patient placed in a sidelying position.

• The uppermost arm is draped across the patient's chest and the scapula allowed to translate laterally on the torso.

• As much as 2–3 inches of additional access may be achieved and the previous steps may be easily performed.

• This position is especially convenient to use when the patient is unable to reach behind the back.

 MET for rhomboids

• The patient is supine; the practitioner stands next to the rhomboids being assessed and faces the table.

• The patient flexes her elbow and places her arm into horizontal adduction (across chest) as far as is comfortable and assists this position with her opposite hand holding her own elbow.

• It is important to ensure that the patient's torso does not roll as the arm is brought into adduction.

• The practitioner places his caudad hand onto the dorsal surface of the patient's distal upper arm.

• The practitioner's cephalad hand is slid under the patient's scapula so that his finger pads can gain a contact on its medial border.

• The patient is asked to draw the scapula lightly but firmly toward the spine, pressing against the practitioner's finger pads, without any effort coming from the patient's arm.

• After 7–10 seconds the patient is asked to release the effort.

• The patient then adducts the arm further, assisted by the practitioner applying adduction pressure to the flexed arm, while also drawing the scapula away from the spine with the fingers, in order to stretch rhomboids.

Deltoid (Fig. 13.30)

Attachments: From the lateral third of the clavicle, acromion and lateral third of the spine of the scapula to the deltoid prominence (tuberosity) of the humerus
Innervation: Axillary nerve (C5–6)
Muscle type: Phasic (type 2), weakens when stressed

Function: *Anterior (clavicular) fibers*: flexion of humerus, horizontal adduction of the flexed humerus, stabilization of the humeral head during abduction, medial rotation of humerus (questionable) and its most peripheral anterior fibers may adduct the arm
Lateral (acromial) fibers: abduction of humerus, flexion (later phases)
Posterior (spinal) fibers: extension of humerus, stabilization of the humeral head during abduction, lateral movements when the humerus is abducted to 90° (horizontal abduction), prevents downward dislocation when arm is weighted, lateral rotation (unconfirmed) and its most peripheral posterior fibers may adduct the arm
Synergists: *Abduction of humerus*: supraspinatus, upper trapezius, rhomboids
Flexion of humerus: supraspinatus, pectoralis major, biceps brachii, coracobrachialis
Horizontal adduction of humerus: coracobrachialis, clavicular fibers of pectoralis major
Extension of humerus: long head of triceps, latissimus dorsi, teres major
Antagonists: *To translation upward during abduction (by deltoid)*: subscapularis, infraspinatus, teres minor. Anterior and posterior fibers of deltoid are antagonistic to each other

Indications for treatment

• Shoulder pain
• Difficulty or pain with most movements of the arm
• Pain after an impact trauma to the shoulder region

Special notes

The anterior and posterior portions of the deltoid have a fusiform arrangement which sacrifices strength while providing speed. However, the acromial fibers are a multipennate design which provides tremendous strength but not the speed of the other sections. While trigger points in the anterior and posterior fibers occur primarily in the middle of those fibers, trigger points in the multipennate portion appear to be sprinkled throughout the lateral upper arm due to their fiber arrangement.

Numerous muscles and attachments of muscles underlie the deltoid. A portion of infraspinatus may be reached through the posterior (spinal) fibers, while pectoralis major, the tubular tendon of biceps short head and the broad tendon of subscapularis may be addressed through the overlying anterior (clavicular) fibers. The lateral (acromial) fibers overlay the synovial sheath of biceps long head and the subdeltoid and subacromial bursae.

Inflammation in these underlying tissues may not be noticeable on the exterior surface of the thick deltoid until the area has been overworked. The underlying tendons

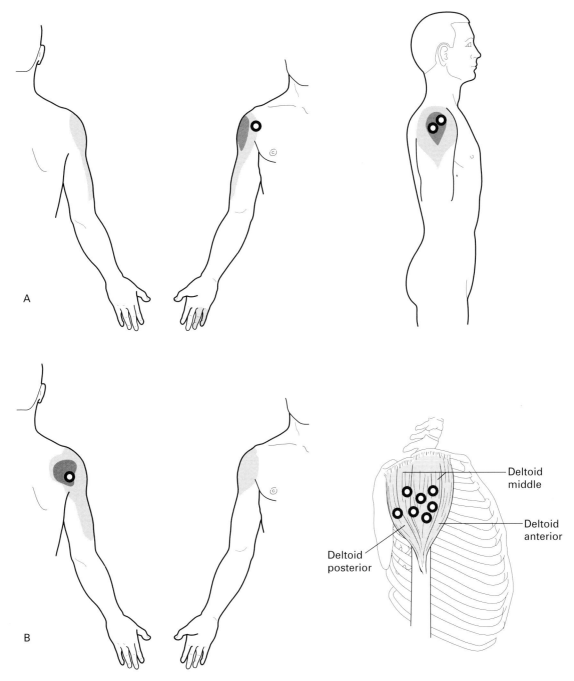

Figure 13.30 A: Deltoid referral patterns encompass most of the upper arm; its lateral fibers are multipennate with an extensive endplate zone. B: The composite pattern of target zones of synergistic lateral rotators.

should be palpated prior to the application of friction or deep gliding strokes to evaluate for appropriate pressure. When moderate or extreme tenderness is found in the underlying tissues, ice and other antiinflammatory treatments should be applied before NMT techniques are used.

NMT for deltoid

• The patient is prone with the arm hanging off the table or the hand is placed next to the face to passively shorten the deltoid fibers so they may be lifted and grasped.

• Each of the three heads of the deltoid may be individually compressed and manipulated in small increments until the full length of the fibers has been treated (Fig. 13.31).

• Broad compression of the tissues will reduce general ischemia of the fibers, while rolling the fibers between

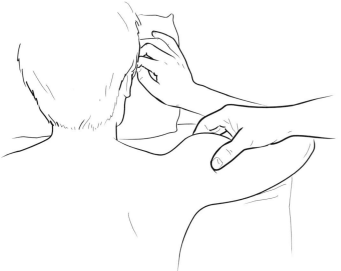

Figure 13.31 Each head of the deltoid can be compressed as shown here on middle fibers.

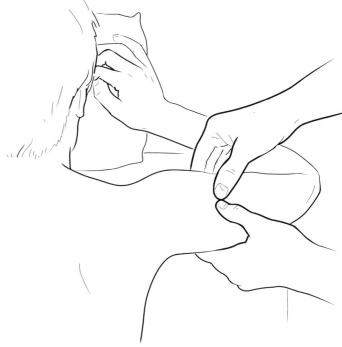

Figure 13.32 Palpation of the deltoid tuberosity where the three heads of the deltoid merge into a common attachment.

the thumb and fingers more precisely will reveal taut bands and nodules characteristic of trigger points often found there.

• Compression techniques or flat palpation may be applied to trigger points in the deltoid fibers for 10–12 seconds while feeling for release of the taut band.

• The position of the arm can be altered to place more or less stretch on taut bands as they are being assessed and released.

• Friction techniques or gliding strokes with the thumbs may be applied along the inferior surface of the spine of the scapula, acromion and clavicle to reveal attachment trigger points.

• The deltoid tuberosity should be examined for tenderness or evidence of inflammation (Fig. 13.32).

• Attachment trigger points may need to be addressed as inflamed tissue which can be caused by tension placed on attachment sites; applications of ice may reduce pain and tenderness.

• With the deltoid lubricated, gliding strokes may be applied with the thumbs in proximal strokes from the deltoid tuberosity to the proximal attachments to further loosen the fibers of the deltoid and soothe the tissues.

• Tenderness found in attachments deep to the deltoid should be noted as the associated muscles should also be examined.

Supraspinatus

Attachments: Medial two-thirds of the supraspinous fossa of the scapula to the superior facet of the greater tubercle of the humerus

Innervation: Suprascapular nerve (C5–6)

Muscle type: Postural (type 1), shortens when stressed

Function: Abducts the humerus (with deltoid), seats the humeral head in the glenoid fossa, stabilizes the head of the humerus during arm movements

Synergists: *Abduction*: middle deltoid, upper trapezius, lower trapezius, serratus anterior (while rhomboids stabilize the scapula during abduction) (Simons et al 1998)

Humeral head stabilization: infraspinatus, teres minor, subscapularis (while serratus anterior stabilizes scapula)

Antagonists: *To abduction*: pectoralis major (lower fibers), latissimus dorsi, teres major

Indications for treatment

• Pain during abduction of the arm or dull ache during rest

• Difficulty or pain in reaching overhead or to the head

• Rotator cuff involvement

Special notes

Supraspinatus, infraspinatus, teres minor and subscapularis are the four rotator cuff muscles, often called the SITS tendons, so named from the combined first letters of their names. These four tendons directly overlie the joint and their fibers often blend with the joint capsule.

Since the articulation surface of the glenohumeral joint is shallow, excessive translation in all directions makes it necessary for these muscles to constantly check the position of the humeral head and stabilize the joint during all arm movements.

Supraspinatus assists deltoid in abduction while infraspinatus, teres minor and subscapularis counteract the tendency of the humeral head to upslip when deltoid contracts by pulling the humerus down the glenoid fossa and seating it into the fossa. Supraspinatus is involved in all phases of abduction while infraspinatus and teres minor rotate the humerus laterally and subscapularis rotates it medially. All four stabilize the humeral head against the glenoid fossa and also support the weighted arm so that the head of the humerus is not pulled downward by the weight. This positioning role is true for supraspinatus even when the arm is not loaded, as the weight of the arm itself could cause downward pull on the humeral head.

In the coronal plane, pure humeral abduction ends at 90° when the greater tubercle impacts the inferior aspect of the acromioclavicular joint. Beyond this point, the humerus must be externally (laterally) rotated so that the greater tubercle passes posteriorly to the acromion (Cailliet 1996, Hoppenfeld 1976) (Fig. 13.33). When sufficient lateral rotation does not occur, especially when the lateral rotators are not functioning properly due to ischemia or trigger points or when the overhanging structures compromise the space in some other manner, such as when luggage is carried over the shoulder, the tendon of supraspinatus may be compressed or repeatedly abused against the overhanging acromion. This process of abuse, particularly when combined with repetitive overuse, overloading or some other strain, may lead to supraspinatus tendinitis and eventually to calcification of the tendon. This process is well explained in *Shoulder pain* (Cailliet 1991). Simons et al (1998) report that, with inactivation of trigger points in supraspinatus, early calcific deposits at the insertion site may resolve.

Supraspinatus is the most frequently ruptured rotator cuff muscle (*Gray's anatomy* 1995), although portions of the conjoined tendon (infraspinatus and teres minor) or the subscapularis may be damaged as well. If partial or complete tear is suspected, range of motion tests or stretching procedures should be delayed until the extent of tearing is known (Simons et al 1998), as these steps could lead to further tearing of the SITS tendons.

The supraspinatus fibers lie deep to the trapezius and its tendon attachment lies deep to the deltoid. Therefore, supraspinatus is not directly palpable except in some cases where displacement of the upper trapezius allows a small amount of access. However, tenderness and trigger points within this muscle may be addressed through the overlying trapezius if the fibers are not too tender to be pressed.

Assessment for supraspinatus dysfunction

- The practitioner stands behind the seated patient, with one hand stabilizing the shoulder on the side to be assessed while the other hand reaches in front of the patient to support the flexed elbow and forearm.
- The patient's upper arm is adducted to its easy barrier and the patient then attempts to abduct the arm.
- If pain is noted in the posterior shoulder region, supraspinatus dysfunction is suspected and because it is a postural muscle, shortness is implied.

Assessment for supraspinatus weakness

- The patient sits or stands with arm abducted 15°, elbow extended.
- The practitioner stabilizes the shoulder with one hand while the other hand offers a resistance contact at the distal humerus which, if forceful, would adduct the arm further.
- The patient attempts to resist this and the degree of effort required to overcome the patient's resistance is graded as weak or strong (see grading scale, p. 306).

 ## NMT treatment of supraspinatus

The patient is prone with the arm resting on the table or sidelying with the arm resting on the lateral surface of the body and the practitioner stands cephalad to the shoulder.

- The top of the shoulder is lubricated from the acromioclavicular joint to the upper angle of the scapula.
- Gliding strokes may be applied in both lateral and medial directions 7–8 times in the region of the supraspinous fossa to reveal thickened or tender areas.
- Deeper pressure through the overlying trapezius, if appropriate, will treat the supraspinatus muscle belly.
- Often the trapezius will need extensive treatment to reduce upper and middle trapezius tension and associated trigger points before deeper pressure can be used.

The trapezius, when softened and its fiber ends approximated, may sometimes be displaced posteriorly to allow access to a small portion of supraspinatus which lies deep to it. This displacement procedure will usually only allow a small portion of supraspinatus to be compressed directly. However, this procedure is worthwhile in those cases where displacement is possible.

If trigger points are found in supraspinatus, gliding massage techniques may be applied from the center of its fibers outwardly toward the ends to elongate sarcomeres and reduce attachment tension from taut fibers. Trigger point pressure release may also be applied through the trapezius. Since this muscle underlies the thick trapezius

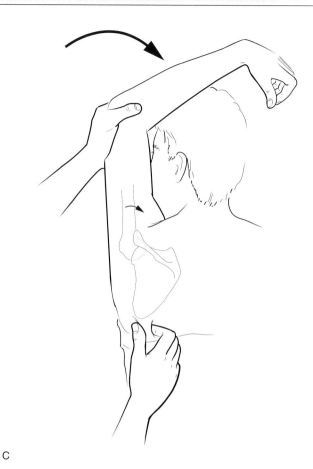

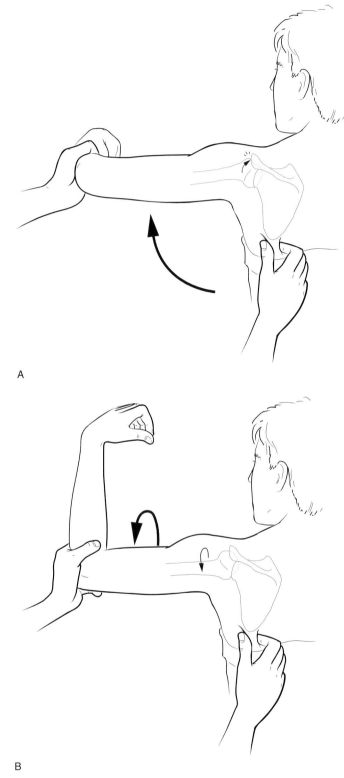

A

C

B

Figure 13.33 Pure glenohumeral abduction is increased to full range of 180° only with lateral rotation of the humerus to avoid impaction of the greater tubercle against the acromion.

which effectively obscures palpation, it may be a candidate for trigger point injections when manual methods of release fail to be effective.

A finger tip or the tip of the beveled pressure bar may be pressed (caudally) straight into the tissues directly medial to the acromioclavicular joint to treat the tendon of supraspinatus through the trapezius fibers. Static pressure is held for 10–12 seconds. This procedure is avoided if a supraspinatus tear, subacromial (or subdeltoid) bursitis or bicipital or supraspinatus tendinitis is suspected.

The tendon attachment of supraspinatus is addressed with the SITS tendons (in a sidelying position) after the infraspinatus and teres minor muscles have been treated. See description in the teres minor section of this text on pp. 346 and 348.

MET treatment of supraspinatus
(see p. 315, Fig. 13.14)

• The practitioner stands behind the seated patient, with one hand stabilizing the shoulder on the side to be treated while the other hand reaches in front of the patient to support the flexed elbow and forearm.

• The patient's upper arm is adducted to its easy barrier and the patient then attempts to abduct the arm using 20% of strength against practitioner resistance.

• After a 10-second isometric contraction the arm is taken gently toward its new resistance barrier into greater adduction with the patient's assistance.

• Repeat several times, holding each painless stretch for not less than 20 seconds.

 ## MFR for supraspinatus (Fig. 13.34)

• The practitioner palpates the dysfunctional muscle, seeking an area of local restriction, fibrosis, 'thickening'.

• This may lie above the spine of the scapula or on the greater tuberosity of the humerus.

• Having located an area of altered tissue texture which is sensitive and after the patient has abducted the arm to about 30°, a firm thumb contact should be made slightly lateral to the dysfunctional area.

• The patient is then asked to slowly but deliberately adduct the arm as far as possible, while the thumb contact (reinforced by the other hand, if necessary) is maintained.

• This process takes the myofascial tissue from a shortened position to its longest and modifies the tissue's status under the thumb.

• This process should be repeated between three and five times.

Infraspinatus

Attachments: Medial two-thirds of the infraspinous fossa of the scapula to the middle facet of the greater tubercle of the humerus

Innervation: Suprascapular nerve (C5–6)

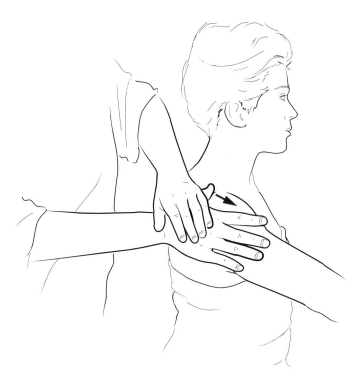

Figure 13.34 Myofascial release of supraspinatus.

Muscle type: Postural (type 1), shortens when stressed

Function: Laterally rotates the humerus, stabilizes the head of the humerus in the glenoid cavity during arm movements

Synergists: *Lateral rotation*: teres minor, posterior deltoid *Humeral head stabilization*: supraspinatus, teres minor, subscapularis (while serratus anterior stabilizes the scapula)

Antagonists: *To lateral rotation*: pectoralis major, latissimus dorsi, anterior deltoid

Indications for treatment

• Pain sleeping on side
• Difficulty hooking bra behind back or putting hand into back pocket
• Scapulohumeral rhythm test positive (see p. 303)
• Identification of shortness (see tests below).

Special notes

Infraspinatus and teres minor have almost identical actions and are so closely related that their tendons are often fused together (Cailliet 1991, *Gray's anatomy* 1995, Platzer 1992). Overlying fascia envelopes the two muscles together as if they are one. However, their innervations are different.

When infraspinatus trigger points are active, the patient finds it difficult to reach behind her back to tuck in a shirt or fasten a bra, comb her hair or scratch her back. Trigger points in infraspinatus often produce deep shoulder pain, suboccipital pain and referral patterns just medial to the vertebral border of the scapula, an area of common complaint. Trigger points in infraspinatus respond favorably to massage applications and manual release methods (Simons et al 1998).

The humeral attachment of infraspinatus is addressed with the SITS tendons (in a sidelying position) after the remaining rotator cuff muscles have been treated. However, as with supraspinatus, if partial or complete tear is suspected, range of motion tests and stretching procedures should be delayed until extent of injury is known.

Assessment for infraspinatus shortness/ dysfunction

• The patient is asked to touch the upper border of the opposite scapula by reaching with the forearm behind the head.

• If this effort is painful, infraspinatus shortness should be suspected.

• Visual evidence of shortness is obtained by having the patient supine, her humerus at right angles to the trunk with the elbow flexed so that the pronated forearm is parallel with the trunk pointing caudally.

• This brings the arm into internal rotation and places infraspinatus at stretch (see p. 314, Fig. 13.12).

• The practitioner ensures that the shoulder remains in contact with the table during this assessment by applying light compression onto the anterior shoulder.

• If infraspinatus is short the lower arm will not be capable of resting parallel with the floor, obliging it to point somewhat toward the ceiling.

Assessment for infraspinatus weakness

• The patient is prone with head rotated toward the side being assessed.

• The patient's arm is abducted to 90° at the shoulder and flexed 90° at the elbow.

• The forearm hangs over the edge of the table and the elbow is supported on a pad, folded towel or cushion to maintain it in the same plane as the shoulder and to prevent undue pressure from the edge of the table.

• The practitioner provides slight stabilizing compression just proximal to the elbow to prevent any extension at the shoulder and offers resistance to the lower forearm as the patient attempts to bring the forearm from its starting position pointing to the floor to one where it is parallel with the floor, palm downwards.

• The relative strength of the efforts of each arm is compared.

• Note that in this, as in other tests for weakness, there may be a better degree of cooperation if the practitioner applies the force and the patient is asked to resist as much as possible. Force should always be built slowly and not suddenly.

NMT for infraspinatus

The patient is prone with the arm resting on the table or sidelying with the arm resting on the lateral surface of the body. The infraspinous fossa of the scapula is lightly lubricated and gliding strokes are applied (both medially and laterally) under the inferior edge of the spine of the scapula where infraspinatus attaches. The gliding strokes are repeated 7–8 times in each direction to examine the attachment site. The thumbs are moved caudally and the gliding process repeated, in rows, until the entire surface of the scapula has been covered. Gliding strokes are also applied in a diagonal and vertical pattern as there are many directions of fibers in this muscle and varying the direction of the glides will reveal taut fibers more clearly.

Central trigger points form in the center of the various fibers' bellies. An especially tender trigger point with a strong referral pattern may be found in the center of the most lateral fibers. The practitioner's thumbs are placed against the lateral edge of the muscle and pressure gradually applied into these often very tender fibers (Fig. 13.35). Tender areas or central trigger points are

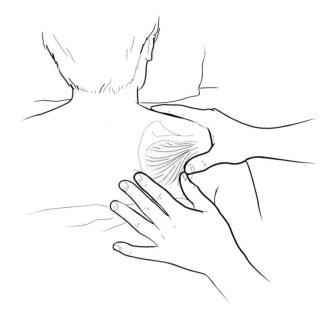

Figure 13.35   Palpation of the most lateral fibers of infraspinatus.

treated with static pressure for 8–12 seconds as thumb pressure meets and matches the tension found within them.

Attachment trigger points often form under the inferior aspect of the spine of the scapula. The beveled pressure bar tip is placed parallel to the spine of the scapula and angled at 45° underneath the inferior aspect of the scapula's spine which often has an overhanging ledge. Gentle friction is used to assess the attaching fibers for taut bands and tender spots. Static pressure is used to commence treatment of any trigger points found there. If extreme tenderness is found, ice massage may be applied to reduce inflammation which often exists at attachment sites.

MET treatment of short infraspinatus (and teres minor) (Fig. 13.36)

• The patient is supine, upper arm at right angles to the trunk, elbow flexed so that the lower arm is parallel with the trunk, pointing caudad with the palm downwards.

• This brings the arm into internal rotation and places infraspinatus at stretch.

• The practitioner applies light compression to the anterior shoulder to ensure that it does not rise from the table as rotation is introduced since this would give a false appearance of stretch in the muscle.

• The practitioner applies mild resistance just proximal to the dorsum of the wrist for 10–12 seconds as the patient attempts to lift it toward the ceiling so introducing external rotation of the humerus at the shoulder.

• On relaxation, the forearm is taken toward the floor (combined patient and practitioner action), which

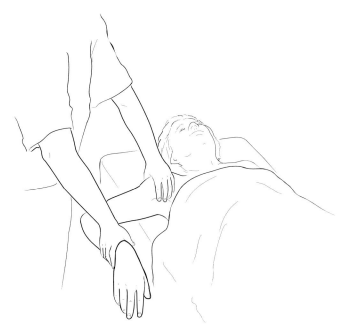

Figure 13.36   MET treatment of infraspinatus.

increases internal rotation at the shoulder and stretches infraspinatus (mainly at its shoulder attachment).

MFR treatment of short infraspinatus (Fig. 13.37)

• The patient is prone and the practitioner palpates and locates areas within the muscle with pronounced tension, contraction or fibrosis.

• The patient lies with the arm on the affected side flexed at the elbow and close to the side of the body in order to bring the muscle into a shortened state.

• The practitioner applies a firm, flat compression contact (thenar eminence or thumb) to an area of the muscle just superior and lateral to the dysfunctional area.

• The patient initiates a slow abduction of the shoulder, extension of the elbow followed by flexion of the shoulder to its fullest limit, which will bring the distressed soft tissues under the practitioner's pressure contact.

• As the movement is performed, a degree of internal rotation should be included so that at the end of the range, the patient's upper arm should be alongside the head, thumb downwards.

• The arm is then slowly returned to the starting position and the process is repeated (3–5 times).

PRT treatment of infraspinatus (most suitable for acute problems)

• The patient is supine and the practitioner, while standing or seated at waist level and facing the patient's head, uses the tableside hand to locate an area of marked tenderness in infraspinatus.

• The patient is asked to grade the applied pressure to this dysfunctional region of the muscle as a '10'.

• The practitioner's other hand holds the forearm and slowly positions the patient's flexed arm in such a way as to reduce the score to a '3' or less.

• This will almost always involve the practitioner passively taking the muscle into an increased degree of shortness, involving external rotation together with either

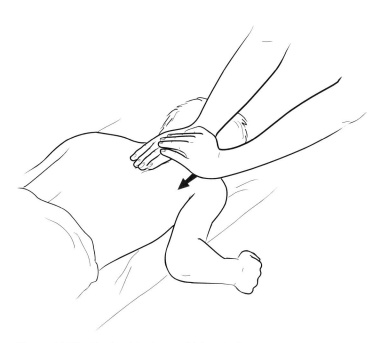

Figure 13.37   Myofascial release of infraspinatus.

abduction or adduction (whichever reduces the 'score' more efficiently), as well as some degree of shoulder extension.

• When the score is reduced to '3' or less, the position of ease is held for 90 seconds before a slow return to neutral.

Triceps and anconeus (Fig. 13.38)

Attachments: *Long head*: infraglenoid tubercle of scapula
Medial head: posterior surface of humerus (medial and distal to the radial nerve) and intermuscular septum
Lateral head: posterior surface of humerus (lateral and proximal to the radial nerve) and lateral intermuscular septum
All three heads: join together to form a common tendon which attaches to the olecranon process of the ulna
Anconeus: dorsal surface of the lateral epicondyle to the lateral aspect of the olecranon and proximal one-fourth of the dorsal surface of the ulna
Innervation: Radial nerve (C6–8)
Muscle type: Phasic (type 2), inhibited or weakens when stressed (Janda 1983, 1988). Triceps may nevertheless require stretching in order to help normalize trigger points located in its fibers
Function: *All three heads*: extension of the elbow
Long head: humeral adduction and extension, counteracts downward pull on head of humerus
Anconeus: extension of the elbow, may stabilize ulna during pronation of the forearm
Synergists: *Extension of the elbow*: anconeus
Humeral adduction and extension: teres major and minor, latissimus dorsi, pectoralis major (adduction)
Antagonists: *To extension of the elbow*: biceps, brachialis
To humeral adduction and extension: pectoralis major, biceps brachii, anterior deltoid
Counteracts downward pull on head of humerus by pectoralis major and latissimus dorsi

Indications for treatment

• Vague shoulder and arm pain
• Epicondylitis
• Olecranon bursitis
• 'Tennis elbow' or 'golfer's elbow'

Special notes

The triceps fills the extensor compartment of the upper arm with the long and lateral head superficial to the medial head in the upper two-thirds of the arm. The medial head is directly available on both the medial and lateral aspects of the posterior arm just above the elbow. The radial nerve lies deep to the lateral head of triceps and is vulnerable to entrapment by taut fibers or

scar tissue. Care should be taken during deep or frictional massage to avoid irritation of the radial nerve.

The anconeus, a small, triangular muscle positioned on the posterolateral elbow, is easily addressed when treating the olecranon attachment of triceps. It is associated with the triceps through their common action of extension of the elbow and may serve to stabilize the elbow joint during pronation of the forearm by securing the ulna. The articularis cubiti (subanconeus muscle) is a small slip of the medial head of the triceps and, when present, may insert into the capsule of the elbow joint.

Assessment for triceps weakness

• Patient is prone with the head resting in a face cradle.
• The patient's arm is flexed at the shoulder, the elbow is flexed and the hand is resting as close to the same side scapula as possible, arm close to the side of the head.
• The practitioner cradles the patient's elbow just proximal to the joint and asks the patient to push the elbow toward the floor.
• The two sides are compared for relative strength of the triceps.
• Note that in this test (as in other tests for weakness), there may be a better degree of cooperation if the practitioner applies the force and the patient is asked to resist as much as possible. Force should always be built slowly and not suddenly.

 NMT for triceps (see also p. 384)

The patient is prone with the arm hanging off the side of the table so that the upper arm is supported by the table surface. The posterior aspect of the upper arm is lubricated and proximal gliding strokes are applied in thumb-width rows to cover the entire surface of the posterior upper arm to assess the (superficially positioned) lateral and long heads. The radial nerve lies deep to the lateral head and is vulnerable to compression with deep pressure. If an electric-like sensation is felt down the arm, the hands are repositioned or lighter pressure used to avoid compression of the nerve.

The medial head of triceps lies deep to the other two heads except for just above the elbow, where it lies superficial on both the medial and lateral sides. The practitioner increases the pressure, if appropriate, and repeats the proximal gliding process to address the medial head through the lateral and long heads. A double-thumb gliding technique may also be used by simultaneously gliding up both medial and lateral aspects of the medial head (deep to the other two heads) with pressure from each thumb directed toward the midline of the posterior humerus.

The attachment of the long head of triceps is isolated on the infraglenoid tuberosity of the scapula and treated

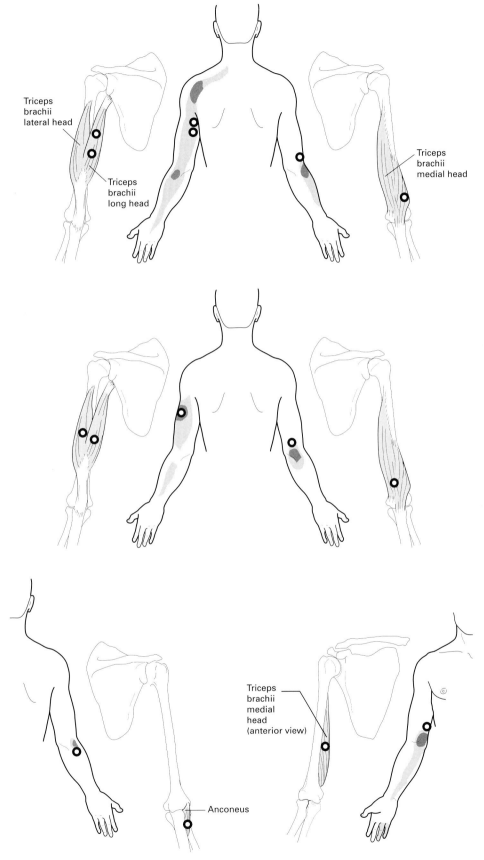

Triceps
brachii
lateral head

Triceps
brachii
long head

Triceps
brachii
medial head

Triceps
brachii
medial
head
(anterior view)

Anconeus

Figure 13.38 Referral patterns for triceps trigger points.

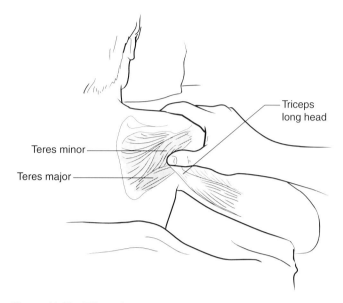

Figure 13.39 Triceps long head attachment on infraglenoid tubercle.

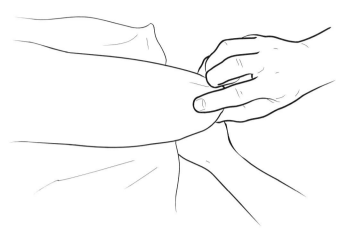

Figure 13.40 Finger friction of triceps tendon at the olecranon process. Avoid pressing on the ulnar nerve.

with static pressure or mild friction (Fig. 13.39). The practitioner applies resistance to elbow extension while simultaneously palpating the tendon attachment to assure its location. It may be advantageous to muscle test and isolate the two teres muscles as well, since the triceps passes between the teres major and minor before attaching onto the scapula. The olecranon attachment of the triceps is treated with finger friction or friction which is carefully applied with the beveled pressure bar (Fig. 13.40). Pressure should be applied directly on the tendon to avoid compressing neural structures on each side of this tendon.

MET treatment of triceps (to enhance shoulder flexion with elbow flexed) (Fig. 13.41)

- Patient is prone with the head resting in a face cradle.
- The patient's arm is flexed at the shoulder, the elbow

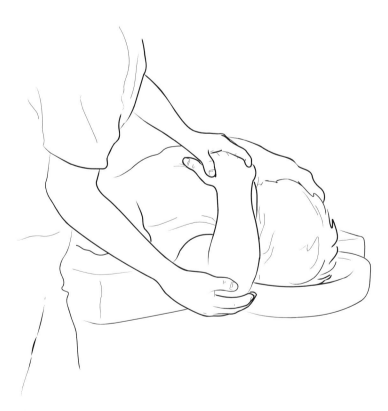

Figure 13.41 MET treatment position of triceps.

is flexed and the hand is resting as close to the ipsilateral scapula as possible with the arm placed close to the side of the head.

• The practitioner cradles the patient's elbow just proximal to the joint and asks the patient to push the elbow toward the floor for 10 seconds, using no more than 20% of strength as resistance to movement is offered.

• Following this isometric contraction, the patient is asked to stretch the hand further down the scapula, assisted by the practitioner. The stretch should be held for not less than 20 seconds.

 ## NMT for anconeus (see also p. 384)

The anconeus lies just lateral and distal to the olecranon process. It is easily isolated by placing an index finger on the olecranon process and the second finger on the lateral epicondyle with the practitioner's hand flat against the patient's forearm. The anconeus lies between the two fingers. Short gliding strokes are applied between the ulna and radius (in the space between what the fingers have outlined) to assess this small muscle which is often involved in elbow pain.

Note: The following muscles are addressed with the person placed in a sidelying position (see Repose in cervical region, p. 229). The patient's uppermost arm is often placed in a supported position so that the practitioner has both hands free. Alterations can be made in this position, including supporting the arm on the practitioner's shoulder, in many cases.

Teres minor

Attachments: Upper two-thirds of the dorsal surface of the most lateral aspect of the scapula to the lowest (third) facet on the greater tubercle of the humerus

Innervation: Axillary nerve (C5–6)

Muscle type: Not established

Function: Laterally rotates the humerus, stabilizes the head of the humerus in the glenoid cavity during arm movements

Synergists: *Lateral rotation*: infraspinatus, posterior deltoid
Humeral head stabilization: supraspinatus, infraspinatus, subscapularis (while serratus anterior stabilizes the scapula)

Antagonists: *To lateral rotation*: teres major, pectoralis major, latissimus dorsi, anterior deltoid, subscapularis, biceps brachii (Platzer 1992)

Indications for treatment

• Rotator cuff dysfunction
• Teres minor should always be considered as a possible contributor to upper arm or elbow pain

Special notes

CAUTION: **If rotator cuff tear is suspected, range of motion testing, stretches and any therapeutic intervention which could risk further damage to the tissues are not recommended until a full diagnosis discloses the extent and exact location of the tear. Only the most gentle assessment and technique steps may be used until diagnosis is clear.**

Teres minor is the third posterior rotator cuff muscle. Along with infraspinatus and posterior deltoid, it antagonizes medial rotation as well as providing stability of the humeral head during most arm movements. Teres minor and infraspinatus also act together to counteract the upward pull of the deltoid during abduction of the humerus to prevent upslip of the humeral head. With their downward tension, the humeral head may then rotate into abduction rather than slide superiorly, which might result in capsular damage but will most certainly result in mechanical dysfunction.

The long head of triceps passes between teres minor and teres major and is palpated by placing a thumb between these two muscles to contact the infraglenoid tubercle of the scapula. Muscle testing of teres minor and teres major with resisted lateral and medial rotation of the humerus, respectively, helps to distinctly identify these two muscles.

Assessment for teres minor weakness

• Patient is seated, elbow flexed to 90° with the arm touching the side of the body and the humerus internally rotated.

• The practitioner cups and stabilizes the elbow with one hand while the palm of the other hand holds just proximal to the wrist to maintain the humerus in internal rotation.

• The patient is asked to externally rotate the humerus ('Twist your upper arm against my resistance' or 'I am going to try to turn your arm inwards and you should resist, against my hand on your wrist, as strongly as you can') and the practitioner grades the relative strength of the action and compares one side with the other.

• Note that in this test (as in other tests for weakness), there may be a better degree of cooperation if the practitioner applies the force and the patient is asked to resist as much as possible. Force should always be built slowly and not suddenly.

 ## NMT for teres minor

The patient is placed in a sidelying position with the arm to be treated lying uppermost. The arm is placed in passive flexion at 90° and is supported there by the patient. This position is hereafter referred to as the supported arm position (see sidelying supported arm position, p. 229).

The practitioner stands, kneels or sits caudad to the extended arm. He uses both hands (or the caudad hand) to grasp the posterior aspect of the axilla with a pincer compression as close to the head of the humerus as possible. His fingers are placed on the posterior surface of the teres minor while the thumbs rest on the anterior (axillary) surface (Fig. 13.42).

The practitioner's grasp encompasses the teres major and latissimus dorsi fibers but does not compress them as the thumb and fingers are placed precisely on and capture the teres minor. Muscle testing with mildly resisted lateral rotation will produce contraction of teres minor to assure direct palpation (Fig. 13.43A). The muscle is relaxed before treating it.

Pressure is applied with precision and local twitch responses monitored from both sides of the muscle. As the tissue releases and softens, a light stretch may be applied until taut fibers are again distinctive. A firm nodule (or nest of them) within a taut band is often present near the center of the fibers. Pressure which matches the tension in the tissue and reproduces the patient's pain pattern confirms the presence of a trigger point, which often can be effectively released with trigger point pressure release.

Compression, friction or snapping palpation is used on the full length of teres minor and its scapular attachments unless a tear is suspected, which would warrant more caution. It attaches to the third facet of the greater tubercle of the humerus, which is often tender to palpation.

The patient's arm is draped forward to lie passively

across her chest. The practitioner assesses the scapular attachment of teres minor by sliding a thumb along the upper two-thirds of the lateral (axillary) border of the scapula (Fig. 13.44). If appropriate, static pressure or light friction is applied to any tender points or trigger points in the attachment site or, if inflammation is suspected, ice therapy is applied. The teres major attachment is located on the remaining lower one-third of this border and may be addressed in a similar manner.

To treat the SITS tendons, the arm remains draped across the patient's chest. When the humerus is so positioned, the humeral head is in flexion combined with extreme horizontal adduction and medial rotation. This position rotates the greater tubercle of the humerus posterior to the acromioclavicular joint and makes the facet attachment of supraspinatus available to palpation (through the deltoid). The attachment of supraspinatus faces directly toward the practitioner along with the second and third facet attachments of infraspinatus and teres minor, respectively (Fig. 13.45).

Unless contraindicated by extreme tenderness or suspicion of rotator cuff tear, the practitioner cautiously applies friction or static compression directly to the insertion of each of the SITS tendons. The tendon attachment of the fourth rotator cuff muscle, subscapularis, is treated later on the anterior surface of the joint capsule (see Fig. 13.79).

MET for teres minor is the same as for infraspinatus described above.

PRT for teres minor (most suitable for acute problems) (Fig. 13.46)

- The patient is supine and the practitioner (standing or sitting at waist level and facing the patient's head) uses the tableside hand to locate an area of marked tenderness in teres minor on the lateral border of the scapula close to the axilla.
- The patient is asked to grade the applied pressure to this dysfunctional region of the muscle as a '10'.
- The practitioner's other hand holds the forearm and slowly positions the patient's flexed arm in such a way as to reduce the score to a '3' or less.
- This will almost always involve the practitioner passively taking the muscle into an increased degree of shortness, involving a degree of shoulder flexion, abduction and external rotation.
- When the score is reduced to '3' or less, the position of ease is held for 90 seconds before a slow return to neutral.

Teres major (Fig. 13.47)

Attachments: Oval area on the dorsal surface of the

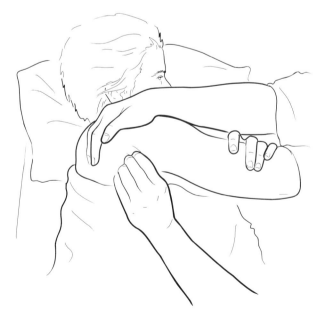

Figure 13.42 The thumb and fingers grasp around the teres major and latissimus fibers to precisely compress teres minor.

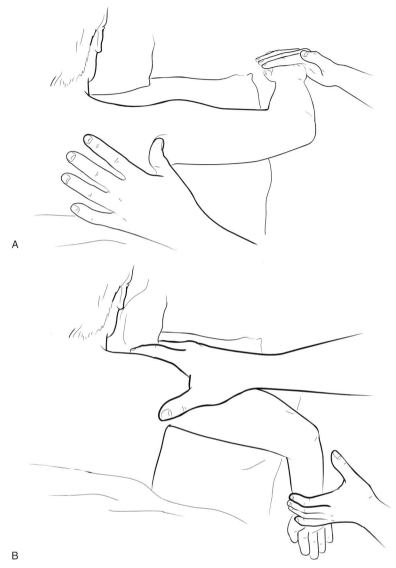

Figure 13.43 The palpating thumb feels fibers of teres minor (A) contract with resisted lateral rotation while teres major (B) contracts with medial rotation.

scapula (near the inferior angle) to the medial lip of the intertubercular sulcus of the humerus

Innervation: Lower subscapular nerve (C5–7)

Muscle type: Phasic (type 2), weakens when stressed

Function: Assists medial rotation and extension of the humerus against resistance, adducts the humerus, particularly across the back

Synergists: *Medial rotation*: latissimus dorsi, long head of triceps, pectoralis major, subscapularis

Extension of humerus: latissimus dorsi, posterior deltoid and long head of triceps

Antagonists: *To medial rotation*: teres minor, infraspinatus, posterior deltoid

To extension of humerus: pectoralis major, biceps brachii, anterior deltoid, coracobrachialis

Indications for treatment

- Pain upon motion
- Pain at full overhead stretch.

Special notes

Teres minor, teres major and latissimus dorsi together form the posterior axillary fold. Muscle testing with resisted medial rotation causes the fibers of teres major to contract and distinguishes it from teres minor but not latissimus dorsi, which 'cradle' teres major as they course medially around the humerus to attach anteriorly to it.

Teres major and latissimus dorsi fibers can be more easily distinguished by separation of their fibers rather than through muscle testing since they perform the same

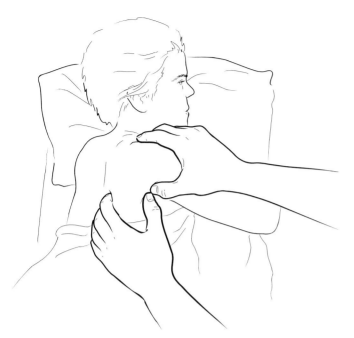

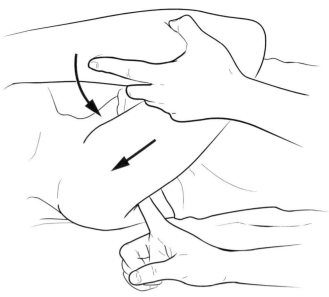

Figure 13.46 Strain-counterstrain (PRT) for teres minor.

Figure 13.44 Teres major and teres minor attachments of the lateral (axillary) border of the scapula are often 'surprisingly' tender.

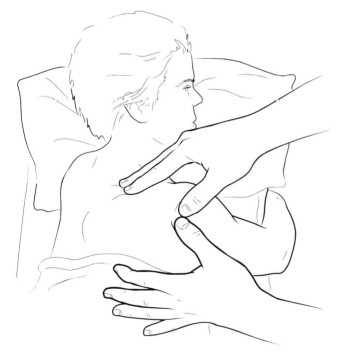

Figure 13.45 The SIT tendons are easily accessed posterior to the acromion when the patient is sidelying and the arm is draped across the chest.

action. Distinction is usually easily made since the fibers of latissimus dorsi continue past the scapula while the teres major fibers end there. However, occasionally teres major may be fused with latissimus dorsi (Platzer 1992), especially near the scapular portion (*Gray's anatomy* 1995),

or a slip of it may join the long head of triceps (*Gray's anatomy* 1995).

 ## NMT for teres major

The patient remains in a sidelying supported arm position (see p. 229). The practitioner stands caudad to the extended arm and uses one or both hands to grasp the posterior aspect of the axilla with a pincer palpation similar to that used for teres minor. The palpating fingers are positioned 1–2 inches toward the free border of the posterior axillary fold and directly contact teres major (Fig. 13.48). Muscle testing with resisted medial rotation will help distinguish teres major fibers from those of teres minor, which is relaxed (inhibited) during medial rotation. Latissimus dorsi will also activate during medial rotation along with teres major and should be distinguishable from it (see Fig. 13.43B).

The practitioner applies pincer compression, friction or snapping palpation onto the entire length of teres major. If appropriate, the teres fibers may be slightly stretched by moving the humerus into further flexion. The fibers of latissimus dorsi are usually distinguished from teres major since they continue past the scapula and into the lower back (see Fig. 13.47).

The patient's arm is draped forward to lie passively across her chest. The practitioner stands in front of the patient and assesses the scapular attachment of teres major by sliding a thumb along the lower third of the lateral (axillary) border of the scapula. The scapular attachment is often tender, therefore a lighter pressure is used before increased pressure is applied. Trigger points in the attachment sites require that the associated central trigger point is deactivated. If inflammation is

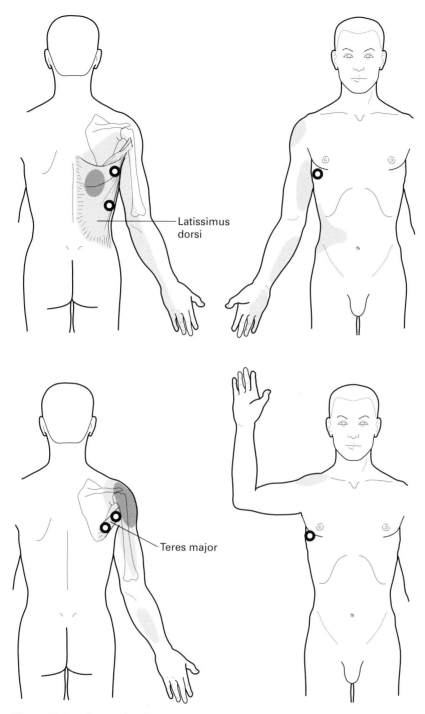

Figure 13.47 Composite trigger point target zones for medial rotators.

suspected, ice therapy is applied. The teres minor attachment is located on the remaining upper two-thirds of this border and may be addressed in a similar manner.

PRT for teres major (most suitable for acute problems) (Fig. 13.49)

• The patient is seated and the practitioner, while standing behind, locates an area of marked tenderness in teres major close to its attachment on the lower lateral surface of the scapula.

• The patient is instructed to grade the applied pressure to this dysfunctional region of the muscle as a '10'.

• The practitioner's other hand holds the forearm, bringing the arm backwards, internally rotating the humerus and slowly positioning the patient's extended arm in such a way as to reduce the 'score' markedly.

• The position is a virtual 'hammerlock' position.

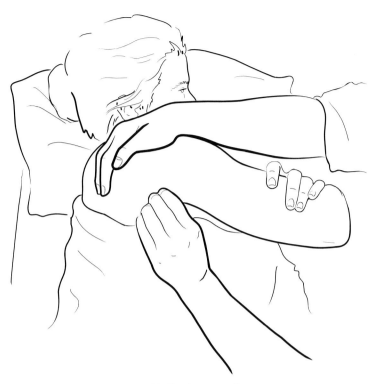

Figure 13.48 Compression of belly of teres major.

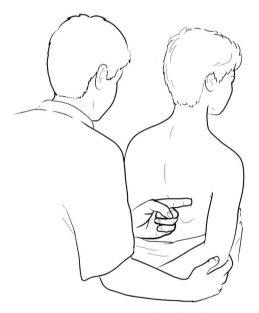

Figure 13.49 Strain-counterstrain (PRT) position for teres major.

• This will almost always involve the practitioner passively taking the muscle into an increased degree of shortness which involves shoulder extension, adduction and internal rotation.

• Long-axis compression toward the shoulder, through the humerus, may provide additional ease to the painful tender point.

• When the score is reduced to '3' or less, the position of ease is held for 90 seconds before a slow return to neutral.

Latissimus dorsi

Attachments: Spinous processes of T7–12, thoracolumbar fascia (anchoring it to all lumbar vertebrae and sacrum), posterior third of the iliac crest, 9th–12th ribs and (sometimes) inferior angle of scapula to the intertubercular groove of the humerus

Innervation: Thoracodorsal (long subscapular) nerve (C6–8)

Muscle type: Postural (type 1), shortens when stressed

Function: Medial rotation when arm is abducted, extension of the humerus, adducts the humerus, particularly across the back, humeral depression; influences neck, thoracic and pelvic postures and (perhaps) forced exhalation (Platzer 1992)

Synergists: *Medial rotation*: teres major, pectoralis major, subscapularis, biceps brachii

Extension of humerus: teres major and long head of triceps

Adduction of humerus: most anterior and posterior fibers of deltoid, triceps long head, teres major, pectoralis major

Depression of shoulder girdle: lower pectoralis major, lower trapezius

Antagonists: *To medial rotation*: teres minor, infraspinatus, posterior deltoid

To extension of humerus: pectoralis major, biceps brachii, anterior deltoid

To humeral head distraction: stabilized by long head of triceps, coracobrachialis

To depression of shoulder girdle: scalenes (thorax elevation), upper trapezius

Indications for treatment

- Mid-back pain in referred pattern not aggravated by movement
- Identification of shortness (see tests below).

Special notes

If latissimus dorsi is short it tends to 'crowd' the axillary region, internally rotating the humerus and impeding normal lymphatic drainage (Schafer 1987).

Portions of latissimus dorsi attach to the lower ribs on its way to the lower back and pelvic attachments. Latissimus dorsi powerfully depresses the shoulder and therefore can influence shoulder position and neck postures as well as influencing pelvic and trunk postures by its extensive attachments to the lumbar vertebrae, sacrum and iliac crest (Simons et al 1998).

Latissimus dorsi can place tension on the brachial plexus by depressing the entire girdle and should always be addressed when the patient presents with a very 'guarded' cervical pain associated with rotation of the head or shoulder movements. This type of pain often feels 'neurological' when the tense nerve plexus is further stretched by neck or arm movements. Relief is often immediate and long lasting when the latissimus contractures and myofascial restrictions are released, especially if they were 'tying down' the shoulder girdle.

Assessment for latissimus dorsi shortness/ dysfunction

- The patient lies supine, knees flexed, with the head 1.5 feet (45 cm) from the top edge of the table, and extends the arms above the head, resting them on the treatment surface with the palms facing upward.
- If latissimus is normal, the arms should be able to easily lie flat on the table above the shoulder. If the arms are held laterally, elbow(s) pulled away from the body, then latissimus dorsi is probably short on that side.

or

- The standing patient is asked to flex the torso and allow the arms to hang freely from the shoulders as she holds a half-bent position, trunk parallel with the floor.
- If the arms are hanging other than perpendicular to the floor, there is some muscular restriction involved and if this involves latissimus, the arms will be held closer

to the legs than perpendicular (if they hang markedly forward of such a position, then trapezius or deltoid shortening is possible).

- To assess latissimus in this position (one side at a time), the practitioner stands in front of the patient (who remains in this half-bent position). While stabilizing the scapula with one hand, the practitioner grasps the arm just proximal to the elbow and gently draws the (straight) arm forward.
- If there is not excessive 'bind' in the tissue being tested, the arm should easily reach a level higher than the back of the head.
- If this is not possible, then latissimus is shortened.

 NMT for latissimus dorsi (Fig. 13.44)

The patient remains in a sidelying position with the arm supported as in the treatment of teres major. Myofascial release may be easily applied before or immediately following these techniques (Fig. 13.50).

The practitioner sits (or stands) caudal to the supported arm and grasps the latissimus dorsi, which is the remaining muscular tissue in the free border of the posterior axillary fold. Pincer compression is used in a similar manner to that used for teres major. Beginning near the humerus, the practitioner assesses the latissimus dorsi's long fibers at hand-width intervals until the rib attachments are reached. These upper fibers 'tie' the humerus to the lower ribs. Ischemic bands are often found in this portion of the muscle and central trigger points are found at mid-fiber region of this most lateral portion of the muscle, which is approximately halfway between the humerus and the lower ribs.

The practitioner stands with the (sidelying) patient's arm placed over his upper shoulder to elevate the latissimus dorsi and lift its lower fibers (somewhat) away from the thorax, which makes them easier to grasp. In this position, control of the arm is easily maintained while moving it into varying positions to stretch the fibers and define taut bands for location and palpation. Sometimes the fibers are more defined and respond more quickly in a stretched position but less pressure is usually needed when the tissue is treated in a stretched position. Once located, the fibers may be more easily lifted away from the torso (and manually stretched) if tension on them is reduced. Hence, varying the position of the humerus will assist the practitioner in discovering the best position for accessing and also for treating the latissimus fibers.

The attachments onto the spinous processes, sacrum and iliac crest may be addressed with friction, glides or static pressure, depending on tenderness level. The beveled pressure bar can be used to apply friction or static pressure techniques throughout the lamina groove and sacrum while thumbs are best used along the top of the iliac crest. These portions of the latissimus dorsi are

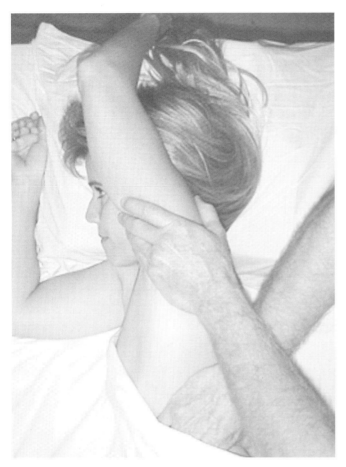

Figure 13.50 A broad application of myofascial release to the axillary region.

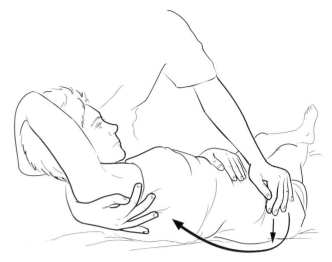

Figure 13.51 Body and hand positions for MET treatment of latissimus dorsi.

discussed more thoroughly in Volume 2 of this text (lower body) as this muscle is very often associated with pelvic distortions.

⚘⚘ MET treatment of latissimus dorsi
(Fig. 13.51)

• The patient lies supine with the leg crossed over the other one at the ankle.
• The practitioner stands on the side opposite the side to be treated at waist level and faces the table.
• The patient slightly sidebends the torso contralaterally (bending toward the practitioner).
• With the legs straight, the patient's feet are placed just off the side of the table to help anchor the lower extremities.
• The patient places the ipsilateral arm behind her neck as the practitioner slides his cephalad hand under the patient's shoulders to grasp the axilla on the treated side, while the patient grasps the practitioner's arm at the elbow.
• The practitioner's caudad hand is placed lightly on the anterior superior iliac spine on the side to be

treated, in order to offer stability to the pelvis during the subsequent contraction and stretching phases.
• The patient is instructed to very lightly take the point of that elbow toward her sacrum as she also lightly tries to bend backwards and toward the treated side. The practitioner resists this effort with the hand at the axilla, as well as the forearm which lies across the patient's upper back. This action produces an isometric contraction in latissimus dorsi.
• After 7 seconds the patient is asked to relax completely as the practitioner, utilizing body weight, sidebends the patient further and, at the same time, straightens his own trunk and leans caudad, effectively lifting the patient's thorax from the table surface and so introducing a stretch into latissimus (as well as quadratus lumborum).
• This stretch is held for 15–20 seconds, allowing a lengthening of shortened musculature in the region.
• Repeat once or twice more for greatest effect.

⚘⚘ PRT for latissimus dorsi (most suitable for acute problems) (Fig. 13.52)

• The patient is supine and lies close to the edge of the table. The practitioner is tableside, at waist level, facing cephalad.
• Using his tableside hand, the practitioner searches for and locates an area of marked localized tenderness on the upper medial aspect of the humerus, where latissimus attaches.
• The patient is instructed to grade the applied pressure to this dysfunctional region of the muscle as a '10'.
• The practitioner's non-tableside hand holds the patient's forearm close to the elbow and eases the humerus into slight extension or compression, ensuring (by 'fine tuning' the degree of extension) before the next movement that the 'score' has reduced somewhat.

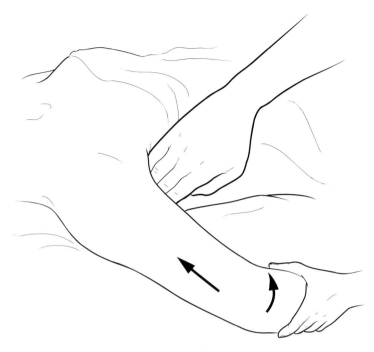

Figure 13.52 Strain-counterstrain position for treatment of latissimus dorsi.

• The practitioner then internally rotates the humerus while also applying light traction or compression in such a way as to reduce the pain 'score' more.

• When the score is reduced to '3' or less, the position of ease is held for 90 seconds before a slow return to neutral.

Subscapularis (Figs 13.53, 13.54)

Attachments: Subscapular fossa (costal surface of scapula) to the lesser tubercle of the humerus and the articular capsule

Innervation: Superior and inferior subscapular nerves (C5–6)

Muscle type: Postural (type 1), shortens when stressed

Function: Medial rotation and adduction of humerus, stabilization of humeral head

Synergists: *Medial rotation*: latissimus dorsi, pectoralis major, teres major
Adduction of humerus: most anterior and posterior fibers of deltoid, triceps long head, teres major, pectoralis major
Humeral head stabilization: supraspinatus, infraspinatus, teres minor

Antagonists: *To medial rotation*: infraspinatus, teres minor
To adduction: deltoid, supraspinatus

Indications for treatment

• Loss of lateral rotation and abduction of the humerus, 'frozen shoulder' syndrome

• Difficulty in reaching as if to throw a ball overarm
• Identification of shortness (see test below).

Special notes

Subscapularis is a rotator cuff muscle whose job is to stabilize the humeral head and seat it deeply into the glenoid fossa. It is a powerful medial rotator of the humerus and is responsible for countering downward tension on the head of the humerus when the initial action of abduction forces the humerus upward, toward the overhanging acromion process (Simons et al 1998).

When hypertonicity or trigger points in subscapularis cause excessive tension within the muscle, it holds the humeral head fast to the glenoid fossa, creating a 'pseudo' frozen shoulder (Simons et al 1998). That is, the humeral head appears immobile, as in true frozen shoulder syndrome, but without associated intrajoint adhesions. Ultimately, however, long-term reduced mobility and capsular irritation from subscapularis dysfunction may result in adhesive capsulitis (Cailliet 1991). Additionally, the subscapularis lies in direct relationship with serratus anterior within the scapulothoracic joint space. Myofascial adhesions of these tissues to each other may contribute to full or partial loss of scapular mobility.

The tendon of subscapularis passes over the anterior joint capsule and lies horizontally between the two almost vertical tendons of biceps brachii. It may be injured or torn when the person falls backwards and throws the hands back to bear the body's weight. This impact will

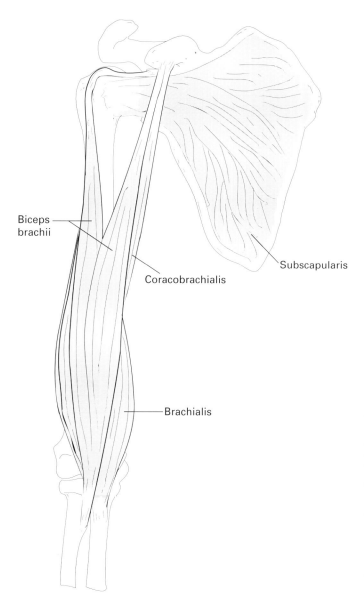

Figure 13.53 The muscles overlying the anterior aspect of the glenohumeral joint.

force the head of the humerus anteriorly against the joint capsule and the tendon of subscapularis, which overlies the anterior joint capsule (Cailliet 1991). The subscapular bursa lies between the tendon and the joint capsule and communicates with the capsule between the superior and middle glenohumeral ligaments while the subcoracoid bursa lies between the subscapularis and the coracoid process. Both bursae communicate with the shoulder joint cavity and therefore may play a role in true frozen shoulder syndrome if they become inflamed (Cailliet 1991, McNab & McCulloch 1994, Simons et al 1998). Ice may be applied if inflammation of the tendon or bursa is suspected or if the region is found to be excessively tender.

Assessment of subscapularis dysfunction/ shortness

- Direct palpation of subscapularis is an excellent means of establishing dysfunction in it, since pain patterns in the shoulder, arm, scapula and chest may all derive from it.
- The practitioner's fingernails must be cut very short.
- With the patient supine, the practitioner stands on the side to be treated and uses the cephalad side hand to position the humerus by grasping it just above the elbow. The patient's arm is positioned so that the fully flexed elbow points toward the ceiling and the patient's hand rests on the top of the ipsilateral shoulder.
- The practitioner places the fingers of the caudad (treating) hand so that they lie between the scapula and the torso with the finger pads in contact with the anterior (inner) surface of the scapula and the dorsum of the hand facing the ribs. The hand will (eventually) slide deeper into the subscapular space (Fig. 13.55A).
- Once the fingers are 'prepositioned', the patient is asked to slowly reach toward the anterior surface of the contralateral shoulder. While the patient slowly moves the hand, the practitioner gently releases the humerus and slides the cephalad hand under the torso to 'hook' the fingers onto the vertebral border of the scapula.
- The scapula is tractioned laterally by the cephalad hand as the caudal hand slides further medially on the ventral surface of the scapula and presses onto the subscapularis (Fig. 13.55B).
- There may be a marked reaction from the patient when this muscle is touched, indicating acute sensitivity.

Observation of subscapularis dysfunction/ shortness (see p. 315)

- The patient is supine with the arm abducted to 90°, the elbow flexed to 90° and the forearm in external rotation, palm upwards.
- The whole arm is resting at the restriction barrier, with gravity as its counterweight.
- If subscapularis is short the forearm will be unable to rest easily, parallel with the floor, but will be somewhat elevated, with the hand pointing toward the ceiling.
- Care is needed to prevent the shoulder lifting from the table, so giving a false-negative result (i.e. allowing the forearm to achieve parallel status with the floor by means of the shoulder lifting).

Assessment of weakness in subscapularis

- The patient is prone with humerus abducted to 90°, the elbow flexed to 90° and the humerus internally rotated so that the forearm is parallel with the torso and the palm facing toward ceiling.

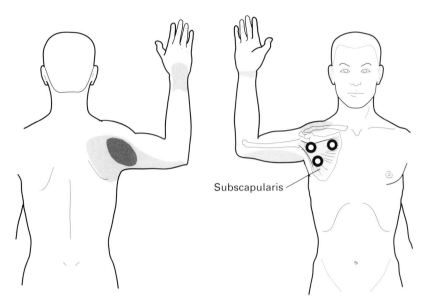

Figure 13.54 Subscapularis referral patterns to the posterior shoulder and into the anterior and posterior wrist.

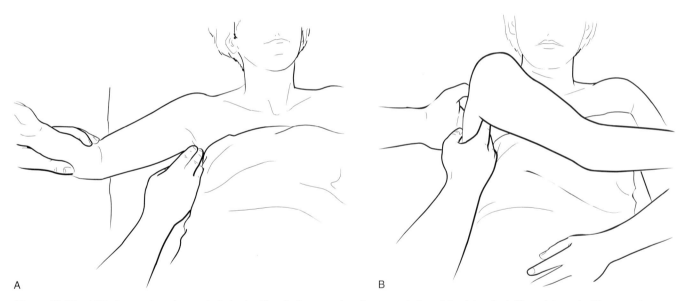

A

B

Figure 13.55 A&B: Access to subscapularis is significantly increased as the scapula translates laterally (with assistance) with proper arm positioning.

• The practitioner stabilizes the scapula with one hand and with the other applies pressure (toward the floor) to the patient's distal forearm to externally rotate the humerus against the patient's resistance.

• The strength of the two sides should be compared.

 NMT for subscapularis

The patient is placed in a sidelying position (see p. 229) with the arm supported by the patient or placed on top of the practitioner's shoulder when the practitioner is seated in front of the patient at the level of the patient's

chest. The patient's arm is tractioned directly forward as far as possible to translate the scapula laterally and allow maximum palpable space on the ventral (anterior) surface of the scapula.

The practitioner's cephalad hand lies on the posterolateral portion of the shoulder and can be used to support the shoulder's position. The bellies of teres major and latissimus dorsi comprise the posterior axillary fold. Subscapularis resides medial to both of these muscles and fills the subscapular fossa on the ventral surface of the scapula. The practitioner locates the lateral edge of the scapula (medial to teres major and latissimus dorsi)

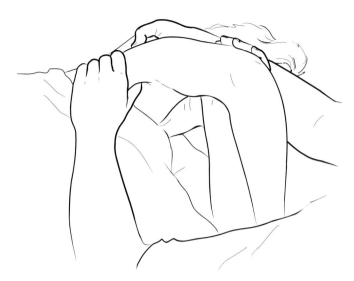

Figure 13.56 A small portion of subscapularis may be reached in the sidelying position.

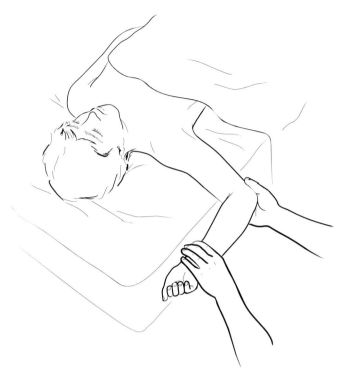

Figure 13.57 MET treatment of subscapularis.

with the thumb of the caudal hand and slides the thumb medially onto the anterior surface of the scapula where subscapularis resides. The elbow of the practitioner's treating arm must remain low to assure the proper angle of the thumb (Fig. 13.56).

Since this muscle is often extremely tender, mild pressure is initially used and increased only if appropriate. The practitioner applies static pressure for 10–12 seconds at thumb-width intervals onto all accessible portions of subscapularis. If not too tender, repeat the process while increasing the static pressure or by applying a snapping (unidirectional) transverse friction. Repeat the entire process 3–4 times during the session while allowing short breaks in between applications of pressure.

The humeral attachment and a portion of the tendon of subscapularis may be treated between the two bicipital tendons on the anterior surface of the humeral head; this is discussed with biceps brachii (p. 376). Recurrent bicipital tendinitis and frozen shoulder may both improve considerably after the (horizontal) subscapularis tendon is treated between the two (vertical) biceps tendons.

 MET for subscapularis (Fig. 13.57)

• The patient is supine with the arm abducted to 90°, the elbow flexed to 90° and the forearm in external rotation, palm upwards.
• The whole arm is resting at the restriction barrier, with gravity as its counterweight.
• Care is needed to prevent the anterior shoulder from becoming elevated in this position (moving toward the ceiling) and so giving a false-normal picture.
• The patient raises the forearm slightly, rotating the shoulder internally, pivoting at the elbow against

light resistance offered by the practitioner on the lower forearm, and holds the resistance for 7–10 seconds.
• Following relaxation, gravity or slight assistance from the practitioner takes the arm into external rotation and through the soft tissue resistance barrier, where it is held for at least 20 seconds.

PRT for subscapularis (most suitable for acute problems)

• The patient is supine and lying so that the arm being treated is close to the edge of the table.
• The practitioner locates an area of marked tenderness on the anterior border of the scapula, using the procedure outlined above for direct palpation assessment.
• The patient is instructed to grade the applied pressure to this dysfunctional region of the muscle as a '10'.
• The practitioner's other hand holds the arm above the elbow and eases it into slight extension and asks the patient for a score. If no reduction is reported, 'fine tuning' of the degree of extension is carried out to achieve this.
• Once a reduction in the score is reported, the practitioner then internally rotates the humerus in such a way as to reduce the 'score' further.
• When the score is reduced to '3' or less, the position of ease is held for 90 seconds before the arm is slowly returned to neutral.

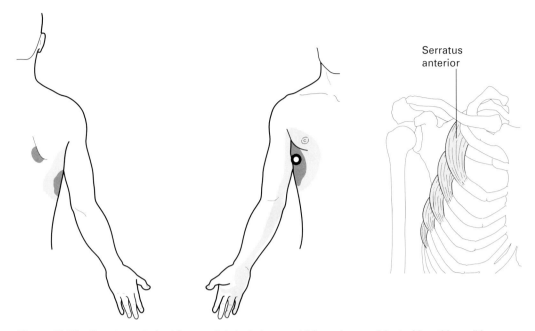

Figure 13.58 Serratus anterior trigger points include one which produces a 'short of breath' condition as well as an often familiar interscapular pain.

Serratus anterior (Fig. 13.58)

Attachments: *Superior part*: outer and superior surface of ribs 1 and 2 and intercostal fascia to the costal and dorsal surfaces of the superior angle of the scapula
Intermediate part: outer and superior surface of ribs 2, 3 and (perhaps) 4 and intercostal fascia to the costal surface along almost the entire medial border of the scapula
Inferior part: outer and superior surface of ribs 4 or 5 through 8 or 9 and intercostal fascia to the costal and dorsal surfaces of the inferior angle of the scapula

Innervation: Long thoracic nerve (C5–7), which lies on the external surface of the muscle

Muscle type: Phasic (type 2), weakens when stressed

Function: Stabilization of the scapula during flexion and abduction of the arm; rotates the scapula laterally to make the glenoid fossa face upward; abducts the scapula and therefore protracts the shoulder girdle; assists in elevating the scapula; presses the scapula to the thorax, counteracting 'winging' of the scapula; may be an accessory muscle of inspiration during abnormal or demanding breathing patterns

Synergists: *Protraction of scapula*: pectoralis minor and upper fibers of pectoralis major
Upward rotation of the glenoid fossa: trapezius
Elevation of scapula: levator scapula, upper trapezius, rhomboids
Fixation of scapula during arm movements: rhomboids, middle trapezius

Antagonists: *To protraction*: rhomboids, latissimus dorsi, middle trapezius

To upward rotation of the glenoid fossa: latissimus dorsi, pectoral muscles, levator scapula, rhomboids

Indications for treatment

- Shortness of breath due to trigger points
- 'Winging' of the scapula (reflexive, inhibited weakness)
- Scapula fixation flat to the thorax (tense fibers)
- Loss of expansion of rib cage during inhalation
- Disrupted scapulohumeral rhythm
- Restriction of adduction of the scapula

Special notes

Serratus anterior is an accessory breathing muscle, recruited during demanding situations rather than normal breathing patterns. Whether its fibers are activated and how much they are activated will vary depending upon the conditions. When it is inhibited, unusual demand may be placed on other respiratory muscles, such as the scalenes and sternocleidomastoid, when the serratus would normally be used. This overload may lead to associated trigger point formation in these and other respiratory muscles, although it is not always clear which comes first – the abnormal respiratory pattern or the trigger points (Simons et al 1998).

The long thoracic nerve, which innervates serratus anterior, lies vertically on the surface of the muscle in the line of the axillary fold and is therefore vulnerable during palpation. Additionally, portions of this nerve supply may pass through the scalenus medius muscle, where it may be entrapped. Damage to or compression of this nerve would produce excessive 'winging' of the scapula in which the medial border of the scapula stands out away from the thorax. However, since 'winging' can sometimes be relieved when trigger points in this muscle are inactivated (Simons et al 1998), the condition may be a result of a combination of activation of antagonists (reflex facilitation) and weakness induced within the serratus since it is a phasic muscle and weakens when stressed (Janda 1996a, Simons et al 1998). Weakness in the serratus anterior would affect the patient's ability to raise the arm as well as push away with the arm.

Herpes zoster lesions often run the course of intercostals nerves, forming on the skin surface superficial to the serratus anterior. These lesions are extremely painful, have a long recovery process and often recur. Care should be taken to avoid stimulating them through examination of this muscle, particularly during the early stages of this condition when they are the most tender and prone to spread into further eruptions. During the early stages of eruption, herpes zoster pain may mimic that of serratus or intercostal trigger points and herpes viruses are likely to aggravate and perpetuate myofascial trigger points as well (Simons et al 1998).

CAUTION
Caution must be exercised in the deep axillary regions as lymph nodes are present and should be avoided, especially if enlarged. If enlarged lymph nodes or other masses are found, the patient should immediately be referred to the proper health-care professional to confirm or rule out breast cancer, thoracic or systemic infections or other serious pathologies.

Trigger points in serratus anterior, as well as the diaphragm and external oblique, may produce a 'stitch in the side' complaint, especially when a high demand is placed on it for excessive breathing. The pain may be accompanied by the inability to take a full breath as serratus anterior and surrounding tissues restrict movement of the ribs. Injection of these trigger points should only be attempted when manual methods of release have failed and then only by the most highly skilled practitioner, due to the risk of thoracic puncture (Simons et al 1998).

Assessment for weakness of serratus anterior

- The patient adopts a position on all fours with weight placed mainly onto the arms rather than knees.
- On slightly flexing the elbows, the scapulae are observed to see whether they wing or deviate laterally, which indicates weakness of serratus anterior (there is some influence from lower trapezius in this assessment but it focuses mainly on serratus).

- The implication, according to Lewit (1985) and Janda (1996a), is that excessive tone in the upper fixators of the shoulder and accessory breathing muscles is probably inhibiting these lower fixators.

NMT for serratus anterior

The patient remains in a sidelying position with the arm resting in the supported arm position without forward pull on the arm. The practitioner stands caudad to the extended arm and uses the thumb of the most caudal hand to perform the therapy. The patient's arm may be placed on the practitioner's shoulder for support and elevation, which will also allow better access to portions of the serratus anterior which lie deep to the scapula (Fig. 13.59).

The practitioner palpates the fibers of serratus anterior on the lateral chest wall to determine the level of tenderness and whether friction or gliding strokes are appropriate to apply. Treatment begins high in the axilla and progresses down the lateral surface of the thorax.

Each palpable segment of serratus anterior is wider than the one before, forming a triangular treatment area with the vertex of the triangle in the axilla. As the treatment progresses down the lateral thorax, the vertical (often extremely tender) fibers of the pectoralis minor are encountered on the most anterior aspect. The scapula forms the posterior border of the palpable region and may be lifted away from the thorax so as to reach as much of the muscle as possible by sliding the treating thumb under the lateral aspect of the scapula to apply friction or gliding strokes onto the rib cage.

If the muscle fibers are not excessively tender, light

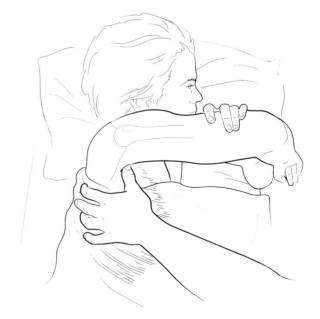

Figure 13.59 When serratus anterior is exquisitely tender, gentle lubricated gliding strokes may be substituted for frictional techniques.

friction is applied in between and on the ribs to assess and treat the serratus anterior. If extremely tender, light-pressure gliding strokes (anterior to posterior) are applied to an area which begins at the top of the lateral chest (in the axilla) and ends at the bottom of the rib cage. The more tender the muscle is, the lighter the pressure should be. If the lightest pressure is still too much, cryotherapy (ice applications) may be substituted and the treatment attempted again at a future session. Progressively more pressure may be applied as the tenderness subsides with treatment, unless osteoporosis or recent rib fractures contraindicate pressure techniques.

The friction or gliding techniques may be repeated at thumb-width intervals, from the pectoralis minor to as far posteriorly as possible and from the axilla to the 9th rib. Allowing the tissue to rest between applications of gliding strokes or friction will often produce dramatic reduction of tenderness.

Myofascial release techniques may also be used on the lateral surface of the body.

Box 13.10 MFR

MFR stands for myofascial release. A number of different approaches are clustered under this heading.

1. John Barnes (1996) describes MFR as the application of passive (practitioner active, patient passive) gentle pressure to restricted myofascial structures, in the direction that will stretch the tissues as far as 'their collagenous barrier'. Sustained pressure results in the 'creep' phenomenon (see Chapter 1), a gradual elongation and ultimately 'freedom from restriction'.
2. Mark Barnes (1997) states: 'Myofascial release is a hands-on soft tissue technique that facilitates a stretch into the restricted fascia. A sustained pressure is applied into the restricted tissue barrier; after 90–120 seconds the tissue will undergo histological length changes allowing the first release to be felt. The therapist follows the release into a new tissue barrier and holds. After a few releases the tissue will become softer and more pliable'.
3. Mock (1997) offers a different, more active (both practitioner and patient) form of myofascial release methodology. 'Adhesions' (described as 'ropy', 'leathery', 'fibrous', 'nodular', etc.) are identified in soft tissues by means of palpation. Various release methods are described, the most active involving compression of the dysfunctional tissues as the muscle in which it is found is taken, four or five times at one treatment session, either passively or actively, through a range of movement from its shortest to its longest length. This effectively 'drags' the 'adhesion' under the compressive contact and 'releases' it.

Note: MET applied to the upper fixators of the shoulder (if they test as short), notably upper trapezius, to release hypertonicity would automatically increase tone in serratus anterior.

Facilitation of tone in serratus anterior using pulsed MET (Ruddy 1962)

This technique is used for rehabilitation and proprioceptive reeducation of a weak serratus anterior.

- The patient is seated or standing and the practitioner places a single-digit contact very lightly against the lower medial scapula border, on the side of the upper trapezius being treated. The patient is asked to attempt to ease the scapula (at the point of digital contact) toward the spine.
- The request is made, 'Press against my finger with your shoulder blade, toward your spine, just as hard (i.e. very lightly) as I am pressing against your shoulder blade, for less than a second'.
- Once the patient has managed to establish control over the particular muscular action required to achieve this subtle movement (which can take a significant number of attempts) and can do so for 1 second at a time, repetitively, she is ready to begin the sequence based on Ruddy's methodology (see Chapter 10).
- The patient is told something such as, 'Now that you know how to activate the muscles which push your shoulder blade lightly against my finger, I want you to do this 20 times in 10 seconds, starting and stopping, so that no actual movement takes place, just a contraction and a stopping, repetitively'.
- This repetitive contraction will activate the rhomboids, middle and lower trapezii and serratus anterior, all of which are probably inhibited if upper trapezius is hypertonic. The repetitive contractions also produce an automatic reciprocal inhibition of upper trapezius.
- The patient should be taught to place a light finger or thumb contact against her own medial scapula (opposite arm behind back) so that home application of this method can be performed several times daily.

Pectoralis major (Figs 13.60, 13.61)

Attachments: *Clavicular portion*: sternal half of the anterior surface of the clavicle
Sternal portion: sternum
Costal portion: costal cartilage of ribs 2–6 (or 7)
Abdominal portion: superficial fascia of external oblique and (sometimes) upper part of rectus abdominis; all portions converge into a tendon attaching to the lateral lip of the intertubercular sulcus of the humerus at its greater tubercle
Innervation: Medial and lateral pectoral nerves (C5–T1)
Muscle type: Postural (type 1), shortens when stressed
Function: Adduction (and horizontal adduction), medial rotation of the humerus, flexion of the humerus (clavicular), extension of the flexed shoulder (sternal, costal), brings the trunk toward the humerus when the humerus is fixed (such as in pull-ups), lowers the raised arm (sternal, costal, abdominal), pulls the shoulder girdle down and forward (sternal, costal) or up and forward (clavicular), accessory in deep (forced) respiration
Synergists: *Adduction*: teres major (and perhaps minor), anterior and posterior deltoid, subscapularis, triceps (long head), latissimus dorsi

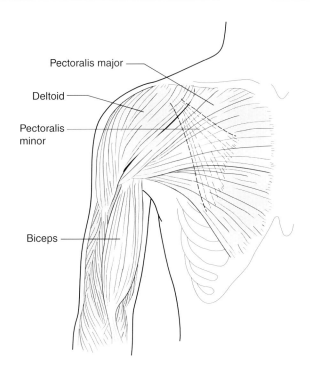

Figure 13.60 Pectoralis major and minor.

Medial rotation: latissimus dorsi, teres major, subscapularis

Flexion of humerus: supraspinatus, anterior deltoid, biceps brachii, coracobrachialis

Protraction of shoulder: subscapularis, pectoralis minor, serratus anterior, subclavius

Depression of shoulder: latissimus dorsi, lower trapezius, serratus anterior

Assist clavicular section: anterior deltoid, coracobrachialis, subclavius, scalenus anterior, sternocleidomastoid

Assist lower fibers: subclavius, pectoralis minor

Antagonists: *To sternal section*: rhomboidii, middle trapezius

To adduction: supraspinatus, deltoid

To medial rotation: teres minor, infraspinatus, posterior deltoid; the clavicular and costal fibers antagonize each other in raising and lowering the arm to horizontal

Indications for treatment

- Back pain between the scapulae
- Pain in front of the shoulder, in the chest and/or down the arm
- Intense chest pain
- Breast pain
- Symptoms of vascular thoracic outlet syndrome

Special notes

The pectoralis major is one of the most complex muscles of the shoulder region, having four sections, a spiraling twist to its laminated layers and crossing three joints (sternoclavicular, acromioclavicular, glenohumeral) to influence several movements of the upper extremity. The complex arrangement of its layers of laminae is best viewed from behind (as shown exquisitely by Simons et al (1998) in Figure 42.5) as an anterior view primarily encompasses only the superficial layers. To form the anterior axillary fold, the dorsal layers fold under the ventral layers in a spiral so that the lowest fibers attach highest on the humerus.

Pectoralis major is one of many muscles whose trigger points can refer pain that mimics true cardiac pain. While it is important to rule out these trigger points as the source of false angina, it is even more important to rule out ischemic heart disease as the source of viscerosomatic chest pain. If trigger points are a source of a mimicking angina pattern and the pattern is abolished, an underlying true cardiac condition may still exist even though the external pain pattern has been eliminated. Similarly, once a cardiac condition is stabilized and chest pain still exists, trigger points may be found to be the source of the long-lasting (and fear-provoking) pain (Simons et al 1998), long after the source of the pain has been removed.

Pectoralis major or underlying intercostal fibers may contain trigger points associated with cardiac arrhythmias, a somatovisceral referral which causes irregular heart beats. The associated trigger points are found between the 5th and 6th ribs on the right side while trigger points in a similar position on the left side mimic ischemic heart disease.

In the condition of thoracic outlet syndrome, the pectoralis major and subclavius should be treated due to their downward pull on the clavicle. This tension, coupled with upward pull of the 1st and 2nd ribs by the scalene muscles, can close the subclavicular space, leading to impingement of the neurovascular and/or lymphatic structures serving the upper extremity, which by definition is thoracic outlet syndrome (Simons et al 1998). Additionally, the pectoralis minor may produce a similar result a few inches further inferolaterally along the neurovascular course and the scalene muscles may entrap the cervical nerves as they exit the vertebral column (especially when breathing patterns are abnormal).

Chronic shortening of pectoralis major and minor produces rounded shoulder, slumping posture which is usually accompanied by a forward head position. Treatment of the pectoral muscles, diaphragm, upper rectus abdominis and other muscles which influence this dysfunctional posture is important in an effort to regain proper alignment. Further, the rhomboids and lower trapezius are often inhibited and weak, which allows the forward slumping. A postural retraining program should be implemented which incorporates lengthening, strengthening and awareness exercises to avoid recurring

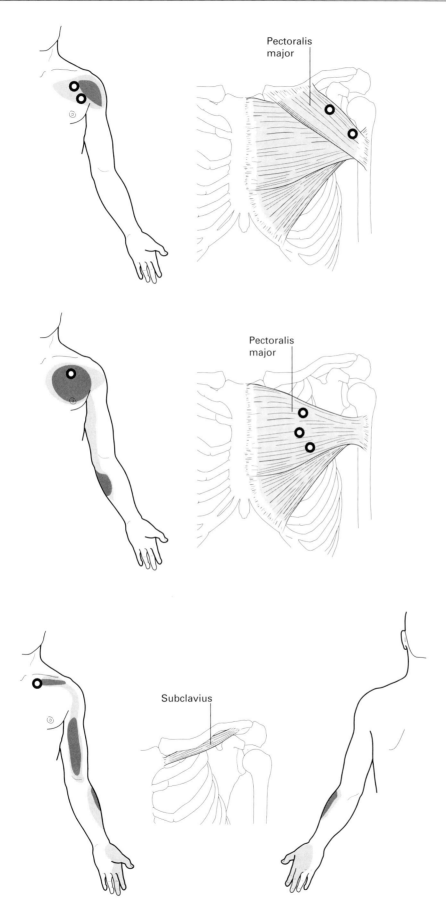

Figure 13.61 Trigger point patterns of pectoralis major and subclavius.

dysfunctional postural patterns which are often induced by chronic work positions and recreational habits.

Overlying the pectoralis major are mammary tissues and the nipple of the breast. In both genders, but significantly in a higher percentage of females, breast cancer is a condition for which surgical removal, various types of reconstruction and significant tissue damage may be presented; 99% of breast cancer cases occur in women. Fifty years ago a woman's chance of developing breast cancer was 1 in 20 while today's chances are 1 in 8 (DeLany 1999, Fitzgerald 1998). It is the second leading cause of cancer deaths in women and is the leading cause of all death in women aged 40–55. Postmastectomy care is a condition often presented to the manual practitioner for rehabilitation of the upper extremity and chest muscles.

Since breast cancer is a life-threatening condition, it is critically important that a comprehensive treatment plan with a qualified health-care professional be initiated as soon as a breast cancer diagnosis has been made. Traditional treatments include surgery, radiation, chemotherapy and tamoxifen (DeLany 1999, Fitzgerald 1998). Each of these treatments has its own post treatment side effects and special precautions must be taken in each case. Consultation with the patient's physician(s) and a clear understanding of her particular condition and treatment plan is recommended before beginning myofascial therapy.

Great care must be used when addressing postmastectomy tissues, especially with reconstruction efforts or lymph node removal (Chikly 1999). The myofascial tissues of the area may be extremely tender and the site of incision may not have healed completely. In the case of radiation therapy, extreme caution must be taken with any tissue which was irradiated as its capillaries are often more fragile. Aggressive therapies, such as friction, skin rolling or even myofascial release, may result in permanent injury to the capillary vessels.

Special care is advised with postmastectomy cases to avoid increasing lymph congestion within the extremity (Chikly 1999), to avoid stretching the incision tissue until well healed and to avoid working with certain techniques when edema or inflammation already exist. Unless otherwise contraindicated, lymph drainage and antiinflammatory techniques, such as cryotherapy, may be applied to these tissues until the tissue conditions change to allow massage applications. Special training may be needed to safely apply lymphatic drainage and other techniques in cancer recovery therapy.

Other less aggressive techniques, such as myofascial release or mild stretching techniques, may be applied to associated muscles until the questionable tissues can be safely treated with NMT. Extreme tenderness to even mild touch, redness, swelling and heat within the tissues all indicate an inflammatory response which could be intensified or spread with NMT applications. Consultation with the patient's physician is strongly advised and

special training in postmastectomy care is suggested, especially if the practitioner's experience is limited in this area.

Assessment for shortness in pectoralis major

- The patient lies supine with the head several feet from the top edge of the table and is asked to extend the arms above the head and rest them on the treatment surface with palms facing up.
- If pectoralis major is normal the arms should be able to easily reach horizontal (parallel with the floor) while being directly in contact with the surface of the table for the entire length of the upper arms. There should be no arching of the back or twisting of the thorax.
- If an arm cannot rest with the dorsum of the upper arm in contact with the table surface, without effort, then pectoral fibers are almost certainly short.
- Assessment of the sternal portion of pectoralis major involves abduction of the arm to 90° (Lewit 1985). In this position the tendon of pectoralis major at the sternum should not be found to be unduly tense even with maximum abduction of the arm, unless the muscle is short.
- For assessment of costal and abdominal attachments the arm is brought into elevation and abduction as the muscle as well as the tendon on the greater tubercle of the humerus is palpated.
- Tautness will be visible and tenderness of the tissues under palpation will be reported, if the sternal fibers have shortened.

Assessment for strength of pectoralis major (Fig. 13.62)

- Patient is supine with arm in abduction at the shoulder joint and medially rotated (palm is facing down) with the elbow extended.
- The practitioner stands at the head and secures the opposite shoulder with one hand to prevent any trunk torsion and contacts the dorsum of the distal humerus with the other hand.
- The patient attempts to lift the arm and to bring it across the chest, against resistance, as strength is assessed in the sternal fibers.
- Different arm positions can be used to assess clavicular and costal fibers.
- For example, with an angle of abduction/elevation of 135°, costal and abdominal fibers will be involved and with abduction of 45°, the clavicular fibers will be assessed.
- The practitioner should palpate to ensure that the 'correct' fibers contract when assessments are being made.

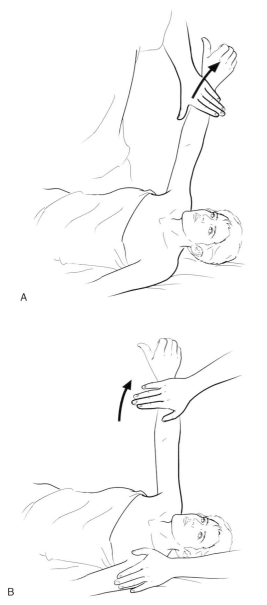

A

B

Figure 13.62 Test for strength of pectoralis major. A: incorrect procedure. B: correct procedure (because shoulder is stabilised).

 ## NMT for pectoralis major

The patient remains in a sidelying position. The arm to be treated is uppermost and rests in the supported arm position without forward pull on it. The practitioner is seated caudad to the extended arm at the level of the patient's waist and grasps the fibers of the axillary portion of pectoralis major with the cephalad (treating) hand. The patient's arm may be placed on the practitioner's shoulder for support and elevation, which may also allow better access to the area, or it may be supported by the patient. The arm is pulled forward until the pectoralis major 'pulls away' from the chest wall. The breast tissues will displace themselves toward the therapy table and away from the mid-belly region of the pectoralis major where the central trigger points can be found. Though he could be standing to perform this technique, a seated position for the practitioner is recommended to decrease wrist stress and avoid bending at the waist (which may produce low back strain). If the practitioner finds that the wrist feels strained, he should reposition himself in such a way that the wrist rests in a neutral position, which usually involves moving toward the patient's feet.

Pincer palpation is used to isolate and assess each section of the muscle (in small portions) while avoiding intrusion onto breast tissues. If not too tender and unless otherwise contraindicated, each of the three sections of pectoralis major is manipulated by rolling the fibers between the thumb and fingers of the examining hand. Taut bands which are adhered to one another may separate and can then be addressed more independently.

The practitioner continues to examine the fibers in thumb-width segments while moving toward the humeral insertion (Fig. 13.63). Repeat the process for all divisions of pectoralis major. Thickness usually associated with trigger points is often found in the mid-fiber region. When nodules, exquisitely tender spots or taut fibers are found, the practitioner locates and isolates the trigger points and applies static compression for 8–12 seconds

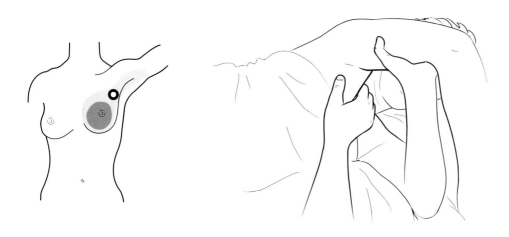

Figure 13.63 The breast tissue self-displaces toward the treatment table which allows excellent access to pectoralis major's lateral portions.

which may provoke classic referral patterns into the breast tissues, onto the chest and down the arm. Additionally, a light stretch placed on the fibers may make the taut fibers more palpable and also may augment the release.

To treat the clavicular attachment of pectoralis major and subclavius (see p. 361) which lies deep to it, the patient remains in a sidelying position and the practitioner stands cephalad to the patient's head. The patient's supported arm is pulled as far forward as possible to distract the clavicle from the chest. The fingers of the 'face-side' (treating) hand are 'curled' onto the inferior surface of the clavicle and friction is applied to the entire length of the inferior aspect of the clavicle to treat the clavicular attachment of pectoralis major and subclavius (Fig. 13.64). The supraclavicular fossa is avoided as the brachial plexus and blood vessels lie here and may be damaged by excessive pressure. Pectoralis major is usually thick and pressure may need to be increased to influence subclavius which lies deep to it. However, the pressure should be directed onto the inferior surface of the clavicle and not deeply into the torso as the neurovascular bundle serving the upper extremity courses through the subclavicular area as well. When addressing subclavius in this position, the arm should be pulled so far forward that the patient almost rolls forward, which will pull the clavicle even further away from the chest wall and help to protect the neurovascular structures.

Following the treatment of pectoralis minor in the sidelying position (see p. 367), the patient moves to a supine position. The sternal and costal attachments of pectoralis major and sternalis are assessed by the practitioner who stands at the level of the chest on the side being treated. Lubricated gliding strokes, friction or myofascial release may be applied to the remaining portions of pectoralis major while care is taken not to intrude on breast tissue. The patient's hand may be used to displace and protect the breast while the practitioner examines the attachments along the sternum and the portion of the muscle which lies caudal to the breast.

Slow, transverse friction is applied to the sternum to examine for a sternalis muscle or trigger points within the fascia covering the sternal area. These trigger points may refer a deep ache to the chest and pain down the upper arm (details regarding sternalis are found on p. 371).

The practitioner locates the top of the xiphoid process or where the two sides of the ribs meet if the xiphoid is not palpable. The practitioner's palpating finger moves laterally onto the right side (approximately 2 inches, depending upon body size) and into the rib space between the 5th and 6th ribs. The practitioner palpates on the ribs and in between the ribs on pectoralis major and intercostal muscle fibers for tenderness and trigger points. These 'cardiac arrhythmia' trigger points may refer into the heart and cause disturbances in its normal rhythm (Simons et al 1998) (Fig. 13.65). Though the trigger point is located on the right side, the corresponding points on the left side should also be treated to eliminate contralateral referrals which may perpetuate these volatile trigger points.

 ## MET for pectoralis major

• The patient lies supine with the arm abducted in a direction which produces the most marked evidence

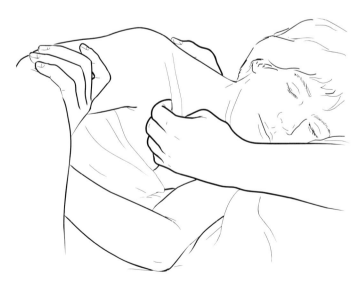

Figure 13.64 The arm is tractioned forward to pull the clavicle away from the underlying neurovascular structures.

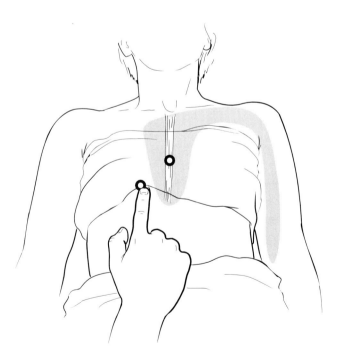

Figure 13.65 The sternalis has a frightening 'cardiac-type' pain pattern independent of movement while the 'cardiac arrhythmia' trigger point (see finger tip) contributes to disturbances in normal heart rhythm without pain referral.

of pectoral shortness (assessed by palpation and visual evidence of the particular fibers involved).

• The more elevated the arm (i.e. the closer to the head), the more focus there will be on costal and abdominal fibers.

• With a lesser degree of abduction, to around 45°, the focus is more on the clavicular fibers.

• Between these two extremes lies the position which influences the sternal fibers most directly.

• The patient lies as close to the side of the table as possible so that the abducted arm can be brought below the horizontal level in order to apply gravitational pull and passive stretch to the fibers, as appropriate.

• The practitioner stands on the side to be treated and grasps the humerus while the other hand contacts the insertion of the shortened fibers (on a rib or near the sternum or clavicle, depending upon which fibers are being treated and which arm position has been adopted).

• The thenar and hypothenar eminence of the contact hand stabilizes the area during the contraction and stretch, preventing movement of it but not exerting any pressure to stretch it.

• The patient's hand should be placed on the contact area so that the practitioner can place his hand over it, allowing it to act as a 'cushion'. This hand placement is for physical comfort and also prevents physical contact with emotionally sensitive areas, such as breast tissue.

• All stretch is achieved via the positioning and leverage of the arm; the contact hand on the thorax (whether directly or 'through' the patient's hand) acts as a stabilizing contact only.

• As a rule, the long axis of the patient's upper arm should be in a straight line with the fibers being treated.

• A useful hold, which depends upon the relative sizes of the patient and the practitioner, involves the practitioner grasping the anterior aspect of the patient's flexed upper arm just above the elbow, while the patient cups the practitioner's elbow and holds this contact throughout the procedure (Fig. 13.66).

• Starting with the patient's arm in a position which takes the affected fibers to just short of their restriction barrier, the patient introduces a light contraction (20% of strength) involving adduction against resistance from the practitioner, for 7–10 seconds.

• If a trigger point has previously been identified in pectoralis major, the practitioner should ensure, by means of palpation if necessary or by observation, that the fibers housing the triggers are involved in the contraction.

• As the patient exhales following complete relaxation of the area, a stretch through the new barrier is activated by the patient and maintained by the practitioner.

• The stretch needs to be one in which the arm is first pulled away (distracted) from the thorax, before the stretch is introduced which involves the humerus being taken below the horizontal.

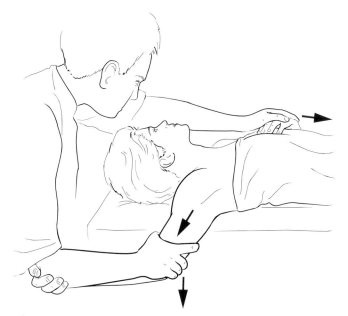

Figure 13.66 MET treatment of pectoralis major, supine position.

• During the stretching phase it is important for the entire thorax to be stabilized. No rolling or twisting of the thorax in the direction of the stretch should be permitted.

• The stretching procedure should be thought of as having two phases:
1. the slack being removed by distracting the arm away from the contact/stabilizing hand on the thorax
2. movement of the arm toward the floor, initiated by the practitioner bending his knees.

• Stretching should be repeated 2–3 times in each position.

• All attachments should be treated, which calls for the use of different arm positions, as discussed above, as well as different stabilizing ('cushion') contacts as the various fiber directions and attachments are stretched.

Alternative MET for pectoralis major
(Fig. 13.67)

• Patient is prone with face in a face hole or cradle.

• Her right arm is abducted to 90° and the elbow flexed to 90°, palm towards the floor, with upper arm supported by the table.

• The practitioner stands at waist level facing cephalad and places his non-tableside hand palm to palm with the patient's so that the patient's forearm is in contact with the ventral surface of the practitioner's forearm.

• The practitioner's tableside hand rests on the patient's right scapula area, ensuring that no trunk rotation occurs.

• The practitioner eases the patient's arm into extension at the shoulder until he senses the first sign of resistance from pectoralis. It is important when extending

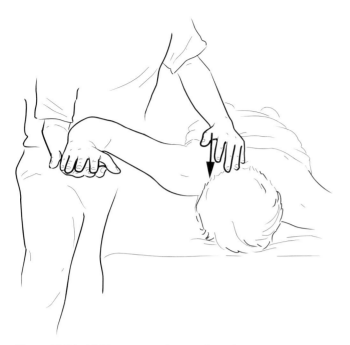

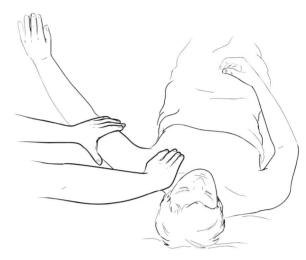

Figure 13.68   Palpation of pectoralis major for MFR application.

Figure 13.67   MET treatment of pectoralis major, prone position.

the arm in this way to ensure that no trunk rotation occurs and that the anterior surface of the shoulder remains in contact with the table throughout.

• The patient is asked, using no more than 20% of strength, to bring her arm towards the floor and across her chest, with the elbow taking the lead in this attempted movement, which is completely resisted by the practitioner.

• The practitioner ensures that the patient's arm remains parallel with the floor throughout the isometric contraction.

• Following release of the contraction effort and on an exhalation, the arm is taken into greater extension, with the patient's assistance, and held at stretch for not less than 20 seconds.

• This procedure is repeated 2–3 times, slackening the muscle slightly from its end-range before each subsequent contraction, to reduce discomfort and for ease of application of the contraction.

• Variations in pectoralis fiber involvement can be achieved by altering the angle of abduction; with a more superior angle (around 140°), the lower sternal and costal fibers, and with a lesser angle (around 45°), the clavicular fibers will be committed.

🖐 🖐 **MFR for pectoralis major** (Fig. 13.68)

• Patient is supine with arm in abduction at the shoulder joint and medially rotated so that the palm is facing down and the elbow is extended.

• The practitioner palpates and assesses pectoralis major until areas of restriction, congestion or fibrosis are discovered.

• The arm is then brought into adduction to slacken the muscle fibers.

• The slackening process is further encouraged by means of light compression from the upper humerus toward the lower sternum.

• A broad flat (fingerpads or thumb) digital contact is then made just distal to the dysfunctional tissues.

• The patient is then asked to move the arm to its fullest abduction and then back into adduction, lengthening and shortening the muscle, and so intermittently dragging the dysfunctional tissues under the compressive force of the practitioner's fingers or thumb.

• 3–5 repetitions are normally adequate for each contact area.

• Different arm positions can be used to treat the various pectoral fibers in the same manner.

Pectoralis minor

Attachments: Outer and upper surfaces of 3rd through 5th ribs (sometimes 2nd through 4th) and fascia of adjoining intercostals to the medial aspect of the coracoid process

Innervation: Medial and lateral pectoral nerves (C5–T1)

Muscle type: Not determined

Function: Draws the shoulder down and forward, rotates the scapula (depressing the glenoid), accessory in deep (forced) respiration, lifts the inferior angle and medial border of the scapula away from the ribs

Synergists: *Deep respiration*: diaphragm, scalenes, intercostals, levator scapula, sternocleidomastoid, upper trapezius

Shoulder depression: pectoralis major, latissimus dorsi, lower trapezius

Forward pull and rotation of scapula: pectoralis major

Downward rotation: rhomboids, levator scapula

Antagonists: *To protraction and rotation of scapula*: lower trapezius
To shoulder depression: upper trapezius, levator scapula

Indications for treatment

- Chest pain similar to cardiac pain
- Restricted humeral movements (particularly in reaching overhead)
- Constriction of nerve or blood flow when reaching overhead or sleeping with the arms resting overhead (neurovascular entrapment syndrome)

Special notes

Postural implications of pectoralis minor have been discussed previously with the overlying pectoralis major. Widely prevailing slumping postures created by tightness in pectoralis minor are readily noticeable (along with forward head position) when viewing the body from the side (coronal plane). Kyphosis often accompanies the 'depressed' look of this postural position, as do repressed breathing patterns.

Impingement of neurovascular structures which course deep to pectoralis minor may create duplication of symptoms of thoracic outlet syndrome. In such a case, the patient will report loss of feeling in the hand or a tendency to drop objects, particularly when reaching up to a shelf to retrieve them. Additionally, the radial pulse (which is being simultaneously palpated) will disappear as the axillary artery becomes occluded when the practitioner administers the Wright maneuver, a positioning which places the arm in hyperabduction or, in some cases, by merely abducting the humerus to 90° with lateral rotation (see Simons et al 1998, p. 350, Fig. 43.4).

Trigger points in pectoralis minor can refer into the breast, creating pain and hypersensitivity of the breast and nipple, into the chest and anterior shoulder, down the ulnar side of the arm and into the last three fingers and palmar hand.

Whereas scalenus anticus is more likely to produce hand edema and finger stiffness by entrapment of the subclavian vein, the author's clinical experience indicates that fascial restrictions and scar tissue, due to surgery or other traumas, near the coracoid process may also occlude lymph drainage of the upper extremity. This consideration is especially important if lymph node removal was necessary, particularly from the subclavicular area. (See additional information regarding the lymphatic system on p. 18.) Simons et al (1998) note that pectoralis major can occlude lymphatic drainage of the breast and that trigger points which form in posttraumatic scar tissue in the regions of pectoralis minor's coracoid attachment are relieved by trigger point injection. However, extreme caution is advised when injecting thoracic muscles to avoid penetration into the thoracic cavity.

Additional slips of the muscle are sometimes noted, varying in number and level (*Gray's anatomy* 1995, Platzer 1992, Simons et al 1998) including fibers extending to the greater tuberosity of the humerus (Simons et al 1998). More rare variations include pectoralis minimus (coracoid process to the first rib) (*Gray's anatomy* 1995) and pectoralis intermedius (from rib cartilages to the fascia covering biceps brachii and coracobrachialis) (Simons et al 1998). Though rarely absent, pectoralis minor may be present or absent when pectoralis major is missing (*Gray's anatomy* 1995).

NMT for pectoralis minor

The patient is placed in a sidelying position with the arm supported by the patient or placed on top of the practitioner's shoulder when the practitioner is seated at the level of the patient's chest. The arm is pulled forward sufficiently to allow the thumb of the practitioner's caudal hand to be placed posterior to pectoralis major and directly on the caudal end of pectoralis minor. The practitioner presses onto the lateral head of pectoralis minor at its 5th rib attachment to assess for tenderness. Static pressure may be used for 8–12 seconds or, if not too tender, light-pressure transverse friction may be applied. This muscle, when non-tender or only mildly tender, responds well to a unidirectional snapping friction which transverses its fibers.

The practitioner's treating thumb is moved up the muscle at thumb-width intervals and applies static pressure and/or crossfiber friction to the entire length of pectoralis minor (Fig. 13.69). This muscle may become significantly wider at the 4th and then at the 3rd rib attachments. The treatment techniques are stopped approximately 2 inches caudal to the coracoid process to avoid

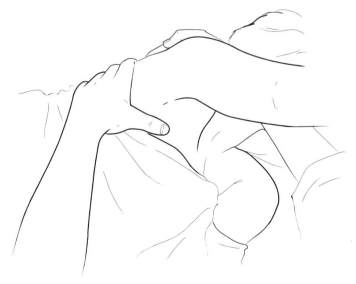

Figure 13.69 When pectoralis minor is extremely tender, mild static pressure is substituted for frictional techniques.

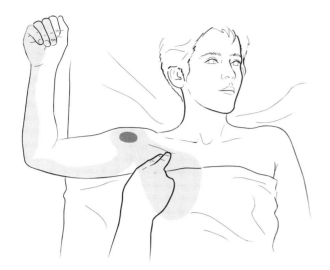

Figure 13.70 Trigger point target zones for pectoralis minor.

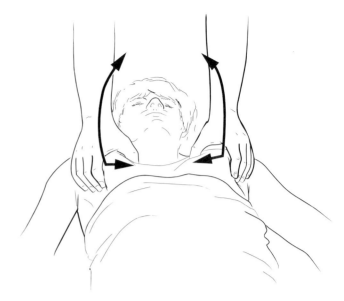

Figure 13.71 Direct myofascial stretch for pectoralis minor.

compressing the neurovascular bundle which supplies the arm. If pectoralis minor is not too tender, these steps are repeated (gently) 2–3 more times. Often, static compression will release the fibers more readily, especially after the light friction has been applied at least once.

With the patient in the supine position, pectoralis minor may be further addressed through pectoralis major. With the elbow flexed to 90°, the arm is placed in an abducted, externally rotated ('Hi') position (Fig. 13.70). Myofascial release may be used superficial to pectoralis minor (through pectoralis major). The pressure should be toward the clavicle rather than toward the breast to avoid stretching the fascia and ligaments which support the breast tissue. This step may also help to bring the shoulders back into coronal alignment. Gentle friction may also be applied through pectoralis major while transversing the fibers of pectoralis minor, coracobrachialis and short head tendon attachment of biceps brachii as long as the supporting structures of the breast mentioned above and neurovascular structures deep to the coracoid are respected. Biceps tendon and coracobrachialis lie laterally and perpendicularly oriented to pectoralis minor in this arm position.

The muscle fibers are all stretched when the arm is in this position of extreme lateral rotation and less pressure is used to avoid tearing the fibers or provoking a reflexive spasm.

MET and MFR treatments of pectoralis major (pp. 364–366) would also involve (to an extent) pectoralis minor.

Direct (bilateral) myofascial stretch of shortened pectoralis minor (Fig. 13.71)

- The patient is supine with the arms comfortably at the side.

- The practitioner, while standing at the head of the table, internally rotates his arms and places the palms of his hands (having ensured nails are well clipped) into the axilla, palms touching the medial humerus, thumb side of index fingers touching the axilla.

- At this stage the dorsum of the finger pads are located under the lateral border of each pectoralis minor.

- The practitioner now slowly externally rotates his arms and, using gentle pressure, insinuates the finger tips (index, middle and ring – the small finger and thumb play no part in this method) under the lateral border of the muscle.

- The hands, the palms of which are now facing medially, are then drawn lightly toward each other (medially) until all the slack in pectoralis minor has been removed.

- The practitioner's hands then slowly, deliberately and painlessly lift the tissues toward the ceiling, easing the muscle away from its attachments, until all slack has been removed (i.e. no actual stretching is taking place at this stage, merely a removal of all slack).

- The practitioner should then transfer body weight backwards to introduce a lean which removes the slack further, by tractioning in a superior direction (toward the head).

- The muscle fibers will now have been eased medially, anteriorly and superiorly and should be held at these combined barriers as they slowly release over the next few minutes.

- If correctly applied, this should not be painful or prove invasive to breast tissue. The procedure is normally both well accepted and effective in releasing tensions at the lower end of the thoracic inlet.

Subclavius

Attachments: From the first rib at its junction with its costal cartilage to the middle third of the clavicle on its caudad surface
Innervation: Subclavian nerve (C5–6)
Muscle type: Not determined

Function: Assists in bringing the shoulder down and forward, seats the clavicle onto an articular disc at the sternoclavicular joint
Synergists: *Protraction of the shoulder*: pectoralis major, subscapularis, pectoralis minor, serratus anterior
Antagonists: Trapezius, rhomboidii

Box 13.11   Shoulder and arm pain due to neural impingement

- Tissues which surround neural structures, and which move independently of the nervous system, are called the mechanical interface (MI) (e.g. supinator muscle is the MI to the radial nerve, as it passes through the radial tunnel).
- Any pathology in the MI may produce tension on the neural structure, with unpredictable results, e.g. disc protrusion, osteophyte contact, carpal tunnel constriction.
- Symptoms are more easily provoked in active movement rather than passive tests.
- Pathophysiological changes resulting from inflammation or from chemical damage (i.e. toxic) are noted as commonly leading on to internal mechanical restrictions of neural structures in a different manner to mechanical causes, such as those imposed by a disc lesion, for example.
- Adverse mechanical tension (AMT) changes do not necessarily affect nerve conduction (Butler & Gifford 1989) but Korr's (1981) research shows it to be likely that axonal transport would be affected.
- Maitland (1986) suggests that treatment (placing the neural structures at tension, in the test positions) involves 'mobilization' of the neural structures, rather than simply stretching them, and recommends that these tests be reserved for conditions which fail to respond adequately to normal mobilization of soft and osseous structures (muscles, joints and so on), for example by use of techniques such as NMT or MET.

Notes

1. When a tension test is positive (i.e. pain is produced by one or another element of the test – initial position alone or with 'sensitizing' additions) it only indicates that AMT exists somewhere in the nervous system.
2. The restriction is not, however, necessarily at the site of reported pain.
3. When tissues housing myofascial trigger points are stretched, pain may result. This can add a degree of confusion when evidence derived from use of the tension tests is being evaluated.

GENERAL PRECAUTIONS AND CONTRAINDICATIONS

- **Care should be taken when introducing sideflexion of the neck during the upper limb tension test.**
- **If any area is sensitive care should be taken not to aggravate existing conditions during the performance of tests.**
- **If obvious neurological problems exist special care should be taken not to exacerbate the condition by vigorous or strong stretching.**
- **Similar precautions apply to diabetic, MS or recent surgical patients or where the area being tested is much affected by circulatory deficit.**
- **The tests should not be used if there has been recent onset or worsening of neurological signs or if there is any cauda equina or cord lesion.**

General advice regarding use of these methods
- Usually treatment positions which encourage release of

mechanical restrictions impinging on neural structures involve replication of the test positions.
- Butler (1991) suggests that initial stretching should commence well away from the site of pain in sensitive individuals and conditions.
- Retesting regularly during treatment is useful, in order to see whether there are gains in range of motion or lessening of pain provoked during testing.
- Any sensitivity provoked by treatment should subside immediately following application of a test position/stretch. If it does not the technique/test should be stopped to avoid irritation of the neural tissues involved.
- Additional tests to assess for shortened muscle structures and joint restrictions would also be appropriate, as these may be the cause of adverse tension in the nervous system.

Upper limb tension tests (ULTT)

Both versions of the ULT test described below should be used in cases involving thoracic, cervical and upper limb symptoms, even if this involves only local finger pain.

ULTT 1

1. Patient is supine and the practitioner places the tested arm into abduction, extension and lateral rotation of the glenohumeral joint.
2. Once these positions are established supination of the forearm is introduced together with elbow extension.
3. This is followed by addition of passive wrist and finger extension.

If pain is experienced at any stage during the positioning into the test position or during addition of sensitization maneuvers (below), particularly reproduction of neck, shoulder or arm symptoms previously reported, the test is positive, this confirms a degree of mechanical interference affecting neural structures.
    Additional sensitization is performed by:

- adding cervical lateral flexion away from the side being tested, or
- introduction of ULTT 1 on the other arm simultaneously, or
- the simultaneous use of straight leg raising, bi- or unilaterally, or
- introduction of pronation rather than supination of the wrist.

ULTT 2

Butler maintains that ULTT 2 replicates the working posture involved in many instances of upper limb repetition disorders.

1. To perform right-side ULTT 2, the patient lies close to right side of the couch, i.e. scapula is free of the surface.
2. Trunk and legs are angled towards the left foot of the couch.
3. The practitioner stands to right side of the patient's head facing the feet with his left thigh depressing her right shoulder girdle.
4. The patient's fully flexed right arm is supported at both elbow and wrist.
5. Variations in the degree and angle of shoulder depression ('lifted' towards ceiling, held towards floor) may be used.

Box 13.11 *(cont'd)*

6. Holding the shoulder depressed, the practitioner's right hand grasps the patient's right wrist while the elbow is held by the practitioner's left hand.

Sensitization options include:

- shoulder internal or external rotation
- elbow flexion or extension
- forearm supination or pronation

A combination of shoulder internal rotation, elbow extension and forearm pronation is the most sensitive

The practitioner then slides his right hand down onto the patient's open hand, with his thumb between the patient's thumb and index finger and introduces supination or pronation, ulnar or radial deviations or stretching of fingers/thumb.

Further sensitization may involve:

- neck movement (e.g. sidebend away from tested side) or
- altered shoulder position, such as increased abduction or extension.

Notes

- Butler (1991) reports that where mechanical interface restrictions are present, cervical lateral flexion away from the tested side increases arm symptoms in 93% of people and cervical lateral flexion towards the tested side increases symptoms in 70% of cases.
- ULTT mobilizes the cervical dural theca in a transverse direction.

 Box 13.12 Modified PNF spiral stretch techniques

Proprioceptive neuromuscular facilitation (PNF) methods have been incorporated into useful assessment and treatment sequences (McAtee & Charland 1999). These ideas have been modified to take account of MET principles (Chaitow 1996b).

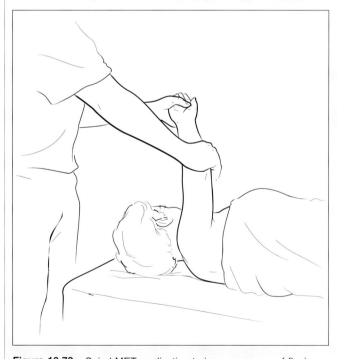

Figure 13.72 Spiral MET application to increase range of flexion, adduction and external rotation of shoulder.

1 Stretch into extension

- To increase the range of motion in flexion, adduction and external rotation.
- The patient lies supine and ensures that her shoulders remain in contact with the table throughout the procedure and turns her head left.
- She flexes, adducts and externally rotates her (right) arm fully, maintaining the elbow in extension (palm facing the ceiling).
- The practitioner stands at the head of the table and supports the patient's arm at proximal forearm and hand.
- The patient is asked to begin the process of returning the arm to her side, in stages, against resistance.
- The amount of force used by the patient should not exceed 25% of her strength potential.
- The first instruction is to pronate and internally rotate the arm ('Turn your arm inwards so that your palm faces the other way'), followed by abduction and then extension ('Bring your arm back outwards and to your side').
- All these efforts are combined by the patient into a sustained effort which is resisted by the practitioner so that a 'compound' isometric contraction occurs involving infraspinatus, middle trapezius, rhomboids, teres minor, posterior deltoid and pronator teres.
- On complete relaxation, the practitioner, with the patient's assistance takes the arm further into flexion, adduction and external rotation, stretching these muscles to a new barrier.
- The same procedure is repeated 2–3 more times.

2 Stretch into flexion

- To increase the range of motion in extension, abduction and internal rotation.
- The patient lies supine and ensures that her shoulders remain in contact with the table throughout the procedure.
- She extends, abducts and internally rotates her (right) arm fully, maintaining the elbow in extension (wrist pronated).
- The practitioner stands at the head of the table and supports the patient's arm at distal forearm and elbow.

Box 13.12 *(cont'd)*

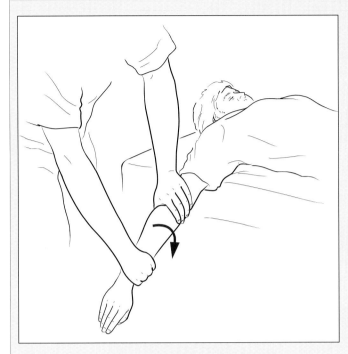

- The patient is asked to begin the process of returning the arm to her side, in stages, against resistance.
- The amount of force used by the patient should not exceed 25% of her strength potential
- The first instruction is to supinate and externally rotate the arm ('Turn your arm outwards so that your palm faces the other way'), followed by adduction and then flexion ('Bring your arm back towards the table and then up to your side').
- All these efforts are combined by the patient into a sustained effort which is resisted by the practitioner, so that a 'compound' isometric contraction occurs involving the clavicular head of pectoralis major, anterior deltoid, coracobrachialis, biceps brachii, infraspinatus and supinator.
- On complete relaxation, the practitioner with the patient's assistance takes the arm further into extension, abduction and internal rotation, stretching these muscles to a new barrier.
- The same procedure is repeated 2–3 more times.

Figure 13.73 Spiral MET application to increase range of extension, abduction and internal rotation of shoulder.

Indication for treatment

- Pain under clavicle and down the arm

Special notes

This muscle has a short, thick tendon and is difficult to palpate or access for electromyography. It may be absent but that would be difficult to determine manually since it underlies the thick clavicular head of pectoralis major. Some of its fibers may be influenced through pectoralis major if care is taken to avoid intruding on the neurovascular complex which lies deep to a portion of it.

The pain pattern for subclavius is significant as it is one of numerous muscles referring a pattern which mimics ischemic cardiac disease. As discussed in other areas of this book, referral to a physician is advised to rule out cardiac involvement.

NMT techniques for subclavius are presented with pectoralis major (p. 364).

 MFR for subclavius

- The muscle lies deep to pectoralis major, between the first rib and the clavicle.
- The patient abducts and internally rotates the arm.
- The practitioner makes digital contact with the muscle by applying broad flat finger pad pressure as

far under the clavicle as possible, without causing undue discomfort.

- The patient is then asked to adduct and externally rotate the shoulder slowly and deliberately while firm digital pressure is maintained.
- This should be repeated 3–5 times.

Sternalis

Box 13.13 Sternalis and chest pain
Chest pain referred from this muscle [sternalis] has a terrifying quality that is remarkably independent of body movement. (Simons et al 1998)

Attachments: A vertical slip ascending from the sheath of rectus abdominis, fascia of the chest or costal cartilages of the lower ribs to merge with the fascia of upper chest, attach to the sternum or blend with sternocleidomastoid

Innervation: Varies considerably, but usually intercostal nerves or the medial pectoral nerve

Muscle type: Not determined

Function: Unknown

Synergists: Not applicable

Antagonists: Not applicable

Indications for treatment

- Soreness on surface of the sternum
- Deep, intense pain internally deep to the sternum

Special notes

Sternalis remains one of the great mysteries of modern anatomy. Since function is unknown and no apparent movement has been determined, the evolution of this muscle continues to intrigue those who study the locomotor system. To add to the mysterious nature of this anomalous muscle, its presence is highly variable, it may be unilateral or, if bilateral, may not be symmetrical in length or size and its attachments as well as innervation are unpredictable.

It is present on average 4.4% of the time but cadaver studies range from 1.7% to 14.3% (Simons et al 1998). It is half as likely to be bilateral as unilateral though, when present, is likely to develop trigger points following acute myocardial infarction or angina pectoralis and needlessly prolong the fear associated with the pain of heart attack (Simons et al 1998).

NMT techniques for sternalis are presented with pectoralis major (p. 364).

Coracobrachialis (Fig. 13.74)

Attachments: From the coracoid process to mid-way along the medial border of the humeral shaft (between the triceps and brachialis muscle)
Innervation: Musculocutaneous nerve (C6–7)
Muscle type: Postural (type 1), shortens when stressed
Function: Flexes the arm forward and adducts it, seats the humeral head into the glenoid fossa during abduction, may assist in returning the arm to neutral position
Synergists: *Flexion of humerus*: anterior deltoid, biceps brachii (short head), pectoralis major
Antagonists: *To flexion*: latissimus dorsi, posterior deltoid, teres major, triceps (long head)

Indications for treatment

- Pain in front of shoulder and down the posterior arm
- Pain when reaching across the lower back

Special notes

This muscle's position allows it to be stretched with both medial and lateral rotation of the humerus. It assists in adduction and may (uniquely) assist in hyperabduction as well by pulling the arm toward the mid-line in both of these vertical positions.

Approximately half of its belly can be touched directly beneath the skin before it courses deep to pectoralis major

on its way to the coracoid process. The practitioner's thumb may slide under pectoralis major to touch an additional small portion of this muscle. The practitioner must exercise caution on the inner surface of the upper humerus to avoid pressing on the neurovascular bundle which courses posterior to coracobrachialis by palpating for the arterial pulse and remaining anterior to the pulse.

Assessment for strength of coracobrachialis (Janda 1983)

- Patient is seated, arm alongside trunk, internally rotated, elbow flexed.
- The practitioner offers a stabilizing contact to the shoulder from above, hand resting directly over the joint.
- The practitioner's other hand is placed on the distal aspect of the upper arm, above the elbow, offering counterforce/resistance as the patient attempts to flex the upper arm to 90°.
- Both sides should be tested and compared for relative strength.

 ## NMT for coracobrachialis

With the patient resting supine, her arm is abducted to 90° with the forearm supinated and the upper arm supported by the table. This position will allow access to the medial aspect of the upper arm and allow room for the practitioner's hands to glide proximally when they are correctly positioned.

To assess coracobrachialis, the thumbs are placed on the medial surface of the upper humerus at mid-level and posterior to the biceps brachii while avoiding the neurovascular bundle mentioned previously (Fig. 13.75). A muscle test of horizontal adduction (resisted above the elbow as the upper arm is raised toward the ceiling) will help define the lower fibers of coracobrachialis for palpation. The practitioner applies proximal gliding strokes 7–8 times directly on the portion of coracobrachialis which is available. As pectoralis major is encountered, the thumbs slide deep to it to continue gliding as high as possible on coracobrachialis.

Trigger point pressure release methods may be used by pressing the muscle against the humeral shaft. However, care must be taken to avoid the artery and nerves coursing posterior to the muscle. Palpation of the pulse and then positioning the hands to avoid the pulse is required to safely treat this muscle.

The coracoid attachment of coracobrachialis has been discussed with pectoralis minor in the supine position (p. 367). In that procedure, friction is applied through pectoralis major while transversing the fibers of pectoralis minor, coracobrachialis and short head tendon attachment of biceps brachii while avoiding the neurovascular structures deep to these tissues.

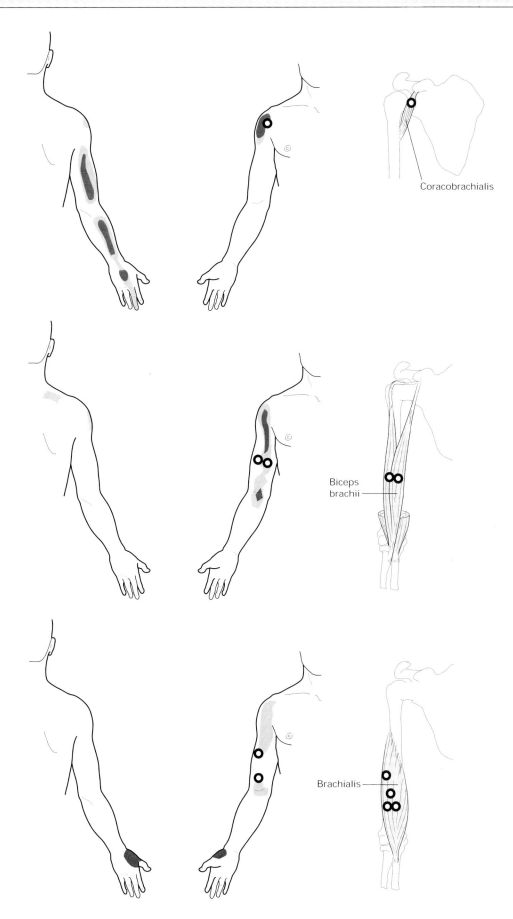

Figure 13.74 Biceps and brachialis both refer similar patterns to the anterior upper arm while brachialis also extends to the thumb.

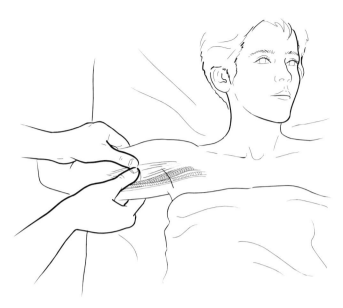

Figure 13.75 The neurovascular structures located nearby are avoided by muscle testing for location of coracobrachialis.

 MFR for coracobrachialis (Fig. 13.76)

• An area of restriction or fibrotic change is palpated for and identified in the accessible part of the muscle, i.e. in its distal third mid-way along the medial border of the humeral shaft (between the triceps and brachialis muscles).

• A flat thumb contact is made by the practitioner slightly distal to the dysfunctional tissues.

• The patient lies close to the edge of the table with the elbow flexed and the shoulder externally rotated.

• The practitioner's thumb introduces slight but firm compression, as the patient slowly and deliberately extends both the elbow and the humerus at the shoulder, before returning to the commencement position.

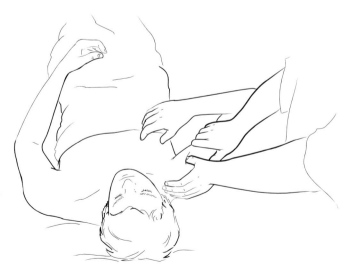

Figure 13.76 Myofascial release of coracobrachialis.

• The lengthening of the muscle during the extension aspect of this movement will draw the dysfunctional tissue under the compressive thumb contact.

• The procedure is repeated 3–5 times.

 PRT for coracobrachialis

• Patient is seated with the practitioner standing behind.

• The practitioner identifies a point of tenderness on the anteromedial aspect of the coracoid process.

• The palpating hand cups the shoulder while a finger of that hand makes contact on the tender point and applies pressure to it, sufficient to have the patient ascribe a value of '10' to the discomfort.

• With his other hand the practitioner eases the ipsilateral arm into extension and introduces internal rotation at the shoulder, with the dorsum of the patient's hand being placed flat against her back.

• The patient is asked to report the pain score and fine tuning of the arm position is carried out to achieve a reduction in the pain score of at least 50%.

• Fine tuning is then increased, for example the patient's flexed elbow may be eased anteriorly, increasing internal rotation at the shoulder, to further reduce the reported score.

• Additional fine-tuning methods to reduce pain scores further might include:

1. the hand on the shoulder applying light (1 lb maximum) inferomedial 'crowding' of the shoulder contact towards the painful point or
2. crowding of the acromioclavicular joint by long-axis compression of the humerus in a cephalad direction (1 lb force at most).

• Once pain is reduced by 70%, the position is held for not less than 90 seconds, before a slow return of the arm to a neutral position and a reassessment of function and tenderness is performed.

Biceps brachii

Attachments: *Short head*: Apex of the coracoid process
Long head: supraglenoid tubercle of the scapula at the apex of the glenoid cavity to a common tendon merging the two heads and attaching to the posterior surface of the radial tuberosity with additional expansions (bicipital aponeurosis) blending into the deep fascia of the forearm on the ulnar side
Innervation: Musculocutaneous nerve (C5–6)
Muscle type: Postural (type 1), shortens when stressed
Function: Supination of the forearm (when elbow is at least slightly flexed), elbow flexion (strongest with the forearm supinated), assists flexion of the shoulder joint (when medially rotated), stabilizes the humeral head against upward translation when deltoid contracts and against downward translation when the dependent

arm is weighted, assists abduction of the arm (when laterally rotated), horizontal adduction of the arm, eccentric (lengthening) contractions when extending the weighted forearm, brings the humerus toward the forearm when the forearm is fixed (such as in pull-ups)

Synergists: *Supination*: supinator

Elbow flexion: brachialis and brachioradialis

Flexion of shoulder: anterior deltoid, pectoralis major

Abduction of the arm: middle deltoid, supraspinatus

Adduction of the arm: pectoralis major (clavicular portion), coracobrachialis

Antagonists: *To supination*: pronator teres, pronator quadratus

To elbow flexion: triceps brachii

To flexion of shoulder: posterior deltoid, triceps brachii (long head)

To adduction of the arm: middle deltoid, supraspinatus

To abduction of the arm: pectoralis major (clavicular portion), coracobrachialis

Indications for treatment

- Shoulder pain (superficial anterior)
- Pain when supinating or when forearm flexion is overloaded
- Snapping or crackling sounds as the arm is abducted
- Pain or weakness when elevating the hand higher than the head

Special notes

The biceps brachii is discussed here with the shoulder and is followed by a full discussion of the elbow joint since it crosses both of these joints. Additionally, note that the triceps also crosses both joints and is discussed briefly with the elbow (supine position). The reader is referred to p. 342 for a full discussion of the triceps brachii.

The biceps brachii is a complex shoulder muscle as it crosses three joints (glenohumeral, humeroulnar, humeroradial) and consists of two heads (sometimes three) whose shape and length are different from each other. A third head anomaly is noted by some authors as present in 1–10% of cases (*Gray's anatomy* 1995, Platzer 1992, Simons et al 1998).

The long, narrow tendon of the lateral head lies in the intertubercular groove and courses through the joint capsule enclosed in a double tubular sheath which is continuous with the joint capsule. It is held in the groove by the transverse humeral ligament. When this ligament is torn free, the long head tendon may 'pop' as it dislocates from the groove during lateral and medial rotation. When the tendon ruptures completely, the humeral head rises conspicuously and the muscle belly bulks on the anterior surface of the arm.

The short head tendon is thick and flattened. It does not attach to or pierce the joint capsule but instead runs slightly diagonally (anterior to the subscapularis tendon) to attach at the coracoid process with the coracobrachialis and pectoralis minor. It lies deep to the deltoid and pectoralis major's usually thick mass.

Passive supination of the forearm and slight lateral rotation of the humerus places biceps brachii in the most ideal position for palpation. The long head tendon may be more easily felt with full lateral rotation of the humerus. Additionally, strumming laterally across the medial tendon (short head) and medially across the lateral tendon (long head) will help the practitioner to more consistently feel them through the often thick mass of overlying deltoid muscle.

A portion of the tendon of subscapularis may be addressed between the two proximal bicipital tendons and can be a source of pain when recurrent bicipital tendinitis has been diagnosed. A bursa lies horizontally between the tendon and the joint capsule and communicates with the capsule between the superior and middle glenohumeral ligaments. Ice applications may be needed on the anterior shoulder if inflammation of the subscapular or bicipital tendons is suspected. Subscapularis is further discussed on p. 353.

Assessment for strength of biceps brachii

- Janda (1983) reports: *'It must be remembered that biceps brachii is the most important [elbow] flexor. Differentiation … is a means of deciding on future treatment and the arm should therefore be positioned so that biceps brachii can act as the principal flexor … A slight weakness of biceps brachii only shows on testing if the movement starts from maximal extension'.*
- Patient is supine with arm outstretched, abducted and externally rotated from the shoulder to 90°, palm upwards.
- The practitioner places one hand, palm upwards, on the posterior surface of the distal upper arm, above the elbow.
- The other hand is placed palm downwards on the proximal forearm, above the wrist.
- The practitioner introduces *light* hyperextension of the patient's elbow, utilizing the contact on the lower arm for leverage.
- The patient is asked to introduce flexion at the elbow against this resistance.
- Relative strength of biceps brachii is compared on each side.

Assessment for shortness and MET treatment of biceps brachii

- The patient sits on the treatment table, with the practitioner seated alongside, on the side of the dysfunctional arm.

- The practitioner supports the elbow with the hand nearest the patient while the other hand holds the patient's proximal wrist area (patient's forearm supinated), introducing slight elbow extension (the slack is removed, this is not a forced extension).
- If there is biceps brachii shortness elbow extension will be limited and possibly painful.
- To treat this shortness using MET, the patient is asked to attempt to flex the elbow for 7–10 seconds, using minimal effort, resisted by the practitioner.
- Following the contraction the degree of extension is increased with patient assistance and the stretch held for not less than 20 seconds.
- The process is repeated 2–3 times more.

 ### NMT for biceps brachii

The patient is lying supine with the arm resting on the table for support and the forearm passively supinated. The anterior humerus is lightly lubricated and the thumbs are used to glide proximally, in thumb-width segments, from the crease of the elbow to the head of the humerus to address the entire belly of the biceps brachii. Medially placed gliding strokes address the short head while laterally placed strokes assess long head fibers and are repeated 7–8 times on each segment while evidence of tenderness, thickness or taut fibers is assessed within the bellies of the biceps brachii.

Gently applied transverse friction can be used on both bicipital bellies to assess for muscular nodules and taut bands, both characteristics of trigger points. When thickness, taut fibers or trigger point nodules are located, pincer compression can be used to lift and differentiate the biceps brachii from the brachialis, which lies deep to it (Fig. 13.77). Trigger points found within its bellies may be treated with compression techniques, either by lifting and compressing the fibers or by pressing them against the deeper belly of brachialis.

With the forearm passively supinated, the groove between the ulna and radius is located and the patient is asked to mildly flex the elbow against resistance while the practitioner contacts the tendon area with a thumb or finger (Fig. 13.78). Contraction of the radial attachment of the biceps brachii and the ulnar attachment of brachialis will make their location obvious. The patient should relax the arm before the tendon is treated with static pressure or mild friction. A bicipitoradial bursa protects the tendon from the radial tuberosity (see discussion of the elbow joints next).

To address the proximal tendons of the biceps brachii (through the deltoid), the short head tendon on the anterior upper humerus and the long head tendon on the lateral upper humerus are both located (Fig. 13.79). These tendons feel very tubular and are slightly larger in diameter than the shaft of a pencil. The strumming

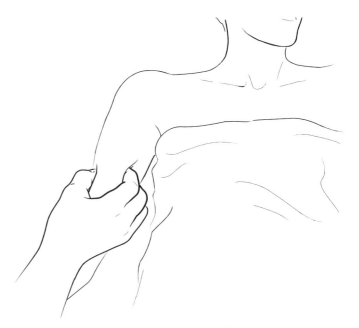

Figure 13.77 The biceps and brachialis may be grasped individually and compressed between the thumb and fingers.

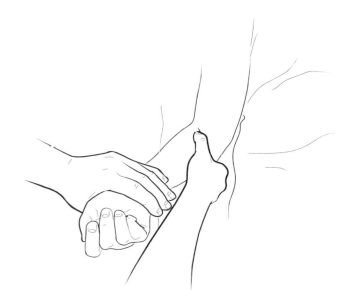

Figure 13.78 Lightly resisted flexion with the forearm supinated will contract the tendon of biceps to identify its specific attachment so as to avoid the neurovascular structures nearby.

techniques used to locate the tendons (mentioned above) may also be used as a treatment step or transverse (snapping) friction may be used if the tissue is not inflamed. Additionally, gliding strokes are applied proximally to soothe the tissues following the frictional techniques. Short gliding strokes are applied (through the deltoid) between the bicipital tendons to address the subscapularis tendon which lies between the two bicipital tendons and deep to the deltoid.

Biceps brachii and triceps brachii cross both the shoulder

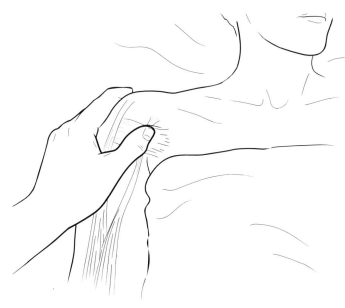

Figure 13.79 The short and long tendons of biceps are identified with transverse palpation. Subscapularis tendon fills the space between the two.

and the elbow joints. Triceps brachii is discussed on p. 342 and an additional supine approach is given (see p. 384) after the discussion of the elbow joint.

 MET for painful biceps brachii tendon (long head) (Fig. 13.80)

- Patient is seated with practitioner behind.
- The patient is asked to take her hand behind her back

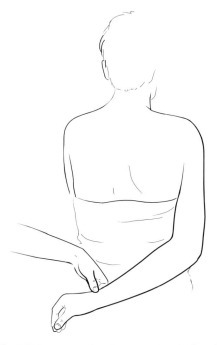

Figure 13.80 MET treatment for biceps tendon dysfunction.

and to place the dorsum of that hand against the contralateral buttock.
- The practitioner holds the patient's hand and gently takes it into pronation, taking out the slack.
- The patient is asked to attempt to lightly turn the hand into a supinated position against resistance offered by the practitioner.
- After 7–10 seconds the patient ceases the effort and the practitioner (assisted by the patient) increases the degree of pronation at the same time as extending the elbow and further adducting the arm.
- This stretch is held for at least 20 seconds.
- The process is repeated 2–3 times.

PRT for biceps brachii

There are two tender points associated with biceps brachii: in the bicipital groove (long head) and on the inferolateral surface of the coracoid process (short head).

Long head

- The practitioner locates an area of tenderness in the bicipital groove and applies sufficient pressure to have the patient ascribe a value of '10' to the discomfort.
- The practitioner eases the patient's arm into a position in which it rests, elbow flexed, with the dorsum of the lower arm against the patient's forehead.
- The practitioner fine tunes this position until the reported tenderness score is reduced by at least 70%.
- A greater degree of 'score' reduction is usually possible by the addition of a small degree of pressure (0.5 kilos, 1 lb maximum) applied from the elbow through the long axis of the humerus to 'crowd' the shoulder joint.

Short head

- The practitioner locates an area of tenderness on the inferolateral surface of the coracoid process and applies sufficient pressure to have the patient ascribe a value of '10' to the discomfort.
- The position of ease which reduces the pain score in this tender point is found by the practitioner taking the patient's internally rotated arm, flexed at the elbow, into adduction.
- Once pain is reduced by 70% in either of these positions, it is held for not less than 90 seconds, before a slow return of the arm to a neutral position and a reassessment of function and tenderness is performed.

ELBOW

The mechanical advantages which the shoulder joint offers include the ability to achieve an amazing range of positions. The elbow has a more limited ability but its use is absolutely critical to normal daily functioning. Its bending action allows food to be brought to the mouth, the upper body to be scratched and many other daily activities which are performed literally without thought. This joint's design also permits the hand and forearm to be rotated, which allows us to turn doorknobs, use screwdrivers and open jar lids.

The two distinct functions of the elbow joint – flexion/ extension and supination/pronation – are discussed individually though they are often used in combination during real movement. For instance, for food to be placed in the mouth, the arm begins in extension with pronation and ends in flexion with supination. Eating would indeed look different if either of these actions were not possible.

INTRODUCTION TO ELBOW TREATMENT

Before beginning treatment of the elbow, postural distortions of the body's framework should be observed and a distinction made between structural and muscular causes. Inability of the arm to hang straight at the side, loss of range of motion at the elbow joint, functional arm length differences and vertical plane deviations of the torso all suggest biomechanical challenges for which the elbow (and other joints) may be compensating. For instance, when shoulder motion is restricted, compensations might involve more distal portions of the extremity, placing undue stress on the elbow, wrist or hand.

The patient should be asked to demonstrate to the practitioner the sort(s) of work activities and positions, seated and standing, which are performed on a daily basis. Long hours without breaks are often spent at office and home office desks with little attention given to ergonomic (postural) design of the workspace. The postural and use causes of repetitive stress disorders involving the forearm muscles and strains of the arm, wrist, shoulder, neck and torso need to be addressed if long-lasting relief is to be achieved. Frequent breaks, coupled with stretches and movement therapy, should be part of both recovery and preventive programs.

When addressing pain in the elbow, forearm and hand, it is important to treat trigger points in the torso and shoulder girdle muscles as well as nerve compression possibilities at the spinal level and potential entrapment sites along the nerve's path. The cervical region should be assessed in all hand, arm or shoulder pain patterns, including the thoracic outlet and subclavicular area (such as pectoralis minor, which should be tested for potential encroachment upon neurovascular space).

STRUCTURE AND FUNCTION

The elbow joint is the intermediate joint of the arm, which links the forearm to the upper arm and allows the upper extremity to bend and the forearm to rotate. The proximal radioulnar joint, the humeroradial joint and the humeroulnar joint together form the compound joint usually referred to as the elbow. These three joints work in combination together to provide:

- flexion/extension – by the humeroradial and humeroulnar joints
- pronation/supination – by the humeroradial and radioulnar joints.

Stability of these joints is provided by bony support of the apposition of the trochlea of the humerus and the trochlear notch of the ulna and also the ligamentous support of the annular and collateral ligaments. Additionally, a joint capsule encloses the structure, housing all three joints within the capsule.

Humeroulnar joint

This joint is formed where the trochlea of the humerus, a spoon-shaped surface, is met by the trochlear notch of the ulnar. The longitudinal ridge of the ulnar head fits into the channel of the trochlea while the concave surfaces on either side of the ridge correspond to the lips of the trochlea The ulnar head's anterior edge, the coronoid process, and its posterior edge, the olecranon process, slide within the channel during flexion and extension, this joint's only movement. Posteriorly, on the distal end of the humerus, the olecranon fossa receives the protrusive olecranon process of the ulna when the elbow is fully extended.

Humeroradial joint

This joint is formed where the capitulum of the humerus, a hemispherical surface, is met by the concave fovea of the radial head. This ball and socket joint allows for flexion and extension as well as rotational movements. The radial head is stabilized by the annular ligament. This ligament, which encircles the radial head and attaches at both ends to the ulna, allows rotation and flexion/ extension while forbidding lateral and medial excursions of the head of the radius. By stabilizing the ulna and radius together, the annular ligament ensures that these two joints act as one during flexion and extension.

Radioulnar joint

This pivotal joint is formed where the rounded circumference of the radial head fits against the radial notch of the ulna. While the proximal ulna remains stable during pronation and supination, the radius spins inside the annular ligament against the ulna and against the ball-shaped distal surface of the capitulum of the humerus. During this spinning action, the shaft of the radius rotates around the ulna which flips the forearm and hand over. Pronation and supination can occur at any point during flexion and extension if these radial joints are functional.

The interosseous membrane provides a continuing fibrous joint between the radius and ulna for the full length of the two bones. This membrane prevents upslip or displacement of the two bones and also acts to transmit pressure stresses from one bone to the other. It is an extremely strong fibrous network which provides a place for muscular attachment as well as tremendous structural support for the forearm. In fact, during structural distress, the radius and ulna are prone to fracture before the fibers of the membrane are torn (Platzer 1992).

Assessment of bony alignment of the epicondyles (Fig. 13.81)

- Patient's arm is hanging at her side.
- Practitioner, standing behind, places thumb on medial epicondyle, index finger on olecranon, middle finger on lateral epicondyle.
- When elbow is fully extended the three contacts should form a straight line.
- When the elbow is flexed to 90° they should form an inverted triangle.
- Traumatic insults, for example to radioulnar articulation, may alter these alignments.

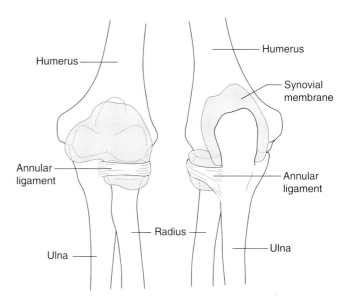

Figure 13.82 The head of the radius 'spins' inside the confines of the annular ligament (anterior and posterior views).

The ligaments of the elbow

- The *joint capsule* is thin and lax and is continuous with the *annular ligament*, a strong band which encircles the head of the radius.
- The *medial ligament (ulnar collateral ligament)* is a thick triangular band, comprising an anterior and posterior band which unite at a thin intermediate portion.
- The *anterior* part attaches superiorly, via its apex, to the medial epicondyle of the humerus and inferiorly, via its base, to the medial margin of the coronoid process.
- The *posterior* part is also triangular which attaches superiorly to the posterior aspect of the medial epicondyle and inferiorly to the medial margin of the olecranon.
- The *intermediate* fibers run from the medial epicondyle to an *oblique band* which joins the olecranon and the coronoid processes.
- The *lateral ligament (radial collateral ligament)* is attached superiorly to the distal aspect of the lateral epicondyle of the humerus and inferiorly to the annular ligament.

Assessment for ligamentous stability

- Patient is seated or supine.
- Practitioner holds patient proximal to the wrist, to avoid undue stress on the joints (this is the practitioner's 'motive hand') while the other hand cups the distal humerus ('stabilizing hand').
- The patient is asked to slightly flex the elbow (i.e. the procedure is not performed in hyperextension) and the practitioner introduces a translation action at the elbow by means of a medial push with the motive hand and a simultaneous lateral push with the stabilizing hand, followed by a reversal of these two directions of push.

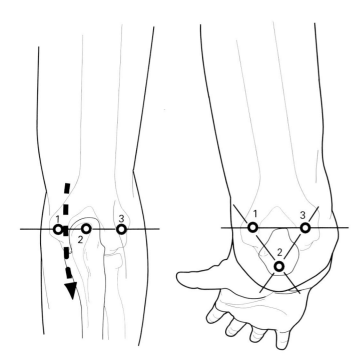

Figure 13.81 1. Medial epicondyle. 2. Olecranon. 3. Lateral epicondyle. Horizontal bony alignment becomes equilateral triangle during elbow flexion.

● As these side-shift – translation – movements are gently and repetitively carried out, the stabilizing hand notes whether a normal degree of slight gapping is taking place as the valgus and varus stresses are applied.

EVALUATION

CAUTION: Avoid testing (active or passive) for range of motion if there exists the possibility of dislocation, fracture, advanced pathology or profound soft tissue damage (tear).

There are three important reflex tests which help to evaluate the neural integrity of the upper extremity. They are placed here with the elbow since they are examined at the elbow, but they are commonly also used when evaluating the shoulder and cervical region.

Biceps reflex

● This evaluates the integrity of nerve supply from C5 level.
● The seated patient's forearm is placed so that it rests on the practitioner's forearm.
● The practitioner cups the medial aspect of the patient's elbow so that his thumb can be placed in the cubital fossa.
● The patient's arm must be relaxed.
● The practitioner taps his own thumbnail with a neurologic hammer and the biceps should jerk slightly to the extent that it is both visible and palpable.

Brachioradialis reflex

● This evaluates the integrity of nerve supply from C6 level.
● The arm is supported in precisely the same manner as in the biceps reflex test above.
● The brachioradialis tendon at the distal end of the radius is tapped (the tendon is tapped, not the practitioner's thumbnail) with the neurologic hammer and a palpable and visible jump should occur in brachioradialis.

Triceps reflex

● This evaluates the integrity of nerve supply from C7 level.
● The arm is supported in precisely the same manner as in the biceps reflex test above.
● The triceps tendon where it crosses the olecranon fossa is tapped (the tendon is tapped, not the practitioner's thumbnail) with the neurologic hammer and a palpable and visible jump should occur in triceps.
● Note:
  1. an increase in normal reflex activity may indicate upper motor neuron disease

  2. a decrease in normal reflex activity may indicate a lower motor neuron lesion (such as a herniated disc).

RANGES OF MOTION OF THE ELBOW

The neutral position of reference for the elbow joint occurs when the forearm and upper arm are in a straight line (Fig. 13.83). Hence, the range of motion for true extension of the elbow is actually 0°, since the forearm does not extend beyond neutral, except in a few subjects with hyperextension conditions due to ligamentous laxity. However, the term 'relative extension' is used when the forearm is returned toward a neutral position from any point of flexion.

The forearm is flexed when it is brought toward the anterior aspect of the upper arm. Active flexion produces a range of 135–145° (Hoppenfeld 1976, Kapandji 1982) with an additional 15° available with passive assistance. During active flexion, various muscles will contract, depending upon the rotational position of the forearm.

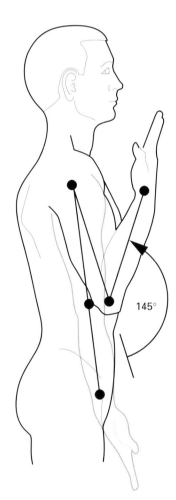

Figure 13.83 From neutral to full range of flexion of the elbow joint. Relative extension returns the forearm back to neutral while true extension of the elbow (beyond neutral) is termed hyperextension.

Both active and passive range of motion tests may be used to assess limits of movement of the elbow joint. Bilateral comparison is possible by both sides performing action simultaneously. If active testing shows normal range without pain or discomfort, passive tests are usually not necessary but with elbow flexion an additional 15° of flexion may be achieved with assistance.

Restrictions which have a hard end-feel during passive range of motion assessment are usually joint related. Restrictions which have a softer end-feel, with slight springiness still available at the end of range, are usually due to extraarticular soft tissue dysfunction.

Range of motion and strength tests

• Range of motion tests are performed both actively and passively involving flexion (135–145°), extension (0°), forearm pronation and supination (90° each).
• Strength is tested with the practitioner (standing in front of the patient) cupping the flexed (to 90°) elbow with one hand ('stabilizing hand') while the other hand holds the patient proximal to the wrist.
• As the patient attempts to extend the elbow, the relative strength of triceps and anconeus is being evaluated. Neural supply to these muscles is from C7 and C8.
• The patient begins with the forearm pronated and the practitioner restricts this position as the patient attempts to supinate against resistance. This evaluates relative strength of biceps, supinator and possibly brachioradialis. Neural supply is from C5 and C6.
• The patient begins with the forearm supinated and the practitioner restricts this position as the patient attempts to pronate against resistance. This evaluates the relative strength of pronator teres, pronator quadratus and flexor carpi radialis. Neural supply is from C6–8 and T1.

Elbow stress tests

• Patient is seated or supine.
• Practitioner holds patient's arm proximal to the wrist, to avoid undue stress on the wrist joints (this is the practitioner's 'motive hand') while the other hand cups the distal humerus ('stabilizing hand').
• With the arm relaxed, normal range of motion is assessed involving flexion, extension, pronation and supination.
• Any pain or restriction of motion should be noted.
• These symptoms could involve tendinitis, joint pathology or contractures.
• If these tests are negative (i.e. if no pain or restriction is noted), the same movements are then carried out against resistance. The practitioner notes which soft tissues are being lengthened (stretched) if pain or restriction is noted. And these tissues are investigated further by means of active patient movements and/or by palpation.

• The same movements are also observed with the patient actively and slowly performing them (more than once to gain insight into normal behavior). The practitioner notes which soft tissues are reported as being painful and these structures are subsequently palpated for dysfunction or assessed for shortness.

Strains or sprains

• Bicipital attachment to the radius may be traumatized on hyperextension injuries. Palpation of the tendon will reveal extreme tenderness. Rest (in a sling) for a few days, plus appropriate sprain therapy (ice, etc.), is advised.
• Hyperpronation or hypersupination injuries may result in limitation to rotation and pain. The radial head may actually dislocate.
• If forced abduction or adduction occurs rupture of the capsular apparatus, including ligamentous attachments to humerus, radius or ulna, is possible.
• If a fall occurs in which the outstretched arm absorbs the compression injury, damage to the dorsiflexed wrist (stretching the ventral soft tissues), the extended elbow or the shoulder is possible. The age of the individual – and therefore tissue elasticity – will usually influence where damage occurs (e.g. wrist fracture in elderly, distal humerus in younger individuals).
• With hyperextension strain of the elbow, the following could all be swollen and tender on palpation: posterior capsule, bicipital tendon, olecranon fossa, medial and lateral collateral ligaments, flexor attachments at medial epicondyle. Pain will usually be eased by moving the tissues in a direction which would reproduce the strain – see positional release notes on pp. 147, 388 and 407.
• With hyperabduction strain, tenderness of the ulnar collateral ligament, below the lateral epicondyle, is usual. Pain is usually eased by taking the joint in a direction which would reproduce the strain – see positional release notes on pp. 147, 388 and 407).
• With hyperadduction strain, tenderness of the radial collateral ligament, below the medial epicondyle, is usual. Pain is usually eased by taking the joint in a direction which would reproduce the strain – see positional release notes on pp. 147, 388 and 407).

INDICATIONS FOR TREATMENT (DYSFUNCTIONS/SYNDROMES)
Carpal tunnel syndrome

Carpal tunnel syndrome is caused by compression of the median nerve within the carpal tunnel. Compression of the nerve may be the result of:

• subluxation of carpal bones (lunate in particular)
• entrapment by scar tissue
• excessive pressure within the tunnel due to enlarged flexor tendons

- abnormal tissue, such as osteophytes or tumors, within the canal
- excessive fluid retention.

Unfortunately, in recent years, carpal tunnel syndrome has become a collective diagnosis for many hand and wrist dysfunctions without precise testing of median nerve dysfunction. Since many trigger points in shoulder, neck and forearm muscles duplicate the symptoms of carpal tunnel syndrome, a full evaluation, assessment and treatment of these various muscles is indicated.

While carpal tunnel syndrome remains the most common nerve entrapment syndrome of the upper extremity, cubital tunnel syndrome runs a close second place (Simons et al 1998), due to increased computer usage with resultant poor hand and arm positioning.

The cubital tunnel, positioned on the posterior aspect of the medial epicondyle, is formed by the cubital groove (floor of the tunnel) and an aponeurotic band (roof of the tunnel) which stabilizes the nerve during movement (Fig. 13.84). During flexion, the retinacular band becomes more taut and closes in on the tunnel's space. This may irritate or compress the ulnar nerve as it passes through the tunnel. Additionally, if the wrist is extended and the shoulder is held is less than ideal position, pressure may be further increased within the tunnel. Resting the elbow of the pronated arm on the desk while working may also irritate this superficial portion of the ulnar nerve.

A few inches more proximally, the nerve passes under the 'arcade of Struthers' as the nerve enters deep to the medial head of the triceps. This dense fascial arch is another possible site of ulnar nerve entrapment and may produce similar symptoms to cubital tunnel syndrome, such as a medial epicondylar ache with accompanying shooting points to the little finger and ulnar portion of the hand (Cailliet 1996). The flexor carpi ulnaris may entrap the ulnar nerve as it lies deep to this muscle and superficial to the flexor digitorum profundus. Additionally, an anomalous muscle, the anconeus epitrochlearis (Simons et al 1998), may cause ulnar nerve compression when it is present.

Radial nerve entrapment

This may be produced by the long head of the triceps, the supinator and extensor carpi radials brevis as well as an anomalous flexor carpi radialis brevis muscle.

Median nerve entrapment

This may be produced by the pronator teres, flexor digitorum superficialis or the anomalous flexor digitorum superficialis indicis. Impingement of the nerve within the carpal tunnel may be due to subluxation of carpal bones, scar tissue or enlarged flexor tendons.

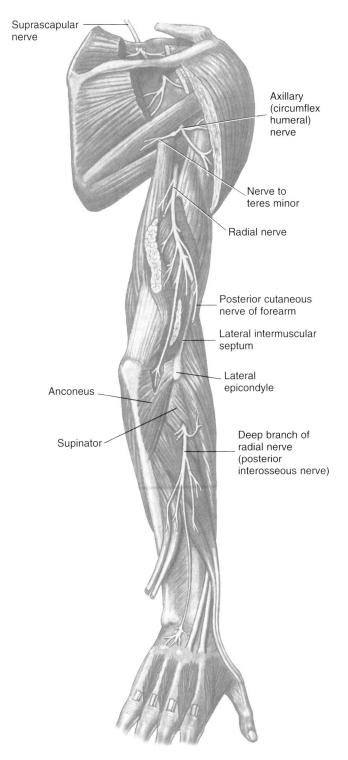

Figure 13.84 Nerve pathways of the upper limb, anterior aspect (reproduced, with permission, from *Gray's anatomy* (1995)).

Tenosynovitis ('tennis elbow' and/or 'golfer's elbow')

- This painful condition involves damage, inflammation and dysfunction associated with the epicondyles of the humerus.

• It may involve epicondylitis and/or radiohumeral bursitis.

• The cause is thought to be repetitive trauma to the joint involving supination or pronation of the wrist together with elbow extension (for 'tennis elbow').

• The result of repetitive stress of this type is for contraction to occur involving the extensor-supinator muscles of the forearm.

• It is possible for the radial nerve to be entrapped as part of the etiology.

• The medial epicondyle may also be involved in which case the flexor-pronator muscles of the forearm are implicated (a condition known as 'golfer's elbow' – see MET treatment recommendation for shortness of flexors of the wrist below).

• It is possible for calcification at the margin of the joint to occur or for lateral epicondyle erosion to take place. X-ray evidence would be needed to confirm these changes.

• Symptoms of lateral epicondylitis would usually include: severe, lancating, often radiating pain on extension of the elbow; residual dull aching pain at rest; squeezing actions produce cramp-like pain; inflammation evidence – heat and swelling – may be noted at the epicondyle; supination and pronation as well as grip strength will be diminished.

Assessments for tenosynovitis and epicondylitis

1. *Cozens test*. The practitioner stabilizes the patient's pronated forearm by cupping the elbow. The patient extends her clenched fist and the practitioner's other hand holds this and attempts to flex the wrist against the patient's resistance. If tenosynovitis exists there will be pronounced sudden pain reported at the lateral epicondyle as the contracting tendons provoke irritation at a very likely site of enthesitis.

2. *Mills test*. The patient clenches her fist, flexes the elbow and wrist, and pronates the arm. The practitioner offers resistance as the patient then attempts to supinate and extend the forearm and wrist. Pain noted at the lateral epicondyle confirms radiohumeral epicondylitis.

3. *Medial epicondyle test ('golfer's elbow')*. Patient flexes elbow to 90° and supinates the hand. The practitioner offers resistance as the patient then attempts to extend the elbow. If pain is noted, medial epicondylitis is suggested.

Box 13.14 Definition of enthesitis

Enthesitis: 'Traumatic disease occurring at the insertion of muscles where recurring concentrations of muscle stress provoke inflammation with a strong tendency toward fibrosis and calcification'. (Simons et al 1998)

TREATMENT

As previously discussed, biceps brachii and triceps brachii cross both the shoulder and elbow joints and should be assessed with joint dysfunctions of either of these joints. Since biceps brachii lies superficial to brachialis, it should be treated prior to the assessment of the deeper muscle (see p. 374).

Brachialis

Attachments: Distal half of the anterior surface of the humerus and intermuscular septa to the ulnar tuberosity, coronoid process and the joint capsule of the elbow
Innervation: Musculocutaneous and radial nerve (C5–6)
Muscle type: Postural (type 1), shortens when stressed
Function: Flexion of the forearm at the elbow joint
Synergists: *Flexion*: biceps brachii, brachioradialis, supinator
Antagonists: Triceps brachii

Indications for treatment

• Soreness of the thumb (referred zone)
• Anterior shoulder pain

Special notes

While most muscles perform more than one function, brachialis is one of the few muscles which provides only a single motion, that being flexion of the forearm. It provides this function whether the arm is supinated, pronated or resisted. It is quiet (no activity) when the arm is loaded in a fully dependent position and works best when the elbow is flexed to 90°.

Brachialis has the ability to entrap the radial nerve (cutaneous branch) and thereby causes symptoms of tingling, numbness and dysesthesia of the thumb and the webbed space beside it. These symptoms may also be referred from trigger points in brachioradialis, supinator and other muscles of the thumb, which should be treated as part of an overall examination.

NMT for brachialis

With the patient resting supine, the arm being treated is slightly passively flexed and tucked under the practitioner's arm. This position will allow room for the practitioner's hands to glide proximally when they are correctly positioned. The practitioner places one thumb on the medial side of the exposed portion of the brachialis and the other thumb on the lateral side of the exposed portion of the brachialis. The thumbs will be deep to the belly of the biceps and opposite each other on the sides of the anterior upper arm (Fig. 13.85).

With lubrication, the practitioner glides the thumbs

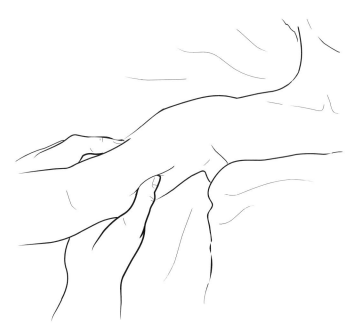

Figure 13.85 With both thumbs deep to the biceps, brachialis may be compressed as gliding strokes are applied simultaneously with both thumbs.

proximally, while simultaneously pressing them toward each other. This 'double-thumb' technique will entrap the brachialis as pressure is applied. The gliding process is repeated 7–8 times from the distal end until the deltoid is reached. Caution is exercised to avoid pressing on the neurovascular bundle on the medial upper arm by ending the stroke with both thumbs near the deltoid tuberosity as brachialis shifts laterally on the humerus.

The biceps brachii can usually be displaced slightly on both the medial and lateral aspects to allow access to a small portion of brachialis fibers. The forearm should be passively flexed and supinated for best access. Short, gliding strokes or pressure release methods may then be applied directly onto the brachialis muscle. Pressure applied through the biceps bellies will address the central portion of brachialis and can be used if the biceps brachii is not too tender.

Triceps and anconeus

A full discussion of triceps is offered on p. 342. Triceps is also placed here to offer an additional supine position treatment and to remind the reader that it should be assessed with all elbow dysfunctions as well as the previous shoulder conditions.

Tests for strength of triceps are given earlier in this chapter on p. 342.

NMT for triceps (alternative supine position)

The patient is supine and the practitioner stands cephalad to the shoulder to be treated. The shoulder may be placed in flexion with or without flexion of the elbow. If both joints are simultaneously moderately flexed, the triceps may be placed under excessive tension and may respond as extremely tender, especially at its attachment sites. It is therefore better to maintain one or both of these joints in partial flexion rather than full flexion.

The practitioner applies lubricated gliding strokes in segments to cover the entire surface of the posterior upper arm to assess the lateral and long heads of triceps brachii. The radial nerve lies deep to the lateral head and is vulnerable to entrapment by triceps (Simons et al 1998). The practitioner should avoid compression of the nerve while treating it.

The proximal glides may be repeated with increased pressure, if appropriate, to address the medial head of the triceps, which lies deep to the lateral and long heads. Additionally, the medial head lies superficial on both the medial and lateral aspects of the posterior arm just above the elbow and can be addressed in a manner similar to brachialis by using a 'double-thumb' technique.

To isolate the attachment of the long head of triceps on the infraglenoid tuberosity of the scapula, the thumb is slid proximally along the tendon which courses between teres major and teres minor. When the scapular attachment is reached, static pressure or mild friction can be used to assess and treat the attachment. Elbow extension is resisted to assure direct tendon contact. It may be necessary to muscle test for the two teres muscles as well since triceps passes between them before attaching to the scapula.

The olecranon attachment of the triceps is examined with finger friction or the small pressure bar. Pressure is placed directly on the tendon while the areas medial and lateral to the tendon are avoided due to vulnerable nerve passage.

NMT for anconeus (see also p. 344)

The anconeus, a small, triangular muscle positioned just lateral and distal to the olecranon process, is easily addressed when treating the olecranon attachment of triceps. It extends the elbow and may serve to stabilize the elbow joint during pronation of the forearm by securing the ulna. The articularis cubiti (subanconeus muscle) is a small slip of the medial head of the triceps and, when present, may insert into the capsule of the elbow joint.

The anconeus is easily isolated by placing an index finger on the olecranon process and the second finger on the lateral epicondyle with the practitioner's hand flat against the patient's forearm. The anconeus lies between the two fingers, which are moved when treatment is applied. Short glides between the ulna and radius (in the space between what the fingers have outlined) will address this small muscle which is often involved in elbow pain.

MET for triceps is described earlier in this section on p. 344.

Brachioradialis

Attachments: Proximal two-thirds of the lateral supracondylar ridge of the humerus and intermuscular septum to the (proximal) lateral surface of the styloid process of the radius
Innervation: Radial nerve (C5 and C6)
Muscle type: Postural (type 1), shortens when stressed
Function: Flexes the elbow and stabilizes it during extension, brings it to neutral position (semisupinated)
Synergists: Biceps brachii, brachialis
Antagonists: Triceps

Indications for treatment

- Limited forearm movement
- Weakness
- Pain

Special notes

Brachioradialis is a forearm flexor in neutral position, acting on only one joint, the elbow. Controversy about its actions began when it was wrongly named supinator longus as its action was thought to supinate the forearm (Simons et al 1998). While its supposed function to return the arm to neutral from either a supinated or a pronated position has inspired debate, it does help prevent distraction of the elbow joint during rapid elbow movements.

While functioning as a flexor of the elbow, brachioradialis is sometimes grouped with the extensors of the wrist due to its proximity to them and its innervation by an extensor nerve. Its trigger point activity, somewhat like the wrist extensors, is into the elbow, forearm and the hand (web of the thumb) (see p. 410). It often becomes tender in association with the supinator and their similar pain patterns require examination of both when either is suspect. Its superficial location makes this muscle easily palpable and therefore successfully addressed with massage and stretching techniques.

Assessment for strength of brachioradialis

- The patient is supine with the arm at her side, elbow flexed to 75°, forearm semisupinated.
- The practitioner cups the patient's elbow with one hand to support it and offers resistance on the anterolateral aspect of the distal forearm.
- The patient is asked to resist the practitioner's effort to push the forearm into extension.
- The relative strength of each brachioradialis is tested.

 ## NMT for brachioradialis

With the forearm in a relaxed, semisupinated position and passively flexed at the elbow to near 90°, brachioradialis is grasped with pincer compression near its humeral attachment. Taut bands within the muscle are compressed between the thumb and fingers for 8–12 seconds and the compression techniques are applied at thumb-width intervals as far distally as possible. If tension and referred pain are discovered and compression is applied to the associated tissues, the patient should feel the discomfort fade as the pressure is sustained. If the discomfort or referred sensation does not fade within 8–12 seconds, the techniques are applied again with slightly less pressure. A deeper grasp may also address the extensor carpi radialis longus and brevis which lie deep to brachioradialis and are discussed with the forearm and wrist on p. 410.

The muscle fibers may also be rolled between the thumb and fingers to discover taut bands and nodules characteristic of trigger points. Trigger points are treated with pressure release techniques followed by stretching of the involved tissues.

The practitioner follows the manipulation of the fibers with lubricated gliding strokes from the styloid process to the humeral attachment. Hydrotherapy applications may precede or follow these procedures. Inflammation of the supinator muscle and epicondyles of the humerus should be ruled out before applying heat to the elbow region. Ice therapy may be applied to any of the muscles following therapy.

 ## MFR for brachioradialis

- The patient is seated with the arm at the side, elbow flexed, fist closed, thumb uppermost.
- The practitioner identifies brachioradialis by having the patient flex the elbow against resistance.
- The patient releases the fist, relaxes the muscle and palpation is performed to identify areas of contraction, fibrotic change or other evidence of altered tissue status.
- The practitioner applies a broad, flat, thumb compression a thumb width distal to the dysfunctional tissues, and with this thumb contact, slight soft tissue traction is introduced, from the attachments above the lateral epicondyle, to lengthen the fibers slightly.
- With the arm relaxed and semisupinated, the patient is asked to extend it fully (drawing the dysfunctional tissues under the compression force of the thumb) and then to return to the neutral starting position, while the firm compression contact is maintained.
- This procedure is repeated 3–4 times more

Supinator (see p. 409)

Attachments: Supinator crest of the ulna, lateral epicondyle of the humerus and the ligaments and joint capsule of the elbow to the lateral surface of the proximal third of the radius

Innervation: Radial nerve – deep (posterior interosseous) branch (C5 and C6, sometimes C7)

Muscle type: Postural (type 1), shortens when stressed

Function: Supinates the forearm by spinning the radius; forceful elbow flexion

Synergists: *Supination*: biceps brachii
  Elbow flexion: biceps brachii, brachioradialis

• **Antagonists**: *To supination*: pronator quardratus, pronator teres
  To elbow flexion: triceps, anconeus

Indications for treatment

• Elbow pain, such as in tennis elbow and golfer's elbow
• Lateral epicondylitis
• Pain when supinating, such as to twist a doorknob, open a jar or use a screwdriver
• Elbow pain when using the elbow in any movement
• Pain in the web of the thumb (referral zone)

Special notes

The supinator muscle comprises two flat layers of muscles which spiral around the radius to attach to the ulna. Contraction of its fibers will spin the radius against both the humerus (proximally) and the ulna (located to its medial side) to turn the palm and forearm toward the ceiling. Coursing between these two layers of muscle is the deep branch of the radial nerve, which lies vulnerable to entrapment by the supinator's fibers (Simons et al 1998). Weakness in the supinator itself is not likely to be caused by this particular entrapment syndrome since innervation to the supinator branches off the radial nerve before it enters the muscle.

Supinator trigger points and ischemic fibers are often created with overuse or strain of this muscle. Common supinator symptoms may be initiated by manual use of a screwdriver, either with a difficult-to-turn screw (strain) or with numerous screws (repetitive), sorting envelopes by flipping them into stack trays or postal boxes or straining to open a stuck jar lid or doorknob that is difficult to turn. Supinator very rapidly may become overly tender following an overuse or strain, while tending to rather urgently exhibit inflammatory symptoms and weakness (very likely from trigger points).

Weakness in the muscles innervated by the radial nerve, when not accompanied by pain, suggests nerve entrapment and may be caused by a tumor pressing on the nerve or some other lesion along its path (Simons et al 1998). While pain in the supinator area (tennis elbow) suggests a myofascial cause, including trigger points or enthesitis, it may or may not be accompanied by weakness of

muscles supplied by the radial nerve. When both pain in the supinator area and weakness of muscles supplied by the radial nerve are present, the cause is most likely myofascial trigger points with nerve entrapment due to taut bands within the muscle (Simons et al 1998).

Assessment for strength of supinator

• The patient is seated with elbow flexed to 90°, forearm pronated fully.
• The practitioner stabilizes the patient's arm against her trunk at the elbow and applies a resistance contact with the other hand to the distal forearm (Daniels & Worthingham 1980).
• The patient is asked to supinate the forearm as the practitioner evaluates the relative strength and compares one side with the other.

 ## NMT for supinator

The brachioradialis and extensor carpi muscles are displaced laterally and lubricated gliding strokes are applied directly on the supinator, which lies deep to it (Fig. 13.86). The superficial muscles are displaced medially and the gliding strokes repeated on the remainder of the supinator muscle. Only a small piece of the muscle may be reached

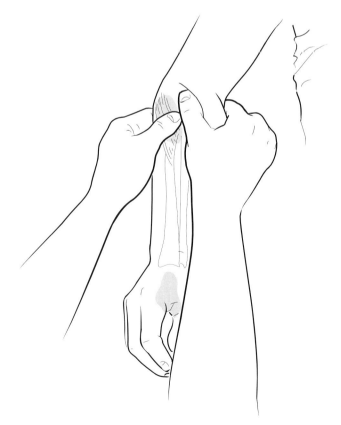

Figure 13.86 Supinator can entrap the radial nerve as well as refer to the elbow and web of thumb.

from each side of the overlying muscles. However, repeated gliding techniques, assisted pronation stretches and post-treatment ice applications usually achieve a degree of improvement.

MET for supinator shortness

- The patient is seated with elbow flexed to 90°, forearm pronated fully.
- The practitioner stabilizes the patient's arm against her trunk at the elbow and applies a resistance contact with the other hand to the proximal forearm.
- The patient is asked to supinate the forearm against resistance for 7–10 seconds using minimal force.
- After the isometric contraction the patient relaxes the arm completely and then attempts, with the practitioner's assistance, to pronate the forearm further.
- This stretch is held for at least 20 seconds.
- This treatment can be usefully self-applied, especially in cases of 'tennis elbow'.

MFR for supinator

- The practitioner palpates the supinator from the lateral epicondyle to its radial attachments and locates areas of dysfunction, fibrotic change or contraction.
- The patient's arm is flexed at the elbow and pronated and a flat thumb contact is made distal to the restricted soft tissue area.
- A light traction is applied to the soft tissues via the thumb along the long axis of the muscle and, while this is sustained, the patient is asked to slowly and deliberately move the forearm from pronation to supination while extending the elbow and then to return to the starting position (pronated forearm, flexed elbow).
- This is repeated 3–4 times.

Pronator teres

Attachments: *Humeral head*: medial epicondyle of humerus (common flexor tendon) and medial intermuscular septum
Ulnar head: coronoid process of the ulna to a common tendon at the pronator tuberosity of the radius approximately mid-shaft on the lateral surface of radius
Innervation: Median nerve (C6–7)
Muscle type: Not established
Function: Pronates the forearm by spinning the radius and contributes to flexion of the elbow against resistance
Synergists: Pronator quadratus, brachioradialis (assistance to a neutral position)
Antagonists: Supinator, biceps brachii

Indications for treatment

- Deep pain on radial side of the anterior surface of the wrist

- A diagnosis of carpal tunnel syndrome
- Pain upon full supination, especially if accompanied by extension of the elbow and cupping of the hand

Special notes

Pronator teres assists pronator quadratus (below) during rapid or forceful pronation of the forearm. In 83% of cases (*Gray's anatomy* 1995), the median nerve passes between the two heads of pronator teres as it enters the forearm and in some cases pierces the humeral head (Simons et al 1998). Sometimes the ulnar head is absent (Platzer 1992).

Assessment for strength of pronator teres

- The patient is supine with forearm in pronation.
- The patient's elbow is close to the trunk and is flexed to 60°.
- The practitioner stabilizes the patient's elbow against her trunk so that no abduction occurs during the test.
- With the other hand the practitioner holds the proximal lower forearm, close to the wrist, and asks the patient to resist as he attempts to supinate her forearm.
- Relative strength of pronator teres is assessed and compared on each side.

NMT for pronator teres

The arm is placed in passive supination with partial flexion of the elbow. The practitioner palpates below the crease of the elbow for pronator teres as it courses diagonally from the medial epicondyle to the mid-shaft of the radius. The muscle is wider near the epicondyle and narrows considerably before coursing deep to the brachioradialis and the radial wrist flexors. Resisted pronation will assist the practitioner in locating the fibers.

The practitioner applies unilateral transverse friction at thumb-width intervals from the proximal end of the muscle (Fig. 13.87) to the point at which its belly is no longer accessible. Static compression may also be applied to its fibers, if needed.

The distal attachment is sometimes palpable on the lateral shaft of the radius. Inflammation of the common flexor tendon may warrant ice applications to the medial epicondyle.

MFR for pronator teres

- The practitioner palpates and identifies an area of fibrotic or contracted tissues in pronator teres.
- He places a broad, flat thumb contact distal to the dysfunction, applying traction to the tissues along their fiber direction.
- To maintain firm and precise compression contact, the other thumb may be superimposed on the first.

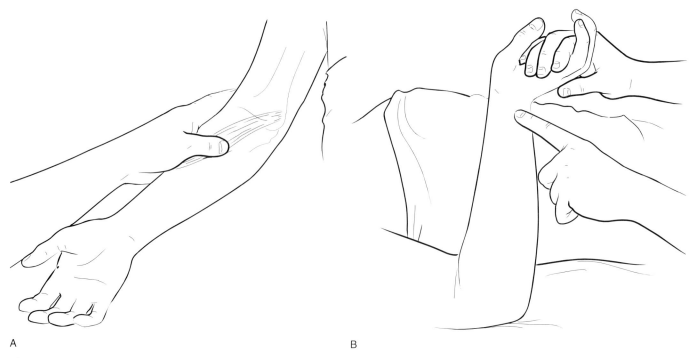

A   B

Figure 13.87   A: Pronator teres is palpated with transverse friction. B: Strain-counterstrain for wrist problems which often accompany pronator dysfunction (see p. 407).

• The patient is asked to slowly and deliberately fully pronate and then supinate her forearm.
• This is repeated 4–5 times for each area of dysfunction.

 ## PRT for pronator teres

• The patient is supine and the practitioner palpates for an area of tenderness anterior to the medial epicondyle of the humerus.
• Pressure is applied to this tender point, sufficient for the patient to register this as an intensity of '10'.
• While pressure is maintained on this point, the practitioner holds the proximal forearm and flexes the elbow until the pain 'score' drops appreciably.
• Fine-tuning maneuvers to reduce the score further include assessing the effect of various degrees of pronation and internal rotation of the humerus.
• Additional ease and therefore reduction in the pain score may be achieved by means of application of a light (half pound) compressive force, from the contact hand on the forearm through the long axes of the radius and ulna, toward the elbow joint.
• Once the pain score has dropped to 3 or less, the position is held for at least 90 seconds before a slow return to a neutral position and reassessment of function and discomfort.

Pronator quadratus

Attachments: Distal quarter of the anterior surface of the ulna to the distal quarter of the anterior surface of the radius
Innervation: Median nerve (C8–T1)
Muscle type: Not established
Function: Pronates the forearm by spinning the radius
Synergists: Pronator teres, brachioradialis (assistance to a neutral position)
Antagonists: Supinator, biceps brachii

Indications for treatment

• Pain upon full supination
• Weakness or inability to fully supinate

Special notes

Pronator quadratus is the primary pronator of the forearm and is assisted by pronator teres during rapid movements or when pronation is resisted. It occupies the deepest layer in the distal anterior forearm, occasionally has fibers reaching more proximal than noted or reaching distally to the carpal bones and is sometimes absent (Platzer 1992). Its trigger point patterns have not yet been established.

NMT for pronator quadratus

Pronator quadratus is the deepest of the anterior forearm muscles and lies directly against the interosseous membrane. A small portion of the muscle may be reached on both the radius and ulna by sliding the fingers or thumb (one or both sides at a time) under the more superficial muscles and applying friction to the distal 2–3 inches of the anterior shaft of the ulna and the radius. Caution should always be exercised to avoid compression of the radial artery and median nerve at the anterior wrist.

FOREARM, WRIST AND HAND

While the shoulder and elbow place the hand in a variety of positions and at various distances relative to the body, the fingers of the hand are designed for precise functional use in a seemingly endless number of ways. Kapandji (1982) offers: *'The human hand, despite its complexity, turns out to be a perfectly logical structure, fully adapted to its multiple functions. Its architecture reflects Occam's principle of universal economy. It is one of the most beautiful achievements of nature'.*

William of Occam (14th century) stated the principle of scientific parsimony thus: *'The assumptions introduced to explain a thing must not be multiplied beyond necessity'* (*Stedman's medical dictionary* 1998). We have attempted to provide an understanding of the simplest use of the hand and fingers while remaining astounded by its complexity. Among the numerous texts available on hand structure and function, Cailliet (1994), Hoppenfeld (1976), Simons et al (1998), Platzer (1992), *Gray's anatomy* (1995), Kapandji (1982) and Ward (1997) provided references to many of the components of this section.

FOREARM

Pronation and supination of the forearm occurs in the elbow region with the articulation of the radioulnar and radiohumeral joints, while the radius and ulna articulate distally with each other as well as with the proximal end of the hand, the carpal bones. The radius and ulna, along with their interosseous membrane, provide attachment sites for the extrinsic muscles of the hand and wrist and influence the ability to flex, extend and rotate at the elbow joint as well as allowing wrist flexion, extension and deviations. The ulna and radius therefore play a major role in the functional use of the hand.

Most of the muscles which lie in the forearm are extrinsic muscles of the hand. While some of these muscles provide movements of the wrist joint (positioning the whole hand) others provide mobility to the fingers or thumb which facilitates the power of the tennis grip,

the accuracy and delicacy of strokes on piano keys and the precision of the brain surgeon.

Postural distortion can create altered shoulder positioning, which may reflect in compensation patterns affecting the elbow, wrist and finger joints. Janda points out that as the upper body slumps and the shoulders round, the angle at which the humerus meets the glenoid fossa changes. The resulting alteration in the direction of the axis of the glenoid fossa causes the humerus to require stabilization by additional levator scapula and upper trapezius activity, with increased activity from supraspinatus as well. Additionally, there will be biomechanical adaptive changes involving the arm, elbow and wrist joints. Similarly, any inability to fully pronate the hand may demand considerable shoulder, torso and/or wrist repositioning. These examples give emphasis to the need to constantly keep in mind the larger picture, out of which the local dysfunction may have emerged. It also underlines the need for reeducation of patterns of posture and use, as a part of all rehabilitation, even if the problem is as localized as a wrist disorder.

When addressing pain in the forearm, wrist and hand, it is important to treat trigger points in the torso and all shoulder girdle muscles, not only due to their potential trigger point referred patterns, but also for their potential to negatively influence shoulder function or create compensatory usage patterns.

WRIST AND HAND

The carpus, the true wrist joint, is an ellipsoid synovial radiocarpal joint formed by the distal end of the radius

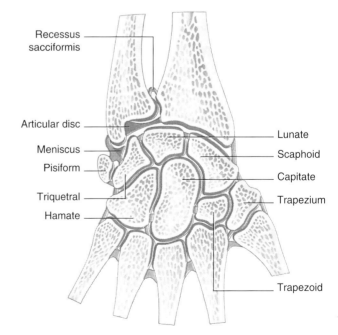

Figure 13.88 Coronal section through carpal bones (reproduced, with permission, from *Gray's anatomy* (1995)).

and the articular disc of the radioulnar joint and their articulation with three proximal carpal bones (Kappler & Ramey 1997). This disc separates the true wrist joint from the distal radioulnar joint and prevents the carpal bones from touching the distal end of the ulna, while still moving in relation to it. To each side of the wrist extends the styloid processes of the ulna and radius, with the latter being longer. Fracture of the styloid process of the radius, (Colles' fracture) is the most common fracture of the wrist.

The carpus contains two rows of small bones which are arranged so that the proximal row forms a palmar arch whose proximal end is convex and whose distal end is concave. Though four bones lie in the proximal row, only three articulate with the radius (scaphoid, lunate and triquetral bones). The fourth, the pisiform, functions as a sesamoid bone in the tendon of flexor carpi ulnaris and articulates only with the palmar surface of the triquetral.

In the second row of carpal bones lie the trapezium, trapezoid, capitate and hamate, which articulate proximally with the first row and distally with the metacarpal bones. The cartilaginous surfaces of each of the eight bones articulate with other bones while the rougher volar and dorsal surfaces accept ligamentous attachments. The two rows slide upon each other to a small degree (mid-carpal joint) and collectively upon the radius and articular disc. The distal row of carpal bones is bound tightly to metacarpal heads as well as to each other, making them together a functional unit.

The metacarpus consists of five miniature long bones (metacarpals) which have a base, shaft and distal rounded heads which articulate with the proximal phalanges to form what is commonly called the knuckles. Their palmar surfaces are longitudinally concave which allows space for the palmar muscles. Though they appear to be parallel, they actually radiate from the carpal bones, with the first metacarpal (thumb) placed more anteriorly, proximally and rotated medially approximately 90° so that its palmar surface faces medially (toward the other metacarpals) (Gray's anatomy 1995), a condition which allows the thumb to have opposition with the fingers and which makes the human hand the remarkable instrument it is.

The metacarpal joint of the thumb (trapezium with first metacarpal) is a saddle joint which is highly mobile due to the design of its articular surfaces. In contrast, the metacarpal joints of the remaining digits are limited, as are the intermetacarpal articulations, each permitting slight gliding to allow some flexion, extension and rotation. These minor movements are especially important when opposing the thumb and small finger, grasping an object or when reaching precisely with individual fingers, as when playing a violin.

The terminology used in various texts in relation to wrist movement is confusing. The terms 'flexion', 'extension' and 'ulnar and radial deviation', of the wrist seem to offer the simplest and most accurate choices and

have been used in this section regarding movement of the hand, though occasionally other terms are used as well.

Within the carpus, flexion (palmar flexion) of the wrist provides 85° of movement while extension (dorsi or volar flexion) of the wrist (from neutral) also allows 85°. The hand may also be placed in ulnar deviation (adduction) of approximately 40–45° or radial deviation (abduction) of 15° (Gray's anatomy 1995, Kapandji 1982) (see Fig. 13.90).

Capsule and ligaments of the wrist (Fig. 13.89)

- The *articular capsule* of the radiocarpal (true wrist) joint has a synovial lining which is strengthened by the palmar radiocarpal, ulnocarpal, dorsal radiocarpal, radial and ulnar collateral ligaments.
- The *palmar radiocarpal* ligament attaches to the anterior margin of the distal radius and its styloid process, passing medially to connect to the anterior surfaces of the scaphoid, lunate and triquetral bones.
- The *palmar ulnocarpal* ligament runs from the base of the styloid process of the ulna and the anterior margin of the articular disc of the distal radioulnar joint to attach to the lunate and triquetral bones.
- The palmar ligaments have apertures which accommodate passage of blood vessels and have a functional relationship with the tendons of flexor pollicis longus and flexor digitorum profundus.
- The *dorsal radiocarpal* ligament attaches proximally to the posterior border of the distal radius, traveling obliquely medially to attach to the dorsal surfaces of the scaphoid, lunate and triquetral bones, where it is continuous with the *dorsal intercarpal* ligaments. There is a functional relationship with the extensor tendons of the fingers and wrist. Anteriorly it blends with the inferior radioulnar articulation.
- The *ulnar collateral* ligament attaches to the end of the styloid process of the ulna, dividing into two fasciculi, one of which attaches to the medial aspect of the triquetral and the other to the pisiform bone.
- The *radial collateral* ligament extends from the tip of the styloid process of the radius to the radial aspect of the scaphoid bone, with some fibers continuing to the trapezium. The radial artery separates the ligament from the tendons of abductor pollicis longus and extensor pollicis brevis.

Ligaments of the hand

- *Dorsal and palmar* ligaments run transversely and connect the scaphoid, lunate and triquetral bones in the proximal row of carpal bones. The dorsal ligaments are stronger than the palmar ones. In the distal row of carpal bones the dorsal and palmar ligaments extend transversely between the trapezium and the trapezoid, the trapezoid and the capitate, and the capitate and hamate bones. At

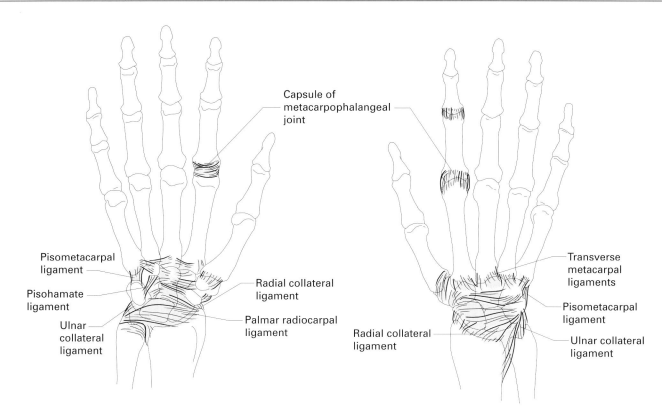

Figure 13.89   Bony structures and ligaments of the wrist.

the mid-carpal joint, on the palmar surface, the fascicles radiating from the head of the capitate to the surrounding bones are known as the *radiate carpal* ligament.

• In the proximal row of the carpal bones, the *interosseous* ligaments connect the lunate and scaphoid bones to each other and the lunate to the triquetral, forming part of the convex articular surface of the radiocarpal joint. In the distal row the interosseous ligaments are thicker; one connects the capitate and the hamate, a second unites the capitate and the trapezoid and a third the trapezium and the trapezoid. The second and third are frequently absent.

• Additional interosseous ligaments are the *pisohamate* and *pisometacarpal* ligaments which, together with the fibrous capsule, connect the pisiform with the palmar surface of the triquetral bone. These ligaments also connect the pisiform with the hamate and the base of the 5th metacarpal bone and are continuations of the tendon of flexor carpi ulnaris (and, according to *Gray's anatomy*, 35th edition p. 437, are therefore misnamed).

• The *radial and ulnar collateral* ligaments of the mid-carpal joint are short. The *radial collateral* connects the scaphoid and the trapezium, and the *ulnar-collateral* connects the trapezium with the triquetral, and the hamate. These ligaments are continuous with the corresponding ligaments of the wrist joint.

The 'true' elbow and the 'true' wrist joints are connected functionally to the radius by means of the synovial joints

(distal and proximal) as well as by an interosseous structure which binds and supports the bones of the forearm. This interosseous membrane forms what is in effect the fibrous middle radioulnar joint. This fibrous 'joint' provides stability for the forearm, reducing stress on ligaments as adduction or abduction of the ulna occurs. This interosseous membrane helps to spread compressive forces on the forearm structures, whether they are transmitted downwards from the shoulder or upwards from the hand.

If examination of elbow, forearm or wrist dysfunction fails to investigate for, or to treat, patterns of dysfunction in the interosseous membrane, results may be disappointing. Kappler & Ramey (1997) state, *'Interosseous membrane dysfunction can perpetuate elbow or wrist disability long after orthopedic care and apparently complete healing of strains, sprains, or fractures of the elbow or wrist should have taken place'.*

Kuchera & Kuchera (1994) describe the relationship between the radius, the ulna and the radiocarpal joints as that of a parallelogram.

• The ulna is part of the elbow joint, relatively fixed at the ulnohumeral joint.

• The radius is part of the wrist joint, relatively fixed at the radiocarpal joint.

• The radius has a greater degree of movement than the ulna due to its rotational component.

• Adduction or abduction of the ulna leads to reciprocal

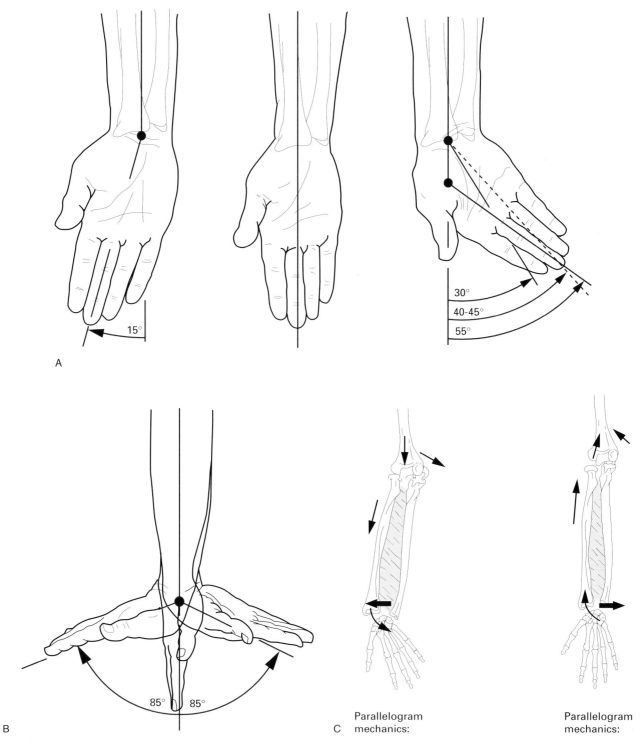

Figure 13.90 The range of movement of the wrist joint. A: Ulnar and radial deviation. B: Flexion and extension. C: Parallelogram mechanics of wrist and ulnar movements.

repositioning of the hand; for example, when the ulna abducts, the radius glides distally, forcing the wrist into increased adduction. The reverse occurs during ulna adduction, which automatically creates an abducted wrist.

• When pronation of the hand occurs, the distal radius crosses over the ulna as the distal end moves anteriorly and medially and toward the end of pronation, the radial head glides posteriorly (dorsally) on the carpal bones.

• When supination occurs, the distal radius crosses back over the ulna as the distal end moves posteriorly (laterally) and, at the extreme of supination, the radial head moves anteriorly.

Palpation exercise

The practitioner supports the flexed elbow so that his thumb is resting on the radial head. At the same time, the other hand grasps the forearm just proximal to the wrist and alternately pronates and supinates it. The movements described above are felt for near the end of full pronation (radial head moves posteriorly) and supination (radial head glides anteriorly). This palpation should be performed on a 'normal' as well as on a 'dysfunctional', symptomatic forearm so that the differences in the movements described above can be noted.

Key (osteopathic) principles for care of elbow, forearm and wrist dysfunction
(modified from Kappler & Ramey 1997)

• Minor restriction (for example, in gliding potential) is commonly the only symptom of dysfunction in this area. Passive bilateral comparison of minor gliding motions is an accurate means of identifying sites of dysfunction.

• Dysfunction of the ulnohumeral joint is commonly the primary feature, with radioulnar dysfunction being secondary, seldom primary, in elbow dysfunction.

• Any dysfunctional state of any joint in the arm will cause adaptive demands on all other joints of the arm, leading to compensatory problems.

• If wrist symptoms are reported, the elbow should be examined.

• If elbow flexion is restricted after all ulnohumeral features have been treated and if inflammation is absent, the radioulnar joints (usually the proximal joint) may require attention.

• Posterior radial head dysfunction is common following a fall forward onto the palm of an outstretched hand, whereas an anterior radial head dysfunction is common following a fall backward onto the palm of the outstretched hand of the extended arm.

Active and passive tests for wrist motion

CAUTION: Avoid testing (active or passive) for range of motion if there exists the possibility of dislocation, fracture, advanced pathology or profound soft tissue damage (tear).

Both active and passive range of motion tests may be used to assess limits of movement of the wrist joint. Bilateral comparison is possible, performing action on each side simultaneously in most cases. If active testing shows normal range without pain or discomfort, passive tests are usually not necessary. Remember the evidence and advice offered in Chapter 11, p. 169, that whereas a single movement in a test situation may not produce symptoms or evidence of dysfunction, repetitive motions replicate 'real life' and are more likely to be informative.

Active and passive range of motion testing for the wrist should show:

• flexion (85°)
• extension (85°)
• ulnar deviation (45°)
• radial deviation (15°).

Assessment tips

• Restrictions which have a hard end-feel during passive range of motion assessment are usually joint related.

• Restrictions which have a softer end-feel, with slight springiness still available at the end of range, are usually due to extraarticular soft tissue dysfunction.

• Kaltenborn (1985) states that if a passive movement and an active movement *in the same direction* produce painful symptoms, this suggests an osseous problem.

• If, however, a *passive* movement in one direction and an *active* movement in the *opposite* direction produce symptoms (pain, for example), this suggests a soft tissue problem.

Supination and pronation tests of the forearm are listed with the elbow on p. 381.

Reflex and strength tests

Strength testing

• The patient clenches the fist and takes it into a flexed position. The practitioner stabilizes the proximal wrist with one hand and covers the clenched fist with the other, as the practitioner attempts to extend the wrist against resistance. This evaluates strength of flexor carpi radialis and flexor carpi ulnaris. Neural supply is from C7, C8 and T1 (Fig. 13.91A).

• The practitioner holds the patient's extended clenched fist (Fig. 13.91B) and resists as the patient attempts to extend this. This evaluates strength of extensor carpi radialis longus and brevis and extensor carpi ulnaris. Neural supply is from C6 and C7 (Fig. 13.91B).

Wrist stress tests

• The practitioner supports the wrist in one hand and with the other, takes the hand, fingers relaxed, into flexion and extension. If pain results, a wide range of possibilities exist including: sprain, fracture, tendinitis, arthritic change or subluxation. If no pain is reported and the same movements are repeated with the patient offering resistance and if pain then results, a soft tissue dysfunction probably exists (strain, tendinitis, etc.). The reader is reminded of the previous advice (p. 169) regarding repeating tests several times, in order to reproduce 'real-life' situations. Such tactics are more informative than performing tests once only.

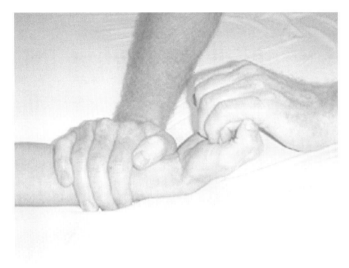

A

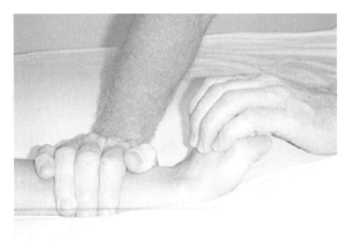

B

Figure 13.91 Strength tests for (A) carpal flexors and (B) extensors.

• The practitioner supports the wrist in one hand and with the other takes the hand into radial and ulnar deviation (abduction and adduction). If pain results a wide range of possibilities exist including: sprain, fracture, tendinitis, arthritic change or subluxation. If no pain is reported and the same movements are repeated with the patient offering resistance and pain then results, a soft tissue dysfunction probably exists (strain, tendinitis, etc.).

• Kappler & Ramey (1997) suggest that translation (gliding) restrictions are often the only evidence of dysfunction, either producing pain or when the joint in one hand/wrist demonstrates a limitation when compared with the same joint on the other hand/wrist. The metacarpophalangeal and interphalangeal joints can usefully be passively tested for anteroposterior glide, mediolateral glide and internal and external rotation potentials, none of which can be initiated by direct muscular action.

• The most common dysfunction affecting carpometa-

carpal joints (apart from that of the thumb), according to Kappler & Ramey (1997), is evidenced by a restriction in the ability to glide ventrally, such as would occur if the digit were moving into extension.

Ganglion

The development of a cyst-like swelling in association with a tendon sheath or joint is thought to result from a protective process related to repetitive stress or to trauma (Schafer 1987). Cysts in the region of the hand or wrist (also, rarely, found on the ankle or foot) are commonly known as ganglions and comprise a tough outer fibrous coat and an inner synovial layer surrounding a thick fluid. Symptoms, which will depend on location and whether the cyst is interfering with normal function or circulation, include aching discomfort, weakness (perhaps of grip strength) and an unsightly swelling. Spontaneous dispersion sometimes occurs. Traditionally, a firm blow with the family Bible was recommended in old texts, to break the cyst and disperse the swelling. The authors do NOT recommend this approach but have no specific non-invasive recommendations. Aspiration of the ganglion is often temporary whereas excision is more permanent. Cyriax (1982) notes that those occurring between the 2nd and 3rd metacarpal bones are often mistaken for rheumatoid arthritis and, regarding those particular ganglions, states: 'Acupuncture affords permanent relief; I have yet to meet a recurrence'.

Carpal tunnel syndrome

Carpal tunnel syndrome is defined as compression of the median nerve within the carpal tunnel. Compression of the nerve may be caused by:

• subluxation of carpal bones (lunate in particular)
• scar tissue
• excessive pressure within the tunnel due to enlarged flexor tendons
• abnormal tissue, such as osteophytes or tumors within the canal
• excessive fluid retention.

Occupational therapist Barbara Ingram-Rice (1997) lists the following risk factors in the development of carpal tunnel syndrome.

• Computer use (or any work requiring repetitive finger dexterity) for more than 2–4 hours/day.
• Infrequent rest breaks (suggests 3–5 minutes every 30 minutes to stretch the neck, shoulders and upper extremity).
• Hypermobile joints, as their instability makes these joints more susceptible to injury.
• Poor posture, including rounded shoulders and forward head, which encourages nerve entrapment.

- Poor technique with activity/work, such as holding the phone to the ear with the shoulder, poor sitting postures or a computer screen set at a less than ideal angle.
- Sedentary lifestyle, leading to overall decreased fitness level.
- Stressful work environment, leading the person to work harder, not smarter.
- Arthritis, diabetes, thyroid disease or other serious medical conditions can accentuate the individual's response to repetitive strain.
- Long fingernails, causing awkward use of finger tips.
- Excessive alcohol or tobacco consumption, decreasing the body's ability to repair tissue damage.
- Overweight, as increased adipose tissue may decrease tunnel space and the overweight person is less likely to properly fit the furniture associated with their job.

Ingram-Rice (1997) points out that prevention is the best course of action and stresses the need to ergonomically design the workspace, including the height of desk, relationship of the chair to the desk, placement of the computer and phone (use headset if possible), and use of footstool. She also suggests:

Another excellent tool for computer operators is a [computer] program called ExcerciseBreak. This program will stop the work at predetermined intervals and take the individual through a predetermined set of exercises. In this way the individual does not forget to exercise.[1]

Ergonomic screensavers are available (often free) and a websearch should offer the reader the chance to access and acquire such a program.[2]

Unfortunately, in recent years, carpal tunnel syndrome has become a collective diagnosis for many hand and wrist problems without precise testing of median nerve dysfunction to confirm this finding. Additionally, since many trigger points in the shoulder, neck and forearm muscles are capable of duplicating the symptoms of carpal tunnel syndrome, these areas deserve evaluation. While carpal tunnel syndrome remains the most common nerve entrapment syndrome of the upper extremity, cubital tunnel syndrome (see p. 382) runs a close second (Simons et al 1998) due to increased computer usage, with resultant poor hand and arm positioning.

Causes of carpal tunnel syndrome

- The most widely accepted explanation is that this condition results from a neural compression condition involving the median nerve.

---

[1] Exercise Break, Hopkins Technology, 421 Hazil Lane, Hopkins, MN 55343, 1–800–397–9211
[2] At the time of this publication an ergonomic computer screensaver is available at no charge from www.aota.org. (American Occupational Therapy Association)

- In this model, causes are thought to vary from increased structural volume of the nerve to a narrowing of the tunnel size. There is commonly a history of trauma to the area.
- Other etiological suggestions include:
1. cervical arthritis as a precursor to carpal tunnel syndrome (Hurst 1985), suggesting that cervical mechanics should always be evaluated, and treated, if appropriate
2. venous and lymphatic congestion (Sunderland 1976), suggesting that blood and lymph flow should be normalized by means of attention to soft tissues as well as to excessive sympathetic tone, possibly by correction of upper thoracic and rib dysfunction
3. altered vasomotion as a result of upper thoracic dysfunction (Larson 1972)
4. interference with axoplasmic flow (see Box 3.1, p. 31) as a result of minor compression somewhere along the course of the median nerve, leading to the evolution of distant denervation changes and symptoms (Upton & McComas 1973).

Symptoms

- Symptoms include pain and numbness, worse at night, weakness, swelling and muscular hypertrophy. The thenar eminence may display atrophy.
- There may be difficulty in pronating and supinating the forearm.
- Direct manual compression or percussion of the carpal tunnel (Tinel's sign) commonly provokes symptoms but these can be confused with normal response to percussion of a nerve and are now considered by some to be an unreliable test (Cailliet 1994).
- When holding the wrist at a full flexed position

Box 13.15   Nerve entrapment possibilities

Ulnar nerve entrapment may be produced by the 'arcade of Struthers', a dense fascial arch near the elbow, which may produce similar symptoms to cubital tunnel syndrome, such as a medial epicondylar ache with accompanying shooting points to the little finger and ulnar portion of the hand (Cailliet 1996). The flexor carpi ulnaris may entrap the ulnar nerve as it lies deep to this muscle and superficial to the flexor digitorum profundus. Additionally, an anomalous muscle, the anconeus epitrochlearis (Simons et al 1998), may cause ulnar nerve compression when it is present.

Radial nerve entrapment may be produced by the long head of triceps, the supinator and extensor carpi radialis brevis as well as an anomalous flexor carpi radialis brevis muscle.

Median nerve entrapment may be produced by pronator teres, flexor digitorum superficialis or the anomalous flexor digitorum superficialis indicis. Impingement of the nerve within the carpal tunnel may be due to subluxation of carpal bones, scar tissue or enlarged flexor tendons.

causes tingling and numbness (paresthesia) of the median nerve distribution (fingers of the radial side of hand), this is considered a more reliable sign (see also Phalen's test below) for carpal tunnel syndrome.

• The diagnosis is confirmed by nerve conduction and EMG tests.

• If such tests are negative and symptoms persist, one of the other etiological patterns, as listed above, may be operating.

Tests for carpal tunnel syndrome

1. *Phalen's test*. Patient places the dorsum of both flexed wrists against each other and applies pressure (light) for a full minute. Symptom increase (pain, numbness, etc.) is a positive sign (Fig. 13.92A).

2. *Tinel's test*. Patient has elbow flexed and hand supinated. The practitioner taps the volar surface of the wrist with a broad reflex hammer or the tip of an index finger (nail trimmed). If pain is noted in all fingers apart from little finger, carpal tunnel syndrome is strongly indicated (Fig. 13.92B).

3. *Oriental prayer test*. The patient fully extends abducted fingers and thumb of each hand and places palms together. If thumbs cannot touch, this indicates paralysis of abductor pollicis brevis due to median nerve palsy resulting from carpal tunnel syndrome (Fig. 13.92C).

Associated wrist tests

1. *Oschner's test*. Patient is asked to interlock fingers by placing palms together and interlacing the fingers, so that their palmar surfaces rest on the dorsum of the contralateral hand. If the index finger on the suspected side cannot flex in this way, median nerve paralysis is indicated. The lesion is likely to be at or above where

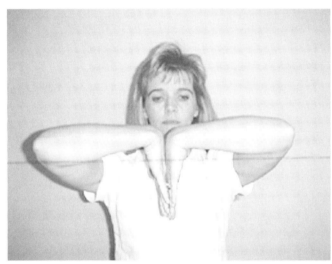

A

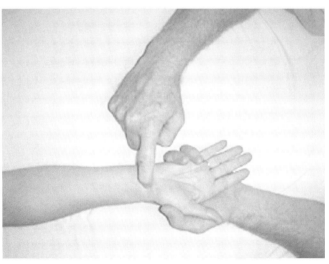

B

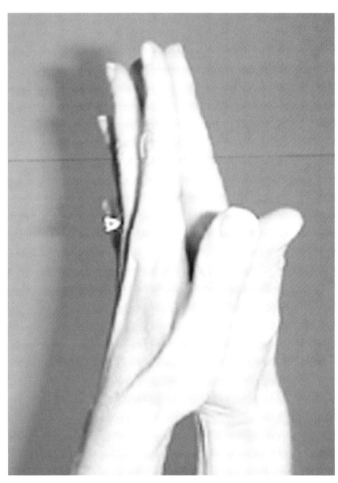

C

Figure 13.92 Tests for carpal tunnel syndrome. A: Phalen's test. B: Tinnel's test. C: Oriental prayer position.

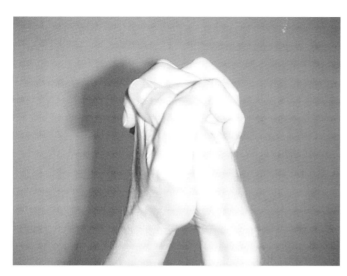

Figure 13.93 Oschner's test. Median nerve paralysis may be indicated if the index finger cannot flex.

branching of the nerve to flexor digitorum superficialis occurs (Fig. 13.93).

2. *Froment's test.* If the ulnar nerve is paralyzed the patient will be unable to form an '0' with thumb and index finger.

3. *'Pinch' test and ulnar nerve entrapment signs.* If the ulnar nerve is entrapped there will be weakness of the ability to 'pinch'; weak thumb abduction ('hitcher's thumb' position); and an inability to actively flex the metacarpophalangeal joints. Interosseous atrophy may be apparent.

4. *Bracelet test.* The practitioner encircles the patient's wrist with thumb and index finger and applies firm compression to the distal radius and ulna. If sharp pain is reported arising in the wrist and/or radiating to the hand or forearm, rheumatoid arthritis is suspected.

PHALANGES

Movements of the fingers are described in relation to the axis of the hand and not that of the whole body. In other words, the hand has its own mid-line, which lies longitudinally along the 3rd metacarpal bone and the middle digit (ray). Adduction and abduction of the fingers and thumb are in relation to the mid-line, so that separating the fingers from each other is abduction and approximating them is adduction.

The metacarpophalangeal joints are composed of an irregularly convex surface articulating with a 'socket' that is shallow, which allows for considerable movement. The phalanges, however, are hinge joints and are limited to flexion and extension.

Like the metacarpals, the phalanges have a proximal base, shaft and (distal) head, which are conveniently designed to stack one upon the other. The fingers are

composed of three phalanges laid end to end while the thumb has two.

- The proximal end of the proximal phalanx carries a concave, oval facet which conforms to its convex associated metacarpal head.
- The distal end (head) of the proximal phalanx is smoothly grooved (like a pulley) to receive the base of the middle phalanx.
- The base of the middle phalanx has two concave facets which have a smooth ridge between them to conform to the above groove.
- The head of the middle phalanx is similar to the head of the proximal one, with a pulley-like groove to receive the distal phalanx.
- The distal phalanx conforms to the above groove while presenting a non-articular head which carries a

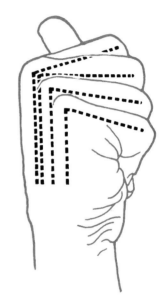

A

B

Figure 13.94 A&B: Range of flexion and extension of metacarpophalangeal joints (reproduced, with permission, from Kapandji (1998)).

rough palmar tuberosity for the attachment of the pulps of the finger tips.

Carpometacarpal ligaments (2nd, 3rd, 4th, 5th)

• Dorsal ligaments connect carpal bones with metacarpals on dorsal surface, passing transversely from one bone to another.
• Palmar ligaments connect carpal bones with metacarpals on the palmar surface, passing transversely from one bone to another.
• Interosseous ligaments connect contiguous distal margins of capitate and hamate bones with adjacent surfaces of 3rd and 4th metacarpals.
• Synovial membrane is often a continuation of the intercarpal joints.

Metacarpophalangeal ligaments

• The *palmar* ligaments are thick fibrous structures on the palmar surfaces of the joints between the collateral ligaments with which they are connected. They are also blended with the *deep transverse* ligaments of the palm.
• The *deep transverse metacarpal* ligaments are made up of three short, wide bands which connect the palmar ligaments of the 3rd, 4th and 5th metacarpophalangeal joints.
• The collateral ligaments are strong, rounded cords lying at the sides of the joints attached to the tubercle on the side of the head of the metacarpal bones, passing obliquely distally to attach to the ventral aspect of the base of the phalanx.

Range of motion

Metacarpophalangeal ranges of motion (of fingers) should be:

• flexion – approximately 90°, with the index finger falling just short of 90° and each finger increasing progressively
• extension – from a few degrees to up to 40° of active movement and up to 90° passive movement in individuals with lax ligaments (Kapandji 1982)
• adduction – relatively small, negligible in flexion
• abduction – relatively small, negligible in flexion
• circumduction – represents a combination of the above four which produces a cone of circumduction
• passive rotation – 60°
• active rotation – limited during flexion-extension; greatest in the smallest finger.

Interphalangeal ranges of motion (of fingers) should be:

• flexion:
  1. proximal interphalangeal joint – greater than 90° (increases from 2nd to 5th fingers)
  2. distal interphalangeal joint – slightly less than 90° (increases from 2nd to 5th fingers)
• extension:
  1. proximal interphalangeal joint – none
  2. distal interphalangeal joint – none or very small
• slight passive side-to-side movement.

THUMB

Five bony structures (scaphoid, trapezium, a metacarpal and two phalanges) make up the osteoarticular column of the thumb. The combined four joints in the column

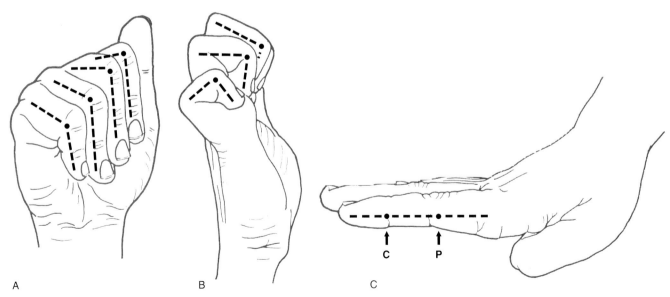

Figure 13.95 A–C: Range of motion of phalangeal joints (reproduced, with permission, from Kapandji (1998)).

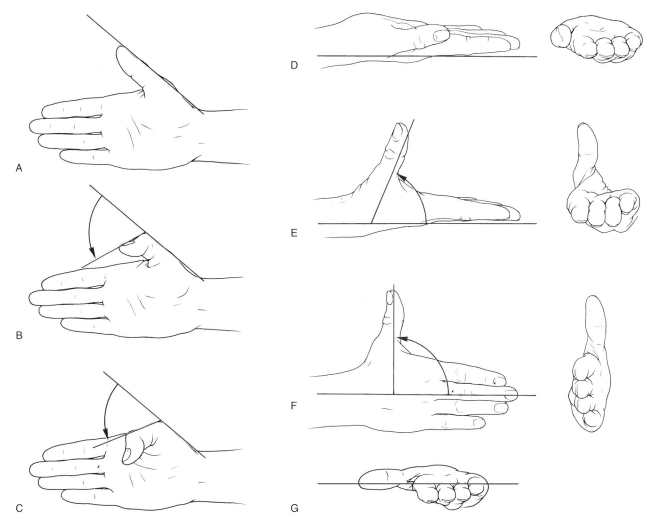

Figure 13.96 A: Thumb in neutral position. B: Interphalangeal joint flexion. C: Interphalangeal and metacarpophalangeal joint flexion. D: Radial adduction. E: Palmar abduction. F and G: Radial abduction.

allow for flexion-extension, abduction-adduction, rotation and circumduction. Additionally, the thumb is attached far more proximally to the hand than the fingers, giving it a tremendous architectural advantage.

Kappler & Ramey (1997) summarize the extraordinary potential of the thumb:

The carpometacarpal joint of the thumb is ... a saddle-type joint, having both a concave and a convex articular surface. This configuration permits angular movements in almost any plane with the exception of limited axial rotation. Only a ball and socket joint has more motion than the carpometacarpal joint of the thumb. Because it has very good motion, it is more likely to have compression strain or sprain of the ligaments than to have a somatic dysfunction.

Thumb ligaments

• The metacarpal bone of the thumb connects to the trapezium by the *lateral*, *palmar* and *dorsal* ligaments, as well as by the *capsular* ligament.

• The thumb's most common dysfunctional pattern relates to compression strain or sprain of its ligaments.

Range of motion at the joints of the thumb

• Metacarpal flexion 50° – movement is parallel to the plane of the palm so that the ulnar side of the thumb sweeps across the palm
• Metacarpal extension 0° – 'relative extension' moves the thumb back to neutral from any point of flexion but the thumb should not be extended beyond neutral
• Metacarpophalangeal flexion 50°
• Metacarpophalangeal extension 0°
• Interphalangeal flexion 90°
• Interphalangeal extension 20°
• Palmar abduction 70° – takes place at the carpometacarpal joint and is perpendicular to the plane of the palm
• Palmar adduction 0°

- Radial abduction 90° – is parallel to the plane of the palm
- Radial adduction 0°
- Opposition is a composite movement of circumduction of the first metacarpal, internal rotation of the thumb (as a whole) and maximum extension of the interphalangeal joint and varying degrees of the metacarpophalangeal joint.

Testing thumb movement

- The patient is asked to touch the tip of the thumb to the base of her little finger and to each finger tip and to abduct the thumb as far as possible.
- If any joint restriction is noted, the muscles controlling the thumb should be palpated.
- In addition, both thumb joints should be assessed passively, in all directions of motion, including gliding (translation).

Dysfunction and evaluation

Thumb dysfunction includes (among others) sprains associated with falls, hitting with clenched fist, bowling (which can also produce neural damage to the digital nerve from the edge of the hole of the ball) and chronic strains which may be associated with excessive use involved in playing video games. Schafer (1987) reports that the commonest trigger point in the region is that of adductor pollicis.

With any such presenting problems, careful evaluation of joint restrictions is essential; evaluation of muscular changes (including fibrotic infiltration, weakness and shortness modifications of flexors and extensors, respectively) and the influence of related joints (elbow, shoulder, upper thoracic and cervical regions) will assist in formulating a treatment plan.

PREPARING FOR TREATMENT

The carpal and digital flexors (along with the pronators previously discussed in connection with the elbow region, p. 387) all lie on the anterior (flexor) surface of the forearm in two layers. The superficial layer flexors have their origins primarily on the medial epicondyle of the humerus while the deeper layer flexors arise from the ulna and radius. The most superficial layer includes the flexor carpi ulnaris and radialis, pronator teres, palmaris longus and flexor digitorum superficialis. Note: The flexor digitorum superficialis is included in the superficial layer even though it is covered almost completely by the other superficial muscles. The deeper layer is composed of the flexor digitorum profundus, flexor pollicis longus and pronator quadratus (discussed with the elbow).

The extensors occur in two layers on the posterior surface, many of which arise from the lateral epicondyle of the humerus. The superficial posterior forearm includes brachioradialis and anconeus (both discussed with the elbow), extensor carpi radialis longus and brevis, extensor carpi ulnaris, extensor digitorum and extensor digiti minimi. The deeper layer contains supinator (discussed with the elbow), extensor pollicis longus and brevis, abductor pollicis longus and extensor indicis.

The forearm muscles should also be considered in terms of function. For instance, even though the pronators and supinator of the forearm lie within the forearm they are considered primary to the elbow, since the movements they perform occur within that joint. Since they are encountered during forearm palpation, the pronators and supinators are discussed in relation to the other muscles of that region. They should be evaluated and, if necessary, treated in relation to dysfunctions of the wrist or hand since normal elbow function is necessary for normal use of the hand. Additionally, trigger points lying in the pronators or supinators (and those of brachialis, brachioradialis and many shoulder cuff muscles) have been shown to have target zones in the wrist, thumb or hand (Simons et al 1998).

Terminology

The remaining forearm muscles are easily identified by function since their names denote the work they do. Unfortunately for the reader who is struggling to identify the anatomy, it can at times seem as though the forearm muscles all have the same name. Understanding why they are named as they are assists in demystifying the apparent confusion as the names start to make sense. In fact, knowledge of the sometimes lengthy names should assist the practitioner in readily identifying and locating the muscles.

The following terminology is basic to the nomenclature of the forearm and while this listing might appear simplistic, combinations of these terms will be found to result in a muscle's name which not only usually identifies its function but often also its location and whether it has an assistant (as with longus and brevis).

- *Carpi* muscles move only the wrist (extensor carpi radialis longus may weakly flex the elbow)
- *Digitorum* muscles move the fingers (and assist with the wrist since they cross that joint as well)
- *Pollicis* pertains to the thumb
- *Indicis* refers to the index finger
- *Digiti minimi* is the smallest finger
- *Radialis* muscles lie on the radial (thumb) side of the forearm
- *Ulnaris* muscles lie on the ulnar side of the forearm
- If there is a *longus*, there is surely a *brevis* (shorter version of muscle with similar function to 'longus')
- If there is a *flexor*, there is also an *extensor* (although if there are two flexors, there are not necessarily two extensors)

When the muscle names are considered, one can quickly decipher what each term means for that muscle. For instance:

- flexor carpi ulnaris occurs on the ulnar side of the flexor (anterior) surface of the arm and serves to flex the wrist
- extensor carpi radialis longus lies on the radial side of the extensor (posterior) surface of the forearm to serve the wrist and (somewhere) has a companion, the brevis.

Since most of the flexors attach to the medial epicondyle and the extensors to the lateral epicondyle, one can quickly identify the anatomy by considering the terms used. This concept is more true for the forearm musculature than any other region of the body.

Neural entrapment

The medial and ulnar nerves can each be entrapped by anterior forearm muscles, including (for ulnar nerve) flexor carpi ulnaris, flexor digitorum superficialis and profundus and (for median nerve) pronator teres and flexor digitorum superficialis. Entrapment of the radial nerve is (rarely) caused by an anomalous flexor carpi radialis brevis muscle (Simons et al 1998).

Distant influences

It is important when addressing hand and wrist pain and dysfunction to include examination of function and dysfunction of (including the presence of trigger points) the cervical, shoulder, upper arm and elbow regions and to consider combined patterns of several trigger points rather than seeking just one trigger point which may be producing the entire pattern (or syndrome). The combined trigger point target zones for the neck and upper extremity muscles leave virtually no part of the distal arm untouched, as many of them have wrist, thumb or hand target zones. Simons et al (1998) offer (at the beginning of each section) regional charting of areas of pain together with a list of the muscles which refer into those regions. These lists can be used as a shortcut to consider which muscles are most likely to be referring pain to a particular area and are particularly helpful when time is limited. A more thorough, detailed examination and treatment plan should also include assessment of the synergists and antagonists of muscles housing trigger points, as well as range of motion assessments and postural considerations.

ANTERIOR FOREARM TREATMENT

The muscles of the superficial layer of the anterior forearm are addressed together and, unless contraindicated, followed by treatment of the deeper layer. Identification

of dysfunctional muscles may require tests for strength and weakness and in some cases for length. Joints associated with the muscles under review require evaluation for their influence on patterns of use and presenting symptoms. Manual palpation, including NMT assessment methods, offers a direct means for the localization of altered tissue status, whether this be tense, flaccid, fibrotic, edematous or indurated, and for the presence (or lack) of active trigger points, so allowing treatment to target the most involved structures, as well as distant influences on them.

Palmaris longus (Figs 13.97, 13.98)

Attachments: From the common flexor tendon on the medial epicondyle to the palmar fascia (aponeurosis or pretendinous fibers) and the transverse carpal ligament (flexor retinaculum)
Innervation: Median nerve (C7–8 or T1)
Muscle type: Postural (type 1), shortens when stressed
Function: Tenses the palmar fascia to cup the hand; flexes the wrist; may assist pronation against resistance and (weakly) assist elbow flexion (Simons et al 1998)
Synergists: *For cupping the hand*: thenar and hypothenar muscles
For wrist flexion: flexor carpi ulnaris, flexor carpi radialis, flexor digitorum superficialis and profundus
Antagonists: *To wrist flexion*: extensor carpi ulnaris, extensor carpi radialis brevis and longus, extensor digitorum, smaller finger and thumb muscles

Indications for treatment

- Prickling to palm and anterior forearm
- Diagnosis of Dupuytren's contracture (see below)
- Tenderness in the palm, especially when working with a hand tool

Special notes

Palmaris longus courses from the medial epicondyle to the palm, directly superficial to the flexor digitorum superficialis, with its tendon remaining outside the flexor retinaculum (the only tendon which does). To some degree, it separates the anterior forearm into ulnar and radial aspects, as the carpi muscles are found one on each side of the palmaris longus. The muscle attaches broadly onto the palmar fascia which, in turn, directs fibers into five groups with longitudinal orientation, each of which projects toward a digit (ray).

The palmaris longus tendon courses directly through the mid-line of the wrist. It may be absent on either arm and, when absent on one arm, is twice as likely to be absent bilaterally than unilaterally. When the muscle is present, its tendon may be more easily distinguished

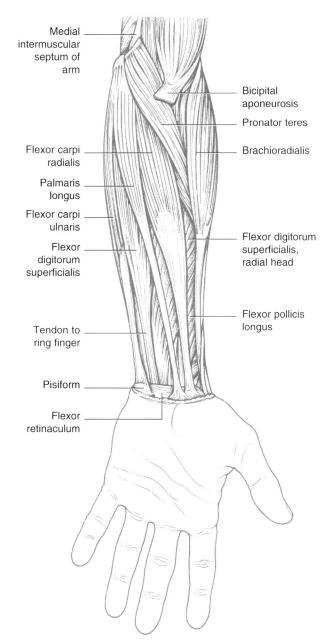

Figure 13.97 The superficial layer of the anterior forearm (reproduced, with permission, from *Gray's anatomy* (1995)).

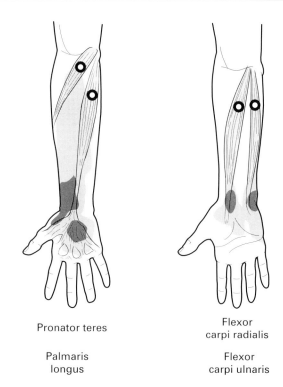

Figure 13.98 Common trigger points of anterior forearm.

from flexor carpi radialis by having the patient place all five digit pads together, with the metacarpophalangeal joints flexed and the phalanges extended (as if picking up a marble with all five digits). The wrist may be flexed simultaneously, which may make palmaris longus even more distinct and/or cause the flexor carpi radialis to stand out as well. If the metacarpophalangeal joints are then extended (fingers in neutral, wrist flexed), the palmaris tendon softens and the flexor carpi radialis becomes more obvious. Even when the muscle is absent, its palmar fascia is still present (Platzer 1992).

Trigger points in this muscle may simulate Dupuytren's contracture, a condition in which the palmar fascia thickens and shortens with resultant flexion contracture of the fingers. Taleisnik (1988) classifies the disease as follows.

Dupuytren's contracture characteristics

Stage 1: A nodule of the palmar fascia that does not include the skin, with no change in the fascia.
Stage 2: A nodule in the fascia with involvement of the skin.
Stage 3: Same as stage 2 but with a flexion contracture of one or more fingers.
Stage 4: Same as stage 3, plus tendon and joint contractures.

Cailliet (1994) notes that, while surgical excision of the fascia and skin bands may be necessary, the hand may lose up to 25% of its grip power as a result. He also notes a non-surgical intervention of injection of trypsin, chymotrypsin A, hyaluronidase and lidocaine, coupled with forceful finger extension. Since the progression is often very slow, observation and minimal or no treatment are often indicated.

Simons et al (1998) point out that heredity is a factor in Dupuytren's contracture and suggest ruling out trigger points as part of the problem. A distinguishing feature is that while Dupuytren's may cause a painful palm, only trigger points in palmaris longus produce the prickling sensation. Simons et al describe a spray and stretch technique which covers the anterior forearm and hand, which may be beneficial.

Flexor carpi radialis

Attachments: From the common flexor tendon on the medial epicondyle of the humerus and from the antebrachial fascia and intermuscular septa to the base of the 2nd and 3rd metacarpals
Innervation: Median nerve (C6–7)
Muscle type: Postural (type 1), shortens when stressed
Function: Flexes the wrist; deviates the hand toward the radius (thumb)
Synergists: *For flexion*: flexor carpi ulnaris, flexor digitorum superficialis and profundus, palmaris longus
For deviation: extensor carpi radialis brevis and longus
Antagonists: *To flexion*: extensor carpi ulnaris, extensor carpi radialis brevis and longus
To deviation: flexor and extensor carpi ulnaris

Flexor carpi ulnaris

Attachments: From the common flexor tendon on the medial epicondyle of the humerus and from the medial border of the olecranon to the pisiform bone and by ligamentous fibers to the hamate and 5th metacarpal. A few fibers blend with flexor retinaculum
Innervation: Ulnar nerve (C7–8)
Muscle type: Postural (type 1), shortens when stressed
Function: Flexes the wrist; deviates the hand toward the ulna
Synergists: *For flexion*: flexor carpi radialis, flexor digitorum superficialis and profundus, palmaris longus
For deviation: extensor carpi ulnaris
Antagonists: *To flexion*: extensor carpi radialis brevis and longus, extensor carpi ulnaris
To deviation: flexor carpi radialis and extensor carpi radialis brevis and longus

Indications for treatment of wrist flexors

- Loss of range or pain upon extension
- Medial epicondylitis
- Carpal tunnel syndrome (some symptoms may be from wrist flexor trigger points)

Flexor carpi ulnaris and radialis work together to powerfully flex the wrist while they unilaterally work with their extensor counterpart(s) to produce radial and ulnar deviation of the hand at the wrist. Since these two muscles arise from the common tendon of the medial epicondyle, they should be evaluated and, if necessary, treated when epicondylar inflammation or tenderness is found.

As with many forearm trigger points, those in the flexor carpi radialis and ulnaris tend to refer to the portion of the joint which the muscle serves, in this case the radial and ulnar aspects of the flexor surface of the wrist, respectively. These trigger points, especially when combined with others, such as those in subscapularis, will present many of the common complaints associated with carpal tunnel syndrome and should always be examined in association with that diagnosis. Trigger points and inflammation found in attachment sites (such as the medial epicondyle) will often resolve unaided if central trigger points associated with them are deactivated (Simons et al 1998).

Flexor digitorum superficialis (Fig. 13.99)

Attachments: *Humeroulnar head*: from the common tendon of the medial epicondyle of the humerus, the coronoid process of the elbow and (radial head) from the oblique line of the radius in a common tendon sheath through the carpal canal to end in four tendons attaching (after splitting for profundus) to the sides of each middle phalanx
Innervation: Median nerve (C7–T1)
Muscle type: Postural (type 1), shortens when stressed
Function: Flexes the middle phalanx on the proximal one, flexes the proximal phalanx on the metacarpal and flexes the hand at the wrist
Synergists: *For finger flexion*: flexor digitorum profundus, palmaris longus
For flexion of MCP joint: flexor digitorum profundus, palmaris longus, lumbricales, palmar and dorsal interossei
For wrist flexion: flexor carpi radialis and ulnaris, flexor digitorum profundus, palmaris longus
Antagonists: *To finger flexion*: extensor digitorum
To flexion of MCP joint: extensor digitorum, extensor indicis, extensor digiti minimi

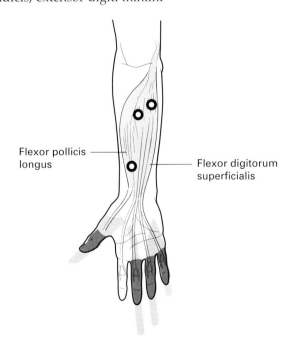

Flexor pollicis longus

Flexor digitorum superficialis

Figure 13.99 Trigger points of digital flexors seem to extend beyond the tips of the digits, like lightning (Simons et al 1998).

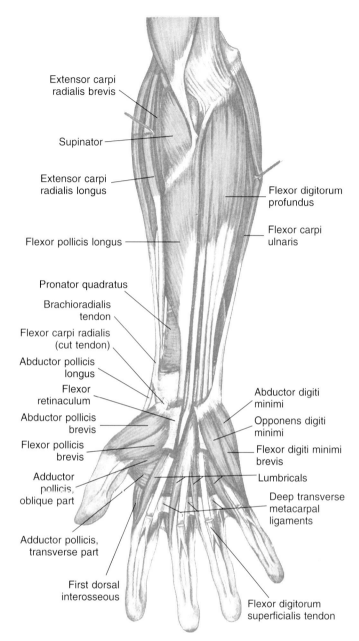

Figure 13.100 The deepest anterior forearm muscles (reproduced, with permission, from *Gray's anatomy* (1995)).

Flexor digitorum profundus (Fig. 13.100)

Attachments: From the proximal 3/4 of the medial and anterior surfaces of the ulna (from brachialis to pronator quadratus) and interosseous membrane and from the coronoid process of the elbow and aponeurosis, shared with the flexor and extensor carpi ulnaris to become four tendons, each attaching to the base of a distal phalanx of a single finger after perforating the tendon of flexor digitorum superficialis

Innervation: Median and ulnar nerves (C8–T1)

Muscle type: Postural (type 1), shortens when stressed

Function: Flexes all joints it crosses, including the wrist, mid-carpal, metacarpophalangeal and phalangeal joints

Synergists: *For finger flexion*: flexor digitorum superficialis, palmaris longus (perhaps)

For flexion of MCP joint: flexor digitorum superficialis, palmaris longus, lumbricales, palmar and dorsal interossei

For wrist flexion: flexor carpi radialis and ulnaris, flexor digitorum superficialis, palmaris longus

Antagonists: *To finger flexion*: extensor digitorum

To flexion of MCP joint: extensor digitorum, extensor indicis, extensor digiti minimi

Indications for treatment of finger flexors (both layers)

- Loss of extension of the fingers (especially when the wrist is also extended)
- 'Explosive pain that "shoots right out the end of the finger like lightning"' (Simons et al 1998)
- Difficulty using scissors or shears
- Difficulty grasping with ends of fingers, such as when curling the hair
- Trigger finger (locking finger)

Special notes

Flexor digitorum superficialis (sublimis) lies in the superficial layer of the anterior forearm, although it is covered for the most part by the remaining muscles of the superficial layer, while the profundus (perforatus) lies deep to it in the second layer of the forearm. Near its distal attachment to the middle phalanx, each superficialis tendon splits and the profundus passes through it to terminate on the distal phalanx (Fig. 13.101). Profundus acts alone to flex the distal interphalangeal joint but is assisted by superficialis for flexion of other hand and finger joints. While together they provide powerful and speedy movements of the fingers, gentle digital flexion is provided by the profundus alone.

Trigger finger

Trigger finger (locking finger) is a condition in which the movement of the finger (or thumb) stops for a moment during flexion or extension movements and then continues with a jerk. Simons et al (1998) suggest loading the locked finger by having the person (slightly) flex it more and applying active resistance while the person pulls it, against the resistance, to its resting position. They note: 'Sometimes firm pressure applied to the tender spot where locking occurs will restore normal function, as if the tendon or tendon sheath had become edematous locally and needed help to return to normal'. They also suggest injection (1.5 ml of 0.5% procaine solution) 'apparently deep in the restricting fibrous ring around the

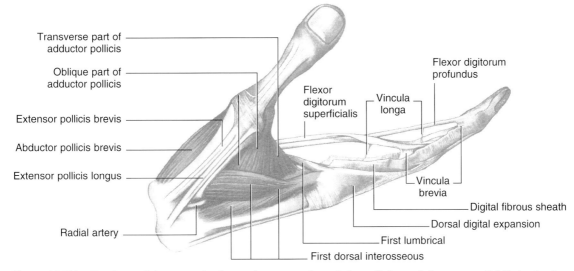

Figure 13.101 The flexor digitorum profundus tendon passes through the split flexor digitorum superficialis tendon to attach to the most distal phalange (reproduced, with permission, from *Gray's anatomy* (1995)).

flexor tendon' and offer supporting evidence of its effectiveness in relieving trigger finger, though the return to normal function may be delayed by a few days. See also Mulligan's 'mobilization with movement' method, described on p. 408.

Flexor pollicis longus

Attachments: From the anterior surface of the radius (from distal to the tuberosity to the pronator quadratus), interosseous membrane and sometimes from the coronoid process or medial epicondyle of the humerus to the base of the distal phalanx of the thumb on its palmar surface
Innervation: Median nerve (C7–8 or T1)
Muscle type: Postural (type 1), shortens when stressed
Function: Flexes the interphalangeal, metacarpophalangeal and carpometacarpal joints of the thumb. May mildly abduct the thumb (Platzer 1992)
Synergists: Flexor pollicis brevis, adductor pollicis
Antagonists: Extensor pollicis longus and brevis, abductor pollicis longus

Indications for treatment

- Difficulty with fine work requiring control of the thumb, such as sewing, fine painting or writing
- Pain in the thumb and extending beyond the tip
- Trigger thumb

Special notes

Flexor pollicis longus courses through the carpal tunnel and between the two heads of flexor pollicis brevis before terminating at the distal phalanx of the thumb. It

is sometimes connected to either flexor digitorum muscle (*Gray's anatomy* 1995, Platzer 1992) and may be partially or completely absent (*Gray's anatomy* 1995).

Trigger thumb

Trigger thumb (like trigger finger) presents with locking in flexion and the inability to straighten the thumb without assistance (Simons et al 1998) and is usually caused by enlargement of the tendon (nodule) where it passes through a fibrous sheath. Cailliet (1994) notes (regarding trigger fingers) that steroid injection to expand the sheath may allow passage of the nodule, surgical intervention to slit the sheath may be necessary and that 'Excision of the nodule invariably causes formation of a new and often bigger nodule'.

NMT for anterior forearm

The patient is seated comfortably opposite the practitioner with a table placed between them on which to support the arm. The forearm to be treated is supinated with the hand in neutral position and rests comfortably on the table with the fingers directed toward the practitioner. This treatment may also be performed with the person supine as long as the table provides enough support for the arm.

- The superficial layer of muscles is addressed first with lubricated gliding strokes along the course of the muscle, from the wrist to the medial epicondyle. The gliding strokes are repeated 6–8 times on each muscle until the entire surface of the anterior forearm has been treated. The order of treatment is not important but when learning to identify these muscles, the following order may be helpful.

- From the midline of the wrist to the medial epicondyle will address the palmaris longus.
- On the ulnar side of this landmark 'mid-line', a portion of the flexor digitorum superficialis is available and next to it (medially) on the most lunar portion of the anterior forearm lies the flexor carpi ulnaris.
- On the radial side of the 'mid-line' lies the flexor carpi radialis.
- Directing inferolaterally across the most proximal portion of flexor carpi radialis is the pronator teres (see p. 387), which can be palpated transversely while pronating the forearm.
- The most lateral (radial) aspect of the anterior forearm will include brachioradialis, radial wrist extensors and the supinator, which are sometimes called the radial muscles, a portion of which is visible from the posterior aspect as well.
- Near the anterior elbow region, the short pronator teres may be easily palpated, as it lies diagonally across the central aspect of the uppermost portion.
- Gliding strokes may again be applied with increased pressure (if appropriate) to influence the flexor digitorum superficialis, flexor digitorum profundus and the flexor pollicis longus.

As the practitioner applies the gliding strokes to the opposite arm to treat or to compare the tissues, a hot

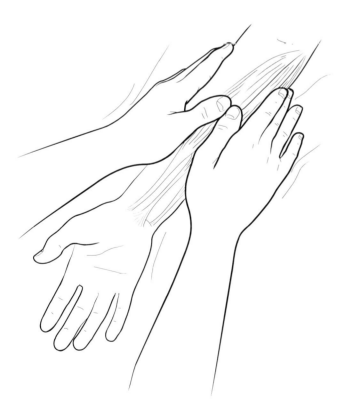

Figure 13.102 Superficial gliding strokes address the wrist and hand flexors while deeper pressure (if appropriate) treats the digital flexors.

pack (if appropriate) may be applied to the arm which has been treated. The gliding strokes are then repeated. If the muscles are moderately uncomfortable with appropriate gliding strokes, inflammation may be present, especially with repetitive use conditions. In this case, heat would be contraindicated and an ice pack used instead.

Once the lubricated gliding strokes have been sufficiently applied to warm and elongate the myofascial tissue, individual palpation of the muscles may easily distinguish the superficial muscles, though the deeper bellies are usually not as distinct. Knowledge of the musculature will be the practitioner's greatest asset when attempting to locate these muscles. While active muscle testing may also assist in locating them, several muscles are likely to be activated by the same movement, which could be confusing unless the anatomy is familiar.

Transverse, snapping palpation may be applied with the thumb or fingertips to identify taut bands within any of these muscles. Since trigger points occur within taut bands, examination of any taut fibers found should be included, especially at the center of the fiber where central triggers occur. The superficial layer of muscles have lengthy tendons, making their endplate zone (where central trigger points occur) lie in the middle of the upper half of the forearm.

Tender attachment sites are often associated with a central trigger point and will usually resolve with little treatment needed, if the central trigger point is released (Simons et al 1998). Trigger points and tender areas may be treated with sustained pressure, spray and stretch techniques, injection, dry needling and possibly through movement techniques such as active myofascial release (as described below). Clinical experience has shown that trigger points are more easily deactivated following lymphatic drainage of the area.

The medial epicondyle is often a site of tenderness and irritation due to tension placed on the common tendon which attaches to it. It is deserving of special attention and careful palpation, as its degree of tenderness may be marked. Additionally, central trigger points should be addressed in the five muscles (pronator teres, palmaris longus, flexor carpi ulnaris and radialis and flexor digitorum superficialis) which merge into the tendon. Habitual overuse of the muscles should be decreased, with more frequent breaks from activities which stress them. Ice applications are useful, in 10–15 minute applications several times daily, in cases of chronic and acute distress of these tissues.

When examining tendons and bony surfaces of the anterior wrist area, caution is needed to avoid pressure or friction on the ulnar and radial arteries and the ulnar and median nerve. The pressure bar is an inappropriate tool for this area due to the vulnerability of these structures (see Chapter 9).

🖐🖐 Assessment and MET treatment of shortness in the forearm flexors

A painful medial humeral epicondyle ('golfer's elbow') usually accompanies tension in the flexors of the wrist and hand (Fig. 13.103).

• The patient is seated facing the practitioner, with her flexed elbow supported by the practitioner's fingers.

• The patient's hand is extended at the wrist, so that the palm is upward and finger tips point toward her own ipsilateral shoulder.

• The extended wrist should easily be able to form a 90° angle with the forearm if the flexors of the wrist are not shortened.

• The practitioner guides the wrist into greater extension to an easy barrier, with pronation exaggerated by pressure on the ulnar side of the palm.

• This is achieved by means of the practitioner's thumb being placed on the dorsum of the patient's hand while the fingers stabilize the palmar aspect, finger tips pressing the hand toward the floor on the ulnar side of the patient's palm.

• The patient attempts to gently supinate the hand against resistance for 7–10 seconds following which, after relaxation and on an exhalation, pronation and extension are increased through the new barrier.

• Repeat 2–3 times.

• This method can easily be adapted for self-treatment by the patient applying the counterpressure.

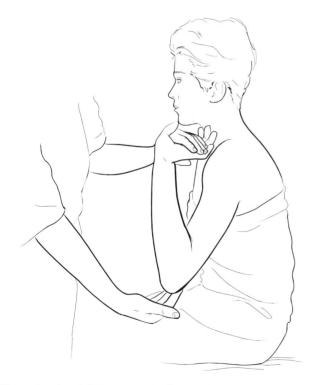

Figure 13.103   MET treatment for forearm flexors.

🖐🖐 MET for shortness in extensors of the wrist and hand

• The patient is seated facing the practitioner, with her flexed elbow supported by the practitioner's fingers.

• The patient's wrist and hand is flexed, so that the palm is facing downward and finger tips point toward her own ipsilateral shoulder.

• The flexed wrist should easily be able to form a 90° angle with the forearm if the extensors of the wrist are not shortened.

• The practitioner places the palm of his other hand onto the dorsum of the patient's hand, his fingers covering her flexed fingers, so that slack is removed and the tissue is taken to its barrier.

• The patient is asked to attempt to take her fingers into extension against the practitioner's resistance for 7–10 seconds, using minimal but steady effort.

• When the patient releases the isometric effort the practitioner, with the patient's assistance, takes the wrist and fingers into greater flexion without force and holds the new position for at least 20 seconds.

• The procedure is repeated 2–3 times more.

• This method can easily be adapted for self-treatment, by means of the patient applying the counterpressure.

🖐🖐 PRT for wrist dysfunction (including carpal tunnel syndrome)

Jones (1985) writes:

Because there are eight bones in the wrist, I had visions of very complicated maneuvers being necessary. I was surprised how easy wrist treatment usually is. I treat it as if it were just one joint ... if the wrist is tender on the dorsal side, I extend [dorsiflex] and rotate. If it is on the palmar side, I flex and rotate. Occasionally I fine tune with sidebending. There are many [patients] with tender spots on the flexor tendons that have been diagnosed [as having] carpal tunnel syndrome, which responds to this type of treatment. I can only guess that they have been misdiagnosed.

• The practitioner palpates and locates an area of extreme sensitivity to light pressure on the dorsum or palmar surface of the hand or wrist (see p. 388, Fig. 13.87B).

• Using sufficient digital pressure to create discomfort which the patient can grade as a '10', the practitioner positions the hand and wrist to remove, as far as possible, the perceived tenderness/pain.

• Tender point pain on the dorsum of the hand is usually relieved by dorsiflexion and slight wrist rotation one way or the other and possibly by additional side-flexion or translation.

• Once the reported pain score has reduced to '3' or less, the position is held for 90 seconds before a slow return to neutral.

Box 13.16 Mulligan's mobilization techniques

Mobilization with movement (MWM) involves a painless, gliding, translation pressure, applied by the practitioner, *almost always at right angles to the plane of movement in which restriction is noted.* At the same time the patient actively (or sometimes the practitioner passively) moves the joint in the direction of restriction or pain.

MWM for flexion restriction of finger joint

- The patient is seated and the practitioner stabilizes the distal end of the proximal bone of the pair which make up the joint, with a finger and thumb hold, one contact on the lateral and one on the medial aspect of the bone.
- The practitioner's other finger and thumb hold the proximal end of the distal bone of the pair making up the joint, again with one contact on the medial and the other on the lateral aspects of the bone. The patient could be asked to do this.
- With these contacts the practitioner is able to easily translate (or glide or shunt) the bones on each other, by gently taking one lateral and the other medial and vice versa.
- The practitioner tests to see which of these options is the least painful, as the finger is flexed.
- Mulligan states that, 'In nearly every case you will find that one direction is painful, and the other is not. You choose the direction which is painless and ask the patient to flex his stiff finger while you sustain the mobilization. This active movement should be pain free and the range should increase'.
- The procedure is repeated several times and the range of movement and pain previously experienced is reassessed.
- Mulligan believes that this method normalizes tracking dysfunctions, such as are known to occur with the patella, but which are not commonly considered to occur in other joints.

 ### MWM for flexion or extension restriction of the wrist

- The patient is seated with the elbow of the (in this example) right arm flexed, forearm pronated.
- The practitioner holds the distal aspects of the radius and ulna with his left hand, so that the web between his finger and thumb lies over the distal aspect of the radius.
- The web between finger and thumb of his right hand is placed on the other side of the hand, covering the proximal row of the carpal bones.
- These contacts allow the practitioner to effectively translate (glide, shunt) the wrist joint so that as one of the practitioner's hands moves medially, the other moves laterally.
- Mulligan states, 'I have found in *every* case the successful glide has been a lateral one [of the carpal bones]'.
- While the practitioner holds the least uncomfortable direction of translation, almost always, according to Mulligan, a lateral translation of the carpals, the patient is asked to actively move the wrist into the restricted direction, flexion or extension.
- 'If the mobilization with movement procedure is indicated the range of movement will improve instantly and painlessly.'
- This is repeated several times.
- If any aspect of the procedure is painful it should be modified until it is painless, possibly by altering the angle of translation very slightly or marginally modifying the practitioner's hand positions.
- Reversing the practitioner's hand positions as illustrated facilitates translation as described above.

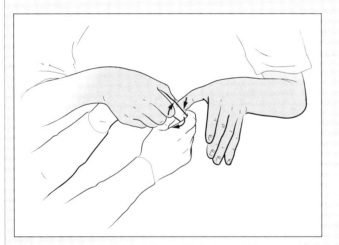

Figure 13.104 Mobilization with movement (Mulligan's method) for interphalangeal dysfunction, with patient holding distal bone of involved joint.

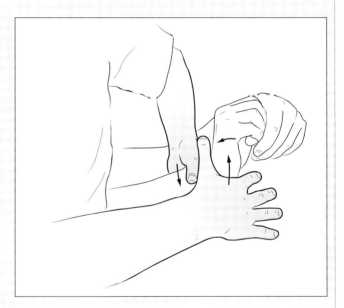

Figure 13.105 Mobilization with movement (Mulligan's method) for wrist dysfunction.

- Tender point pain on the palmar surface is treated in the same way but with flexion instead of dorsiflexion.
- Several tender points can usefully be treated at one session. It is our clinical experience that functional improvement is often immediate (improved range, etc.) but that reduction in existing pain may take several days to manifest following PRT treatment (see notes on PRT, pp. 124 and 147).

 ## MFR for areas of fibrosis or hypertonicity

- The practitioner identifies a localized area of hypertonicity, fibrosis, 'adhesion'.
- The muscles involved are placed in a shortened (i.e. not stretched) position; therefore, if the treatment

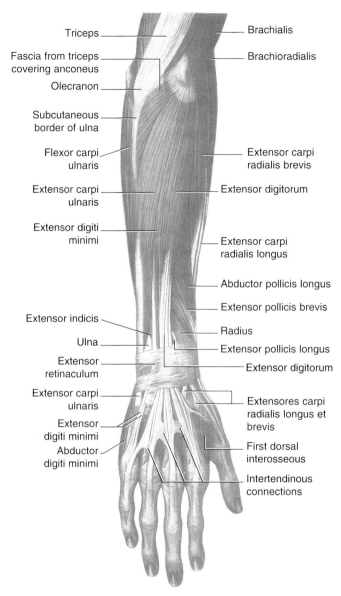

Triceps
Fascia from triceps covering anconeus
Olecranon
Subcutaneous border of ulna
Flexor carpi ulnaris
Extensor carpi ulnaris
Extensor digiti minimi
Extensor indicis
Ulna
Extensor retinaculum
Extensor carpi ulnaris
Extensor digiti minimi
Abductor digiti minimi

Brachialis
Brachioradialis
Extensor carpi radialis brevis
Extensor digitorum
Extensor carpi radialis longus
Abductor pollicis longus
Extensor pollicis brevis
Radius
Extensor pollicis longus
Extensor digitorum
Extensores carpi radialis longus et brevis
First dorsal interosseous
Intertendinous connections

Figure 13.106 Superficial posterior forearm (reproduced, with permission, from *Gray's anatomy* (1995)).

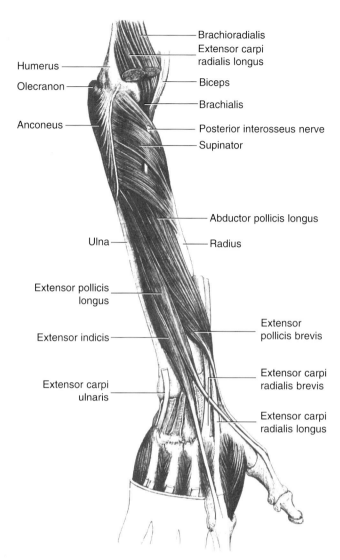

Humerus
Olecranon
Anconeus
Ulna
Extensor pollicis longus
Extensor indicis
Extensor carpi ulnaris

Brachioradialis
Extensor carpi radialis longus
Biceps
Brachialis
Posterior interosseus nerve
Supinator
Abductor pollicis longus
Radius
Extensor pollicis brevis
Extensor carpi radialis brevis
Extensor carpi radialis longus

Figure 13.107 Deep posterior forearm (reproduced, with permission, from *Gray's anatomy* (1995)).

were being applied to the flexors of the forearm, the wrist would be in slight flexion.

• Firm finger or thumb pressure is applied to the tissues, *slightly distal* to the restricted tissues.

• The patient is asked to slowly and deliberately extend and then flex the wrist.

• In this way the flexors are placed at stretch (during wrist extension) and the area of restriction passes under the fixation produced by the practitioner's finger or thumb contact.

• As the wrist is flexed again the muscular and fascial tissues, under pressure, shorten and relax.

• This process is repeated 6–10 times.

• Alternatively, the practitioner can introduce the alternating flexion and extension if the patient is unable to do so.

• Precisely the same method can be used on any tissues which can be compressed manually.

• Self-treatment can be taught to the patient, with cautions as to overtreatment.

POSTERIOR FOREARM TREATMENT

The superficial layer of the posterior forearm contains two muscles of the elbow joint – brachioradialis, anconeus – and five extensor muscles – extensor carpi radialis longus and brevis, extensor digitorum, extensor digiti minimi and extensor carpi ulnaris. The deep extensors include supinator (elbow region), extensor indicis and three thumb muscles – abductor pollicis longus, extensor pollicis brevis and extensor pollicis longus.

Superficial layer

On the most lateral aspect of the forearm lies the radial group – brachioradialis, extensor carpi radialis longus and brevis – and the supinator, as if stacked upon each other. The most superficial and the deepest of these are discussed with the elbow, while the two wrist extensors are included here. These four muscles can be conveniently addressed (palpated and treated) together in the semisupinated forearm with applications of gliding strokes, pincer compression and flat palpation. This 'lateral forearm' position may be varied toward greater pronation or supination to best access or evaluate the muscles. They are also accessible with the arm pronated and a portion can be palpated with the arm in supination.

The lateral epicondyle of the humerus, where many of these muscles share a common tendon attachment, can be readily examined at the same time. When any (or several) of the muscles attaching into the tendon develop contractures, tension will be placed on the common tendon which is capable of provoking an inflammatory response. Commonly called 'tennis elbow', lateral epicondylitis may be initiated, aggravated and perpetuated by hand, wrist and finger extension activities, especially if these are repetitive and/or stressful (Cailliet 1994).

Cailliet (1994) suggests three theories of etiology for symptoms which include deep tenderness accompanied by an ache at the lateral epicondyle, the musculature of which is painful upon palpation:

- tendinitis at the lateral epicondyle
- radial nerve entrapment
- intraarticular or osseous disorders.

He notes that pain is intensified with resisted wrist extension or radial deviation and that tenderness in the posterior interosseous nerve is reported when supination of the extended wrist is resisted.

Treatment for such symptoms may include the following (Cailliet 1994).

Acute

- Rest the wrist and elbow by avoiding the activities which provoke the pain, avoid pronation of the forearm or wrist or finger extension.
- Possible wrist splinting to decrease extension.
- Changes in patterns of use, including sports.
- Possible steroid injection (Cailliet points out that acupuncture has been claimed to be more effective (Brattberg 1983)).

Postacute

- Gentle active and passive range of motion of wrist and elbow.
- Gentle wrist exercises, including extension, radial and ulnar deviations (in pronation and supination), wrist flexion and circumduction, *followed by a period of relaxation.*
- When exercises can be painlessly performed, light weight may be added and gradually increased (in weight and repetitions).

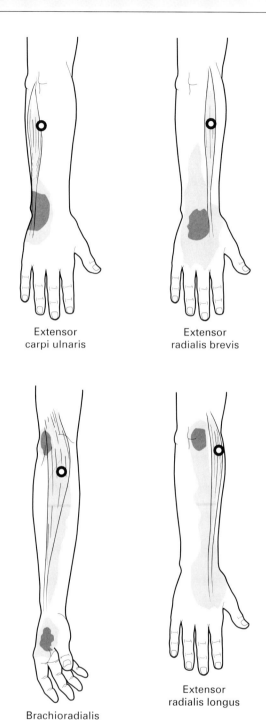

Extensor carpi ulnaris

Extensor radialis brevis

Brachioradialis

Extensor radialis longus

Figure 13.108 Composite of wrist extensors and brachioradialis trigger point patterns.

- Surgical intervention may be considered as a final resort.

We would add to this list – especially in the acute phase – the use of alternating (short) hot and cold applications (see Chapter 10), positional release methods (see Chapter 10) and anti-inflammatory nutritional strategies (see Chapter 7), including increased EPA (fish oil) supplementation and enzymes, such as pineapple bromelaine.

Extensor carpi radialis longus

Attachments: From the distal third of the lateral supra-condylar crest of the humerus and lateral inter-muscular septum (including fibers from the common extensor tendon) to the base of the 2nd metacarpal on the radial side of the posterior surface

Innervation: Radial nerve (C6–7)

Muscle type: Phasic (type 2), weakens when stressed

Function: Extension and radial deviation of the wrist, weakly flexes and influences pronation and supination of elbow (Platzer 1992)

Synergists: *For wrist extension*: extensor carpi radialis brevis, extensor carpi ulnaris, extensor digitorum, extensor digiti minimi

For radial deviation: extensor carpi radialis brevis and flexor carpi radialis

Antagonists: *To wrist extension*: flexor carpi radialis and ulnaris, flexor digitorum superficialis and profundus, palmaris longus

To radial deviation: flexor carpi ulnaris, extensor carpi ulnaris

Extensor carpi radialis brevis

Attachments: From the common extensor tendon of the lateral epicondyle to the base of the 2nd and 3rd metacarpals

Innervation: Deep radial nerve (C7–8)

Muscle type: Phasic (type 2), weakens when stressed

Function: Extension and radial deviation of the wrist

Synergists: *For wrist extension*: extensor carpi radialis brevis, extensor carpi ulnaris, extensor digitorum, extensor digiti minimi

For radial deviation: extensor carpi radialis longus and flexor carpi radialis

Antagonists: *To wrist extension*: flexor carpi radialis and ulnaris, flexor digitorum superficialis and profundus, palmaris longus

To radial deviation: flexor carpi ulnaris, extensor carpi ulnaris

Extensor carpi ulnaris

Attachments: From the common extensor tendon and the posterior border of the ulna to the base of the 5th metacarpal

Innervation: Deep radial (C7–8)

Muscle type: Phasic (type 2), weakens when stressed

Function: Extension and ulnar deviation of the wrist

Synergists: *For wrist extension*: extensor carpi radialis brevis and longus, extensor digitorum, extensor digiti minimi

For radial deviation: flexor carpi ulnaris

Antagonists: *To wrist extension*: flexor carpi radialis and ulnaris, flexor digitorum superficialis and profundus, palmaris longus

To radial deviation: flexor carpi radialis, extensor carpi radialis brevis and longus

Indications for treatment of wrist extensors

- Lateral epicondylar pain (tennis elbow)
- Painful supination
- Weakness of the grip
- Pain in elbow, wrist or web of thumb
- Reduces range of motion in wrist flexion or wrist deviations

Special notes

While all three carpi extensors are active during forceful wrist extension, extensor carpi radialis brevis primarily extends the hand during less demanding use. The wrist extensors are also important during flexion activities where they stabilize the wrist to prevent excessive wrist flexion as the fingers grasp and work and are essential in this role when a power grip is used (Simons et al 1998).

Brachioradialis is sometimes grouped with the extensors of the wrist due to its proximity to them and its innervation by an extensor nerve. Its trigger point activity, somewhat like the wrist extensors, is into the elbow, forearm and the hand (web of the thumb) (see p. 410). Since it is often tender in association when the wrist extensors are tender, it is included together with their examination, which is easily accomplished due to their proximity.

Neural entrapment. Simons et al (1998) point out that the extensor carpi radialis brevis and supinator have both been noted to entrap the radial nerve. Such entrapment may produce motor weakness of the muscles it serves, as well as sensory loss or numbness and paresthesias, depending upon which portion of the nerve is impinged. The ulnar nerve may also be entrapped nearby, at the cubital tunnel, by the flexor carpi ulnaris muscle.

Extensor digitorum

Attachments: From the common extensor tendon of the lateral epicondyle, antebrachial fascia and inter-muscular septa to end in four tendons (which split into three intertendinous connections) which attach to the dorsal surface of the middle phalanx (1) and the base of the distal phalanx (2) of the 2nd–5th fingers (see below)

Innervation: Deep radial (C6–8)

Muscle type: Phasic (type 2), weakens when stressed

Function: Extends the fingers at all phalangeal joints, assists in wrist extension and finger abduction, counteracts finger flexion in a power grip

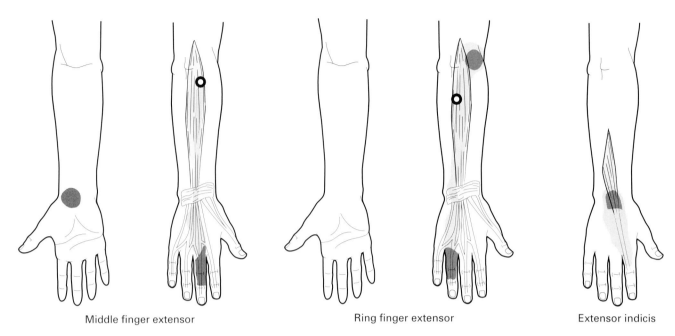

Middle finger extensor

Ring finger extensor

Extensor indicis

Figure 13.109 Composite trigger point referral patterns of finger extensors.

Synergists: *For finger extension*: lumbricales, dorsal inter-ossei, extensor indicis, extensor digiti minimi
For wrist extension: extensor carpi radialis longus, brevis and ulnaris
For finger abduction: dorsal interossei
Antagonists: *To finger extension*: flexor digitorum super-ficialis and profundus, lumbricales, palmar interossei
To wrist extension: flexor carpi radialis and ulnaris
To finger abduction: palmar interossei

Extensor digiti minimi

Attachments: From the common extensor tendon to join with the extensor digitorum at the proximal phalanx to attach to the dorsal expansion of the 5th digit
Innervation: Deep radial (C6–8)
Muscle type: Phasic (type 2), weakens when stressed
Function: Extends the smallest finger, extends the wrist and ulnarly deviates the hand
Synergists: *For finger extension*: extensor digitorum
Antagonists: *To finger extension*: flexor digitorum super-ficialis and profundus, lumbricales, palmar interossei
To wrist extension: flexor carpi radialis and ulnaris
To hand deviation: flexor carpi radialis, extensor carpi radialis brevis and longus

Indications for treatment

- Pain in elbow or fingers
- Weakness of the grip
- Pain at elbow when gripping (such as shaking hands)
- Loss of full flexion of the fingers

- Pain in the elbow, posterior forearm, wrist and fingers due to trigger points

Special notes

The extensor digitorum muscle has an interesting and complex tendon arrangement at its distal attachment, which attaches to the capsules of the metacarpo-phalangeal joints, bases of the proximal phalanges and to the middle and distal phalanges. The interossei and lumbricales participate in the fibrous dorsal expansion of the extensor digitorum tendon, which is described in detail in *Gray's anatomy* (1995) (see Fig. 13.113).

Variations of extensor digitorum include additional bellies (2nd finger), missing bellies (5th finger) and a doubling of the tendons to the individual fingers (Platzer 1992). Simons et al (1998) also note a rare extensor digitorum brevis magnus, which may be misdiagnosed as a ganglion cyst or tumor, and an anomalous extensor digitorum profundus.

The extensor digiti minimi may easily be considered as part of the extensor digitorum since they arise together from the common tendon, are joined at the distal attach-ment and often are fused at the bellies. When the minimi is missing, the digitorum provides an additional tendon to take over its function (Platzer 1992).

 NMT for superficial posterior forearm

With the forearm in a relaxed, semisupinated position and flexed at the elbow to near 90°, the brachioradialis is easily located and treated with pincer compression,

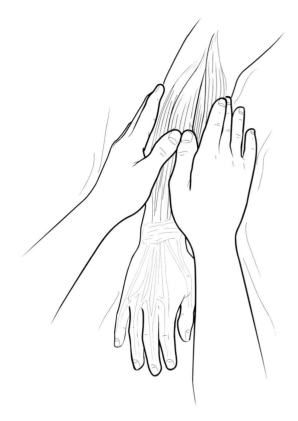

Figure 13.110 Gliding strokes to the posterior forearm help distinguish the superficial layer from the diagonally oriented deeper layer.

lubricated gliding strokes and flat palpation. This muscle should be released before the radial wrist extensors are attended to, since it is superficial to them.

After the brachioradialis is treated, the extensor carpi radialis longus may be grasped with pincer compression, near its humeral attachment, by placing the treating thumb on one side of the muscle and the treating fingers on the other side, while grasping around the brachioradialis. Taut bands within the muscles are examined for trigger points, which may be compressed by flat palpation against the underlying tissue or grasped with pincer compression as previously described. A deeper placement of the fingers may also address the extensor carpi radialis brevis, which lies deep to the longus. A small portion of the supinator may be reached by gliding the thumb on the radial attachment (see p. 386). Only a small portion of supinator may be accessed directly but application of repeated gliding techniques, assisted pronating stretches and posttreatment ice applications usually achieve satisfactory results, especially if the source of the muscular irritation (such as overuse) is eliminated.

Hydrotherapy applications may precede or follow these procedures. Inflammation of the supinator muscle and epicondyles of the humerus should be ruled out before applying heat to the elbow region. Ice therapy may be applied to any of the muscles following therapy.

The patient is seated comfortably opposite the practitioner with a table placed between them on which to support the arm. The forearm and hand to be treated are pronated and rest comfortably on the table with the fingers directed toward the practitioner, as the table provides support for the arm.

• The superficial layer of muscles is addressed first, with lubricated gliding strokes along the course of each muscle, from the wrist to the lateral epicondyle. The gliding strokes are repeated 6–8 times on each muscle until the entire surface of the posterior forearm has been treated. The order of treatment is not important but when learning to identify these muscles, the following order may be helpful.
• From the midline of the wrist to the lateral epicondyle will address the extensor digitorum.
• On the ulnar side of this landmark 'mid-line' lies the extensor digiti minimi and, next to it, the extensor carpi ulnaris.
• On the radial side of the 'mid-line' lies the brachioradialis, extensor carpi longus and brevis and supinator, one stacked upon the other as previously described on p. 409.
• The small anconeus may be palpated just distal to the elbow between the ulna and radius (a line between the olecranon and the lateral epicondyle represents the proximal edge of this small, triangular muscle).
• On the radial side of the distal one-third of the forearm, the deeper layer of muscles lie diagonally oriented, with abductor pollicis longus (proximal) and extensor pollicis brevis being the most palpable. Gliding strokes may again be applied with increased pressure (if appropriate) to influence the bellies of these two muscles, as well as extensor pollicis longus and extensor indicis, which are almost completely covered by extensor digitorum.

As the practitioner applies the gliding strokes to the opposite arm to treat or to compare the tissues, a hot pack (if appropriate) may be applied to the arm which has been treated. The gliding strokes are then repeated. If the muscles are moderately uncomfortable with appropriate gliding strokes, inflammation may be present, especially with repetitive use conditions. In this case, heat would be contraindicated and an ice pack used instead.

Once the lubricated gliding strokes have been sufficiently applied to warm and elongate the myofascial tissue, individual palpation may easily distinguish most of these posterior forearm muscles. Knowledge of the musculature will assist the practitioner in being correctly positioned and active movement of most of these muscles will assist in readily identifying them.

Transverse, snapping palpation may be applied with the thumb or finger tips to identify taut bands within any of these muscles. Since trigger points occur within taut bands, examination of any taut fibers found should be included as part of the NMT treatment/examination, especially at the center of the fiber where central triggers occur. Most of these muscles have lengthy tendons, making their endplate zone (where central trigger points occur) more proximal than one would expect.

Tender attachment sites are often associated with a central trigger point and will usually resolve with little treatment needed if the central trigger point is released (Simons et al 1998). Lewit (1985) states: 'Frequently, like trigger points in muscles, pain points [on the periosteum] are highly characteristic of certain lesions, and therefore have high diagnostic value. Their disappearance (improvement) also serves as a valuable test for the efficacy of treatment'. Since these muscles are readily palpable, trigger point pressure release is easily applied to them. Spray and stretch techniques, injection, dry needling, lymphatic drainage and active myofascial release may also be used to deactivate referral patterns. The tissue should be stretched following treatment using MET, PNF or other appropriate stretching methods.

The lateral epicondyle is deserving of special attention as numerous muscles attach to it (extensor carpi radialis longus and brevis, extensor digitorum, extensor carpi ulnaris, supinator and anconeus). Careful palpation is suggested as it is often very tender, especially associated with wrist and elbow pain. Additionally, central trigger points should be addressed in all the muscles which merge into the common extensor tendon which attaches here. Habitual overuse of the muscles should be decreased and frequent stretching of the forearm muscles employed as 'homework'. Ice packs are useful in 10–15 minute applications several times daily.

Deep layer

The deep layer of the posterior forearm contains supinator (elbow region), extensor indicis and three thumb muscles – abductor pollicis longus, extensor pollicis brevis and extensor pollicis longus. While the supinator is discussed

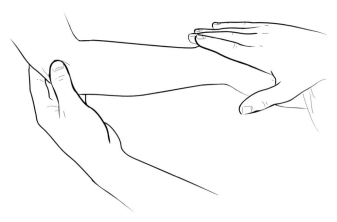

Figure 13.111 Careful palpation of the lateral epicondylar region may reveal inflammation associated with the common tendon attachment shared by several muscles.

with the elbow, the four remaining muscles are addressed in the order in which they lie on the posterior forearm from lateral (radial side) to medial (ulnar aspect). While they are not always distinct, their fiber direction lies diagonally and they are usually palpable when proximal gliding strokes are used and with precisely applied muscle tests.

Abductor pollicis longus

Attachments: From the dorsal surface of the ulna distal to the supinator crest, interosseous membrane and middle third of posterior radius to the base of the first metacarpal and trapezium
Innervation: Deep radial (C7–8)
Muscle type: Phasic (type 2), weakens when stressed
Function: Abducts the thumb, extends the thumb at the carpometacarpal joint
Synergists: *For abduction*: abductor pollicis brevis
For extension: extensor pollicis longus and brevis
Antagonists: *To abduction*: adductor pollicis
To extension: flexor pollicis longus and brevis

Extensor pollicis brevis

Attachments: From the dorsal surface of the ulna distal to abductor pollicis longus, interosseous membrane and middle third of posterior radius to the dorsolateral base of the proximal phalanx of the thumb and sometimes to the distal phalanx
Innervation: Deep radial (C7–8 or T1)
Muscle type: Phasic (type 2), weakens when stressed
Function: Extends and abducts the thumb
Synergists: *For extension*: extensor pollicis longus, abductor pollicis longus
For abduction: abductor pollicis longus
Antagonists: *To extension*: flexor pollicis longus and brevis
To abduction: adductor pollicis

Extensor pollicis longus

Attachments: From the middle third of the dorsal surface of the ulna and the interosseous membrane to the base of the distal phalanx of the thumb
Innervation: Deep radial nerve (C7–8)
Muscle type: Phasic (type 2), weakens when stressed
Function: Extends the distal phalanx of the thumb, extends the proximal phalanx and metacarpal and adducts the first metacarpal. Platzer (1992) notes it dorsiflexes and radially deviates the hand
Synergists: *For extension*: extensor pollicis brevis, abductor pollicis longus
For abduction: abductor pollicis longus
Antagonists: *To extension*: flexor pollicis longus and brevis
To abduction: adductor pollicis

Indications for treatment

- Pain at the base of the thumb
- Loss of range or pain during flexion of the thumb
- Pain with thumb movement
- Tenderness to direct palpation

Special notes

These three thumb muscles, joined by the flexor pollicis longus (deep layer of anterior forearm), work with five intrinsic thumb muscles to provide an amazing mobility which greatly exceeds that of the fingers. When this highly mobile digit interacts with the fingers, simple acts (such as grasping a ball) take on mechanical complexities requiring simultaneous coordinated contraction of multiple muscles. When painfully dysfunctional, the thumb deserves due attention as the actions it performs are indispensable.

The bellies of these thumb muscles lie wholly within the forearm with the long tendons projecting distally to attach to the thumb. When examining for central trigger points (trigger point referral patterns have yet to be established in these tissues), it is useful to remember that central trigger points occur in the fibers only and the tendons are disregarded when considering their locations. The attachments on the forearm are often tender and are palpated through extensor digitorum.

Extensor indicis

Attachments: From the posterior distal third of the ulna and interosseous membrane to the extensor digitorum tendon for the index finger
Innervation: Deep radial (C7–8)
Muscle type: Phasic (type 2), weakens when stressed
Function: Extends the index finger and wrist
Synergists: *For extension of index finger*: extensor digitorum
  For extension of wrist: extensor carpi radialis brevis and longus, extensor digitorum, extensor digiti minimi
  For radial deviation: flexor carpi ulnaris
Antagonists: *To finger extension*: flexor digitorum superficialis and profundus
  To wrist extension: flexor carpi radialis and ulnaris, flexor digitorum superficialis and profundus, palmaris longus

Indications for treatment

- Limitation of flexion of index finger
- Pain in radial side of dorsal wrist extending to but not into finger

 ## NMT for deep posterior forearm

The bellies of abductor pollicis longus and extensor pollicis brevis are palpated with short, 3–4 inch gliding

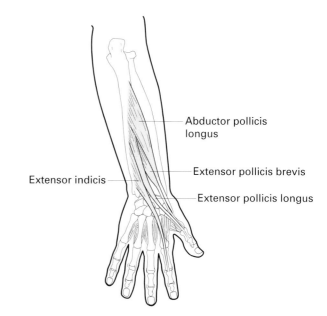

Figure 13.112 Deep posterior forearm.

strokes on the radial side of the distal forearm as the tissues are pressed against the underlying bone. The diagonally oriented fibers are more easily palpated where they overlie the bone and become less distinct after they pass deep to the extensor digitorum. Their attachments along the ulna may be tender and are often palpable when the muscles are tested against resistance.

Abductor pollicis longus and extensor pollicis brevis, as well as extensor pollicis longus and extensor indicis, may also be influenced with gliding strokes which offer increased pressure through the overlying extensor digitorum.

Transverse snapping palpation may be used through the extensor digitorum, provided it is not too tender. Since most muscles of the forearm refer their trigger point patterns toward the joints which they serve, it would

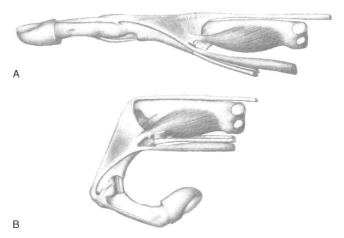

Figure 13.113 A&B: The dorsal extensor expansion forms a 'tendon hood' (reproduced, with permission, from *Gray's anatomy* (1995)).

Box 13.17   Arthritis (Rubin 1997)

Arthritic conditions are broadly divided into inflammatory and non-inflammatory forms, although the latter (such as osteoarthritis) often have periods of inflammatory activity.

Some of the major characteristics of inflammatory arthritis include:

- joints are stiff in the morning, usually with a gradual reduction in stiffness during the day
- the affected joints are swollen and painful
- rest eases the pain and activity exacerbates it
- with rheumatoid arthritis, the commonest form of inflammatory arthritis, there is usually a symmetrical distribution (i.e. both hands and/or elbows and/or knees, etc.).

Examination commonly reveals warmth, redness, a degree of synovial thickening, deformity, swelling, weakness of associated muscles and loss of range of motion.

All diagnosis should be based on evidence which builds a clinical picture and which ultimately confirms the likelihood of a condition. For example, laboratory tests can confirm an arthritic condition but may sometimes be related to conditions other than rheumatic ones.

- Elevated sedimentation rate (present in all types of inflammation and infection including inflammatory arthritis)
- Positive antinuclear antibodies (almost always present in rheumatoid arthritis)
- Abnormal creatine phosphokinase may (or may not) confirm polymyositis
- Rheumatoid factor is commonly found in asymptomatic people over the age of 60

A combination of features, symptoms and tests is therefore required before a suitably qualified and licensed individual can make a diagnosis.

Radiographic evidence

- Inflammatory rheumatic conditions usually show X-ray evidence of erosion, osteopenia, loss of joint substance. In other words, there is a 'subtractive' picture – tissue has 'diminished'.
- Non-inflammatory rheumatic conditions, such as osteoarthritis, tend to display an 'additive' picture, where an increase in bone has taken place (osteophytes, for example).

Inflammatory arthritis variations

- Rheumatoid arthritis affects the joints of the body symmetrically and predominantly affects women of childbearing age. Rheumatoid factor and antinuclear antibodies will usually be found in the blood.
- Seronegative spondyloarthropathies such as ankylosing spondylitis, psoriatic arthritis and Reiter's syndrome have asymmetrical distribution. Rheumatoid factor is not found with these

conditions. They are associated with people who carry the HLA-B27 gene.

- Some researchers have identified a connection between both seronegative spondyloarthropathies and seropositive rheumatic conditions and bowel overgrowth with specific bacteria, for example ankylosing spondylitis is commonly associated with klebsiella overgrowth and rheumatoid arthritis with proteus (which is also commonly associated with bladder infections in women) (Ebringer 1988).
- Infectious arthritis may be caused by gonococcal (or non-gonococcal) bacterial infection and, more rarely, by viral or fungal agents. Usually only one joint is involved and this will be swollen and tender. Other symptoms may include fever, chills and skin lesions. The patient is usually young and sexually active. Infectious arthritis is regarded as a medical emergency although fatal outcomes have declined as physicians have become more aware of the need for rapid fluid drainage from the joint together with appropriate antibiotic therapy.
- Juvenile rheumatoid arthritis may affect only a few joints and is usually characterized by the absence of rheumatoid factor and antinuclear antibodies. Older boys who are also HLA-B27 positive (see ankylosing spondylitis above) may progress to develop AS.
- Crystal-induced arthritis usually occurs in middle age or later. Commonly only a single joint is affected. The condition is either true or pseudo-gout with the diagnosis being made by microscopic examination of the synovial fluid to identify the type of crystal.

Non-inflammatory arthritis

- Osteoarthritis (OA) is usually caused by a combination of joint 'wear and tear' together with an inherited tendency (transmitted by autosomal dominant genes in women) which produces defects in collagen synthesis (Knowlton 1990).
- Primary generalized osteoarthritis affects any (and sometimes all) of the joints of the extremities.
- Sometimes obvious overuse relating to occupational stresses clearly contributes to the sites affected by OA. Leg length discrepancy seems to contribute to the evolution of OA on the long leg side.
- Erosive OA involves self-limiting inflammation affecting the distal interphalangeal joints, producing erosion at the margins and possible fusion.

Treatment

Treatment of arthritic conditions should take account of the presence or otherwise of active inflammation. No manual measures should be utilized during periods of active inflammation apart from gentle lymphatic drainage, positional release and non-stretching use of isometric contractions (e.g. Ruddy's methods, see p. 137). Hydrotherapy to assist in easing swelling and inflammation, as well as nutritional antiinflammatory strategies (see Chapter 8, p. 101), may be usefully introduced.

be reasonable to assume that these would as well, but clear patterns have yet to be established for these muscles.

INTRINSIC HAND MUSCLE TREATMENT

Fine movements of the fingers are controlled by the intrinsic muscles of the hand while gross movements of grip and those which require power are primarily controlled by extrinsic muscles. The intrinsic muscles of the hand are considered in three groups.

1. Thumb muscles – include thenar muscles abductor pollicis brevis, opponens pollicis and flexor pollicis brevis and non-thenar adductor pollicis
2. Hypothenar eminence – includes minimi muscles (abductor digiti minimi, flexor digiti minimi brevis, opponens digiti minimi) and palmaris brevis
3. Metacarpal muscles – lumbricales and interossei (palmar and dorsal)

All of these muscles are served by the ulnar nerve except abductor pollicis brevis, opponens pollicis, superficial head of flexor pollicis brevis and the 1st and 2nd lumbricales, which are innervated by the median nerve. None are normally served by the radial nerve.

The dorsal extensor expansion, a fibrous branching of the extensor digitorum tendon on the posterior aspect of the proximal phalanges, plays an important role in association with the intrinsic muscles. It is into this extension that the interossei, lumbricales and abductor digiti minimi fibers merge, to act upon the fingers. This expansion forms a 'tendon hood' which moves proximally and distally respectively as the finger is extended and flexed to assist in movement of the finger.

Thenar muscles and adductor pollicis

The abductor pollicis brevis arises from the scaphoid tubercle, trapezium, flexor retinaculum and the tendon of abductor pollicis longus to attach to the radial sesamoid bone, base of the first proximal phalanx (thumb) and the dorsal digital expansion of the thumb. It provides palmar abduction, which abducts the thumb at right angles to the palm.

Opponens pollicis, lying deep to abductor pollicis brevis, arises from the flexor retinaculum and tubercle of the trapezium and attaches to the entire length of the first metacarpal's radial margin and its palmar surface. It provides adduction, opposition and flexion of the thumb.

Flexor pollicis brevis, lying medial to abductor pollicis brevis, has a superficial head arising from the flexor retinaculum and trapezium tubercle and a deep head arising from the trapezoid and capitate bones. These two heads merge together into a tendon attaching to the

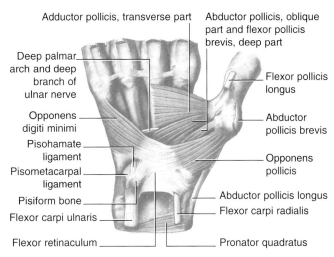

Figure 13.115   Deep hand muscles (reproduced, with permission, from *Gray's anatomy* (1995)).

radial sesamoid bone and base of the first phalanx. It flexes, abducts and adducts the thumb.

Adductor pollicis arises from an oblique head, which attaches to the capitate, bases of 2nd and 3rd metacarpals, palmar carpal ligaments and the tendon sheath of flexor carpi radialis, and a transverse head, which attaches to the distal two-thirds of the 3rd metacarpal. These two tendons converge into a common tendon (which contains a sesamoid bone) shared with the first palmar interosseous muscle, which attaches to the base of the proximal phalanx of the thumb. It adducts and assists in opposition and flexion of the thumb.

In summary, the following muscles contribute to the listed movement.

- Adduction – adductor pollicis, flexor pollicis brevis, opponens pollicis
- Abduction – abductor pollicis brevis, flexor pollicis brevis
- Opposition – opponens pollicis, flexor pollicis brevis, adductor pollicis
- Reposition (return to neutral) – extrinsic thumb muscles (extensor pollicis brevis, extensor pollicis longus, abductor pollicis).

Hypothenar eminence

Palmaris brevis attaches the skin of the ulnar border of the hand to the flexor retinaculum and palmar aponeurosis. It deepens the hollow of the palm by making the hypothenar eminence more prominent.

Abductor digiti minimi arises from the pisiform, tendon of flexor carpi ulnaris and pisohamate ligament and divides into two slips, one of which attaches to the ulnar margin of the base of the 5th proximal phalanx while the other merges into the dorsal digital expansion of the extensor digiti minimi. It serves to abduct the little finger.

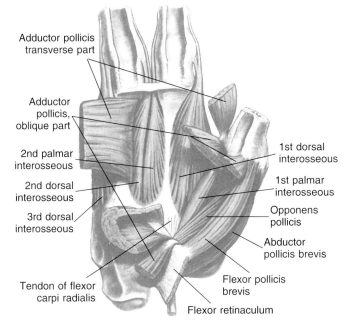

Figure 13.114   Superficial hand muscles (reproduced, with permission, from *Gray's anatomy* (1995)).

Flexor digiti minimi brevis lies next to abductor digiti minimi and arises from the hook of the hamate and the flexor retinaculum to attach to the ulnar margin of the base of the 5th proximal phalanx. It flexes the metacarpophalangeal joint of the 5th digit.

Opponens digiti minimi arises from the hook of the hamate and the flexor retinaculum to attach to the entire ulnar margin of the 5th metacarpal. It brings the 5th digit into opposition with the thumb.

Metacarpal muscles

Dorsal interossei (4) arise each from two adjacent metacarpal bones to insert into the base of the proximal phalanx of the adjacent (medial) finger and its tendon expansion. They flex the metacarpophalangeal joints and extend the interphalangeal joints, abduct the fingers from the midline of the hand and can rotate the digit at the metacarpophalangeal joint.

Palmar interossei (4) arise from the medial aspects of the 1st, 2nd, 4th and 5th metacarpal bones and attach to the extensor expansion (and possibly the base of the proximal phalanx) of the same digit. They flex the metacarpophalangeal joints and extend the interphalangeal joints, adduct the fingers toward the mid-line of the hand and can rotate the digit at the metacarpophalangeal joint.

Lumbricales (4) arise from each of the tendons of flexor digitorum profundus and course to the radial aspect of the metacarpal bone of the same finger, where each attaches to the respective extensor expansion (tendon hood). The lumbricales extend the interphalangeal joint and may weakly flex the metacarpophalangeal joint. In addition, they appear to have a significant role in proprioception based on their numerous muscle spindles and long fiber length (*Gray's anatomy* 1995).

 ## NMT for palmar and dorsal hand

The treatment of the hand may be performed with the patient lying supine or seated across the table from the practitioner. The surface of the table may be needed to support the hand when pressure is applied.

With the hand supine, the thenar eminence is grasped between the thumb and finger of the same hand (Fig. 13.117). This is most easily applied if the thumb is relaxed and mildly, passively flexed. Each of the thenar muscles may be compressed and examined for tenderness in their bellies, at thumb-width intervals. Flat palpation against the underlying tissue and metacarpal is also useful as well as flat compression of the tendon attachments.

The muscles lying in the web of the thumb are most easily compressed with one digit on the palmar surface and the other on the dorsal surface. The compression

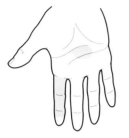

First dorsal interosseous

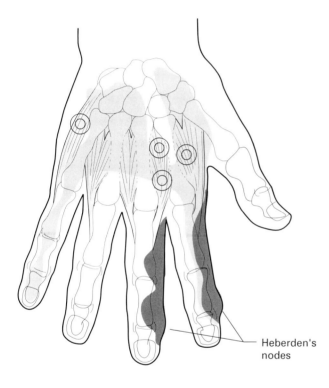

Heberden's nodes

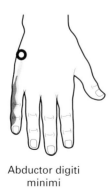

Abductor digiti minimi

Figure 13.116 Heberden's nodes at the distal phalangeal joints may be associated with trigger points in interossei.

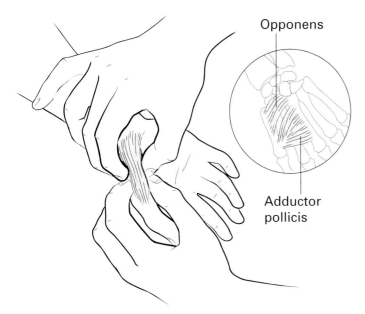

Figure 13.117 The muscles of the thenar eminence may be grasped and compressed as shown or palpated flat against underlying structures.

techniques should be applied alongside the thumb as well as the index finger.

The hypothenar muscles are compressed in a similar manner, using pincer compression and flat compression. Very mildly lubricated, short gliding strokes can be applied to the hypothenar muscles as well as the entire palmar surface of the hand.

The beveled pressure bar is used to examine the interossei muscles by wedging it between the metacarpals and angling it toward the bones (a beveled typewriter eraser may be substituted). Gentle friction is applied at

tip-width intervals to each palmar and dorsal interossei muscle. The small pressure bar may also be used to scrape the palmar fascia and to apply very short, 'scraping' type strokes to each joint of the fingers (unless contraindicated by arthritis, inflammation, infection or pain) (Fig. 13.118).

Myofascial spreads may be applied to the palmar surface of the hand to treat the palmar fascia. Appropriate hydrotherapies may accompany the treatment or may be given as 'homework'. Unless contraindicated (such as with inflammatory arthritis), the hands especially benefit from contrast hydrotherapy, applied by plunging the hands in alternating hot and cold baths of approximately ½–1 minute each for 8–10 repetitions.

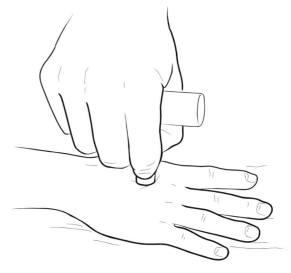

Figure 13.118 The beveled-tip pressure bar can be wedged between the metacarpals to treat the interossei with static pressure or mild friction.

REFERENCES

Barnes J 1996 Myofascial release in treatment of thoracic outlet syndrome. Journal of Bodywork and Movement Therapies 1(1):53–57
Barnes M 1997 Basic science of myofascial release. Journal of Bodywork and Movement Therapies 1(4):231–238
Boyle J 1999 Is the pain and dysfunction of shoulder impingement lesion really second rib syndrome in disguise? Two case reports. Manual Therapy 4(1):44–48
Brattberg G 1983 Acupuncture therapy for tennis elbow. Pain 16:285–288
Butler D 1991 Mobilisation of the nervous system. Churchill Livingstone, Edinburgh
Butler D, Gifford L 1989 Adverse mechanical tensions in the nervous system. Physiotherapy 75:622–629
Cailliet R 1991 Shoulder pain. F A Davis, Philadelphia
Cailliet R 1994 Hand pain and impairment, 4th edn. F A Davis, Philadelphia
Cailliet R 1996 Soft tissue pain and disability, 3rd edn. F A Davis, Philadelphia
Chaitow L 1996a Muscle energy techniques. Churchill Livingstone, Edinburgh
Chaitow L 1996b Positional release techniques. Churchill Livingstone, Edinburgh

Chikly B 1999 Clinical perspectives: breast cancer reconstructive rehabilitation: LDT. Journal of Bodywork and Movement Therapies 3(1):11–16
Cyriax J 1982 Textbook of orthopaedic medicine vol. 1: diagnosis of soft tissue lesions, 8th edn. Baillière Tindall, London
Daniels L, Worthingham C 1980 Muscle testing techniques of manual examination. W B Saunders, Philadelphia
DeLany J 1999 Clinical perspectives: breast cancer reconstructive rehabilitation: NMT. Journal of Bodywork and Movement Therapies 3(1):5–10
Ebringer A 1988 Klebsiella antibodies in ankylosing spondylitis and Proteus antibodies in rheumatoid arthritis. British Journal of Rheumatology 27:72–85
Fitzgerald F 1998 Breast cancer treatments: you do have choices. Nature's Impact August/September: 36–41
Goodheart G 1984 Applied kinesiology workshop procedure manual, 21st edition. Privately published, Detroit
Grays anatomy 1995, 38th edn. Churchill Livingstone, New York
Greenman P 1989 Manual medicine. Williams and Wilkins, Baltimore
Hoppenfeld S 1976 Physical examination of the spine and extremities. Appleton and Lange, Norwalk, Connecticut
Hurst L 1985 Relationship between double crush syndrome and carpal tunnel syndrome. Journal of Hand Surgery 10:202

Ingram-Rice B 1997 Carpal tunnel syndrome: more than a wrist problem. Journal of Bodywork and Movement Therapies 1(3):155–162

Jacob G, McKenzie R 1996 Spinal therapeutics based on responses to loading. In: Liebenson C (ed) Rehabilitation of the spine. Williams and Wilkins, Baltimore

Janda V 1982 Introduction to functional pathology of the motor system. Proceedings of the VII Commonwealth and International Conference on Sport Physiotherapy. Sport 3:39

Janda V 1983 Muscle function testing. Butterworths, London

Janda V 1988 In: Grant R (ed) Physical therapy of the cervical and thoracic spine. Churchill Livingstone, New York

Janda V 1996a Evaluation of muscular imbalance. In: Liebenson C (ed) Rehabilitation of the spine: a practitioner's guide. Williams and Wilkins, Baltimore

Janda V 1996b In: Liebenson C (ed) Rehabilitation of the spine: a practitioner's manual. Williams and Wilkins, Baltimore

Jirout J 1969 Movement diagnostics by X-ray in the cervical spine. Manuelle Medizin 7:121–128

Johnson G, Bogduk N, Nowitzke A et al 1994 Anatomy and actions of the trapezius muscle. Clinical Biomechanics 9:44–50

Jones L 1985 Strain and counterstrain, Jones SCS Inc, Boise, Indiana

Jull G, Janda V 1987 Muscles and motor control in low back pain. In: Twomey L, Taylor J (eds) Physical therapy for the low back. Clinics in physical therapy. Churchill Livingstone, New York

Kaltenborn G 1985 Mobilization of the extremity joints. Olaf Norlis Bokhandel, Oslo

Kapandji IA 1982 The physiology of the joints, vol. 1, 5th edn. Churchill Livingstone, Edinburgh

Kapandji IA 1998 The Physiology of the joints, vol 1. The upper limb. Churchill Livingstone, Edinburgh

Kappler R, Ramey K 1997 Upper extremity. In: Ward R (ed) Foundations for Osteopathic Medicine. Williams and Wilkins, Baltimore

Kendall F, McCreary E, Provance P 1993 Muscles, testing and function, 4th edn. Williams and Wilkins, Baltimore

Knowlton R 1990 Genetic linkage of polymorphism in the type II pro-collagen gene to primary osteoarthritis. New England Journal of Medicine 322:526–530

Korr I 1981 Axonal transport and neurotrophic functions. In: Korr I (ed) Spinal cord as organiser of disease processes, part 4. Academy of Applied Osteopathy, Newark, Ohio, pp 451–458

Kuchera W, Kuchera M 1994 Osteopathic principles in practice, 2nd edn. Greyden Press, Columbus, Ohio

Larson N 1972 Osteopathic manipulation for syndromes of the brachial plexus. Journal of the American Osteopathic Association 72:94–100

Lewit K 1985 Manipulative therapy in rehabilitation of the motor system. Butterworths, London

Lewit K 1991 Manipulation in rehabilitation of the locomotor system, 2nd edn. Butterworths, London

Liebenson C 1990 Active muscular relaxation techniques (parts 1 & 2). Journal of Manipulative and Physiological Therapeutics 12(6):446–451 1989 and 13(1):2–6

Liebenson C 1996 (ed) Rehabilitation of the spine. Williams and Wilkins, Baltimore

Maigne J 1991 Upper thoracic dorsal rami. Surgical and Radiological Anatomy 13:109–112

Maitland G 1986 Vertebral manipulation. Butterworths, London

McAtee R, Charland J 1999 Facilitated stretching, 2nd edn. Human Kinetics, Champaign, Illinois

McNab I, McCulloch J 1994 Neck ache and shoulder pain. Williams and Wilkins, Baltimore

Mitchell F, Moran P, Pruzzo N 1979 Evaluation of osteopathic muscle energy procedure. Privately published, Valley Park, Missouri

Mock L 1997 Myofascial release treatment of specific muscles. Bulletin of Myofascial Therapy 2(1):5–23

Mulligan B 1992 Manual therapy. Plane View Services, Wellington, New Zealand

Nichols A 1996 Thoracic outlet syndrome in athletes. Journal of American Board of Family Practice 9(5):346–355

Norkin P, Levangie C 1992 Joint structure and function: a comprehensive analysis, 2nd edn. F A Davis, Philadelphia

Patriquin D 1992 Evolution of osteopathic manipulative technique: the Spencer technique. Journal of the American Osteopathic Association 92:1134–1146

Platzer W 1992 Color atlas/text of human anatomy: vol. I, locomotor system, 4th edn. Thieme, Stuttgart

Rubin B 1997 Rheumatology. In: Ward R (ed) Foundations of osteopathic medicine. Williams and Wilkins, Baltimore

Ruddy T J 1962 Osteopathic rapid rhythmic resistive technic. Academy of Applied Osteopathy Yearbook, Colorado Springs, pp 23–31

Salmons S 1985 Functional adaptation of skeletal muscle. In: Evarts E (ed) The motor system in neurobiology. Elsevier, Amsterdam

Schafer R 1987 Clinical biomechanics. Williams and Wilkins, Baltimore

Simons D, Travell J, Simons L 1998 Myofascial pain and dysfunction: the trigger point manual, vol 1: upper half of body, 2nd edn. Williams and Wilkins, Baltimore

Spencer H 1976 Shoulder technique. Journal of the American Osteopathic Association 15:2118–2220

Stiles E 1984 Manipulation – a tool for your practice. Patient Care 18:699–704

Sunderland S 1976 The nerve lesion in carpal tunnel syndrome. Journal of Neurology and Neurosurgical Psychiatry 39:615

Taleisnik J 1988 Fractures of the carpal bones. In: Green D P (ed) Operative hand surgery 2. Churchill Livingstone, New York, p 813

Tucker A 1994 Shoulder pain in a football player. Medicine and Science in Sports and Exercise 26(3):281–284

Upledger J, Vredevoogd J 1983 Craniosacral therapy. Eastland Press, Seattle

Upton A, McComas A 1973 The double crush syndrome. Lancet 2:359

Walther D 1988 Applied kinesiology. Synopsis Systems DC, Pueblo, Colorado

Ward R (ed) 1997 Foundations for osteopathic medicine. Williams and Wilkins, Baltimore

Warfel J 1985 The extremities, 5th edn. Lea and Febiger, Philadelphia

14

The thorax

The posterior aspect of the thorax is represented by a mobile functional unit, the thoracic spinal column, through which the sympathetic nerve supply emerges. In addition, the thorax acts as a protective cage for the heart and lungs, inside which respiratory function, with its powerful lymphatic and circulatory influences, occurs. Muscular attachments to the thorax which serve other areas are numerous and include muscles of the shoulder, neck and lower back. The extrinsic thoracic musculature is responsible for positioning the torso and, therefore, also the placement in space of the shoulders, arms, neck and head. The intrinsic thoracic muscles move the thoracic vertebrae or the rib cage (and possibly the entire upper body) and/or are associated with respiration.

The degree of movement in *all* directions (flexion, extension, sideflexion and rotation) allowed by the relatively rigid structure of the thorax is less than that available in the cervical or lumbar spines, being deliberately limited in order to protect the vital organs housed within the thoracic cavity.

STRUCTURE

Structural features of the thoracic spine

- In most individuals the thoracic spine has a kyphotic (forward bending) profile which varies in degree from individual to individual.
- The thoracic spinous processes are especially prominent and therefore easily palpated.
- The angles of orientation of the thoracic spinous processes are increasingly caudad, from T1 to T9, with a modification toward an almost horizontal orientation from T10 to T12.
- The transverse processes from T1 to T10 carry costotransverse joints for articulation with the ribs.
- The thoracic facet joints, which glide on each other and restrict and largely determine the range of spinal movement, have typical plane-type synovial features, including an articular capsule.

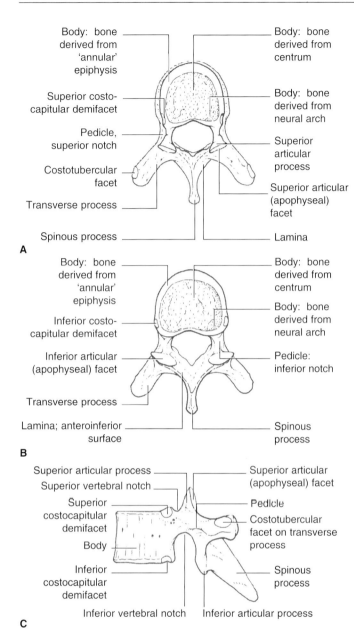

Figure 14.1 Thoracic vertebra. A: Superior view. B: Inferior view. C: Lateral view (reproduced, with permission, from *Gray's anatomy* (1995)).

• Hruby et al (1997) describe a useful method for remembering the structure and orientation of the facet joints: *'The superior facets of each thoracic vertebrae are slightly convex and face posteriorly (backward), somewhat superiorly (up), and laterally. Their angle of declination averages 60° relative to the transverse plane and 20° relative to the coronal plane. Remember the facet facing by the mnemonic, "BUL" (backward, upward, and lateral). This is in contrast to the cervical and lumbar regions where the superior facets face backwards, upwards, and medially ("BUM"). Thus, the superior facets [of the entire spine] are BUM, BUL, BUM, from cervical, to thoracic, to lumbar.'*

• The disc structure of the thoracic spine is similar

to that of the cervical and lumbar spine. The notable difference is the relative broadness of the posterior longitudinal ligament which, together with the restricted range of motion potential of the region, makes herniation of thoracic discs an infrequent occurrence.

• Degenerative changes due to osteoporosis and aging, as well as trauma, are, however, relatively common in this region.

Structural features of the ribs

• The ribs are composed of a segment of bone and a costal cartilage.
• The costal cartilages attach to the costochondral joint of most ribs (see variations below), depressions in the bony segment of the ribs.
• Ribs 11 and 12 do not articulate with the sternum ('floating ribs'), whereas all other ribs do so, in various ways, either by means of their own cartilaginous synovial joints (i.e. ribs 1–7 are 'true ribs') or by means of a merged cartilaginous structure (ribs 8–10, which are 'false ribs').
• The head of each rib articulates with its thoracic vertebrae at the costovertebral joint.
• Ribs 2–9 also articulate with the vertebrae above and below by means of a demifacet.
• Ribs 1, 11 and 12 articulate with their own vertebrae by means of a unifacet.
• Typical ribs (3–9) comprise a head, neck, tubercle, angles and shafts and connect directly, or via cartilaginous structures, to the sternum
• Atypical ribs and their key features include:
1. rib 1 which is broad, short and flat, the most curved. The subclavian artery and cervical plexus are anatomically vulnerable to compression if the 1st rib becomes compromised in relation to the anterior and/or middle scalenes, or the clavicle
2. rib 2 carries a tubercle which attaches to the proximal portion of serratus anterior
3. ribs 11 and 12 are atypical due to their failure to articulate anteriorly with the sternum or costal cartilages.

Structural features of the sternum

There are three key subdivisions of the sternum.

1. The manubrium (or head) which articulates with the clavicles at the sternoclavicular joints. The superior surface of the manubrium (jugular notch) lies directly anterior to the 2nd thoracic vertebrae. The manubrium is joined to the body of the sternum by means of a fibro-cartilaginous symphysis, the sternal angle (angle of Louis) which lies directly anterior to the 4th thoracic vertebrae.

2. The body of the sternum provides the attachment

sites for the ribs, with the 2nd rib attaching at the sternal angle. This makes the angle an important landmark when counting ribs.

3. The xiphoid process is the 'tail' of the sternum, joining it at the xiphisternal symphysis (which fuses in most people during the fifth decade of life) – usually anterior to the 9th thoracic vertebrae.

POSTERIOR THORAX

The thorax can be described both structurally and functionally in order to make sense of its numerous complex features. It can be thought of in terms of a thoracic spinal column as well as a thoracic cage. Each approach will have features and functions which are considered both separately and together.

In regional terms, the thoracic spine is usually divided into (White & Panjabi 1978):

1. *upper* – T1–4 where, at each segment, approximately 4° of flexion and extension, 10° of rotation and no more than 10° of lateral flexion is possible
2. *middle* – T5–8 where, at each segment, approximately 6° of flexion and extension, 6° of rotation and 10–12° of lateral flexion is possible
3. *lower* – T9–12 where, at each segment, approximately 12° of flexion and extension, 3° of rotation and 12–13° of lateral flexion is possible.

- The total range of thoracic flexion and extension combined (between T1 and T12) is approximately 60° (Liebenson 1996).
- The total range of thoracic rotation is approximately 40°. This, of course, is the limit ascribed to the thoracic spine *alone*, not taking account of the rotational component of the lumbar spine on which it rests, which allows an additional 50° and therefore a total of approximately 90° of *trunk* rotation.
- Total range of lateral flexion of the thoracic spine is approximately 50°.
- In addition to the individual degrees of flexion and extension listed above, several degrees of additional coupled flexion occur in the upper thoracics when rotation is introduced. This represents a functional advantage created by the linking of combined vertebral movement potentials during rotation (known as 'coupling'). In this way a few degrees of additional coupled extension also occurs in the lower thoracics during rotation (Grice 1980).

Identification of spinal levels

Hruby et al (1997) state:

A useful way of identifying the thoracic vertebrae involves the 'rule of threes'. This 'rule' is a generalization that is only approximate, but positions the palpating fingers in the estimated positions for location of individual thoracic vertebrae.

- Spinous processes of T1–3 project directly posteriorly so that the tip of each spinous process is in the same plane as the transverse process of the same vertebra.
- The spinous processes of T4–6 project caudally so that the tip of each spinous process is in a plane that is approximately halfway between the transverse processes of its own vertebra and those of the vertebra immediately below.
- The spinous processes of T7–9 project more acutely caudally so that the tip of each spinous process is in the same plane as the transverse processes of the vertebra immediately below.
- T10 spinous process is similar to T7–9 (same plane as the transverse processes of the vertebra immediately below).
- T11 spinous process is similar to T4–6 (in a plane that is approximately halfway between the transverse processes of its own vertebra and those of the vertebra immediately below).
- T12 spinous process is similar to T1–3 (in the same plane as the transverse process of the same vertebra).

This knowledge is particularly useful when using positional release methods, such as the induration technique (see p. 444), in which vertebrae are treated individually, using the spinous process as a point of contact. If the induration technique is being used in treatment of associated rib attachment dysfunction, contact on the appropriate vertebrae would be clinically important.

The sympathetic supply to the organs is as follows.

- T1–4: head and neck
- T1–6: heart, lungs
- T5–9: stomach, liver, gall bladder, duodenum, pancreas, spleen
- T10–11: rest of small intestines, kidney, ureters, gonads, right colon
- T12–L2: pelvic organs, left colon

Spinal segments

The process of facilitation, described in Chapter 6, results in spinal segments – and their paraspinal musculature – becoming dysfunctional in response to nociceptive bombardment from the organs they supply, if the organs become diseased or distressed (Beal 1985). Clinically the practitioner may consider that a paraspinal region involves a facilitation process when the soft tissues fail to respond to normal treatment procedures. In such circumstances consideration of visceral involvement is warranted and organ pathologies may need to be ruled out.

Segmental facilitation example

Myron Beal DO, Professor in the Department of Family Medicine at Michigan State University, College of

Osteopathic Medicine, conducted a study in which over 100 patients with diagnosed cardiovascular disease were examined for patterns of spinal segment involvement (Beal 1983).

Around 90% had 'segmental dysfunction in two or more adjacent vertebrae from T1 to T5, on the left side'. More than half also had left-side C2 dysfunction. Beal reports that the estimation of the intensity of the spinal dysfunction correlated strongly with the degree of pathology noted (ranging from myocardial infarction, ischemic heart disease and hypertensive cardiovascular disease to coronary artery disease). He further reports that the greatest intensity of the cardiac reflex occurred at T2 and T3 on the left. The texture of the soft tissues, as described by Beal, is of interest: 'Skin and temperature changes were not apparent as consistent strong findings compared with the hypertonic state of the deep musculature'.

The major palpatory finding for muscle was of hypertonicity of the superficial and deep paraspinal muscles with fibrotic thickening. Tenderness was usually obvious, although this was not specifically assessed in this study. Superficial hypertonicity lessened when the patient was supine, making assessment of deeper tissue states easier in that position.

Palpation method for upper thoracic segmental facilitation

• With the patient supine, the thoracic spine is examined by the practitioner (who is seated or standing at the head of the table) by sliding the fingers of both hands (one on each side of the spine) under the upper thoracic transverse processes.

• An anterior compressive force is applied with the fingers (see Fig. 14.2) to assess the status of the superficial and deep paraspinal tissues and the response of the transverse process to the 'springing'.

• This compression is performed, one segment at a time, progressively down the spine, until control becomes difficult or tissues inaccessible.

• A positive test (indicating probable facilitation of the segments being tested) would involve a 'wooden', non-elastic response to the springing effort produced by the fingers, involving two or more segments.

• It is also possible to perform the test with the patient seated or sidelying, though neither is as accurate as the supine position.

• It is suggested that such palpation be performed on people with and without known cardiovascular dysfunction, in order to develop a degree of discrimination between normal and abnormal tissue states of this sort.

• It is also suggested that the 'red reflex' assessment method (discussed below) be performed to evaluate its ability to identify areas of reflexively active tissue (possibly facilitated).

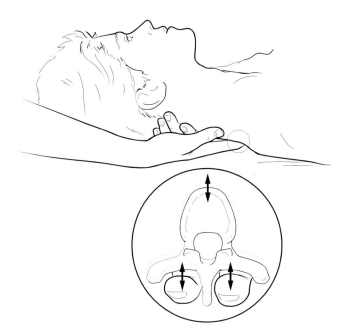

Figure 14.2 Springing assessment for tissue resistance associated with segmental facilitation.

Red reflex assessment (reactive hyperemia)

Late in the 19th century Carl McConnell DO (1962) stated:

I begin at the first thoracic [vertebra] and examine the spinal column down to the sacrum by placing my middle fingers over [each side of] the spinous processes and standing directly back of the patient draw the flat surfaces of these two fingers over the spinous processes from the upper thoracic to the sacrum in such a manner that the spines of the vertebrae pass tightly between the two fingers; thus leaving a red streak where the cutaneous vessels press upon the spines of the vertebrae. In this manner slight deviations of the vertebrae laterally can be told with the greatest accuracy by observing the red line. When a vertebra or section of vertebrae are too posterior a heavy red streak is noticed and when a vertebra or section of vertebrae are too anterior the streak is not so noticeable.

In the 1960s Hoag (1969) wrote:

With firm but moderate pressure the pads of the fingers are repeatedly rubbed over the surface of the skin, preferably with extensive longitudinal strokes along the paraspinal area. The appearance of less intense and rapidly fading color in certain areas, as compared with the general reaction, is ascribed to increased vasoconstriction in that area, indicating a disturbance in autonomic reflex activity. Others give significance to an increased degree of erythema or a prolonged lingering of the red line response.

Upledger & Vredevoogd (1983) suggest:

Skin texture changes produced by a facilitated segment are palpable as you lightly drag your fingers over the nearby paravertebral area of the back. I [Upledger] usually do skin drag evaluation moving from the top of the neck to the sacral area in one motion. Where your fingertips drag on the skin you will probably find a facilitated segment. After several repetitions, with increased force, the affected area will appear redder than nearby areas. This is the 'red reflex'. Muscles and connective tissues at this level will:

1. have a 'shotty' feel (like buckshot under the skin)
2. be more tender to palpation
3. be tight, and tend to restrict vertebral motion, and
4. exhibit tenderness of the spinous processes when tapped by fingers or a rubber hammer.

Korr (1970) described how this red reflex phenomenon corresponded well with areas of lowered electrical resistance, which themselves correspond accurately to regions of lowered pain threshold and areas of cutaneous and deep tenderness (termed 'segmentally related sympatheticotonia'). Korr was able to detect areas of intense vasoconstriction which corresponded well with dysfunction elicited by manual clinical examination.

You must not look for perfect correspondence between the skin resistance (or the red reflex) and the distribution of deeper pathologic disturbance, because an area of skin which is segmentally related to a particular muscle does not necessarily overlie that muscle. With the latissimus dorsi, for example, the myofascial disturbance might be over the hip but the reflex manifestations would be in much higher dermatomes because this muscle has its innervation from the cervical part of the cord.

Hruby et al (1997) describe the thinking regarding this phenomenon:

Perform the red reflex test by firmly, but with light pressure, stroking two fingers on the skin over the paraspinal tissues in a cephalad to a caudad direction. The stroked areas briefly become erythematous and almost immediately return to their usual color. If the skin remains erythematous longer than a few seconds, it may indicate an acute somatic dysfunction in the area. As the dysfunction acquires chronic tissue changes, the tissues blanch rapidly after stroking and are dry and cool to palpation.

The reader is reminded that Hilton's law (see p. 2) confirms simultaneous innervation to the skin covering the articular insertion of the muscles, not necessarily the entire muscle.

Biomechanics of rotation in the thoracic spine

- In the *cervical spine* between C3 and C7 a coupling occurs, in which sidebending and rotation take place toward the same side (type 2).
- There is a great deal of disagreement among experts as to what is 'normal coupling behavior' in the *thoracic spine*.
- The upper four thoracic segments are said by some (Grice 1980) to behave in the same manner as the cervical spine (type 2) when the spine is in neutral (not flexed or extended), that is, rotation and sidebending take place toward the same sides.
- This is contradicted by Grieve (1981) who says that

between T3 and T10, 'in neutral and extension, side-bending and rotation occur to opposite sides (type 1). In flexion, they occur to the same side (type 2)'.
- The mid-thoracic segments also represent a confusing mixture of types in their coupling behavior, so that during sidebending, rotation may occur to either the concave (type 2) or the convex side (type 1), depending on whether the spine is in flexion, extension or neutral.
- The lower thoracic coupling pattern is generally agreed to be similar to the lumbar spine (type 1) in which sidebending and rotation coupling are toward opposite sides (e.g. sidebend right, rotation of vertebral body left).
- Grieve (1981) comes to the rescue of the (by now) confused practitioner, by saying that it is wise 'to allow the joints of individual patterns to speak for themselves, in the prime matter of the nature and direction of the most effective therapeutic movement'. He suggests that, 'individual responses and clinical assessment should take precedence over "theories of biomechanics"'.

Coupling test

In order to establish the specific coupling pattern in an individual segment, the following simple sidebending and rotation palpation procedure is used.

- The patient is seated or standing with arms folded on chest, hands on opposite shoulders.
- The practitioner stands behind and to the side of the patient and passes an arm across the chest to cup the patient's hand which is resting on the opposite shoulder.
- The practitioner's other hand is placed so that the index and middle fingers lie on one side and the ring and small fingers on the other side, with the finger tips pointing cephalad parallel with the thoracic spinal segment under review.
- A horizontal line drawn through the finger tips would place them on a line dissecting the one collectively represented by the spinous processes, although not necessarily the spinous process of the one being assessed due to the inclination of the thoracic spinous processes. These fingers monitor the rotational pattern followed by the segment when it is sidebent.

Box 14.1 Identification of spinal level from spinous process

- The spinous processes of T1, T2, T3 are on the same plane as the transverse process of the same vertebra.
- The spinous processes of T4, T5, T6 are in a plane approximately halfway between the transverse processes of their own vertebra and those of the vertebra immediately below.
- The spinous processes of T7, T8, T9 are in the same plane as the transverse processes of the vertebra immediately below.
- T10 spinous process is similar to T7 to T9.
- T11 spinous process is similar to T4 to T6.
- T12 spinous process is similar to T1 to T3.

• The practitioner introduces slight sideflexion *precisely* at the segment, by means of his contact on the patient's shoulder, and repeats this in both directions as the rotational response, which *has* to accompany sideflexion, is palpated.

• If 'fullness' ('backwards pressure') is noted on the side *toward* which sideflexion is taking place, this represents a type 2 response. If sideflexion is toward the right and the fingers on the right register greater pressure or 'fullness' during this movement, this indicates that the body of that vertebra has rotated toward the right (the concavity) so that the right side of the transverse process is producing the fullness, pressure, on the palpating fingers.

• Alternatively if, on right sideflexion, fullness is noted on the left, this indicates that rotation of the vertebral body is toward the left side (the convexity) and the palpated response therefore represents a type 1 coupling.

• This same assessment can be carried out at each segment and with the spine in relative neutral, as well as flexion and extension, to experience the variations in the biomechanical coupling responses which occur.

• This knowledge is of clinical value when attempting to increase range of motion in restricted segments, as will become clear when specific MET protocols are suggested toward this objective later in this chapter.

• Confirmation of findings in this test is available by observation – see stages 9 and 10 of C-curve observation test, below.

Observation of restriction patterns in thoracic spine (C-curve observation test)

• The patient is seated on the table with the legs fully extended, pelvis vertical, and bends into fullest flexion possible.

• A sequential (C-shaped) curve should be observed when the profile of the spine is viewed from the side with the patient in full flexion.

• No knee flexion should take place and all movement should be spinal.

• Any areas of 'flatness' should be noted as these represent regions where normal flexion of one segment on the other is absent or reduced.

• The patient then sits with knees flexed, thus relaxing hamstrings, and again bends into fullest flexion possible with hands resting on crest of pelvis.

• Observation from the side should indicate which segments remain unable to move fully into flexion.

• If there is a greater degree of flexion possible in this position (knees flexed) as compared to that noted with knees straight, then hamstring restriction is a factor.

• All flat areas should be charted.

• The practitioner should at this time view the spine from the perspective gained by looking at it along its

length, from the head or from the lower lumbar area, while the patient is flexed.

• Segments which are in a rotated state will be easily identified and the direction of their rotation observed, by means of the rotational deviation caused by their transverse processes. The transverse processes and ribs will produce a 'mounding' or fullness on the side toward which the vertebra has rotated. Any such findings can be compared with those of the palpation evaluation (Coupling test described above) which palpates for fullness during sideflexion.

Breathing wave assessment

• The patient should now be placed lying prone, ideally with the face in a cradle or padded hole, for comfort and to avoid cervical rotation.

• The operator squats at the side and observes the 'spinal breathing wave' as deep breathing is performed (see below). Areas of restriction, lack of movement or where motion is not in sequence should be noted and compared with findings from the observation of the C-curve (above).

• Commonly, areas of the spine which appear to move as a block during this evaluation are areas where there is limited flexion potential, as observed during the C-curve assessment.

Breathing wave – evaluation of spinal motion during inhalation/exhalation

• The patient is placed prone and the 'breathing wave' observed.

• When the spine is fully flexible this wave-like motion commences in the lower lumbar region, near the sacrum, and spreads as a wave up to the base of the neck.

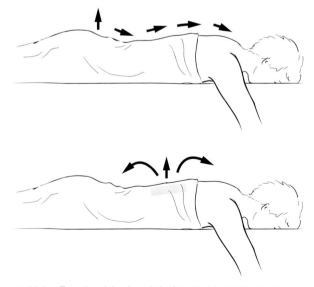

Figure 14.3 Functional (top) and dysfunctional breathing wave movement patterns.

• If there is restriction in any of the spinal segments or if associated muscles of the region are short and tight, the pattern will vary.

• Movement may start somewhere else (the patterns observed will differ as widely as the patterns of restriction in individual spines) so that areas which are lacking in flexibility may be seen to move as a block, rather than as a wave.

The observing practitioner should question:

• Does movement start at the sacrum?
• Does it start elsewhere?
• Does it move caudad, cephalad or in both directions?
• Where does the wave cease – in the mid-thoracic area or as it should, at the base of neck?
• How does this relate to the observations already made and the patient's symptoms?

As spinal, rib or muscular restrictions are removed or improved – by treatment or exercise – the breathing wave should be seen to gradually benefit, with the wave commencing closer to the sacrum and finishing closer to the neck. The breathing wave observation test can therefore be used as a means of monitoring progress; it is not in itself diagnostic.

Passive motion testing for the thoracic spine

Segmental palpation is used to identify specific (rather than general) areas of restriction. The areas of the spine observed in the C-curve which remain 'flat' on flexion are almost certain to palpate as restricted. Such restrictions might be the result of joint dysfunction or of muscular and/or ligamentous restrictions. The nature of the end-feel noted during any spinal palpation exercise (below) offers some guidance as to whether a problem is osseous (hard end-feel) or muscular/ligamentous (softer end-feel).

Flexion and extension assessment of T1–4

• The patient is seated and the practitioner is standing to the side with one hand on top of the patient's head.

• The practitioner's other hand is placed, palmar surface on the patient's posterior upper thoracic region, so that the ring and middle fingers can be placed between the spinous processes of three vertebrae (between T1 and T2 and between T2 and T3, for example).

• The hand on the head guides the neck into unforced flexion and extension until motion is noted by the palpating fingers.

• A normal response in both flexion and extension would be for the most cephalad segment to move before the more caudad one. It is worth recalling that the entire range of flexion/extension in these vertebrae is less than 5°.

• The practitioner evaluates whether there is an appropriate degree of separation of the spinous processes on flexion and of closure on extension and also takes note of the quality of end-feel in these movements.

Flexion and extension assessment of T5–12

• Once the upper four segments (including movement between T4 and T5) have been evaluated for flexion and extension, the palpating fingers are placed between T5 and T6.

• The practitioner passes his other arm across the patient's upper chest to cup the opposite shoulder, enabling flexion and extension to be controlled via this contact (control is further enhanced if the practitioner's axilla can contact the superior aspect of the patient's ipsilateral shoulder).

• It is worth recalling that the entire range of flexion/extension in the lower eight segments ranges from approximately 6° (at T5) to 12° (at T12).

• The spine is sequentially flexed and extended as the practitioner evaluates whether there is an appropriate degree of separation of the spinous processes on flexion and closure on extension and also takes note of the quality of end-feel in these movements.

Sideflexion palpation of thoracic spine

• The assessment method outlined earlier in this section, in which coupling motions were assessed in relation to sideflexion and rotation, forms a basis for similar assessment of rotation and/or sideflexion individually.

• The patient is seated or standing with arms folded across chest and hands resting on her own opposite shoulders.

• For the upper three or four thoracic segments the practitioner uses a light contact on the patient's head to introduce sideflexion. For the lower segments the practitioner stands behind and to the side of the patient and passes an arm across the chest to cup the patient's hand which rests on the opposite shoulder and uses this contact to introduce sideflexion in either direction.

• The practitioner's other hand is placed with the fingers pointing cephalad, so that the index and middle finger pads lie on one side of the spinous process and the ring and small fingers on the other side, with the fingers pointing cephalad.

• As sideflexion is induced to the level being assessed, the practitioner notes whether the transverse processes separate and approximate appropriately, during the different phases of sideflexion.

• Both the range (10–12° is normal) and quality (end-feel) of the movement are noted and a judgment is reached as to the relative symmetry and normality of the segment in its sideflexion potential.

Rotation palpation of thoracic spine

- The assessment method outlined above for sideflexion forms the basis for this assessment of rotation.
- The patient is seated or standing with arms folded on chest, hands on opposite shoulders, as above.
- For the upper three or four thoracic segments the practitioner uses a light contact on the patient's head to introduce rotation down to the level being palpated. For the lower segments, the practitioner stands behind and to the side of the patient and passes an arm across the chest to cup the patient's hand resting on the opposite shoulder and uses this contact to introduce rotation in either direction.
- The practitioner's other hand is placed so that the index and middle fingers lie on one side and the ring and small fingers on the other side, with the tips pointing cephalad, on the transverse processes of the thoracic spinal segment under review.
- As rotation is induced to the level being assessed the practitioner notes the range (10° in the upper, reducing to 3° in the lower segments) and quality of movement (end-feel) of the transverse process on the side toward which rotation is taking place.
- Judgment is reached as to the relative symmetry and normality of the segment in its rotational potential.

Prone segmental testing for rotation

- The patient is prone.
- The practitioner places his thumbs onto the transverse processes of the segment under assessment.
- An anterior pressure is applied with each thumb alternately, taking out the slack and sensing the range of rotation as well as the quality of the end-feel of the movement on each side.
- If a transverse process feels less free in its ability to move anteriorly, the vertebra is rotated in that direction (i.e. if the right transverse process is less yielding in its anterior movement than the left transverse process, this indicates a vertebra which is inappropriately rotated to the right and which cannot easily rotate left).

Comment

Many spinal restrictions are 'held' by soft tissue restrictions and can be normalized by release of the soft tissue component. Almost all the positions of assessment described above can immediately become the commencement positions for the application of muscle energy techniques, via the introduction of isometric contractions, either toward or away from the restriction barrier, or by means of Ruddy's pulsed MET procedures. See MET notes on p. 137 which explain these concepts.

Box 14.2   Lief's NMT of the upper thoracic area (Chaitow 1996a)

- The practitioner stands on the patient's left side at the level of the patient's waist, facing diagonally toward the head of the patient.
- With the right hand resting at the level of the lower thoracic spine where its function is to distract tissue, the left thumb commences a series of strokes cephalad from the mid-thoracic area, immediately to the left of the spinous processes.
- Each stroke covers two or three spinal segments and runs in a cephalad direction, immediately lateral to the spinous process, so that the *angle of pressure* imparted, via the medial tip of the thumb, is roughly toward the contralateral nipple. *Note*: While this series of strokes is cephalad, the pressure exerted by the thumb tip is not toward the floor, rather it angles toward the contralateral side.
- A series of light assessment and deep therapeutic strokes are employed and a degree of overlap is suggested with successive strokes (see Fig. 14.18).
- In this way the first two strokes might run from T8 to T5 followed by two strokes (one light, one deeper) from T6 to T3 and finally two strokes from T4 to T1.
- Deeper and more sustained pressure is exerted upon discovering marked contraction or resistance to the gliding, probing thumb.
- In the thoracic area a second line of upward strokes is employed to include the spinal border of the scapula, as well as one or two searching, laterally directed, probing strokes along the inferior spine of the scapula and across the musculature inferior to and inserting into the scapula.
- Treatment of the right side may be carried out without necessarily changing position, other than to lean across the patient, as long as this causes no distress to the practitioner's back.
- A shorter practitioner should change sides so that, standing half-facing the head of the patient, the right thumb can perform the strokes outlined above.

What may be found?

- Apart from trigger points in the lower trapezius fibers, other trigger points may be sought (while in this assessment/treatment position) in levator scapulae, supra- and infraspinatus (Melzack 1977).
- A series of *tsubo*, or acupressure points, lie symmetrically on either side of the spine and along the mid-line and are said to have great reflex importance (Serizawe 1980).
- The Bladder meridian points lie in two lines running parallel with the spine, one level with the medial border of the scapula and the other mid-way between it and the lateral border of the spinous processes (Mann 1971).
- Goodheart's work suggests that rhomboid weakness indicates liver problems and that pressure on C7 spinous process and a point on the right of the interspace between the 5th and 6th dorsal spinous processes assists its normalization. Latissimus dorsi weakness apparently indicates pancreatic dysfunction. Lateral to the 7th and 8th dorsal interspace is the posterior pressure reflex to normalize this (Walther 1988). These and other reflexes would appear to derive from Chapman's reflex theories and are deserving of further study (Mannino 1979, Owens 1980).
- Viscerosomatic influences which produce dysfunction of the erector spinae group of muscles between the 6th and 12th thoracics indicate liver involvement (Beal 1985).
- Similarly 4th, 5th and 6th thoracic area congestion or sensitivity may involve stomach reflexes and gastric disturbance, whereas facilitation at the levels of T12 and/or L2 indicates possible kidney dysfunction.
- The connective tissue zones affecting the arm, stomach, heart, liver and gall bladder are noted in this region (Ebner 1962) and Chapman's neurolymphatic reflexes relating to the arm, thyroid, lungs, throat and heart are located in the upper thoracic spine, including the scapular area (DiGiovanna 1991).

ANTERIOR THORAX

In earlier chapters emphasis has been given to the profound negative influence on emotions, structure and function when breathing function is disturbed (Chapter 2). In purely structural terms, Lewit (1980) states: 'The most important disturbance of breathing is overstrain of the upper auxiliary muscles by lifting of the thorax during quiet respiration'.

In order to normalize breathing function, a focus is required which evaluates structural and functional elements and which offers appropriate therapeutic and rehabilitation approaches to what is revealed.

Chila (1997) suggests the following in order to evaluate respiration function.

- *Category*: does breathing involve the diaphragm, the lower rib cage or both?
- *Locus of abdominal motion*: does it move as far as the umbilicus or as far as the pubic bone?
- *Rate*: rapid, slow? The rate should be recorded before and after treatment.
- *Duration of cycle*: are inhalation and exhalation phases equal or is one longer than the other?

Respiratory function assessment

Assessment of breathing function should begin by means of palpation and observation with the patient both

---

Box 14.3 Respiratory muscles

Muscles of inhalation

Primary
Diaphragm (70–80%)
Parasternal (intercartilaginous) internal intercostals
Upper and more lateral external intercostals
Levator costae
Scalenii

Accessory
Sternocleidomastoid
Upper trapezius
Serratus anterior (arms elevated)
Latissimus dorsi (arms elevated)
Serratus posterior superior
Iliocostalis thoracis
Subclavius
Omohyoid

Muscles of exhalation

Primary
Elastic recoil of lungs, pleura and costal cartilages

Accessory
Interosseous internal intercostals
Abdominal muscles
Transversus thoracis
Subcostales
Iliocostalis lumborum
Quadratus lumborum
Serratus posterior inferior
Latissimus dorsi

Box 14.4 Respiratory mechanics

Respiratory function is extremely complex and no attempt will be made in this text to fully elaborate on this complexity, other than to highlight those aspects which impact on somatic dysfunction and/or which can be helpfully modified by means of NMT and its associated modalities.
Breathing depends on four areas of influence:

1. efficient ventilation
2. gas exchange
3. gas transportation to and from the tissues of the body
4. breathing regulation.

The status of the muscles and joints of the thorax and the way the individual breathes can influence all of these, to some extent. Ventilation itself is dependent on:

1. the muscles of respiration and their attachments
2. the mechanical characteristics of the airways
3. the health and efficiency of the lungs' parenchymal units.

Inhalation and exhalation involve expansion and contraction of the lungs themselves and this occurs:

1. by means of a movement of the diaphragm, which lengthens and shortens the vertical diameter of the thoracic cavity. This is the normal means of breathing at rest. This diameter can be further increased when the upper ribs are raised during forced respiration, where the normal elastic recoil of the respiratory system is insufficient to meet demands. This brings into play the accessory

breathing muscles including sternocleidomastoid, the scalenes and the external intercostals
2. by means of movement of the ribs into elevation and depression which alters the diameters of the thoracic cavity.

The main purpose of respiration is to assist in providing gas exchange between inhaled air and the blood. Additionally, the actions of the diaphragm enhance lymphatic fluid movement by means of alternating intrathoracic pressure. This produces a suction on the thoracic duct and cisterna chyli and thereby increases lymph movement in the duct and presses it toward the venous arch (Kurz 1986, 1987). Venous circulation is likewise assisted by this alternating pressure between the thoracic and abdominal cavity, suggesting that respiratory dysfunction ('shallow breathing') may negatively impact on venous return from the lower extremities, contributing to conditions such as varicose veins.
Kapandji (1974), in his discussion of respiration, has described a respiratory model. By replacing the bottom of a flask with a membrane (representing the diaphragm), providing a stopper with a tube set into it (to represent the trachea) and a balloon within the flask at the end of the tube (representing the lungs within the rib cage), a crude respiratory model is created. By pulling down on the membrane (the diaphragm on inhalation), the internal pressure of the flask (thoracic cavity) falls below that of the atmosphere and a volume of air of equal amount to that being displaced by the membrane rushes into the balloon, inflating it. The balloon relaxes when the lower membrane is released, elastically recoiling to its previous position, as the air escapes through the tube.
The human respiratory system works in a similar, yet much more

Box 14.4 *(cont'd)*

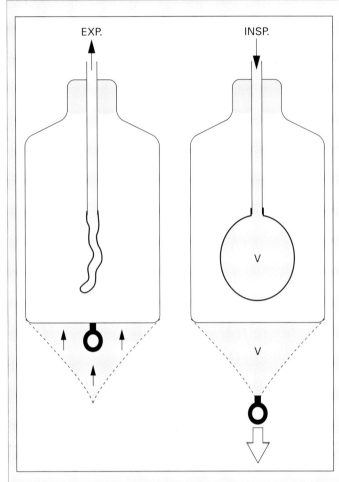

Figure 14.4 A working model with similarities to thoracic air movement is demonstrated by Kapandji (1974).

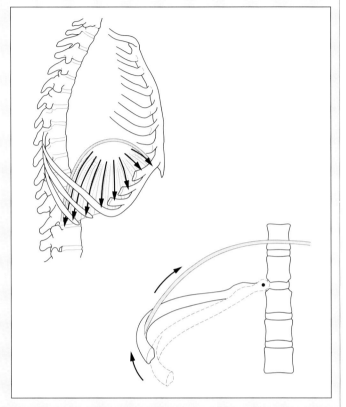

Figure 14.5 Lateral excursion of ribs due to elevation by diaphragm.

complex and highly coordinated manner. During inhalation, the diaphragm displaces caudally, pulling its central tendon down, thus increasing vertical space within the thorax. As the diaphragm descends, it is resisted by the abdominal viscera. At this point, the central tendon becomes fixed against the pressure of the abdominal cavity, while the other end of the diaphragm's fibers pulls the lower ribs cephalad, so displacing them laterally (Fig. 14.5). As the lower ribs are elevated and simultaneously moved laterally, the sternum moves anteriorly and superiorly. Thus, by the action of the diaphragm alone, the vertical, transverse and anteroposterior diameters of the thoracic cavity are increased. If a greater volume of breath is needed, other muscles may be recruited.

• Abdominal muscle tone provides correct positioning of the abdominal viscera so that appropriate central tendon resistance can occur. If the viscera are displaced or abdominal tone is weak and resistance is reduced, lower rib elevation will not occur and volume of air intake will be reduced.
• The posterior rib articulations allow rotation during breathing, while the anterior cartilaginous elements store the torsional energy produced by this rotation. The ribs behave like tension rods and elastically recoil to their previous position when the muscles relax. These elastic elements reduce with age and may also be lessened by intercostal muscular tension (see tests for rib restrictions, p. 433).
• Rib articulations, thoracic vertebral positions and myofascial

elements must all be functional for normal breathing to occur. Dysfunctional elements may reduce the range of mobility and therefore lung capacity.
• Whereas inhalation requires muscular effort, exhalation is primarily a passive, elastic recoil mechanism provided by the tensional elements of the ribs (see above), the elastic recoil of the lung tissues and pleura and abdominal pressure created directly by the viscera and the muscles of the abdomen.
• Being a fluid-filled container, the abdominal cavity is incompressible as long as the abdominal muscles and the perineum are contracted (Lewit 1999).
• The alternating positive and negative pressures of the thoracic and abdominal cavities participate in the processes of inhalation and exhalation, as well as in fluid mechanics, assisting in venous return and lymphatic flow.
• Gravity directly influences diaphragmatic, and therefore respiratory, function. When the individual is upright diaphragmatic excursion has to overcome gravitational forces. When lying down, respiratory function is easier as this demand is reduced or absent. The excursion of the diaphragm is limited during sitting, especially if slumped, because of relaxation of the abdominal muscles.
• When the integrity of the pleural cavity is lost, whether by puncture of its elastic membrane or damage to its hard casing (broken ribs), inflating volume of the lung(s) will decrease, resulting in respiratory distress.
• The intercostal muscles, while participating in inhalation (external intercostals) and exhalation (internal intercostals), are also responsible for enhancing the stability of the chest wall, so preventing its inward movement during inspiration.
• Quadratus lumborum acts to fix the 12th rib, so offering a firm attachment for the diaphragm. If QL is weak, as it may be in certain individuals, this stability is lost (Norris 1999).

Box 14.4   (cont'd)

- Bronchial obstruction, pleural inflammation, liver or intestinal encroachment and ensuing pressure against the diaphragm, as well as phrenic nerve paralysis, are some of the pathologies which will interfere with diaphragmatic and respiratory efficiency.

Since the volume of the lungs is determined by the vertical, transverse and anteroposterior diameters of the thoracic cavity, the ability to produce movements which increase any of these three diameters (without reducing the others) should increase respiratory capacity under normal circumstances (intact pleura, etc.). While simple steps, such as improving upright posture, may influence volume, treatment of the associated musculature, coupled with breathing exercises, may substantially enhance breathing function.

- Vertical dimension is increased by the actions of diaphragm and scalenes.
- Transverse dimension (bucket handle action) is increased with the elevation and rotation of the lower ribs – diaphragm, external intercostals, levatores costarum.
- Elevation of the sternum (pump handle action) is provided by upwards pressure due to spreading of the ribs and the action of SCM and scalenes.

The muscles associated with respiration function can be grouped as either inspiratory or expiratory and are either primary in that capacity or provide accessory support. It should be kept in mind that the role that these muscles might play in inhibiting respiratory function (due to trigger points, ischemia, etc.) has not yet been clearly established and that their overload, due to dysfunctional breathing patterns, is likely to impact on cervical, shoulder, lower back and other body regions.

- The primary inspirational muscles are the diaphragm, the more lateral external intercostals, parasternal internal intercostals, scalene group and the levator costarum, with the diaphragm providing 70–80% of the inhalation force (Simons et al 1998).
- These muscles are supported by the accessory muscles during increased demand (or dysfunctional breathing patterns): SCM, upper trapezius, pectoralis major and minor, serratus anterior, latissimus dorsi, serratus posterior superior, iliocostalis thoracis, subclavius and omohyoid (Kapandji 1974, Simons et al 1998).

Since expiration is primarily an elastic response of the lungs, pleura and 'torsion rod' elements of the ribs, all muscles of expiration could be considered to be accessory muscles as they are recruited only during increased demand. They include internal intercostals, abdominal muscles, transverse thoracis and subcostales. With increased demand, iliocostalis lumborum, quadratus lumborum, serratus posterior inferior and latissimus dorsi may support expiration, including during the high demands of speech, coughing, sneezing, singing and other special functions associated with the breath.

Box 14.5   Some effects of hyperventilation (Timmons 1994)

- Reduction in pCO_2 (tension of carbon dioxide) causes respiratory alkalosis via reduction in arterial carbonic acid, which leads to abnormally decreased arterial carbon dioxide tension (hypocapnia) and major systemic repercussions.
- The first and most direct response to hyperventilation is cerebral vascular constriction, reducing oxygen availability by about 50%.
- Of all body tissues, the cerebral cortex is the most vulnerable to hypoxia which depresses cortical activity and causes dizziness, vasomotor instability, blurred consciousness ('foggy brain') and blurred vision.
- Loss of cortical inhibition results in emotional lability.

Neural repercussions of hyperventilation

- Loss of CO_2 ions from neurons during moderate hyperventilation stimulates neuronal activity, while producing muscular tension and spasm, speeding spinal reflexes as well as producing heightened perception (pain, photophobia, hyperacusis), all of which are of major importance in chronic pain conditions.
- When hypocapnia is more severe or prolonged, it depresses neural activity until the nerve cell becomes inert.
- What seems to occur in advanced or extreme hyperventilation is a change in neuronal metabolism: anaerobic glycolysis produces lactic acid in nerve cells, while lowering pH. Neuronal activity is then diminished so that in extreme hypocarbia, neurons become inert. Thus, in the extremes of this clinical condition, initial hyperactivity gives way to exhaustion, stupor and coma.

---

seated and supine and should be accompanied by a general evaluation of overall posture and especially head, shoulder and torso positioning. Treatment of associated myofascial tissues will be enhanced by the addition of breathing awareness exercises which will, in part, reduce stressful loading of tissues which are assisting in dysfunctional breathing patterns.

Seated

- The patient places a hand on the upper abdomen and another on the upper chest (Fig. 14.6). The hands are observed as the person inhales and exhales several times. If the upper hand (chest) moves superiorly rather than anteriorly and moves significantly more than the hand on the abdomen, this is noted as indicating a dysfunctional pattern of upper chest breathing.
- The practitioner stands behind the seated patient and places his hands gently over the upper trapezius area (midway between base of neck and tip of shoulder). The patient is asked to inhale and the practitioner notes whether his hands move toward the ceiling significantly. If so, scalenes are excessively active and since these are (or may have become – see p. 21) type 1 postural muscles, the indication is that shortening will have occurred.
- The practitioner squats behind the patient and places

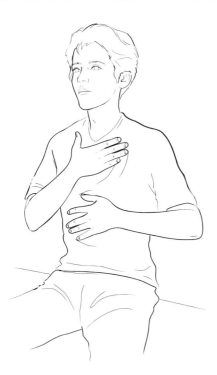

Figure 14.6 Hand positions for breathing function assessment.

his hands onto the lateral aspect of the lower ribs and notes whether there is lateral excursion on inhalation (are the hands pushed apart?) and, if lateral excursion does occur, is it bilateral and/or symmetrical?

Supine

- The breathing pattern is observed.
1. Does the abdomen move anteriorly on inhalation?
2. How much of the abdomen is involved?
3. Does the upper chest move anteriorly or cranially on inhalation while the abdomen retracts?
4. Is there an observable lateral excursion of the lower ribs?

- Shortness in pectoralis major and latissimus dorsi is assessed (arms extended above head; see pp. 351 and 362).

- Chin protrusion ('poking') is observed as the patient moves the neck/head into flexion, trying to place the chin on the chest. If this movement is not possible without 'chin poking' or the position cannot be maintained without protrusion of the chin, sternomastoid is short (see Janda's functional tests, p. 10).

- With folded arms on the chest (or extended in 'sleep-walking' position), knees flexed and feet flat on the table, the patient is asked to raise the head, neck and shoulders from the surface without allowing the feet to leave the surface or the back to arch (see Fig. 5.4). If this is not possible then psoas is considered short (and rectus abdominis weak). Since psoas merges with the diaphragm it should receive attention in any program of breathing rehabilitation.

Sidelying

Quadratus lumborum is assessed by palpation and observation (leg abduction, look or palpate for 'hip hike') (see Janda's functional assessment, p. 61).

Prone

- The practitioner observes the breathing wave – the movement of the spine from the sacrum to the base of the neck on deep inhalation, as described on p. 426.
- Scapula stability is observed as the patient lowers the torso from a push-up position. A normal functional evaluation reveals the scapulae stable and moving medially toward the spine. If, however, winging occurs or if either or both scapulae move significantly cephalad then the rhomboids and serratus anterior are weak and inhibited, which could impact on respiratory function. A further implication of weakness in these lower scapula fixators is that the upper fixators (levator and upper trapezius in particular) will usually be overactive and short.

Palpation for trigger point activity

All muscles which are shown to be dysfunctional in the above assessments (whether shortened or lengthened) should be evaluated for trigger point activity using NMT and/or other palpation methods.

Alternative categorization of muscles

Information was presented in Chapter 2 (Box 2.1) relating to alternative ways of conceiving the muscular imbalances commonly listed as postural and phasic. According to Norris' research (1995a,b,c,d,e, 1998), inhibited/weak muscles often actually lengthen, adding to the instability of the region in which they operate. Muscles which fall into this category are more deeply situated, are slow twitch and have a tendency to weaken and lengthen if deconditioned. These include transverse abdominis, multifidus, internal obliques, medial fibers of external oblique, gluteus maximus and medius, quadratus lumborum, deep neck flexors and, of interest in the region under review, serratus anterior and lower trapezius. These muscles can be correlated, to a large extent (apart from quadratus lumborum), with muscles designated by Lewit (1999) and Janda (1983) as 'phasic'.

The more superficial, fast-twitch muscles, which have a tendency to shortening, include the suboccipital group, sternocleidomastoid, upper trapezius, levator scapula, iliopsoas and hamstrings. These fall into the category of 'postural' muscles as described by Lewit, Janda and Liebenson. Norris calls these mobilizers because they cross more than one joint.

Examples of patterns of imbalance emerge in the thoracic region, as some muscles weaken and lengthen while their synergists become overworked and their antagonists shorten. This can be summarized as follows:

'Weak'/lengthened	Overactive synergist	Shortened antagonist
Lower trapezius	Levator scapula/upper trapezius	Pectoralis major
Serratus anterior Diaphragm	Pectoralis major/minor	Rhomboids Scalenes Pectoralis major

Rib palpation

- With the patient seated, the practitioner, standing behind, palpates the angles of the ribs for symmetry/asymmetry.
- If any rib angles appear more prominent than others or if any individual rib contours seem asymmetrical, these should receive more detailed attention in subsequent tests for elevation or depression (see below).
- Finger pad tracing of the intercostal spaces can reveal areas in which the width of the interspace is reduced. Ideally, the width should be symmetrical along its entire length, from the sternum to the vertebral ends.
- As this palpation proceeds, any tissue changes or sensitivity should be noted. The description of Lief's NMT (p. 447) includes indications as to what might be palpated for in the intercostal spaces. Based on clinical experience the lower aspect of the rib shaft is more easily palpated than the superior border.

Specific 1st rib palpation

- The patient is seated. The practitioner stands behind with fingers covering the upper trapezius close to the base of the neck.
- Trapezius is drawn posteriorly by the practitioner's fingers to allow access for the finger tips to move caudally to make contact with the superior surface of the posterolateral portion of the first rib.
- The rib on one side may be noted to be more cephalad ('higher') than the other side. The higher side will also usually be reported as being more sensitive to the palpation contact.
- Scalene assessment may also indicate greater shortening on the same side.

Test and treatment for elevated and depressed ribs

It is important that the functional freedom of ribs be assessed in any overall evaluation of thoracic structure and function. One of the commonest dysfunctional states involving the ribs is for one or more ribs to be restricted in their normal range of motion (this more commonly occurs in groups rather than single ribs).

1. If ribs do not rise fully on inhalation they are said to be 'depressed', locked in relative exhalation.
2. If ribs do not fall fully on exhalation they are said to be 'elevated', locked in relative inhalation.

Rib motion

- *Pump handle motion*: on inhalation, the anterior aspect of the upper ribs (in particular) moves cephalad, causing an increase in the anteroposterior diameter of the thorax. This action is less apparent in the lower ribs.
- *Bucket handle motion*: on inhalation, the lateral aspect of the lower ribs in particular moves cephalad, causing an increase in the transverse diameter of the thorax. This action is less apparent in the upper ribs.
- Ribs 11 and 12 do not exhibit either pump or bucket handle motion because they lack a cartilaginous attachment to the sternum. These 'floating' ribs move posteriorly and laterally on inhalation and anteriorly and medially on exhalation. Assessment of these ribs' respiratory response is best performed with the patient prone with hands in contact with the rib shafts. On inhalation, a posterior motion should be noted and on exhalation an anterior motion.

Tests for rib motion restrictions (Fig. 14.7)

Palpation and evaluation are performed from the side of the table which brings the dominant eye over the centerline. Examination is performed using full inhalation and exhalation to assess the comparative rise and fall of the ribs on either side (pump handle movement, mainly in the five or six upper ribs) as well as lateral excursion (bucket handle movement mainly in the lower six or seven ribs).

- The patient is supine and the practitioner stands at waist level and places his middle or index fingers on the inferior borders of the clavicle, an inch or so lateral to the sternum.
- The patient inhales and exhales fully as the practitioner observes movement of his fingers overlying the upper ribs during pump handle motion.
- Is movement symmetrical and equal as the inhalation ends and as the exhalation ends?
- Each rib from 1 to 6 is assessed individually in this manner.
- The fingers are then placed on the mid-axillary lines and bucket handle motion is observed in the same manner, looking for asymmetry at the end of the inhalation and exhalation phases.
- Each of the lower ribs, down to the 10th, is assessed individually in this manner.

Box 14.6 Upper ribs and shoulder pain

An association has frequently been shown between thoracic outlet syndrome and 1st rib restriction (Nichols 1996, Tucker 1994). However, a connection between 2nd rib restriction and shoulder pain has not been recorded in the literature until recently.

Boyle (1999) reports on two case histories in which symptoms were present which resembled, in all respects (diagnostic criteria, etc.), shoulder impingement syndrome or rotator cuff partial tear, which responded rapidly to mobilization of the 2nd rib. The patients both had positive tests for shoulder impingement, implicating supraspinatus and/or bicipital tendon dysfunction (see Impingement test description below).

Boyle (1999) describes evidence to support the way(s) in which 2nd rib restrictions (in particular) might produce false-positive test results and give rise to shoulder symptoms.

- The dorsal ramus of the 2nd thoracic nerve continues laterally to the acromion, providing a cutaneous distribution in the region of the posterolateral shoulder (Maigne 1991).
- Rotational restrictions involving the cervicothoracic region have been shown to produce a variety of neck and shoulder symptoms. Since the 2nd rib articulates with the transverse process of T1 (costotransverse joint) and the superior border of T2 (costovertebral joint), rotational restrictions of these vertebrae could produce rib dysfunction (Jirout 1969).
- Habitual overactivity involving scalenus posterior can produce 'chronic subluxation of the 2nd rib at its vertebral articulation' (Boyle 1999). This could result in a superior glide of the tubercle of the 2nd rib at the costotransverse junction.
- Boyle reports that 'true' impingement syndrome is often related to overactivity of the rhomboids which would 'downwardly rotate the scapula', impeding elevation of the humerus at the glenohumeral joint.
- He suggests that rhomboid overactivity might also impact on the upper thoracic region as a whole (T1 to T4), locking these segments into an extension posture. If this situation were accompanied by overactivity of the posterior scalene, the 2nd rib might 'subluxate superiorly on the fixed thoracic segment', leading to pain and dysfunction mimicking shoulder impingement syndrome.
- Boyle hypothesizes that mechanical interference might occur involving 'the dorsal cutaneous branch of the 2nd thoracic nerve … in its passage through the tunnel adjacent to the costotransverse joint'. This nerve might be 'drawn taut, due to the superior anterior subluxation of the 2nd rib', leading to pain and associated restricted movement symptoms.
- The reason for a false-positive impingement test, Boyle suggests, relates to the internal rotation component which adds to the mechanical stress of the dysfunctional rib area. This could also, through pain inhibition, result in rotator cuff muscles testing as weak, suggesting incorrectly that a partial tear had occurred.
- The possibility of a 2nd rib involvement should not disguise the possibility that this coexists with a true impingement lesion.

Palpation

- With the patient prone and the scapula protracted to expose the angle of the rib, practitioner standing at the head of the table, direct thumb pressure (both thumbs) applied at the angle of the rib in an anterocaudad direction will demonstrate relative rigidity, compared with normal rib motion. This palpation will probably produce pain if the rib is dysfunctional.
- The test for assessment of depressed rib function is described on p. 435.

Treatment possibilities and choices

- If the posterior aspect of the 2nd rib is 'subluxated' superiorly, because of a combination of excessive activity and subsequent hypertonicity and shortness of the rhomboids and/or the posterior scalene muscles, NMT attention to these should assist in resolution of the problem.
- If the posterior aspect is 'subluxated superiorly', this will automatically produce a 'depressed' rib appearance anteriorly, i.e. the rib will be relatively locked in its exhalation phase. Positional release and MET methods exist to assist in releasing such restrictions.
- Boyle describes a treatment method (successful in both the cases reported) based on Maitland's (1986) oscillatory mobilization technique.
  1. The patient lies prone, with the scapula on the side to be treated passively protracted.
  2. Thumb pressure (both thumbs adjacent to each other), sufficient to take out all slack, is applied to the angle of the rib in an anterocaudal direction.
  3. Depending on the degree of acuteness, oscillatory movements are applied using a small or a large amplitude. A series of rapid, rhythmic oscillations is executed for 30–60 seconds, repeated three or more times, until retesting indicates improved mobility.
  4. Attention to the musculature, particularly the posterior scalene and possibly serratus anterior muscles, is indicated

Impingement syndrome test

- The patient is supine with her arms at the side with the elbow on the side to be tested flexed to 90° and internally rotated so that the forearm rests on the patient's abdomen.
- The practitioner places one hand to cup the shoulder in order to stabilize it, while the other hand cups the flexed elbow.
- A compressive force is applied through the long axis of the humerus, forcing the humerus against the inferior aspect of the acromion process and glenohumeral fossa.
- If symptoms are reproduced or if pain is noted, supraspinatus and/or bicipital tendon dysfunction is indicated.

- Ribs 11 and 12 are assessed with the patient prone, as described above.

Dysfunctional patterns

- If the ribs (fingers) rise symmetrically on inhalation, completing the excursion at the same time, but on exhalation one seems to continue falling toward its exhalation position after the other has ceased, then the one that ceased moving earlier is regarded as an *elevated* rib, restricted in its ability to exhale, 'locked' in the inhalation phase.

- Conversely, should the ribs commence inhalation together with one ceasing to rise while the other continues, then the one that has ceased to rise is regarded as a *depressed* rib, restricted in its ability to inhale and 'locked' in the exhalation phase.

Treatment hints

- Most rib restrictions are found in groups of two or more, suggesting that they are in this state as a result of an adaptive compensation process (see Chapter 5 for discussion of adaptation patterns).

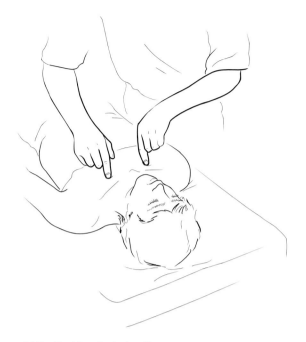

Figure 14.7 Test for rib dysfunction.

- When a single rib is found to be dysfunctional it almost always can be shown to have resulted from direct trauma rather than a compensation process.
- In a group of *depressed* ribs, there is usually no need to release any rib other than the most superior (cephalad) of the group.
- In a group of *elevated* ribs the most inferior (caudad) is usually the key rib requiring treatment. If this is successfully achieved, the others in the group will release automatically.
- This 'key rib' concept has a long tradition in osteopathic medicine.

Discussion

All the rib restrictions described are usually capable of being successfully treated by either positional release or muscle energy approaches. This suggests that the muscular ('soft tissue') component of these restrictions is a major influence on their continued existence.

THORACIC TREATMENT TECHNIQUES

Positioning and movements of the thorax and upper body are strongly influenced by muscles which attach to the lower back and pelvis. These extrinsic muscles of the thorax move it as a unit and offer it many options when postural compensations are necessary. While many osseous elements of the lower body influence upper body posture, such as leg length differential or anterior pelvic tilt, the muscles which most readily adjust the position of the torso for these and other compensations include erector spinae, quadratus lumborum, obliques, psoas and rectus abdominis, all of which are discussed in detail in volume 2 of this text.

Interesting new research shows that many of the muscles supporting and moving the thorax and/or the spinal segments (including erector spinae) prepare to accommodate for subsequent movement as soon as arm or shoulder activity is initiated, with deep stabilizing activity from transversus abdominis, for example, occurring miniseconds *before* unilateral rapid arm activity (Hodges & Richardson 1997). Stabilization of the lumbar spine and thorax has been shown to depend, to a large extent, on abdominal muscle activity (Hodges 1999). These concepts are explored in more detail in volume 2 of this text.

Gait significantly involves the spine in general and the thoracic spinal muscles in particular. Gracovetsky (1997) reports, 'In walking, the hip extensors fire as the toe pushes the ground. The muscle power is directly transmitted to the spine and trunk via two distinct but complementary pathways'.

1. Biceps femoris has its gait action extended by the sacrotuberous ligament, which crosses the superior iliac crest and continues upwards as the erector spinae aponeurosis, iliocostalis lumborum and iliocostalis thoracis (among others).
2. Gluteus maximus force is transmitted superiorly via the lumbodorsal fascia and latissimus dorsi.

Gracovetsky (1997) continues:

As a consequence, firing hip extensors extends and raises the trunk in the sagittal plane. The chemical energy liberated within the muscles is now converted, by the rising trunk, into potential energy stored in the gravitational field. When a person is running, so much energy needs to be stored that the necessary rise in the center of gravity forces the runner to become airborne.

A more detailed review of these and other gait-related influences is to be found in volume 2 of this text.

The intrinsic thoracic muscles are largely responsible for movement of the thoracic spinal column or cage, as well as respiratory function. Though many of these muscles have very short fibers and therefore may appear relatively unimportant, they are strategically placed to provide, or initiate, precisely directed movement of the thoracic vertebrae and/or ribs. They therefore demand due attention in the development of treatment plans.

Posterior superficial thoracic muscles

When viewing the posterior thorax, the trapezius is immediately obvious as it lies superficially and extensively covers the upper back, shoulder and neck. In addition to trapezius, the latissimus dorsi, which superficially covers the lower back, as well as the rhomboids, serratus anterior, and pectoralis major and minor should be assessed and treated prior to the development of a thoracic protocol since they overlie the deeper tissues to be examined and may also be involved. They are all discussed in Chapter 13 which deals with the upper extremity.

A complex array of short and long extensors and rotators lies deep to the more superficial trapezius, latissimus dorsi and the rhomboids.

- Those muscles which support and laterally flex the spinal column (including erector spinae group) are oriented for the most part vertically.
- Those muscles which rotate the column (such as multifidi) are oriented more diagonally.

Platzer (1992) further breaks these two groups into lateral (superficial) and medial (deep) tracts, each having a vertical (intertransverse) and diagonal (transversospinal) component. It is useful to envisage this subdivision, especially when assessing rotational dysfunctions, as the superficial rotators are synergistic with the contralateral deep rotators.

- The lateral (superficial) tract consists of the iliocostalis and longissimus groups and the (cervical) splenii muscles, with the vertical components bilaterally extending the spine and unilaterally sidebending it and the diagonal splenii rotating the spine ipsilaterally.
- The medial (deep) tract includes the spinalis group, the interspinalis (cervical and lumbar) and intertransversarii as the vertical components and the semispinalis group, rotatores and multifidus comprising the deep diagonal group which rotate the spine contralaterally.

Respiratory synkinesis

Numerous combinations of adaptation are possible in the thoracic spine, partly as a result of the compound influences and potentials of the muscles attaching to each segment, as well as the 'interdependent combination of asymmetrical vertebral and upper rib shapes and attachments, and their interaction with cervical muscle extensors and sidebenders that attach as low as T5 and T6' (Hruby et al 1997).

Compensatory patterning seems to be available, and supportable, at any thoracic spinal level. For example, Lewit (1999) has discussed the work of Gaymans (1980) who demonstrated a surprising phenomenon, which he called 'respiratory synkinesis'. This refers, in part, to the alternating inhibitory and mobilizing effects on spinal segments which inhalation and exhalation produce. These follow a predictable pattern in the cervical and thoracic spine during sideflexion, as follows.

- On inhalation, resistance increases to sideflexion in the *even* segments (occiput-atlas, C2, etc., T2, T4, etc.) while in the *odd* segments there is a mobilizing effect (i.e. they are more free).

- On exhalation, resistance increases to sideflexion in the *odd* segments (C1, C3, etc., T3, T5, etc.) while in the *even* segments there is a mobilizing effect (i.e. they are more free).
- The area involving C7 and T1 seems 'neutral' and uninvolved in this phenomenon.
- The restrictive and mobilizing effects at the cervicocranial junction, to inhalation and exhalation respectively, seem to involve not just sidebending but all directions of motion.
- The 'mobilizing influences' of inhalation as described above, diminish in the lower thoracic region.

The clinical value of this information becomes obvious, for example, during mobilization of any of these segments in which sideflexion is a component. In the thoracic region in particular, the value of encouraging the appropriate phase of respiration during application of the induration technique (see p. 444) is easily testable by the practitioner.

Segmental coupling

A more obvious form of adaptation involves the biomechanical coupling of segments during compound movements of the spine. This is based on the fact that during sideflexion an automatic rotation occurs (due to the planes of the facets). In the thoracic spine this coupling process is less predictable than in the cervical region where, from C3 downwards, type 2 (also known as 'non-neutral') is the norm, i.e. sidebending and rotation are to the same side. (These concepts are discussed further in Chapter 11 which covers the cervical spine.)

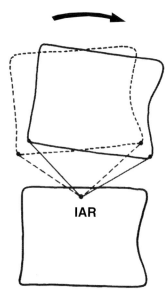

Figure 14.8 During flexion-extension, each lumbar vertebra exhibits an arculate motion in relation to the vertebra below. The centre of the arc lies below the moving vertebra and is known as the instantaneous axis of rotation (IAR) (reproduced, with permission, from *Bogduk* (1999)).

Hruby et al (1997) state:

Upper thoracic coupling is typically [non-]neutral/type 2 [i.e. sidebending and rotation to the same side] and generally occurs as low as T4 … [whereas] … middle thoracic coupling is commonly a mix of neutral/type 1 and non-neutral/type 2 movements, that may rotate to either the formed convexity [type 1] or concavity [type 2]. Lower thoracic coupling is more apt to accompany lumbar neutral/type 1 mechanics.

An assessment exercise is described on p. 425 to enable the practitioner to identify the coupled behavior of specific segments.

Vertical components which lie lateral to the spine include the following (Fig. 14.9).

- Iliocostalis lumborum extends from the iliac crest,

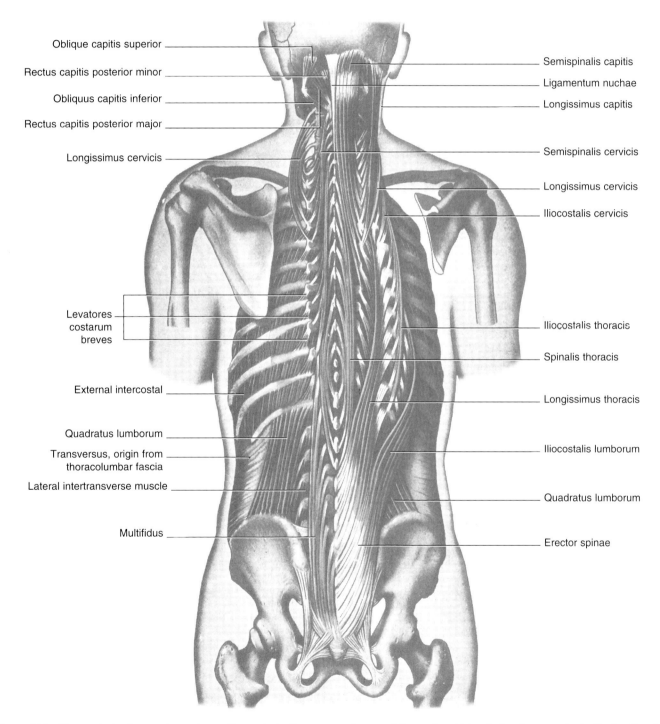

Figure 14.9   The vertical columns of muscles on the posterior thorax serve to powerfully erect and laterally flex the upper body. Dysfunctionally, they produce excessive curvature (lordosis and scoliosis) of the spinal column (reproduced, with permission, from *Gray's anatomy* (1995)).

sacrum, thoracolumbar fascia and the spinous processes of T11–L5 to attach to the inferior borders of the angles of the lower 6–9 ribs.

- Iliocostalis thoracis fibers run from the superior borders of the lower six ribs to the upper six ribs and the transverse process of C7.
- Longissimus thoracis shares a broad thick tendon with iliocostalis lumborum and fiber attachments to the transverse and accessory processes of the lumbar vertebrae and thoracolumbar fascia, which then attaches to the tips of the transverse processes and between the tubercles and angles of the lower 9–10 ribs.

The trigger points for these vertical muscular columns refer caudally and cranially across the thorax and lumbar regions, into the gluteal region and anteriorly into the chest and abdomen (Fig. 14.10).

The erector spinae system is discussed more fully in the second volume of this text due to it substantial role in postural positioning and its extensive attachment to, and influence on, the lumbar and sacral regions. Its thoracic components warrant its mention here and its numerous attachments onto the ribs require that it be released before the deeper tissues are examined. While a more extensive treatment of erector spinae may be necessary, the practitioner can apply NMT strokes (described below) in order to assess tenderness in the muscles and to note if a lengthier treatment is indicated. Later in the protocol, when the intercostal muscles are examined, the practitioner may encounter tender attachment sites which appear to lie in the erectors. Marking each tender spot with a skin-marking pencil may reveal vertical or horizontal patterns of tenderness. Clinical experience suggests that horizontal patterns often represent intercostal involvement, as they are segmentally innervated, while vertically oriented patterns of tenderness usually relate to the erector spinae muscles.

Vertical lines of tension imposed by the erector system can dysfunctionally distort the torso and contribute significantly to scoliotic patterns, especially when unilaterally hypertonic. Leg length differential, whether functional or structural, may need attention in order to sustain any long-term improvement in the myofascial tissue brought about by treatment or exercise.

The posterior fascial lines (of potential tension) which run from above the brow to the soles of the feet (see fascial chains, p. 7) are a critical line of reference to altered biomechanics of the spine and thorax. There may be widespread effects on postural adaptation mechanisms following any substantial release, for example, of the middle portion (erector group) of that posterior line. If the lamina myofascial tissues are also released, the tensegrity tower (the spine) could then more effectively adapt and rebalance. However, the practitioner should note that following such a series of releases, a require-

ment for structural adaptations will be imposed on the body as a whole, as the arms move to new positions of balance and the body's center of gravity is altered. The patient's home-care use of stretching, applied to the neck, shoulder girdle, lower back and pelvis, coupled with postural exercises should be designed to normalize the induced adaptational changes.

🖐 🖐 NMT: posterior thoracic gliding techniques (Fig. 14.11)

Long, gliding strokes may be applied to the posterior thorax with the patient prone and with the practitioner positioned above the head (facing caudally) or near the waist or lower ribs (facing cranially). From above the head, the practitioner can use his own body weight centered (or near centered) over the tissues in order to avoid straining his own back during application of the techniques. The glides may be reapplied in two or three shorter vertical segments, one after the other. Clinically there appear to be postural benefits (for example, in reducing anterior pelvic positioning) when glides are applied toward the pelvis, over lines of normal myofascial tension, such as those provided by the erector group. Lengthening these lines, between the upper thorax and sacroiliac areas, may result in reductions of anterior pelvic tilt, lumbar lordosis and forward head posture.

Each gliding stroke is applied several times while progressively increasing the pressure (if appropriate) before moving the thumbs (palms) laterally, to glide on the next segment of the back, from the first rib through the sacrum, or to the pelvic crest. A flat, palm stroke or one performed by the proximal portion of the forearm (Fig. 14.11a) (not the point of the elbow as it causes too much discomfort when much pressure is applied) may also be used.

These strokes are applied alternately to each side, until each has been treated 4–5 times, while avoiding excessive pressure on the bony protuberances of the pelvis and the spinous processes. Progressive applications usually encounter less tenderness and a general relaxation of the myofascial tissues, especially if heat is applied to the tissues while the contralateral side is being treated. Unless contraindicated (for example, by recent injury, inflammation or excessive tenderness) a hot pack may be moved back and forth between the two sides between the gliding strokes in order to 'flush' the tissues.

The connective tissues may become more supple or the myofascial tensional lines (induced by trigger points, ischemia, connective tissue adaptations) may be released and softened by the gliding strokes, as described above. Trigger points may become more easily palpable as excessive ischemia is reduced or completely released by these gliding strokes. Palpation of the deeper tissues is usually

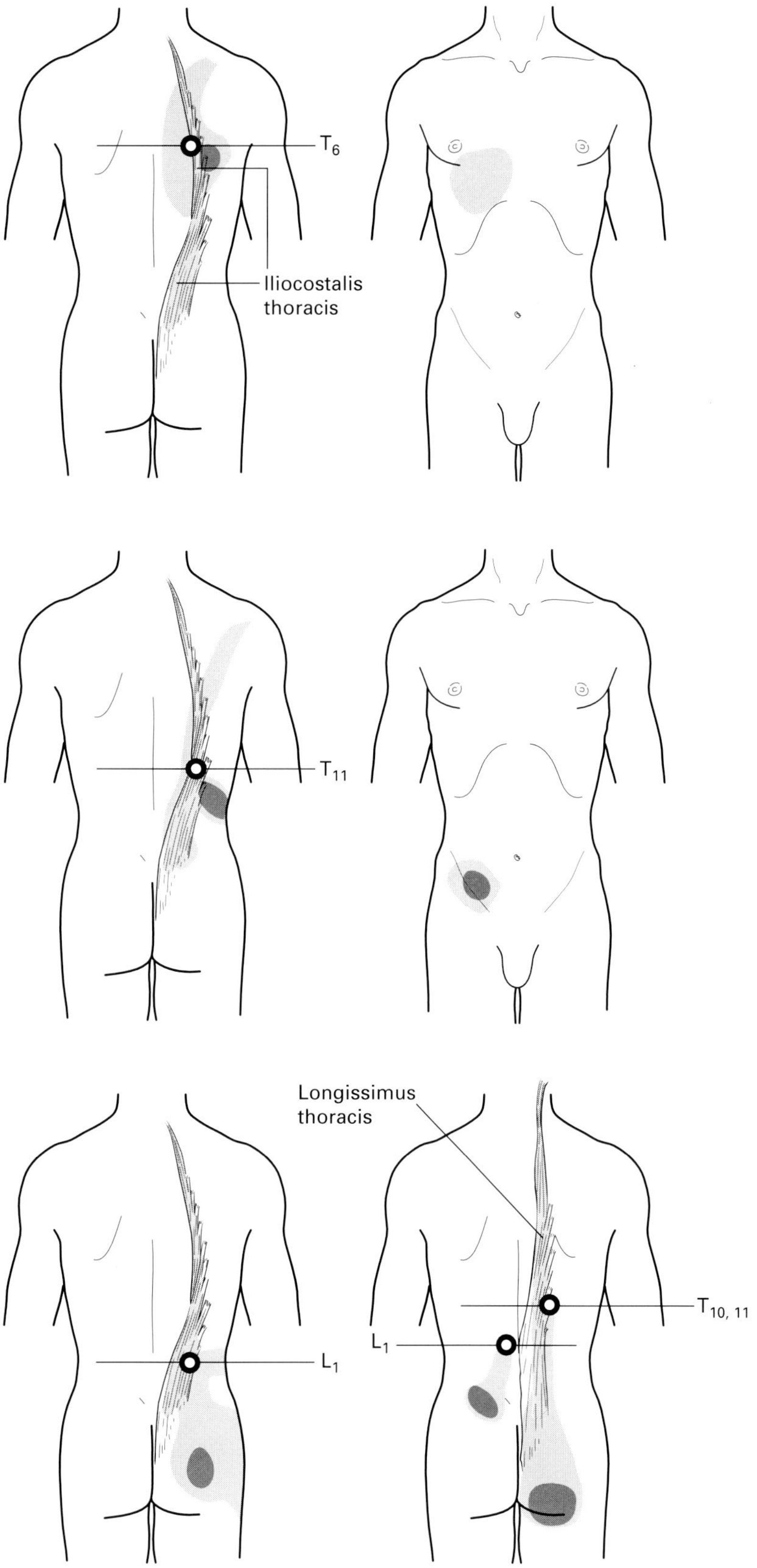

Figure 14.10 Superficial paraspinal muscles collectively known as erector spinae have combined target zones which refer across most of the posterior surface of the body and anteriorly as well.

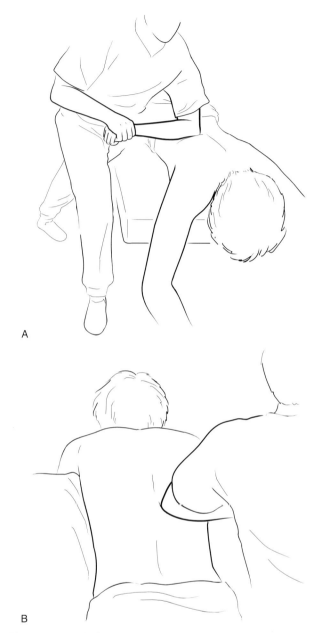

Figure 14.11 A: Gliding strokes applied with the blade of the proximal forearm. B: Avoid olecranon contact with spinous processes.

more defined and tissue response to applied pressure is usually enhanced by this sequence of strokes.

While release of tension might appear to always be desirable, it is important to consider the demands for compensation imposed by induced releases. Local tissues, and the individual as a whole, will be obliged to adapt biomechanically, neurologically, proprioceptively and emotionally. Inducing any substantial release of postural muscles before other areas of the body (and the body as a whole) are prepared may overload compensatory adaptation potentials, possibly creating other areas of pain, structural distress or myofascial dysfunction ('The part

you treated is better, but now I hurt here and here'). Other osseous and myofascial elements may already be adapting to preexisting stresses and may become dysfunctional under such an increased load. However, if treatment has been carefully planned and executed, the process of adaptation to a new situation, following local soft tissue treatment, while almost inevitably producing symptoms of stiffness and discomfort, should be recognized as a probable indication of desirable change and not necessarily 'bad'. The patient should therefore be forewarned to anticipate such symptoms for a day or two following NMT or other appropriate soft tissue manipulation.

NMT for muscles of the thoracic lamina groove

Numerous muscles attach into the thoracic lamina and layer upon each other in a variety of fiber directions. The powerful influence of effluerage strokes, when applied repeatedly to the thoracic and lumbar lamina groove, should not be underestimated. Clinical experience strongly suggests that the application of this form of repetitive NMT effluerage has the ability to significantly influence layer upon layer of fibers, attaching into the lamina. Such strokes are among the most important tools in neuromuscular therapy. Treatment of this sort can beneficially influence segmental spinal mobility, postural integrity and the potential for tensegrity processes to function more effectively in dealing with the stresses and strains to which the body is exposed.

A repeat of these gliding strokes at the end of the session will allow a comparative assessment, which often demonstrates the changes in the tissues (and discomfort levels) to the practitioner as well as the patient.

Many muscular attachments will be assessed with the use of a small pressure bar, or finger friction, applied to the lamina groove, as described below. These attachments may include trapezius, rhomboids, latissimus, splenii, spinalis, semispinalis, multifidus, rotatores and serratus posterior superior and inferior, depending upon which spinal level is being examined. Determining exactly which fibers are involved is sometimes a difficult task and success is based strongly on the practitioner's skill level and knowledge of anatomy, including the order of the multiple layers overlying each other and their fiber directions. Fortunately, the tissue response is not always based on the practitioner's ability to decipher these fiber arrangements (especially in the lamina) and the tender or referring myofascia may prove to be responsive, even when tissue identification is unclear.

Not every muscle attaching to the lamina is discussed below, as some have been detailed together with the descriptions of the upper extremity and/or the cervical region. Because of an overlap in their actions and influences, additional coverage of many of these muscles is to be found in volume 2 of this text, which deals with the lower body. Most of the remaining deeper muscles of the thorax are either discussed here or together with the muscles of respiration.

Spinalis thoracis

Attachments: Spinous process of T11–L2 to the spinous process of T4–8 (variable)
Innervation: Dorsal rami of spinal nerves
Muscle type: Not established
Function: Acting unilaterally, flexes the spine laterally; bilaterally, extends the spine
Synergists: *For lateral flexion*: ipsilateral semispinalis, longissimus and iliocostalis thoracis, iliocostalis lumborum, quadratus lumborum, obliques and psoas
Antagonists: *To lateral flexion*: contralateral semispinalis, longissimus and iliocostalis thoracis, iliocostalis lumborum, quadratus lumborum, obliques and psoas

Semispinalis thoracis

Attachments: Transverse process of T6–10 to the spinous processes of C6–T4
Innervation: Dorsal rami of thoracic nerves
Muscle type: Not established
Function: Acting unilaterally, it rotates the spine contralaterally; bilaterally, it extends the spine
Synergists: *For rotation*: multifidi, rotatores, ipsilateral external obliques and external intercostals and contralateral internal obliques and internal intercostals
For extension: posterior spinal muscles (precise muscles depending upon what level is being extended)
Antagonists: *To rotation*: matching contralateral fibers

of semispinalis as well as contralateral multifidi, rotatores, external obliques and external intercostals and the ipsilateral internal obliques and internal intercostals
For extension: spinal flexors (precise muscles depending upon what level is being extended)

Indications for treatment of spinalis and semispinalis

- Reduced flexion of spine
- Restricted rotation (sometimes painfully)
- Pain along spine
- Tenderness in lamina groove

Multifidi (Figs 14.12, 14.13)

Attachments: From the posterior surface or the sacrum, iliac crest and the transverse processes of all lumbar, thoracic vertebrae and articular processes of cervicals 4–7; these muscles traverse 2–4 vertebrae and attach superiorly to the spinous processes of all vertebrae apart from the atlas
Innervation: Dorsal rami of spinal nerves
Muscle type: Postural (type 1), shortens when stressed
Function: When these contract unilaterally they produce ipsilateral flexion and contralateral rotation; bilaterally, they extend the spine
Synergists: *For rotation*: multifidi, semispinalis, ipsilateral external obliques and external intercostals and contralateral internal obliques and internal intercostals
For extension: posterior spinal muscles (precise muscles depending upon what level is being extended)
Antagonists: *To rotation*: matching contralateral fibers of rotatores as well as contralateral multifidi, semispinalis, external obliques and external intercostals and the ipsilateral internal obliques and internal intercostals

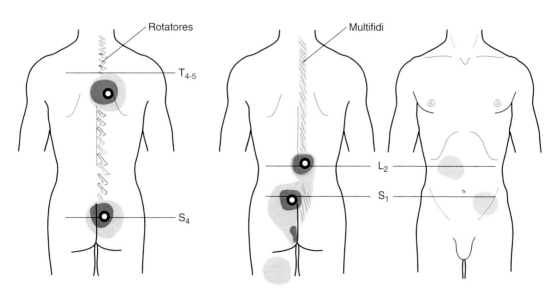

Figure 14.12 Composite trigger point referral patterns of multifidi and rotatores.

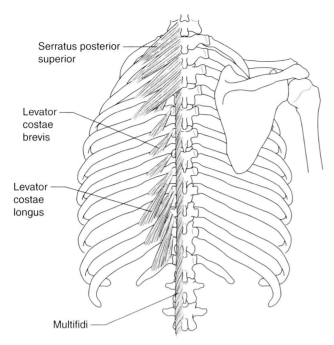

Serratus posterior superior

Levator costae brevis

Levator costae longus

Multifidi

Figure 14.13 Levatores costae elevate and 'spin' ribs during inhalation.

For extension: spinal flexors (precise muscles depending upon what level is being extended)

Indications for treatment

- Chronic instability of associated vertebral segments
- Reduced flexion of spine
- Restricted rotation (sometimes painfully)
- Pain along spine
- Vertebral scapular border pain (referral zone)

Rotatores longus and brevis (see Fig. 14.13)

Attachments: From the transverse processes of each vertebra to the spinous processes of the second (longus) and first (brevis) vertebrae above (ending at C2)

Innervation: Dorsal rami of spinal nerves

Muscle type: Postural (type 1), shortens when stressed

Function: When these contract unilaterally they produce contralateral rotation; bilaterally, they extend the spine

Synergists: *For rotation*: multifidi, semispinalis, ipsilateral external obliques and external intercostals and contralateral internal obliques and internal intercostals

For extension: posterior spinal muscles (precise muscles depending upon what level is being extended)

Antagonists: *To rotation*: matching contralateral fibers of rotatores as well as contralateral multifidi, semispinalis, external obliques and external intercostals and the ipsilateral internal obliques and internal intercostals

For extension: spinal flexors (precise muscles depending upon what level is being extended)

Indications for treatment

- Pain and tenderness of associated vertebral segments
- Tenderness to pressure or tapping applied to the spinous processes of associated vertebrae

Special notes

Multifidi and rotatores muscles comprise the deepest layer of the laminae and are responsible for fine control of the rotation of vertebrae. They exist through the entire length of the spinal column and the multifidi also broadly attach to the sacrum, after becoming appreciably thicker in the lumbar region.

These muscles are often associated with vertebral segments which are difficult to stabilize and should be addressed throughout the spine when scoliosis is present, along with the associated intercostal muscles and pelvic positioning.

Note: Balance mechanisms seem to strongly influence the evolution of scoliosis. Unilateral labyrinthine stimulation (or removal) results in scoliosis, pointing to the relationship between the righting reflexes and spinal balance (Michelson 1965, Ponsetti 1972). In one study, the majority of 100 scoliotic patients were shown to have associated equilibrium defects, with a direct correlation between the severity of the spinal distortion and the degree of proprioceptive and optic dysfunction (Yamada 1971).

Discomfort or pain provoked by pressure or tapping, applied on the spinous processes of associated vertebrae, a test used to identify dysfunctional spinal articulations, also often indicates multifidi and rotatores involvement. Trigger points in rotatores (see Fig. 14.12) tend to produce rather localized referrals whereas the multifidi trigger points refer locally and also to the suboccipital region, medial scapular border and top of shoulder. These local (for both) and distant (for multifidi) patterns of referral continue to be expressed through the length of the spinal column. In fact, the lower spinal levels of multifidi may even refer to the anterior thorax or abdomen.

Local tissue changes in these important muscles (multifidi and rotatores), including chronic hypertonus and ischemia which are precursors to the evolution of trigger points, may result from segmental facilitation (see p. 70).

When segmental facilitation occurs, as a result of either organ disease (i.e. involving viscerosomatic reflexes) or spinal overuse factors, the local musculature becomes hypertonic. Denslow (1944) first described this phenomenon, as follows: 'Motor neuron pools in spinal cord segments related to areas of somatic dysfunction were maintained in a state of facilitation'. He later concluded (Denslow et al 1947): 'Muscles innervated from these segments are kept in a state of hypertonus much of the day with inevitable impediment to spinal motion'.

These concepts were confirmed by research in later years, especially by Korr (1976).

Elkiss & Rentz (1997) summarize:

In the early stages [of facilitation] a continued barrage (nociceptive, proprioceptive, autonomic) and a widening zone of involvement maintain the state of chronic facilitation. With chronic lesions a more lasting mechanism must be at work. Sustained patterns of excitability and synaptic transmission become learned behavior in the spinal cord and brain ... [and there will be] increased signs of somatic dysfunction.

In practice this means that tense, taut paraspinal tissues which are *unresponsive* to normal treatment procedures should always be considered to possibly involve facilitation and to require further investigation as to underlying causes.

Multifidus should co-contract with transversus abdominis to assist in low back stabilization (Richardson & Jull 1995) which suggests that any chronic weakness (or atrophy) is likely to impact strongly on spinal stability. While shortness and tightness are obvious indicators of dysfunction, it is therefore important, when considering muscular imbalances, to also evaluate for weakness. Actual atrophy of the multifidi has been reported in a variety of low back pain settings (see below). Liebenson (1996) observes:

The initial muscular reaction to pain and injury has traditionally been assumed to be an increased tension and stiffness. Data ... indicates inhibition is at least as significant. Tissue immobilization occurs secondarily, which leads to joint stiffness and disuse muscle atrophy.

- Atrophy and fibrosis of multifidus are associated with disc herniation in the lumbar spine (Lehto et al 1989).
- Increased fatty deposits in multifidus ('fatty metaplasia') was a common finding in a population of low back pain patients, when compared with healthy volunteers (Parkkola 1993).
- Hides et al (1994) showed that there was unilateral, segmental wasting of multifidus in acute low back patients. These changes occurred rapidly and were not consistent with 'disuse atrophy'.
- Other researchers have shown type 1 fiber hypertrophy on the symptomatic side and type 2 atrophy bilaterally in multifidus, in chronic low back pain patients (Fitzmaurice 1992).

🖐 🖐 NMT for thoracic (and lumbar) lamina groove muscles

To prepare the superficial posterior thorax for treatment of the tissues which lie deep to them, lubricated gliding strokes may be applied repeatedly with one or both thumbs in the lamina groove and then alongside the lamina from T1 to the sacrum or iliac crest. The thumb nail is not involved in the stroke nor allowed to encounter the skin, as the thumb pads are used as the treatment tool (see p. 113 for hand positioning and cautions in gliding). Each gliding stroke is applied several times from T1 through the sacrum while progressively increasing the pressure (if appropriate) with each new stroke.

The lubricated glides are applied alternately to each side until each has been treated 4–5 times with several repetitions each time. Excessive pressure on the bony protuberances of the pelvis and the spinous processes throughout the spinal column should be avoided. Progressive applications usually encounter less tenderness and a general softening of the myofascial tissues, especially if moist heat is applied to the tissues while the contralateral side is being treated. Unless contraindicated, a hot pack may be placed alternately on each side while the other side is being treated so as to 'flush' the tissues between applications of strokes.

The finger tip (with the nail well trimmed) may be used to friction or assess individual areas of isolated tenderness and to probe for taut bands which house trigger points. Trigger points lying close to the lamina of the spinal column often refer pain across the back, wrapping around the rib cage, anteriorly into the chest of abdomen and frequently refer 'itching' patterns. The trigger points may be treated with static pressure or may respond to rapidly alternating applications of contrasting hot and cold (repeated 8–10 times for 10–15 seconds each), always concluding with cold (see hydrotherapy notes in Chapter 10).

The beveled pressure bar (as described in Box 14.7) may also be used to assess the fibers attaching in the lamina. The tip of the bar is placed parallel to the midline and at a 45° angle to the lateral aspect of the spinous process of T1. In this way it is 'wedged' into the lamina groove where cranial to caudal to cranial friction is applied at tip-width intervals. The assessment begins at T1 and the process continues to (*but not onto*) the coccyx. Each time the pressure bar is moved, it is lifted and placed at the next point, which is a tip width further down the column. The short frictional stroke may also be applied unidirectionally (in either direction), which sometimes more clearly defines the fiber direction of the involved tissue. The location of each involved segment may be marked with a skin-marking pencil so that it may be retreated several times during the session. The 'collection' of skin markings may provide clues as to patterns of involved tissues.

Friction may also be applied between spinous processes (pressure bar or finger tip) in order to treat the supraspinous ligament (throughout the spine) and the interspinalis muscles (lumbar region only). Although the interspinales muscles are also present in the cervical region, the pressure bar is *not* used there as fingers provide a sufficient and more precise treatment (see cervical region, p. 201).

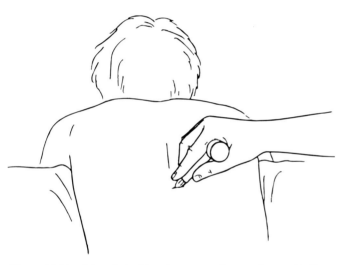

Figure 14.14 A beveled rubber tip pressure bar can be used in the lamina groove to assess the many layers of tissues which attach there.

🖐 🖐 PR method for paraspinal musculature: induration technique (Chaitow 1996b, Morrison 1969)

- The operator stands on the side of the prone patient opposite the side in which pain has been discovered in paraspinal tissues.
- Tender or painful points (lying no more lateral than the tip of the transverse process) are palpated for the level of their sensitivity to pressure.
- Once confirmed as painful, the point is held by firm thumb pressure and the patient is told that the pain being felt represents a score of '10'.
- With the soft thenar eminence of the other hand,

the tip of the spinous process most adjacent to the painful point is very gently eased toward the pain (ounces of pressure only), crowding and slackening the tissues in which the tender point is being palpated until pain reduces by at least 75%.

- Pressure on the spinous process, extremely lightly directed toward the painful point, should lessen the degree of tissue tension and the sensitivity.
- If it does not do so then the angle of 'push' on the spinous process toward the painful spot should be varied slightly, so that, somewhere within an arc embracing a half circle, an angle of push toward the pain will be found to abolish the pain totally and will lessen the objective palpated sense of tension.
- This position of ease is held for not less than 20 seconds after which the next point in the paraspinal musculature is treated.
- If possible, Gaymans' (1980) principles relating to alternate segmental response to inhalation and exhalation, as outlined on p. 436, should be incorporated into the procedure. However, if holding of the breath (in or out) causes the patient any distress, this aspect of the procedure should be ignored.
- If the segment being treated is an odd one (i.e. T3,5,7,9,11), the sidebend, which is being initiated by light pressure on the spinous process toward the painful point, should involve the patient inhaling and holding that *for as long as is comfortable*, during the 20 seconds or so of applied gentle pressure.
- If the segment being treated is an even one (i.e. T2,4,6,8,10,12), the sidebend, which is being initiated by light pressure on the spinous process toward the painful point, should involve the patient exhaling and holding that *for as long as is comfortable*, during the 20 seconds or so of applied gentle pressure.
- For T1 the phase of breathing is irrelevant and the patient should breathe normally during the procedure.

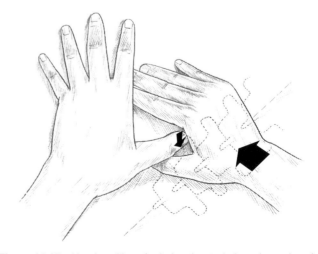

Figure 14.15 Hand positions for induration technique (reproduced, with permission, from Chaitow (1996b)).

• A full spinal treatment is possible using this extremely gentle approach which incorporates the same principles as SCS and functional technique, with the achievement of ease and pain reduction as the treatment focus (see Chapter 10 for details of the principles involved).

• There are no contraindications to this method, which was designed specifically for the fragile and sensitive individual.

Muscles of respiration

The deeper elements of the thoracic musculature represent a remarkable system by means of which respiration occurs. Some of these muscles also provide rotational components which carry similar, spiraling lines of oblique tension from the pelvis (external and internal obliques) through the entire torso (external and internal intercostals), almost as if the ribs were 'slipped into' this supportive web of continuous muscular tubes. Rolfer Tom Myers (1997), in his brilliant 'anatomy trains' concept (p. 7), describes the continuity which occurs between these muscles (obliques and intercostals) as part of his 'lateral line'. Above the pelvic crest this myofascial network creates a series of crossover (X-shaped) patterns.

The obliques tuck into the lower edges of the basket of ribs. Between each of the ribs are the internal and external intercostals, which taken all together form a continuation of the same 'X', formed by the obliques. These muscles, commonly taken to be accessory muscles of breathing, are seen in this context to be perhaps more involved in locomotion [and stability], helping to guide and check the torque, swinging through the rib cage during walking and running.

See Chapter 1 for more of Myers' ideas.

Serratus posterior superior

Attachments: Spinous processes of C7–T3 to attach to the upper borders and external surfaces of ribs 2–5, lateral to their angles
Innervation: Intercostal nerves (T2–5)
Muscle type: Phasic (type 2), weakens when stressed
Function: Uncertain role but most likely elevates the ribs (*Gray's anatomy* 1995)
Synergists: Diaphragm, levatores costarum brevis, scalenus posterior
Antagonists: Internal intercostals

Indications for treatment

• Pain that seems to be deep to the scapula
• Pain may radiate over the posterior deltoid, down the back of the arm, ulnar portion of the hand and to the smallest finger
• Numbness into the ulnar portion of the hand

Special notes

Trigger points for serratus posterior superior lie hidden under the vertebral border of the scapula. When the scapula is in the resting position, the trigger point is unavailable and may be missed during examination. Pressure of the scapula imposed against the trigger point by the patient's sleeping position may irritate and activate the trigger point. Displacement of the scapula to reach the trigger point is imperative and can be accomplished in a seated position (Simons et al 1998) or the sidelying position offered here.

The patient is supported in a sidelying position (see p. 229) with the affected arm uppermost. The arm is draped across the patient's chest and the hand allowed to hang toward the floor so that the scapula translates laterally as far as possible. Having the patient curl the torso into flexion may also assist in exposing more tissue.

Serratus posterior superior's rib attachments may be palpated just lateral to the angles of the ribs and medial to the vertebral border of the scapula. However, this muscle is often relatively thin and its fiber direction is similar to overlying tissues. The practitioner is more likely to locate the exquisite tenderness of any trigger points that may be present, and reproduce their referral patterns, than he is to locate the associated taut bands, although sometimes these may be felt (Fig. 14.16).

Serratus posterior inferior

Attachments: Spinous processes of T11–L3 and the thoracolumbar fascia to the inferior borders of the lower four ribs

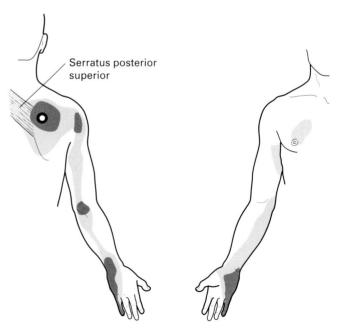

Serratus posterior superior

Figure 14.16 The target zone for serratus posterior superior is significant while its hidden trigger point often remains anonymous.

Innervation: Intercostal nerves (T9–12)
Muscle type: Phasic (type 2), weakens when stressed
Function: Depresses lower four ribs and pulls them posteriorly, not necessarily in respiration (*Gray's anatomy* 1995)
Synergists: Internal intercostals
Antagonists: Diaphragm

Indications for treatment

• Leg length differential
• Rib dysfunction in lower four ribs
• Lower back ache in area of the muscle
• Scoliosis

Special notes

Trigger points in this muscle may produce lower back ache similar to that of renal disease. While its trigger points and attachments should be treated, kidney disease should also be ruled out as the source of viscerosomatic referral, especially when the myofascial pain keeps returning after treatment. The quadratus lumborum muscle, located nearby, should also be examined. This is discussed in more detail in volume 2 of this text and is also considered on p. 61.

CAUTION: As detailed earlier in this chapter, the lower two ribs are 'floating ribs', varying in length, and are not attached anteriorly by costal cartilage. The distal ends of the ribs may be sharp, requiring that palpation is carried out carefully. Additionally, excessive pressure is avoided, especially in patients with known or suspected osteoporosis due to possible fragility of the bones.

The practitioner's thumb can be used to glide laterally along the inferior aspect of each of the lower four ribs (through the latissimus dorsi fibers). The patient will often report tenderness and a 'burning' discomfort as the thumb slides laterally. Repetitions of the stroke usually rapidly reduce the discomfort. Spot tenderness associated with a central trigger point may be found but taut fibers are difficult to feel through the overlying muscles (Simons et al 1998).

Levatores costarum longus and brevis

Attachments: *Longus*: tips of transverse processes of T7–10 to the upper edge and external surface of the tubercle and angle of the 2nd rib below
Brevis: tips of transverse processes of C7–T11 to the upper edge and external surface of the tubercle and angle of the next rib below
Innervation: Dorsal rami of thoracic spinal nerves
Muscle type: Not established
Function: Elevate the ribs; contralateral spinal rotation, ipsilateral flexion and bilaterally extend the column
Synergists: *For rib elevation*: serratus posterior superior, external intercostals, diaphragm, scalenes
Antagonists: Internal intercostals, serratus posterior inferior, elastic elements of thorax

Indications for treatment

• Rib dysfunction
• Breathing dysfunctions, especially ribs locked in elevation
• Vertebral segmental facilitation
• Scoliosis

Special notes

The levatores costarum appears innocuous in its small, short passage from the transverse process to the exterior aspect of the ribs. However, this advantageous placement, directly over the costovertebral joint, puts it in a powerful position to rotate the ribs during inhalation. Simons et al (1998) state, 'They elevate the rib cage with effective leverage. A small upward movement of the ribs so close to the vertebral column is greatly magnified at the sternum'.

These muscles can be difficult to locate precisely and are addressed with the intercostals, if the overlying tissues are not too thick. Additionally, the gliding stroke, described previously for the lamina groove, may also be applied over the costovertebral joints and just lateral to them, in order to assess for tender levatores costarum.

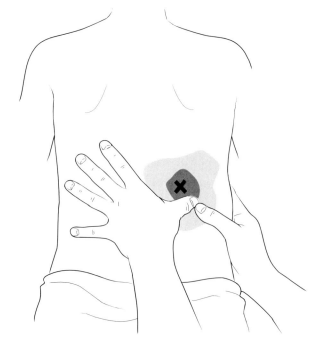

Figure 14.17 Serratus posterior inferior.

Box 14.8 Lief's NMT of the intercostal muscles (Chaitow 1996a)

The intercostal spaces should be assessed for dysfunction.

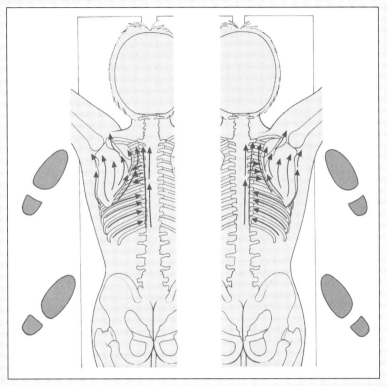

Figure 14.18 Map of suggested NMT stroke patterns for evaluation of lower thoracic area and intercostal spaces (reproduced, with permission, from Chaitow (1996a)).

- The (well-trimmed) thumb tip or a finger tip should be run along both surfaces of the rib margin, as well as in the intercostal space itself.
- In this way the fibers of the internal and external intercostal muscles will receive adequate assessment contacts.
- If there is overapproximation of the ribs, then a simple stroke along the intercostal space may be all that is possible until a degree of rib and thoracic normalization has taken place, allowing greater access.
- The intercostal areas are commonly extremely sensitive and care must be taken not to distress the patient by using inappropriate pressure. Sometimes a 'tickling' element may be eliminated by gently increasing the pressure of the stroke (if appropriate), which will often reveal underlying tenderness in the same tissues.
- At times it is useful to take the patient's hand, have her extend a finger and start the process of stroking through an intercostal space, using her own hand contact, until she desensitizes sufficiently to allow the practitioner's hand to replace her own.
- In most instances the intercostal spaces on the contralateral side will be treated using the finger stroke, as illustrated (Fig. 14.19).
- The tip of a finger (supported by a neighboring digit) is placed in the intercostal space, close to the mid-axillary line, and gently but firmly brought around the curve of the trunk toward the spine.
- The probing digit feels for contracted or congested tissues in which trigger points might be located.
- When an area of contraction is noted, firm pressure toward the center of the body is applied to elicit a response from the patient ('Does it hurt? Does it radiate or refer? If so, where to?').

- Trigger points noted during the assessment may be treated using standard NMT protocols or INIT combination procedures (see p. 123).

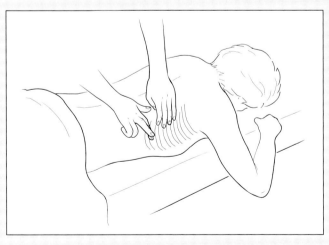

Figure 14.19 Finger strokes as employed in NMT assessment and treatment.

Intercostals (Fig. 14.20)

Attachments: External, internal and innermost lie in three layers, with the innermost outermost, and attach the inferior border of one rib to the superior border of the rib below it. See notes below for direction of fibers
Innervation: Corresponding intercostal nerves
Muscle type: Not established
Function: *For respiration*: external: elevates ribs; internal: depresses the ribs; innermost: unclear function but most likely acts with internal fibers (*Gray's anatomy* 1995)
For rotation: external: rotates torso contralaterally; internal: rotates torso ipsilaterally
Synergists: *For respiration*: external: muscles of inhalation; internal and innermost: muscles of exhalation
For rotation: External: ipsilateral multifidi and rotatores, contralateral internal obliques; internal: contralateral external obliques, multifidi and rotatores
Antagonists: *For respiration*: external: muscles of exhalation; internal and innermost: muscles of inhalation
For rotation: external: contralateral multifidi and rotatores, ipsilateral internal obliques; internal: ipsilateral external obliques, multifidi and rotatores

Indications for treatment

- Respiratory dysfunctions, including dysfunctional breathing patterns and asthma
- Scoliosis
- Rib dysfunctions and intercostal pain
- Cardiac arrhythmia (see pectoralis major, p. 359)

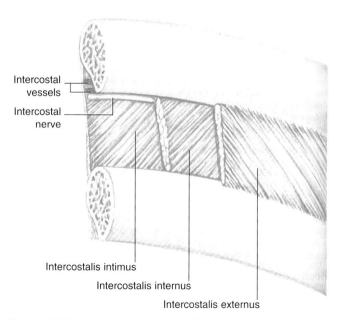

Intercostal vessels
Intercostal nerve
Intercostalis intimus
Intercostalis internus
Intercostalis externus

Figure 14.20 Intercostal muscles provide rotation of the thorax as well as assisting in breathing (reproduced, with permission, from *Gray's anatomy* (1995)).

Special notes

Whereas the internal intercostal muscles attach to the ribs and fully to the costal cartilages, the external intercostals attach only to the ribs, ending at the lateral edge of the costal cartilages with the external intercostal membrane expanding the remaining few inches to the sternum. The external and internal intercostal fibers lie in opposite directions to each other with the external fibers angling inferomedially and the internal fibers coursing inferolaterally when viewed from the front. The reverse is true when viewed from the back.

These fiber directions coincide with the direction of external and internal obliques and provide rotatorial movement of the torso and postural influences in addition to respiratory responsibilities (Simons et al 1998).

Controversy exists as to the role these muscles play in quiet breathing, with some texts suggesting involvement only during forced respiration (Platzer 1992). Simons et al (1998) discuss progressive recruitment depending upon degree of forced respiration. Intercostals may also provide rigidity to the thoracic cage to prevent inward pull of the ribs during inspiration.

The subcostales muscles (when present) are usually only well developed in the lower internal thoracic region. Their fiber direction is the same as that of internal and innermost intercostals and they span across the internal surface of one or two ribs rather than just the intercostal space. They most likely have the same function as the deeper intercostal muscles (*Gray's anatomy* 1995, Platzer 1992, Simons et al 1998).

Since these muscles are segmentally innervated, neuropathies (such as shingles) will be noted to run a course laterally around the torso and may affect one (or more) intercostal spaces along their full length. When shingles (herpes zoster) is present or has been noted in the last six to eight months, applications of NMT are contraindicated. When this segmental pattern of tenderness is noted and the condition of shingles has not been diagnosed, caution should be exercised due to the fact that the tenderness may be the first sign of an oncoming eruption. Though the condition is self-limiting, inappropriate treatment of the tissues may irritate the condition.

A skin marking pen may be used to record tender tissues found during the palpation exercise below. Marking each tender spot may reveal vertical or horizontal patterns of tenderness. Horizontal patterns often represent intercostal involvement while vertically oriented patterns of tenderness are usually indicative of erector spinae muscle dysfunction.

 NMT for intercostals

Fingertip or thumb glides, as described in Box 14.8, are applied to the intercostal spaces of the posterior, lateral and anterior thorax for initial examination as to tenderness and rib alignment. A beveled-tip pressure bar or finger tip may be used to friction the intercostal spaces and more precisely located trigger points or tender tissue, or to address the tissue specific to rib approximation, when the intercostal space is decreased. The pressure bar tip or finger tip can be pressed into the intercostal space (pressure toward the center of the thorax) or angled superiorly or inferiorly against the rib attachments (if space allows).

On the anterior thorax, all breast tissue (including the nipple area on men) is avoided with the intercostal treatment. Specific lymphatic drainage techniques may be applied to the breast area but the frictional techniques used in this procedure are inappropriate for breast tissue. Additionally, the area cephalad to the breast is avoided due to the location of the neurovascular supply to the upper extremity and the pectoralis minor. Lief's NMT incorporates assessment and treatment of the lower inter-costal spaces with the patient supine, as part (usually the commencement) of an abdominal NMT sequence. This is outlined fully in volume 2 of this text.

In the lateral thorax, the region high in the axilla is avoided due to lymph nodes. In the posterior thorax, caution is exercised regarding the floating ribs (noted with serratus posterior inferior). Additionally, in the upper posterior thorax, palpation of the intercostal space is obscured by overlying tissue and location of the intercostals may be unclear.

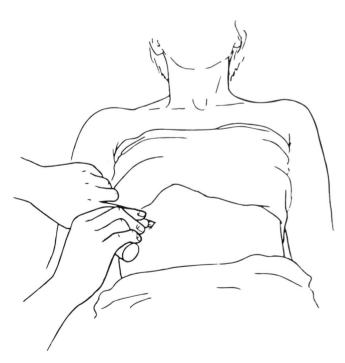

Figure 14.21 The beveled tip pressure bar can be used in intercostal spaces except where the brachial plexus or breast tissue lie.

Influences of abdominal muscles

Like the erector system of the posterior thorax, the abdominal muscles play a significant role in positioning the thorax and in rotating the entire upper body. They are also now known to play a key part in spinal stabilization and intersegmental stability, particularly transversus abdominis (Hodges 1999). The rectus abdominis, external and internal obliques and transversus abdominis are also involved in respiration due to their role in position-ing the abdominal viscera as well as depression of the lower ribs, assisting in forced expiration and especially coughing.

While the abdominal muscles are discussed in detail in volume 2 of this text, the following brief NMT assessment of their uppermost fibers and attachments to the ribs will assist the practitioner in determining if a more thorough examination is warranted. Stretching and strengthening of the abdominal muscles is indicated in many respira-tory and postural dysfunctions as they are often signifi-cantly involved. Additional (to NMT) assessment methods are also detailed in volume 2.

NMT assessment

The practitioner uses lightly lubricated gliding strokes or finger friction on the anterior and lateral aspects of the inferior borders and external surfaces of the 5th through 12th ribs where many of the abdominal muscles fibers attach. Caution is exercised regarding the often sharp tips of the last two ribs.

Palpation of the upper 2 or 3 inches of the fibers which lie over the abdominal viscera may reveal tenderness associated with trigger points or with postural distortions, such as forward slumping postures, which overapproxi-mate these fibers and shorten them. The upper portion of rectus abdominis and the medial upper fibers of the obliques would be softened with short effluerage strokes or by stretching them manually before the treatment of the diaphragm, which will be treated through the overlying muscles. When these overlying muscles are extremely tender, NMT treatment of the diaphragm may need to be postponed until the tissues have been fully treated.

When these overlying muscles are hypertonic, they may prevent penetration into the underlying diaphragm and positional release or muscle energy techniques may be used instead or to prepare for subsequent NMT.

 PR of diaphragm (Fig. 14.22)

- The patient is supine and the practitioner stands at waist level facing cephalad and places his hands over the lower thoracic structures with his fingers along the lower rib shafts.
- Treating the structure being palpated as a cylinder,

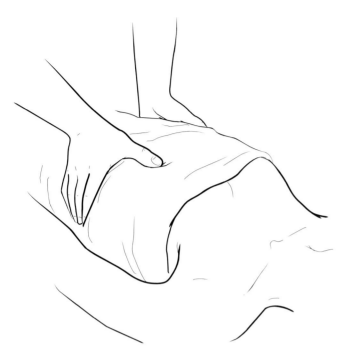

Figure 14.22 Hand positions for assessment of lower thoracic tissue preferences.

the hands test the preference this cylinder has to rotate around its central axis, one way and then the other. 'Does the lower thorax rotate more easily to the right or the left?'

• Once the rotational preference has been established, the preference to sidebend one way or the other is evaluated. 'Does the lower thorax sideflex more easily to the right or the left?'

• Once these two pieces of information have been established, the combined positions of ease, so indicated, are introduced.

• For example, the rotation may well be easier toward the (patient's) right. This is therefore gently introduced by the practitioner, followed, while still in that position, by whichever sidebending preference was indicated during testing, possibly toward the left.

• In this way a compound (stacked) position of ease (or bind) can be established (see functional technique discussion, Chapter 10).

• By holding tissues in their 'loose' or ease positions and waiting for a release (usually 30–90 seconds), the practitioner can encourage changes which will allow more normal diaphragmatic function, accompanied by a relaxation of associated soft tissues.

 MET release for diaphragm

• The same assessment procedure is carried out as for positional release above. However, rather than seeking the direction of ease for rotation and sideflexion

of the thorax, the 'tight' (most restricted) directions are identified.

• This time, by sidebending and rotating *toward the tighter directions*, the combined directions of restriction are engaged, at which time the patient is asked to inhale and hold the breath and to 'bear down' slightly (Valsalva maneuver).

• These efforts introduce isometric contractions of the diaphragm and intercostal muscles.

• On release and complete exhalation and relaxation, the diaphragm should be found to function more normally, accompanied by a relaxation of associated soft tissues.

Interior thorax

Diaphragm

Attachments: Inner surfaces of lower six ribs and their costal cartilages, posterior surface of xiphoid process (or sternum) and the body of the upper 1–4 lumbar vertebrae, vertebral discs and the arcuate ligaments, thereby forming a circular attachment around the entire inner surface of the thorax

Innervation: Phrenic nerves (C3–5) for motor and lower 6–7 intercostal nerves for sensory (*Gray's anatomy* 1995, Simons et al 1998)

Muscle type: Not established

Function: Principal muscle of inspiration by drawing its central tendon downward to stabilize it against the abdominal viscera at which time it lifts and spreads the lower ribs

Synergists: Accessory muscles of inhalation

Antagonists: Elastic recoil of thoracic cavity and accessory muscles of exhalation

Indications for treatment

• Dyspnea or any breathing difficulty
• Dysfunctional breathing patterns
• Chronic respiratory problems (asthma, chronic cough, etc.)
• 'Stitch in the side' with exertion

Box 14.9 McConnell and the diaphragm

Remember that the functional status of the diaphragm is probably the most powerful mechanism of the whole body. It not only mechanically engages the tissues of the pharynx to the perineum, several times per minute, but is physiologically indispensable to the activity of every cell in the body. A working knowledge of the crura, tendon, and the extensive ramification of the diaphragmatic tissues graphically depicts the significance of structural continuity and functional unity. The wealth of soft tissue work centering in the powerful mechanism is beyond compute, and clinically it is very practical. (McConnell 1962)

- Chest pain
- Hiccup

Special notes

The diaphragm is a dome-shaped muscle with a central tendon whose fibers radiate peripherally to attach to all margins of the lower thorax, thereby forming the floor of the thoracic cavity. It attaches higher in the front than either side or back. When this muscle contracts, it increases the vertical, transverse and anteroposterior diameter of the internal thorax (Kapandji 1974) and is therefore the most important muscle in inspiration.

Figure 14.23 shows clearly the structural relationship between the diaphragm, psoas and quadratus lumborum. A brief summary of some of the diaphragm's key attachments and features indicates the complex nature of this muscle.

- The sternal part of the diaphragm arises from the internal surface of the xiphoid process (this attachment is sometimes absent).
- The costal part arises from the internal aspects of the lower six ribs, 'interdigitating with the transverse abdominis' (*Gray's anatomy* 1995).
- The lumbar part arises from two aponeurotic arches (medial and lateral lumbocostal arches or arcuate liga-

ments) as well as from the lumbar vertebrae by means of two crura (pillars).

- The lateral crus is formed from a thick fascial covering which arches over the upper aspect of quadratus lumborum, to attach medially to the anterior aspect of the transverse process of L1 and laterally to the inferior margin of the 12th rib.
- The medial crus is tendinous in nature and lies in the fascia covering psoas major. Medially it is continuous with the corresponding medial crus and also attaches to the body of L1 or L2. Laterally it attaches to the transverse process of L1.
- The crura blend with the anterior longitudinal ligament of the spine, with direct connections to the bodies and intervertebral discs of L1, 2 and 3.
- The crura ascend and converge to join the central tendon.
- With attachments at the entire circumference of the thorax, ribs, xiphoid, costal cartilage, spine, discs and major muscles, the various components of the diaphragm form a central tendon with apertures for the vena cava, aorta, thoracic duct and esophagus.
- When all these diaphragmatic connections are considered, the direct influence on respiratory function of the lumbar spine and ribs as well as psoas and quadratus lumborum becomes apparent.

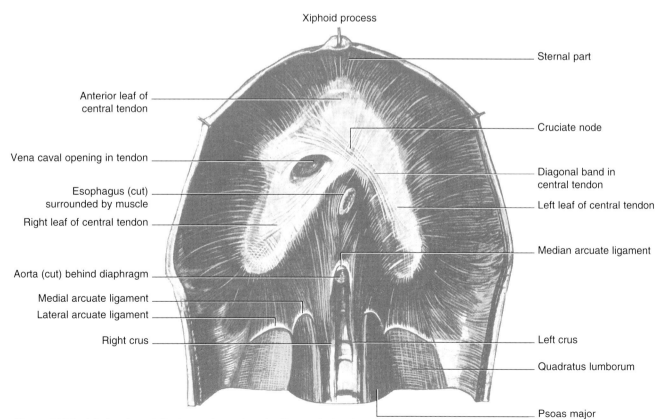

Figure 14.23   Inferior view of diaphragm (reproduced, with permission, from *Gray's anatomy* (1995)).

Patients who suffer from hiatal hernia pain may find that pain is reduced by treatment (and self-treatment) of the diaphragm, as well as by breathing retraining. Simons et al (1998) note that referred pain from trigger points in transversus abdominis may be confused with pain from those associated with the diaphragm and suggest that transversus trigger points will more likely produce pain on deep inhalation, whereas full exhalation (with added compression from the abdomen near the end of exhalation) will reproduce diaphragmatic trigger point referrals. They also note that diaphragmatic trigger points are commonly satellites of primary trigger points found in the ipsilateral upper rectus abdominis.

 NMT for diaphragm (Fig. 14.24)

The patient is supine with the knees flexed and feet resting flat on the table. This position will relax the overlying abdominal fibers and allow a better penetration to the diaphragm. As noted previously, the upper rectus abdominis is treated before the diaphragm. The treatment of the diaphragm is contraindicated for patients with liver and gall bladder disease or if the patient's right side is significantly tender or swollen.

The practitioner stands at the level of the abdomen on the contralateral side and reaches across the person to treat the opposite side of the diaphragm. The fingers, thumbs or a combination of thumb of one hand and fingers of the other may be used.

The practitioner will work with the flow of the breath, sliding the palpating fingers or thumbs under the lower border of the rib cage. As the patient breathes out, the fingers will slide further in. As the patient breathes in, the diaphragm will press against the treating digit(s) and

move the fingers out of position unless the practitioner resists this movement. When penetration appears to be as far as possible, the finger (thumb) tips are directed toward the inner margins of the ribs and static pressure or gentle friction is applied toward the diaphragm's attachment. The treatment may be applied on full exhalation or at half-breath and is repeated to as much of the internal costal margins as can be reached.

While it is uncertain if and how much of the diaphragm's fibers may be reached by this exercise, the connective tissue associated with its costal attachment is probably influenced. Simons et al (1998) describe a similar procedure which ends in an anterior lifting of the rib cage (instead of friction or static pressure) to stretch the fibers of the diaphragm.

Transversus thoracis

Attachments: Inner surface of the body of sternum and xiphoid process superolaterally to the lower borders of the 2nd–6th costal cartilages

Innervation: Intercostal nerves (2–6)

Muscle type: Not established

Function: Depresses the costal cartilages during exhalation, ribs 2–6

Synergists: Muscles of exhalation

Antagonists: Muscles of inhalation

Indications for treatment

- Inadequate lifting of the sternum during inhalation, if shortened
- Inadequate excursion of upper ribs during exhalation ('elevated ribs'), if lax

Special notes

This muscle, also called the sternocostalis or triangularis sternae, lies entirely on the interior chest and is not available to direct palpation. It varies considerably, not only from person to person but also from side to side in the same person (*Gray's anatomy* 1995) and is sometimes absent (Platzer 1992).

Latey (1996) reports that this muscle has the ability to generate powerful sensations, with even light contact sometimes producing reflex contractions of the abdomen or chest with feelings of nausea and choking, as well as anxiety, fear, anger, laughter, sadness, weeping and other emotions. Latey believes that its closeness to the internal thoracic artery is probably significant since when it is contracted, it can exert direct pressure on the artery. He believes that physiological breathing involves a rythmical relaxation and contraction of this muscle and that rigidity is often seen where 'control' dampens the emotions which relate to it (see Chapter 4).

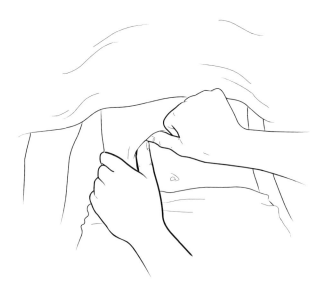

Figure 14.24 Diaphragm – the thumbs or finger tips press through the upper rectus abdominis and under the ribs to influence the diaphragm and associated connective tissues.

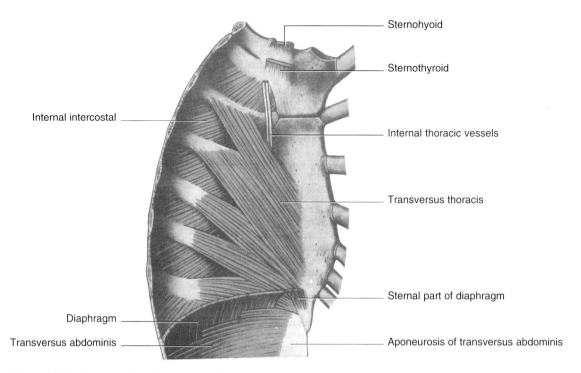

Figure 14.25   Posterior view of transversus thoracis.

REFERENCES

Beal M 1983 Palpatory testing for somatic dysfunction in patients with cardiovascular disease. Journal of the American Osteopathic Association 82:882

Beal M 1985 Viscerosomatic reflexes review. Journal of the American Osteopathic Association 85:786–800

Bogduk N 1999 Clinical Anatomy of the Lumbar Spine and Sacrum. Churchill Livingstone, Edinburgh

Boyle J 1999 Is the pain and dysfunction of shoulder impingement lesion really second rib syndrome in disguise? Two case reports. Manual Therapy 4(1):44–48

Chaitow L 1996a Modern neuromuscular techniques. Churchill Livingstone, Edinburgh

Chaitow L 1996b Positional release techniques. Churchill Livingstone, Edinburgh

Chila A 1997 Fascial-ligamentous release. In: Ward R (ed) Foundations of osteopathic medicine. Williams and Wilkins, Baltimore

DeLany J 1996 American neuromuscular therapy. In: Chaitow L (ed) Modern neuromuscular techniques. Churchill Livingstone, Edinburgh

Denslow J 1944 An analysis of the variability of spinal reflex thresholds. Journal of Neurophysiology 7:207–216

Denslow J, Korr I, Krems A 1947 Quantitative studies of chronic facilitation in human motoneuron pools. American Journal of Physiology 150:229–238

DiGiovanna E 1991 An osteopathic approach to diagnosis and treatment. Lippincott, Philadelphia

Ebner M 1962 Connective tissue massage. Churchill Livingstone, Edinburgh

Elkiss M, Rentz L 1997 Neurology. In: Ward R (ed) Foundations of osteopathic medicine. Williams and Wilkins, Baltimore

Fitzmaurice R 1992 A histo-morphometric comparison of muscle biopsies from normal subjects and patients with ankylosing spondylitis and severe mechanical low back pain. Journal of Pathology 163:182

Gaymans F 1980 Die bedeutung der atemtypen fur Mobilisation der Wirbelsaule. Manuelle Medizin 18:96

Gracovetsky S 1997 A theory of human gait. In: Vleeming A, Mooney V, Sjniders C, Dorman T, Stoekart R (eds) Movement, stability and low back pain. Churchill Livingstone, London

Gray's anatomy 1995 (Williams P, ed) 38th edn. Churchill Livingstone, Edinburgh

Grice A 1980 A biomechanical approach to cervical and thoracic adjusting. In: Haldeman S (ed) Modern developments in the principles and practice of chiropractic. Appleton-Century-Crofts, New York

Grieve G 1981 Common vertebral joint problems. Churchill Livingstone, New York

Hides J, Stokes M, Saide M et al 1994 Evidence of lumbar multifidus muscle wasting ipsilateral to symptoms in patients with acute/subacute low back pain. Spine 19:165

Hoag M 1969 Osteopathic medicine. McGraw Hill, New York

Hodges P 1999 Is there a role for transversus abdominis in lumbo-pelvic stability? Manual Therapy 4(2):74–86

Hodges P, Richardson C 1997 Feedforward contraction of transversus abdominis is not influenced by direction of arm movement. Experimental Brain Research 114:362–370

Hruby R, Goodridge J, Jones J 1997 Thoracic region and rib cage. In: Ward R (ed) Foundations of osteopathic medicine. Williams and Wilkins, Baltimore

Jirout J 1969 Movement diagnostics by X-ray in the cervical spine. Manuelle Medizin 7:121–128

Kapandji I 1974 The physiology of the joints, vol. III, 2nd edn. Churchill Livingstone, Edinburgh

Janda V 1983 Muscle function testing. Butterworths, London

Korr I 1970 The physiological basis of osteopathic medicine. Postgraduate Institute of Osteopathic Medicine and Surgery, New York

Korr I 1976 The spinal cord as organiser of disease processes. Journal of the American Osteopathic Association 76:35–45

Kurz I 1986 Textbook of Dr. Vodder's manual lymph drainage, vol 2: therapy, 2nd edn. Karl F Haug, Heidelberg

Kurz I 1987 Introduction to Dr. Vodder's manual lymph drainage, vol 3: therapy II (treatment manual). Karl F Haug, Heidelberg

Latey P 1996 Feelings, muscles and movement. Journal of Bodywork and Movement Therapies 1(1):44–52

Lehto M, Hurme M, Alaranta H 1989 Connective tissue changes in the multifidus muscle in patients with lumbar disc herniation. Spine 14:302–309

Lewit K 1999 Manipulative therapy in rehabilitation of the motor system, 3rd edn. Williams and Wilkins, Baltimore

Liebenson C 1996 Rehabilitation of the spine. Williams and Wilkins, Baltimore

Mann F 1971 Meridians of acupuncture. Heinemann Medical Books, London

Maigne J 1991 Upper thoracic dorsal rami. Surgical and Radiological Anatomy 13:109–112

Maitland G 1986 Vertebral manipulation, 5th edn. Butterworths, London

Mannino J 1979 Application of neurologic reflexes to treatment of hypertension. Journal of the American Osteopathic Association 79:4

McConnel C 1962 Yearbook. Osteopathic Institute of Applied Technique, Newark, Ohio, pp75–78

Melzack R 1977 Trigger points and acupuncture points of pain. Pain 3:3–23

Michelson J 1965 Development of spinal deformity in experimental scoliosis. Acta Orthopaedica Scandinavica 81 (suppl)

Morrison M 1969 Lecture notes. Research Society for Naturopathy, London

Myers T 1997 Anatomy trains. Journal of Bodywork and Movement Therapies 1(2):91–101

Nichols A 1996 Thoracic outlet syndrome in athletes. Journal of the American Board of Family Practice 9(5):346–355

Norris C M 1995a Spinal stabilisation. 1. Active lumbar stabilisation – concepts. Physiotherapy 81(2):61–64

Norris C M 1995b Spinal stabilisation. 2. Limiting factors to end-range motion in the lumbar spine. Physiotherapy 81(2):64–72

Norris C M 1995c Spinal stabilisation. 3. Stabilisation mechanisms of the lumbar spine. Physiotherapy 81(2):72–79

Norris C M 1995d Spinal stabilisation. 4. Muscle imbalance and the low back. Physiotherapy 81(3):127–138

Norris C M 1995e Spinal stabilisation. 5. An exercise program to enhance lumbar stabilisation. Physiotherapy 81(3):138–146

Norris C M 1998 Sports injuries, diagnosis and managment, 2nd edn. Butterworths, London

Norris C M 1999 Functional load abdominal training. Journal of Bodywork and Movement Therapies 3(3):150–158

Owens C 1980 An endocrine interpretation of Chapman's reflexes. American Academy of Osteopathy, Newark, Ohio

Parkkola R 1993 Magnetic resonance imaging of the discs and trunk muscles in patients with chronic low back pain. Spine 18:830–836

Platzer W 1992 Color atlas/text of human anatomy: vol. l, locomotor system, 4th edn. Thieme, Stuttgart

Ponsetti I 1972 Biomechanical analysis of intervertebral discs and idiopathic scoliosis. Journal of Bone and Joint Surgery 54:1993

Richardson C, Jull G 1995 Muscle control – pain control. Manual Therapy 1(1):2–10

Serizawe K 1980 Tsubo: vital points for Oriental therapy. Japan Publishing, Tokyo

Simons D, Travell J, Simons L 1998 Myofascial pain and dysfunction: the trigger point manual, vol.1, 2nd edn. Williams and Wilkins, Baltimore

Timmons B 1994 Behavioral and psychological approaches to breathing disorders. Plenum Press, New York

Tucker A 1994 Shoulder pain in a football player. Medicine and Science in Sports and Exercise 26(3):281–284

Upledger J, Vredevoogd W 1983 Craniosacral therapy. Eastland Press, Seattle

Walther D 1988 Applied kinesiology. SDC Systems, Pueblo, Colorado

White A, Panjabi M 1978 Clinical biomechanics of the spine. J B Lippincott, Baltimore

Yamada K 1971 A neurological approach to etiology and treatment of scoliosis. Journal of Bone and Joint Surgery 53A:197

Index

Rectus capitis anterior minor *see* Rectus
   capitis anterior
Rectus capitis lateralis, 225–226, 240
   NMT, 226
Rectus capitis major and minor, chronic neck
   pain, 26
Rectus capitis posterior major, 208, 209, 233,
   240
Rectus capitis posterior minor, 207–208, 209,
   233, 240
   proprioceptive dysfunction, 34–35
Red reflex asssessment, 424–425
Red (type I postural) muscles, 18, 21, 22, 53
   chronic back pain, 25
Reference zones, spray and stretch, 135
Referral patterns, trigger points, 69
Referred inhibition, trigger points and, 79
Referred pain, 89
   dermatome C4, 302
   from viscera, 75, **76**, 446
   trigger points, 71–72, 88
   upper crossed syndrome, 56
Reflex effects, muscular pain, 88
Reflex inhibition, 26
Reflex or local pain, 88
Reflex mechanisms, 30, 30–32
Reflex systems, therapeutic rehabilitation
   using, 39
Reflex tests
   elbow assessment, 380
   shoulder assessment, 304
Regeneration phase, inflammatory response,
   86
Rehabilitation, 88, 110–111, 153
   equilibrium, maintaining, 279
   FMS, 136
   goal setting and pacing, 103–104
   summary of sequencing, 111
Reiter's syndrome, 416
Release, meaning of, 238
Remodelling phase, inflammatory response,
   86
Repair process, stages of, **111**
Repetitions, assessment and testing, 169, 170,
   305
   shoulder joint, 299, 301, 302
   wrist movements, 393
Reporting stations, 33
   manipulation of, 35, 39
Reposition, thenar muscles, 417
Residual posture, Latey, 47
Resisted tests, 315
   resistive supination test, 311
   soft tissue or joint pain, 90
Respiration
   abnormal patterns, 357
   and chronic fatigue syndrome, 37
   and lymph movement, 138
   and musculoskeletal dysfunction, 50–53
   posture and adaptation, 44–45
   see also Breathing
Respiratory function assessment, 429, 431–432
Respiratory mechanics, 429–431
Respiratory muscles, 429, 431, 445
Respiratory synkinesis, 436
Restless legs, 101
Restriction barrier, 125
Rheumatic conditions, EPA, 101–102
Rheumatoid arthritis, 416
Rhomboid major and minor, 331–332
   assessment for shortness, 332–333
   assessment for weakness, 332
   MET, 334

NMT, 333–334
   overactivity, 305, 308, 434
Rhythm test, scapulohumeral, 62, 189, 303
Rib motion, 433
   restrictions, 433, 434–435
Ribs, 422
   1st rib palpation, 433
   2nd rib restrictions and shoulder pain,
     304–305, 434
   dysfunction, testing for, **435**
   elevated and depressed, 433
   floating ribs, 422, 433, 446
   lateral excursion, **430**
   palpation, 433
   and shoulder pain, 310
RICE, acute phase inflammatory response,
   86, 110
Right lymphatic duct, 19
Ring finger extensors, trigger points, **412**
Rotation
   cervical region, **176**, 177, 178, 194
   thoracic, 423, 428
Rotation loading, 99
Rotator cuff, 296, 336–337, 339
   assessing, 348
   avascular necrosis and cardiovascular
     problems, 49
   tear, 337, 345
   treatment of SITS tendons, 346
Rotatores longus and brevis, 201, 442–443
Rowe, 'allergic toxemia', 100
Ruddy's reciprocal antagonist facilitation
   (RRAF), 127, 137–138, 180, 359
   see also Pulsed MET (Ruddy's method)
Ruffini end-organs, 33

S

'S' bends, 99
   MFR, masseter, **278**
Sacroiliac joint
   dysfunction, 90
   support from hamstrings, 27
Salivary glands, **291**, 292
   stones, 276
Sarcomere, 21, 22, 68, 70, 74, 80, 112, 118, 190,
   326, 327, 337
Satellite trigger points, 69, **74**
Scalene anticus, 228, **230**
   MET treatment, **232**
Scalene anticus syndrome, 228
Scalene hiatus, 228
Scalene posticus, 229
Scalenes, 171, 226–232, **230**
   indications for treatment, 228
   MET, 230–232
   NMT, 228–230
Scalenus posterior, overactivity, 305, 434
Scalp, 264
   friction, 265
Scapula
   abduction, 305
   elevation, depression and adduction
     protraction, 304, 308
   transverse process attachments, 204
   upper angle, addressing, 330, **331**
   winging of, 332, 358
Scapula stability, breathing assessment, 432
Scapulohumeral dysfunction *see* Capsulitis
Scapulohumeral rhythm test, Janda, 62, 189,
   297–298, 303
Scapulothoracic joint, 296, 297–298

Scar tissue, 3, 6, 11
   trigger points in, 75
   and upper extremity lymphatic drainage,
     367
Schafer, proprioception, 30
Scoliosis, 438, 442
Scope of practice, 302
Secondary trigger points
   activating factors, 74
   spray and stretch, 135
Segmental coupling, 436–437, 438
Segmental facilitation, 70–71, 442–443
   example, 423–424
Segmental neuropathy (shingles), 265, 358,
   448
Selenium, 100
Self-help
   FMS, 136
   TMJ dysfunction, 273
Self-treatment
   TMJ dysfunction, 252, 275
   using SNAGS, 203
   warming compresses, 131
Selye, adaptation, 43–44, 72
Semispinalis capitis, 196, 197, 240
Semispinalis cervicis, 196–197
Semispinalis thoracis, 441
Sensory information, central influences, 32
Sensory receptors, 30
Sequencing, cervical treatment, 187–234
Seronegative spondyloarthropathies, 416
Serratus anterior, 298, 357–358
   assessment for weakness, 358
   NMT, 358–359
   pulsed MET for facilitation of tone, 359
Serratus posterior inferior, 445, 446
   active exhalation phase, breathing, 48
Serratus posterior superior, 445
   trigger points, 332, **333**, 334, 445
Sharpey's fibres, 168
Shearing loading, 99
Sherrington
   proprioception, 30
   Sherrington's law, 22
Shingles, 265, 358, 448
Short head, biceps brachii, 377
Short leg, 58, 71
Short muscles, 59
   FMS, 136
Shortened soft tissue structure, treatment
   options, 180
Shoulder, 295–320
   AP radiograph, **296**
   assessment *see* Shoulder assessment
   key joints, 296–299
   ligaments, **300**, 301
   muscles, evaluations, 313–315
   muscular relationships, 306, 308
   range of motion, 301, 303–305
   structure, 295–299
   three degrees of freedom, 296, **297**
   treatment, 320–377
   trigger points associated with restriction,
     75
Shoulder and arm pain
   common sources, 308–309
   neural impingement, 369–370
Shoulder assessment, 299–320
   cautions, 302
   motion, active and passive tests, 305–306
   muscle evaluations, 313–315
   observation, 303
   reflex tests, 304